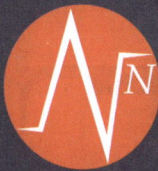
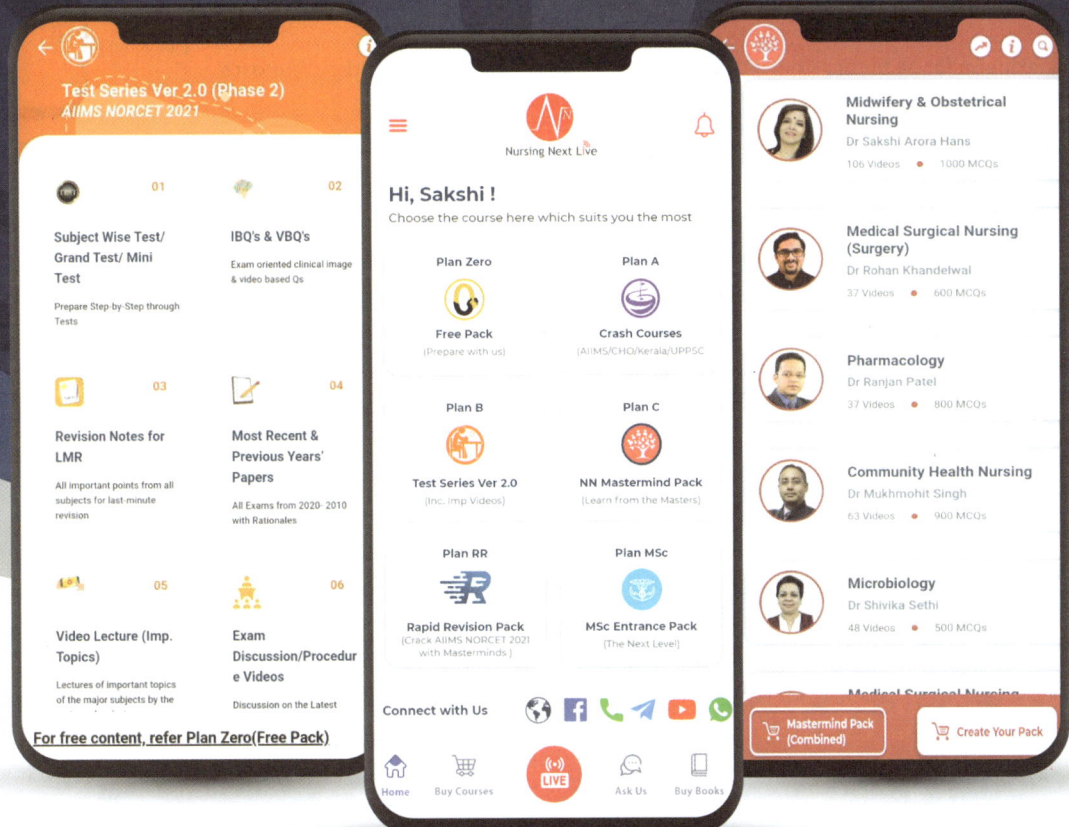

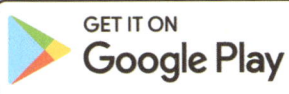
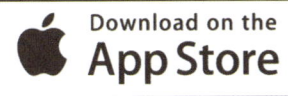

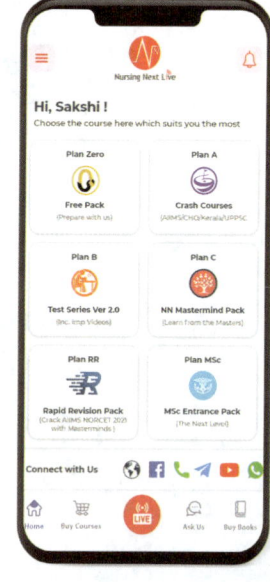

Nursing Next Live has been conceptualized based on the observation that there is a huge gap between the educational services available to the medical graduates and the nursing students. As these two are the strong pillars in providing holistic care to the patients, it is extremely vital that nurses should get equal exposure to access learning. To overcome this issue, we have come forward with the commitment of providing quality education to the nurses in India at their doorstep through Nursing Next Live. And therefore, we say **"We are bringing Learning to the People Instead of People Going for Learning".**

It is India's first and the biggest digital learning platform in the field of Nursing Education. The Nursing Next Live is an interactive self-assessment app, which helps you to build knowledge of nursing specialities any time and anywhere. In a span of one year we have magnified the nursing sector by upscaling it with the strategically designed Quality Content by the Top Medical Faculties of India. We at Nursing Next Live envisage that all students from Kashmir to Kanyakumari should get quality education. We pledge to give the best learning experience to all our students, under one single roof, and that is **"All-in-one and One-in-All platform".**

The Core Values and Principles of Nursing Next Live is:

• First Digital Learning platform for All Nursing Competitive & Undergraduates Exams with Futuristic Approach
• We are bringing Learning to People, Instead of People going for learning!
• Concept Based Teaching by TOP Medical & Nursing Educators (The Masterminds)
• "Quality Content" & "Smart-Study" Approach
• One in All, All in One! Nothing Beyond
• 360 Degree Approach for your complete Preparation
• Most Up to date & updated Content
• Best Guidance & Support at every step
• Best Interface with Unique & Advance Features
• Everything at one Platform ...Buy CBS Nursing Books at Special Discounts/Cashbacks

Nursing Next Live is the fastest-growing Edutech organization in the field of Nursing! With **70k+** downloads, **1200+** total number of selections, **150+** AIIMS NORCET 2020 Selections, and many backend achievements it is the Highest Ranked App on the Play Store. The idea was possible to bring into reality because it was backed by the team of best professionals who did not see time; had One vision and One Goal in Mind of providing the students Nothing but The Best! Their trust towards the vision for the brand and their efforts to continuously make it a success helped Nursing Next to reach to this position

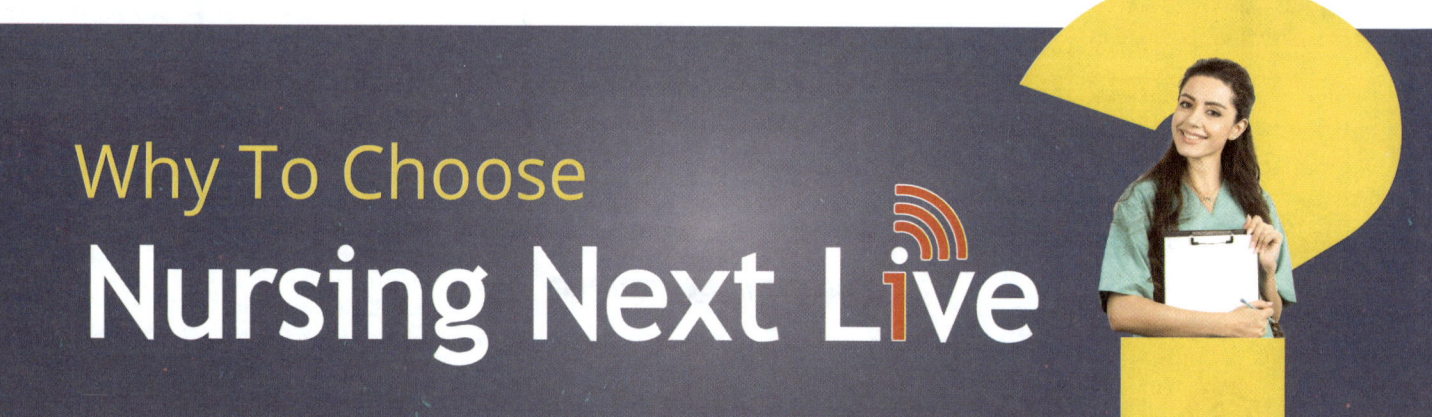

Why To Choose Nursing Next Live

☑ India's 1st Digital Learning Platform for all nursing competitive, nursing undergraduate and nursing postgraduate exams (One-in-All, All-in-One)
☑ User friendly interface with unique & advanced features
☑ Most Up-to-date & Quality Content based on New INC Syllabus
☑ Conceptual learning with an integrated and futuristic approach
☑ Smart Study under the guidance of India's Top Educators who are the masterminds of their subjects
☑ Enhance your learning from Basic To Advance level with a 360-degree approach
☑ Regular Live Doubt Sessions and Live Tests based on real-time exam pattern
☑ TOP Selections in AIIMS NORCET, AIIMS MSc, BFUHS, CHO, SGPGI, JIPMER, RRB, DSSSB etc (From Rank 1 to 1000)
☑ Study Planner that helps you to organize your study
☑ Faculty-Student Meet (Forthcoming) that provides you an opportunity to meet with faculty and get clarify your doubts
☑ Printed Booklet: You will get the printed notes of the video lectures that will save your time in notes making and organize your time in a better way
☑ Customize Study which helps you to create your own pack depending on your needs and wants
☑ Daily dose of information keeps you updated everyday with new information
☑ One-in-all all-in-one: You will get exam oriented plan in the app for whatever exams you are targeting. Simulation Videos

THE COMPLETE PACKAGE

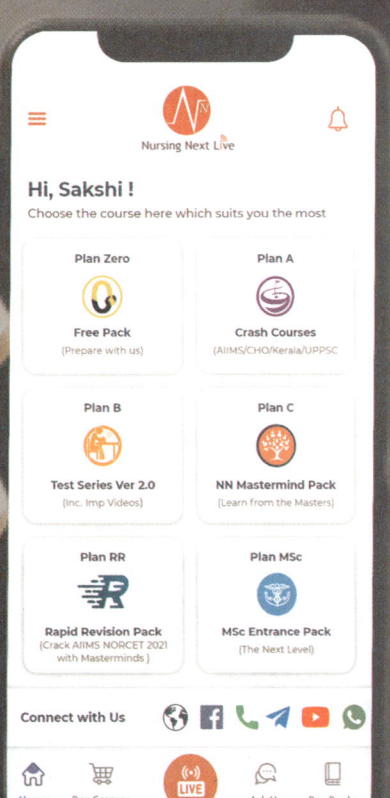

50,000+
MCQs with their Rationale

2000+
Hours of Recorded video lectures (Covering All Subjects/All Topics/ Imp Topics Chanting Videos/Exam Discussions/LMR/IBQ & VBQs Discussions)

150+
Previous years' question papers covering all National & State Level Exams (2021-2010)

Monthly/Weekly/Daily
Live Doubt Sessions & Faculty-Students' Meet (Forthcoming)

200+
Newly Created Subject-wise cum Topic-wise Test, Mini Test & Grand Tests based on all important National Exams like AIIMS, PGIMER, JIPMER, DSSSB, RRB & ESIC, also State level exams like Kerala PSC

1500+
E-Notes/Flash cards of all the subjects for Last-minute Revision

1000+
Image-based Questions with their Rationale

200+
Video-based Questions with their Rationale

Monthly
Special Mega Assessment Tests, National Scholarship Test with up to 100% Scholarship & Reward points

200+
CBS Nursing Books available for purchase

Special Features

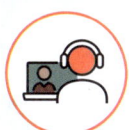
Live Classes

Live Doubt Sessions

Mega Assessment Tests

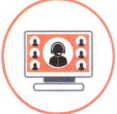
Live Webinars

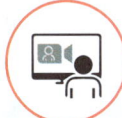
Faculty-Student Meet on Zoom Sessions

Study Plans

Success Stories

Daily Dose of Knowledge

Blogs

National Scholarship Test with upto 100% scholarship

Any Doubt Ask Us

Exam Notifications

Buy CBS Nursing Books

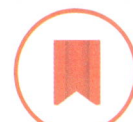
Bookmark Your Imp Topics

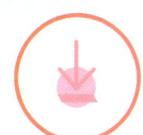
Download Videos/ Notes

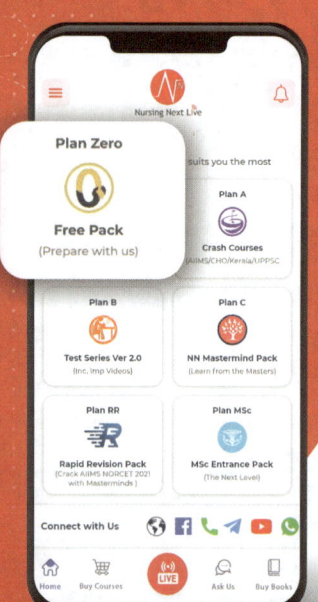

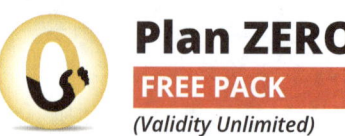

"जांचो, परखो, फिर खरीदो!"

Plan ZERO
FREE PACK
(Validity Unlimited)

Nursing Next Live focuses on providing you the with the best and beyond, nothing less. In Plan ZERO we provide you the glimpse of the content from the various pack that gives you the rights to explore the contents in the App and help in taking the right decisions before selecting the pack.

WHY TO EXPLORE

- Glimpse of the content from the various packs
- TRY-TRUST-OPT. It provides you the rights to first analyze and then go for the best pack
- Enriched content

BEST FOR

- Those who want to explore before selecting the right pack
- Students who have an urge to gain the last momentum by giving a final touch to their preparation.

What all you will get

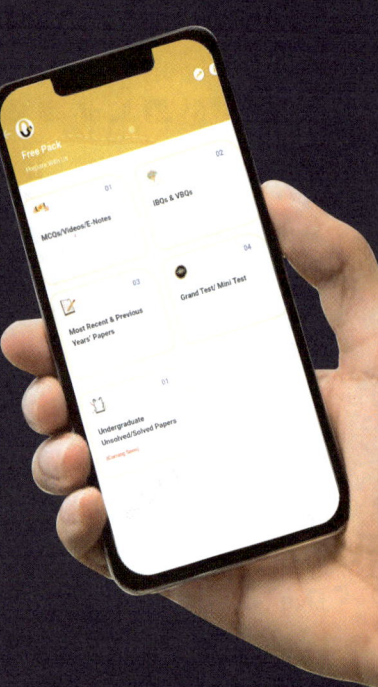

- **2000+** MCQs with Rationale covering All Subjects, Important Topics
- **150+** E-Notes covering All Subjects, Selective important Topics
- **100+** Hours of Lectures covering All Subjects (Topic-wise/Imp Topics/Chanting/Exam Discussions)
- **100+** IBQs & VBQs of All Subjects
- **15** Most Recent/Previous Years Papers with Rationale
- **5+** Grand Test & Bonus Test based on Real Time Exam Pattern
- **5+** National Scholarship test with negaitive marking, National Level Ranking & Cash Rewards
- Daily Dose of Knowledge— Word of the Day, Fact of the Day, Practice Pearls, Question of the Day
- Unsolved & Solved Question Papers of BSc 1st to 4th Year in a consolidated manner covering all Important Universities (Forthcoming)
- Monthly National Scholarship Test with Special Discount for Top Rankers
- How to Prepare for Exams (in the form of Study Planner/Videos)
- Complete Access to Target High Extra Edge Section – which includes additional MCQs & Golden Points in Video Form

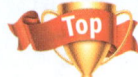

Selections in
Various Competitive Nursing Exams

What our glorified achievers say about **Nursing Next Live**

"लक्ष्य तय है, तो PLAN A सही है!"

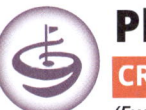

Plan A
CRASH COURSES
(Exam Centric)

If you have a set target and working to achieve it then Plan A is the perfect plan for you. We have come up with this plan to help you prepare for a particular exam that includes exam-centric AIIMS NORCET 2020, SGPGI, CHO & Target Kerala PSC Crash Courses to help you get a hold of every topic in-depth. You get access to in-detailed content of Real-Time Pattern of exams and their latest syllabus. Put your hands on the best!

WHY TO SUBSCRIBE
- Exam specific, it targets the specific exam therefore its pattern syllabus is as per the targeted exam
- Get Acquainted with exam pattern that helps you improve your skills
- Helps in the last minute revision

BEST FOR
- Those who are preparing for specific exams and want to improve their knowledge by practicing
- Those who are working professionals and want to prepare for exams along with their jobs

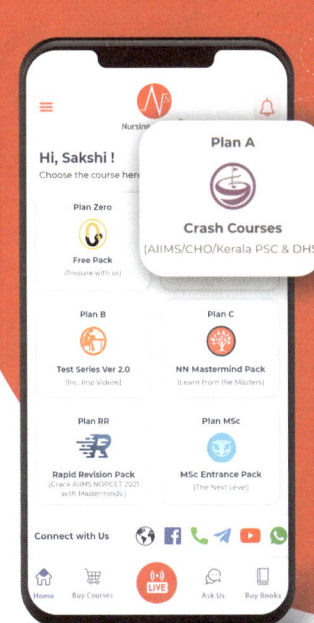

What all you will get

Plan A1
CHO Crash Course

- **35+** Subject-wise Tests & Grand Tests (including Bonus Tests & Previous Years Papers)
- **1500+** Questions with rationale
- **70+** E-notes for last-minute revision covering all the important topics as per the syllabus of CHO
- **30+** (Duration of 30+ Hours) Pre-recorded Videos given by top faculties in Hinglish covering every important topic from exam point of view

MRP ₹689/- | Validity 2 Months

Plan A2
AIIMS NORCET 2020 Crash Course

- **60+** Live Tests Subject-wise based on AIIMS Delhi pattern
- **1500+** Qs with Rationale including MCQs, IBQs, VBQs, Clinical skills, Priority setting, and case study
- **15+** Mock Test, Revision Test, and Grand Tests based on Real-time pattern of AIIMS Delhi with Negative Marking and National Level Ranking
- All Subject-wise Tests & Grand Tests are with Detailed Rationale
- **140+** Last-Minute Revision Notes based on Frequently asked Topics of previous Years
- **12+** Videos on Chanting Session by Top Educators/Subject Experts
- **35+** Multiple videos on special tricks for non-nursing subjects, tips on memory retention, strategies to attempt exams, etc.
- Success Guaranteed as we have had 150+ Selections (Rank 3 to 5k) in AIIMS NORCET 2020.

MRP ₹1499/- | Validity 2 Months

Plan A3
Target Kerala PSC Crash Course

- **60+** Subject-wise/Grand Tests with Rationale
- **320+** E-Notes in the form of Subject-wise synopsis
- **50+** Hours of Videos in English (Important Topics Pre-loaded video + Chanting videos)
- In association with our Best-Selling Title- Target High Staff Nurse Entrance Exam

MRP ₹945/- | Validity 2 Months

Plan A4
UPPSC Staff Nurse Crash Course

- **40+** subject-wise tests which cover the complete syllabus from basics to advance
- **7** Grand Tests Based on real time exam pattern
- **3** Extra Edge Tests covering Important Positions, Important Nursing Procedures, Drug Calculation, suture techniques & COVID special)
- Previous Year Paper Discussion video helps you how to approach the correct answer
- **25+** Quick Revision videos in one-liner form that covers all the important points from the weightage subject
- **1** **"SUCCESS MANTRA"** video to guide you the right approach for preparation

MRP ₹1499/- | Validity 3 Months

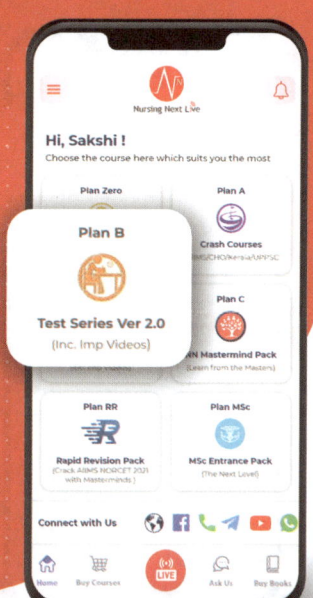

"आज का अभ्यास, आपके कल की सफलता!"

Plan B
Test Series Ver 2.0
(360° Approach)

Test series 2.0, as the name says to excel in any test, you need to base your learnings on two principles 1st is practice, practice, practice, and then 2nd is a 360-degree approach. Variety of subject-wise and topic-wise tests, IBQs, and VBQs that follow the latest exam fashion to help you level up your preparatory work. To give a complete touch to the preparation, we have covered all important national & state level last 15 years papers with important topics/ exam discussion videos.

WHY TO SUBSCRIBE

- Comprehensive test pack with 360 degree approach for those who are targeting any staff nurse examination of National or State level
- Keep track of your progress through test analysis report
- Last-minute revision notes of important topics from all the subjects
- Detailed explanation helps you to enhance your knowledge

BEST FOR

- The students who want to delve into the topic and opt for extensive preparation for any staff nurse entrance exam.
- Who never want to stop learning and always look forward to upgrading their pre-acquired knowledge.
- Working students who don't want to compromise with their preparation and success.

What all you will get

Pre Loaded Content (Phase 1 + Phase 2)

- **190+** Newly Created Subject-wise, Mini Test and Grand Test focusing all important National Exams AIIMS, PGIMER, JIPMER, DSSSB, RRB and ESIC
- **15K+** Qs (MCQs, IBQs, VBQs) with Rationale and updated reference from standard textbooks. All the Tests are designed by the Subject Experts and Topper Students
- **400+** Hours Recorded Video Lectures of Nursing/Non-Nursing Subjects by some of India's best nursing faculties/subject experts. Lectures are in English/Hindi language focusing on concept-based learning.
- **5** Exam Discussion Videos of 2019 Exam papers (Duration 20 Hours)
- **150+** Hours of Recorded Video on Subject-wise Exam Discussion of previous years papers (2017-18) of all nursing exams delivered by subject experts
- **5** Skill Procedure videos demonstrating Nursing Skills in real-time
- **100+** Previous Year Exam Papers of all Nursing Exams from 2020-10 with Rationale (Attempt/View PDF Mode)
- **1500+** Flashcards/E-notes on all the important topics of all the subjects for last minute revision (In 6 months)
- **800+** Image-based Questions with Rationale
- **200+** Video-based Qs with Rationale
- **Complete Access to Plan A-Crash Courses**

New Content (Phase 3) Q Bank Pack

- **8000+** Qs in Q Bank form of all the topics from all the subjects
- **700+** E-Notes covering all subjects/all topics

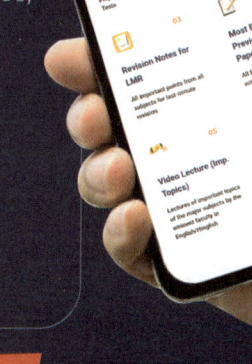

| MRP ₹3497/- | Validity 4 Months | MRP ₹6998/- | Validity 6 Months |

TESTIMONIALS

What our subscribers say about "TEST SERIES PLAN"

RIGHT DECISIONS TO SUCCESS!
"My wise investment in Plan B and continuous practice have proved to be the key to my way to success."
Sabita

LEARNING EFFORTLESSLY!
"Plan B made my understanding better of each vital subject in a very unchallenging manner. I am grateful."
Ritika

GAINING CLARITY WITH PLAN B!
"Plan B covers all the critical and analysis level questions with the rationale that helped me gain clarity of the concepts."
Deeksha Bhatt

THOROUGHLY RECOMMENDED PLAN 101!
"The questions with rationales helped me a lot. Highly recommended for all future nursing officers."
Shilpa Kashyap

ADDING JOY IN LEARNING!
"I am heartily grateful to become a part of Nursing Next Live. The faculty helped me thoroughly in this Pandemic by adding a sense of joy to my studies."
Suman Chauhan

PAVED MY WAY TO SUCCESS!
"More than enough time to practice and brace yourself The MCQs and videos with Rationales and topic-wise LMR have helped me understand the vital subjects in a better way."
Rajkumar James

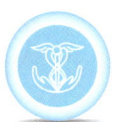

"तैयारी आगे की!"

Plan MSc

MSc Digest

We cant be louder about It, Nursing Next Live is the only growing platform offering MSc preparations to the aspirants. As we say, that your success is our success, so we always look forward to providing the best and beyond study content with a futuristic approach. MSc Digest contains every vital information about the subjects in one place so that it gets easy for all to access the content on one platform.

WHY TO SUBSCRIBE

- Make your preparation easy with your job
- Enriched content helps you to prepare, revise and assess
- Content is prepared by the top Medical & Nursing experts
- Guidance and support

BEST FOR

- Who are always hungry to gain more knowledge from anywhere when they get a chance.
- Who believe in focusing on one topic at a time
- Who want to go further and upgrade their study content to the next level.

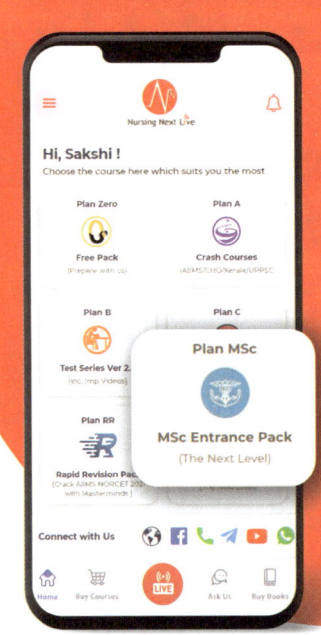

What all you will get

- Subject-wise synopsis covering image base illustrations and interesting Mnemonics to provide an extra edge preparation
- **3500+** MCQs covering the important topics of all subjects
- **800+** IBQs covering all subjects/topics
- **10+** Milestone papers covering more than 1000 MCQs to imbibe the environment of a real examination
- **3** Tests covering 150 IBQs
- **3** Tests covering 75 VBQs
- **10** Previous year papers (2020-2017) covering questions based on important topics/sub-topics from all subjects
- Exam capsules in the form of flashcards & tables
- **400+** LMR flashcards covering all subjects
- Hard copy of notes will be provided

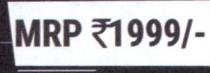

MRP ₹1999/- | **Validity 90 Days**

TESTIMONIALS

What our glorified achievers of MSc Entrance Exam say about Nursing Next Live

ONE APP WITH A COMPLETE GUIDE TO NURSING SUCCESS!
"NNL has helped me a lot in preparing for MSc entrance exam and get a good rank. I will recommend this for every Nursing Aspirant out there."
Sabarni
(AIR Rank-21, AIIMS MSc 2021)

TAKING UNDERSTANDING TO THE NEXT LEVEL!
"It has helped me clear every doubt and that made my understanding of the subjects clearer. Thank you, team!"
Ritika Rajpoot
(AIR Rank-23, AIIMS MSc 2021)

THOROUGHLY RECOMMENDED PLAN 101!
"It was a wonderful experience studying from the top educators and getting counseled by them."
Priti Prajapati
(AIR Rank-39, AIIMS MSc 2021)

NNL FOUND ME WHAT I WAS LOOKING FOR!
"It helped me to polish my subject knowledge and upgraded my preparations. Overall, It is an excellent application for all the Nursing Aspirants."
Pritika Thakur
(AIR Rank-119, AIIMS MSc 2021)

AS EFFICIENT AS THE APP CLAIMS TO BE!
"This app is very helpful if you are looking forward to clearing your doubts in a comprehensive way. The faculty is highly professional and informative."
Aditi Yadav
(AIR Rank-133, AIIMS MSc 2021)

STRESS TURNED INTO THE JOY OF STUDYING!
"NN Live has made me admire the study pattern they follow. The way of teaching of the faculty is very helpful and valuable and filled with enthusiasm."
Shivani Shashni
(AIR Rank-173, AIIMS MSc 2021)

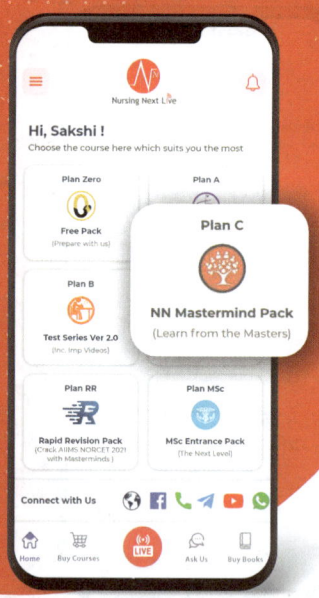

"ज्ञान हो बढ़ाना, तो PLAN C ही लेना!"

Plan C/C Plus
MASTERMIND Pack
(One-in-All, All-in-One)

Nursing Next's One in all, all in one Mastermind pack for complete preparation! Plan C plus is a full package that contains all that you need for your 100% preparation for all the Nursing competitive exams. The content of this package is curated and drafted by the Top-Educators of Nursing Next Live, who are the masterminds of their subjects. NN Mastermind Pack is a gradual phase-wise learning journey with the option of Individual and combined pack and a validity of 12 months!

WHY TO SUBSCRIBE
- Detailed lectures as per the INC syllabus
- Helps you in building the strong foundation
- The MASTERMINDS : India's top medical & nursing faculty is here to guide you
- Sufficient content to cater your undergraduate and entrance exams needs
- Handwritten notes of the lectures that help you to revise the topic
- Question Bank with the topics that help you to assess your understanding in that particular topic

BEST FOR
- Students who are at a good progression level and want to build up their foundation more.
- Those who look forward to studying from the best and beyond educators.
- The students who want to upgrade their knowledge or the one aiming for Staff Nurse Entrance Exam, and also for the Undergraduates.

SPECIAL FEATURES
- Nursing Next's "Mastermind Pack", is a One-Stop solution for all your exam preparation needs for Staff Nurse Entrance Exams & Nursing Undergraduate Exams!
- It is our One-in-All, All-in-One pack for the nursing students of the Digital era!
- NN Mastermind Pack is exactly that 'learning tool' for all the nursing aspirants. It is carefully planned, and strategically designed, under the expertise of TOP Medical/Nursing Educators, just to make learning more authentic and easier for our students.
- Covering All Subjects, All Topics concepts from Basics to Advanced level pattern with the help of Videos/Question Banks & Handwritten Notes
- The Masterminds (TOP EDUCATORS) of NN Live have focused on ALL the upcoming Nursing Exams by giving two convenient options under 'Individual Subject Pack', & 'Combined (NN Mastermind Pack)'
- NN Mastermind Pack is a "road to success" for those who are preparing for any or all staff nurse entrance exams.

What all you will get

Plan C (Including Plan RR)
- **1200+** hours of Video Lectures on All Subject/All Topics
- **11,000+** Questions with Rationale covering All Subject/All Topics
- IBQ/VBQ Video Discussions of All Subjects
- **Monthly Live Doubt Sessions/Live Classes**
- **80+Hours** of Rapid Revision Videos for **AIIMS NORCET**
- **2021** by Mastermind faculty
- **Handwritten Notes** of videos in PDF format integrated in the App
- Focusing on Quality study over quantity study, using the smart-study approach
- Monthly **Mega Assessment** Tests with National LevelRanking
- All upcoming exam's Important Topics & Exam/Discussions will be covered
- Complete **360-degree approach** for preparation
- Unlimited Watch Time, FREE Download Video option, National Level Ranks, Bookmark the content, Pause & Resume video option
- Best Guidance & Support at every stage
- Monthly Live Doubt Sessions/Live Classes/Live Webinars by Mastermind Faculty

Validity: 12 Months
MRP ₹12974/-

Plan C Plus (Including Plan A+B+C+RR)
- Plan A of NN Live (Complete access to Crash Courses—CHO/AIIMS NORCET 2020/KERALA PSC/UPPSC
  +
- Plan B of NN Live (Complete access to Test Series Pack Focusing AIIMS NORCET 2021 & Other Staff Nurse Exams)
  +
- Plan C of NN Live (Complete access to Plan C by the Mastermind Faculty
  +
- Plan RR of NN Live (Complete access to Rapid Revision Pack)

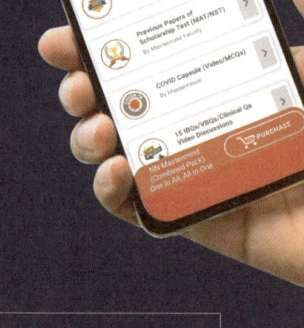

Validity: 6 Months
MRP ₹9995/-

Validity: 12 + 2 Bonus Months
MRP ₹15999/-

Validity: 24 Months
MRP ₹31998/-

Undergraduate Packs (Prof.-wise)

1st Year Students
- ✓ Anatomy
- ✓ Physiology
- ✓ Biochemistry & Nutrition
- ✓ Microbiology
- ✓ Fundamentals of Nursing

2nd Year Students
- ✓ Pharmacology
- ✓ MSN – Medicine
- ✓ MSN – Surgery
- ✓ Community Health Nursing
- ✓ Sociology
- ✓ CET

3rd & 4th Year Students
- ✓ Pediatric Nursing
- ✓ Midwifery & Obstetrical Nursing
- ✓ MSN – Medicine
- ✓ MSN – Surgery
- ✓ Mental Health Nursing
- ✓ Community Health Nursing
- ✓ Nursing Research & Statistics
- ✓ Nursing Management & Administration

Other Mastermind Plans

Mastermind Plan C
For 3rd & 4th Year Students those who are targeting for Staff Nurse Exams

Mastermind Plan C Plus
For Pass out Students those who are targeting for AIIMS NORCET & Staff Nurse Exams

The Masterminds

Learn from the Top Educators of India

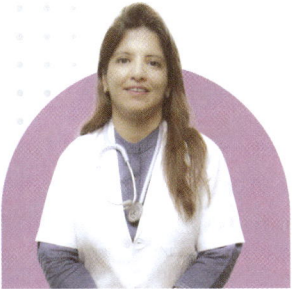

Dr Sakshi Arora Hans

Midwifery & Obstetrical Nursing

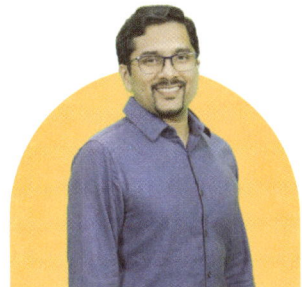

Dr Rohan Khandelwal

MSN - Surgery

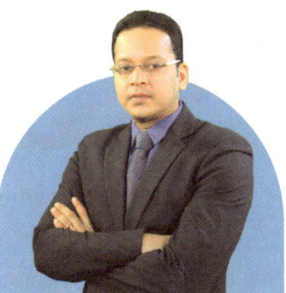

Dr Ranjan Patel

Pharmacology

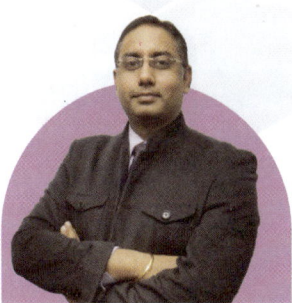

Dr Mukhmohit Singh

Community Health Nursing

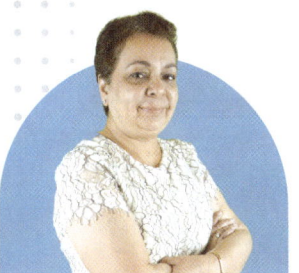

Dr Shivika Sethi

Microbiology

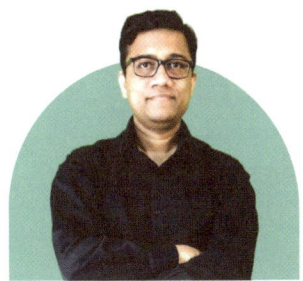

Dr Ashish Kumar

Physiology

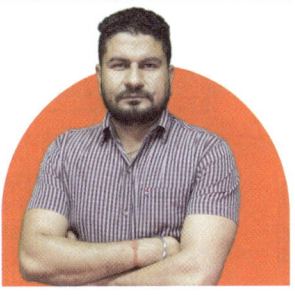

Dr Aman Setiya

MSN - Medicine

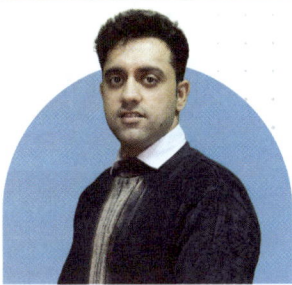

Dr Anand Bhatia

Pediatric Nursing

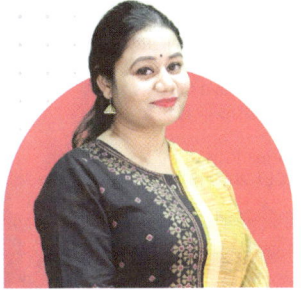

Ms Sabina Ali

Fundamentals of Nursing

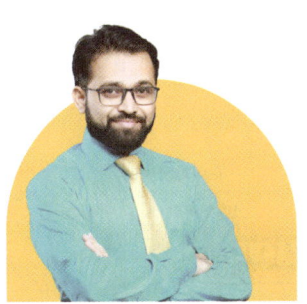

Dr Shrikant Verma

Anatomy

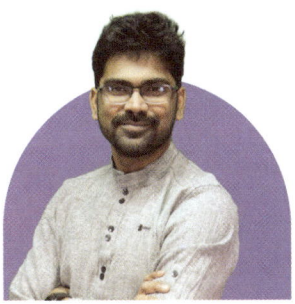

Dr Karthikeyan Pethusamy

Biochemistry & Nutrition

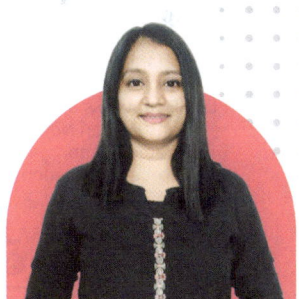

Ms Chetana

Mental Health Nursing

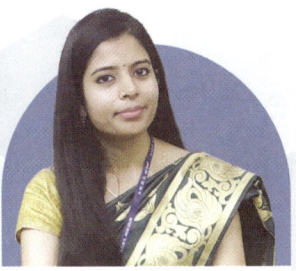

Saumya Srivastava

Nursing Management & Nursing Education

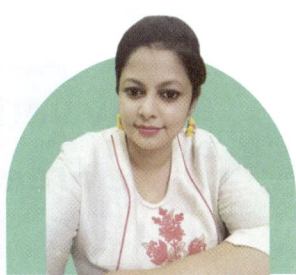

Ms Priyanka Randhir

Sociology & Computers

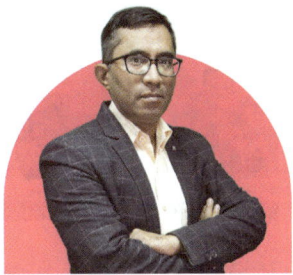

Mr Nitish Dubey

General Arithmetic

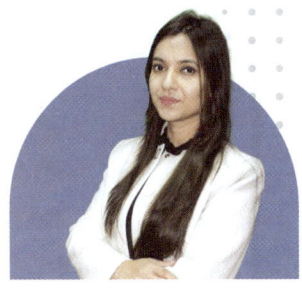

Ms Saloni Sharma

Aptitude & Reasoning

Individual

Midwifery & Obstetrical Nursing

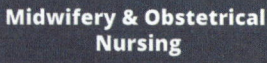

By Dr Sakshi Arora Hans

What all you will get

- **100** hours of Videos on All topics
- IBQs & VBQs Discussion Videos
- **15** hours of Rapid Revision Videos covering Important Topics for AIIMS NORCET 2021
- **1000** Topic-wise MCQs with Rationale
- Live Doubt Sessions/Live Classes
- **88** Hand written Notes in PDF format

Validity: 6 months | **MRP** ₹1994/-

MSN - Surgery

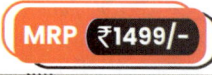

By Dr Rohan Khandelwal

What all you will get

- **50** hours of Videos of All topics
- IBQs & VBQs Video Discussions
- **3** hours of Rapid Revision Videos covering Important Topics for AIIMS NORCET 2021
- **800** Topic-wise Qs with Rationale
- Live Doubt Sessions/Live Classes
- **51** Hand written Notes in PDF format integrated in App

Validity: 6 months | **MRP** ₹1499/-

Pharmacology

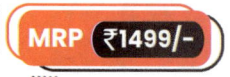

By Dr Ranjan Patel

What all you will get

- **50** hours of Videos of All topics
- IBQs & VBQs Video Discussions
- **10** hours of Rapid Revision Videos covering Important Topics for AIIMS NORCET 2021
- **800** Topic-wise Qs with Rationale
- Live Doubt Sessions/Live Classes
- **71** Hand written Notes in PDF format integrated in App
- **100** Probable Questions of Pharmacology for AIIMS NORCET 2021

Validity: 6 months | **MRP** ₹1499/-

Community Health Nursing

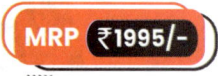

By Dr Mukhmohit Singh

What all you will get

- **90** hours of Videos of All topics
- IBQs & VBQs Video Discussions
- **7** hours of Rapid Revision Videos covering Important Topics forAIIMS NORCET 2021
- **900** Topic-wise Qs with Rationale
- Live Doubt Sessions/Live Classes
- **87** Hand written Notes in PDF format integrated in App
- **300** Probable Questions of CHN for AIIMS NORCET 2021

Validity: 6 months | **MRP** ₹1995/-

Microbiology

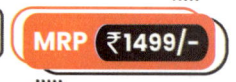

By Dr Shivika J Sethi

What all you will get

- **54** hours of Videos of All topics
- IBQs & VBQs Video Discussions
- **8** hours of Rapid Revision Videos covering Important Topics for AIIMS NORCET 2021
- **800** Topic-wise Qs with Rationale
- Live Doubt Sessions/Live Classes
- **75** Hand written Notes in PDF format integrated in App
- **100** Probable Questions of Microbiology for AIIMS NORCET 2021

Validity: 6 months | **MRP** ₹1499/-

MSN - Medicine

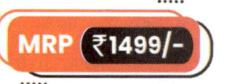

By Dr Aman Setiya

What all you will get

- **90** hours of Videos of All topics
- IBQs & VBQs Video Discussions
- **5** hours of Rapid Revision Videos covering Important Topics for AIIMS NORCET 2021
- **900** Topic-wise Qs with Rationale
- Live Doubt Sessions/Live Classes
- **90** Hand written Notes in PDF format integrated in App
- **400** Probable Questions of MSN - Medicine for AIIMS NORCET 2021

Validity: 6 months | **MRP** ₹1499/-

" जितनी जरूरत उतना पढ़ो !"

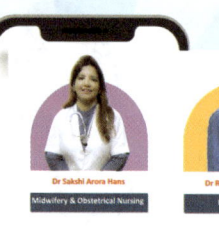
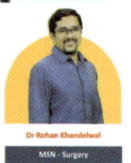
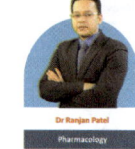
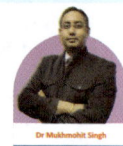
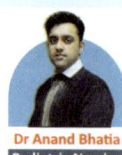

Dr Sakshi Arora Hans — Midwifery & Obstetrical Nursing
Dr Rohan Khandelwal — MSN - Surgery
Dr Ranjan Patel — Pharmacology
Dr Mukhmohit Singh — Community Health Nursing
Dr Anand Bhatia — **Pediatric Nursing**

Now you have
The Freedom to Choose

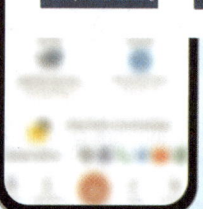

Introducing

CREATE YOUR PACK

Pack

Pediatric Nursing
By Dr Anand Bhatia

What all you will get

- **80** hours of Videos of All topics
- IBQs & VBQs Video Discussions
- **8** hours of Rapid Revision Videos covering Important Topics for AIIMS NORCET 2021
- **900** Topic-wise Qs with Rationale
- Live Doubt Sessions/Live Classes
- **81** Hand written Notes in PDF format integrated in App
- **300** Probable Questions of Pediatric Nursing for AIIMS NORCET 2021

Validity: 6 months | **MRP ₹1994/-**

Anatomy
By Dr Shrikant Verma

What all you will get

- **60** hours of Videos of All topics
- IBQs & VBQs Video Discussions
- **6** hours of Rapid Revision Videos covering Important Topics for AIIMS NORCET 2021
- **605** Topic-wise Qs with Rationale
- Live Doubt Sessions/Live Classes
- **86** Hand written Notes in PDF format integrated in App
- **100** Probable Questions of Anatomy for AIIMS NORCET 2021

Validity: 6 months | **MRP ₹1299/-**

Biochemistry & Nutrition
By Dr Karthikeyan Pethusamy

What all you will get

- **50** hours of Videos of All topics
- IBQs & VBQs Video Discussions
- **3** hours of Rapid Revision Videos covering Important Topics for AIIMS NORCET 2021
- **500** Topic-wise Qs with Rationale
- Live Doubt Sessions/Live Classes
- **45** Hand written Notes in PDF format integrated in App
- **100** Probable Questions of Biochemistry & Nutrition for AIIMS NORCET 2021

Validity: 6 months | **MRP ₹1299/-**

Physiology
By Dr Ashish Kumar

What all you will get

- **60** hours of Videos of All topics
- IBQs & VBQs Video Discussions
- **8** hours of Rapid Revision Videos covering Important Topics for AIIMS NORCET 2021
- **600** Topic-wise Qs with Rationale
- Live Doubt Sessions/Live Classes
- **55** Hand written Notes in PDF format integrated in App

Validity: 6 months | **MRP ₹1299/-**

Fundamentals of Nursing
By Ms Sabina Ali

What all you will get

- **200** hours of Videos of All topics
- IBQs & VBQs Video Discussions
- **14** hours of Rapid Revision Videos covering Important Topics for AIIMS NORCET 2021
- **900** Topic-wise Qs with Rationale
- Live Doubt Sessions/Live Classes
- **200** Hand written Notes in PDF format integrated in App
- **300** Probable Questions of FON for AIIMS NORCET 2021

Validity: 6 months | **MRP ₹1994/-**

Mental Health Nursing
By Dr Dharmendra Singh & Ms Chetana

What all you will get

- **90** hours of Videos of All topics
- IBQs & VBQs Video Discussions
- **6** hours of Rapid Revision Videos covering Important Topics for AIIMS NORCET 2021
- **900** Topic-wise Qs with Rationale
- Live Doubt Sessions/Live Classes
- **300** Probable Questions of MHN for AIIMS NORCET 2021

Validity: 6 months | **MRP ₹1994/-**

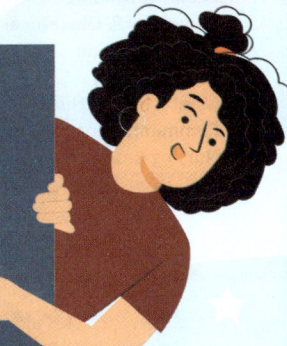

Select any **5 Subjects** by **The Masterminds** and Create Your Own Pack

MRP ₹8450/- | **Validity: 9 Months**

Wondering, HOW? Call us at our helpline number +91-9999117411

Undergraduate Packs

By THE MASTERMINDS

Undergraduate Pack - 1st Year

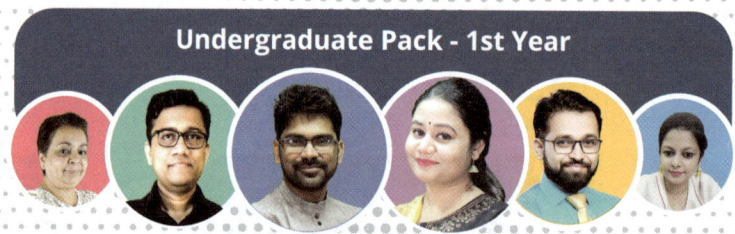

What all you will get

Main Subjects	Video Duration	No. of Questions
Anatomy	60+ Hours	600+ Qs
Physiology	60+ Hours	600+ Qs
Biochemistry & Nutrition	50+ Hours	500+ Qs
Microbiology	50+ Hours	500+ Qs
Fundamentals of Nursing	200+ Hours	400+ Qs

Bonus Subjects:- Computers & Psychology

MRP ₹7997/-

Validity: 18 months

Undergraduate Pack - 2nd Year

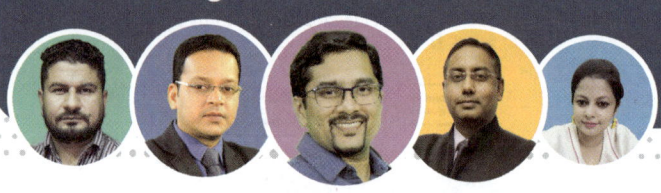

What all you will get

Main Subjects	Video Duration	No. of Questions
Pharmacology	50+ Hours	800+ Qs
MSN - Medicine	90+ Hours	900+ Qs
MSN - Surgery	50+ Hours	600+ Qs
Community Health Nursing	90+ Hours	900+ Qs
Sociology	40+ Hours	250+ Qs

MRP ₹7997/-

Validity: 18 months

Undergraduate Pack - 3rd & 4th Year

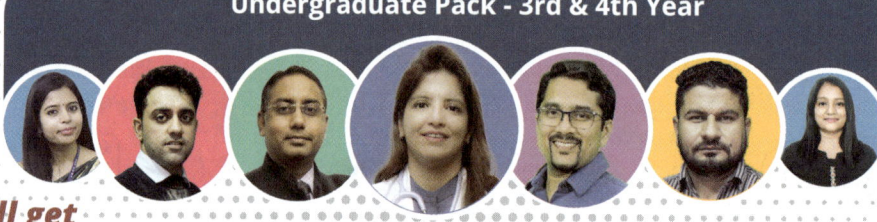

What all you will get

Main Subjects	Video Duration	No. of Questions
Pediatric Nursing	80+ Hours	900+ Qs
Midwifery & Obstetrical Nursing	100+ Hours	1000+ Qs
MSN - Medicine	90+ Hours	900+ Qs
MSN - Surgery	50+ Hours	600+ Qs
Mental Health Nursing	90+ Hours	900+ Qs
Community Health Nursing	90+ Hours	900+ Qs
Nursing Research & Statistics	35+ Hours	400+ Qs

Bonus Subjects:- Nursing Managment & Nursing Education

MRP ₹12992/-

Validity: 24 months

Special Features

- Handwritten Notes of Videos in PDF Format
- IBQs/VBQs Discussion Videos of above mentioned Subjects
- Monthly Mega Assessment Tests
- Monthly Live Doubt Session/Live Classes/Live Webinar by MM Faculty
- Best Guidance & Support
- Get your query directly resolved by MM faculty

"कम समय में जीत पक्की!"

Plan RR

Rapid Revision Pack

(Ready, Steady & Rapid)

We are here to make you a Mastermind for all your Nursing exams, and for that, we believe the last-minute revision works like a wonder. Rapid Revision Pack, as the name says is to make you all ready and rapid for all your Nursing Competetive exams. Learn from basics to advance level and get a hold of every topic. Gain the last-minute momentum with this pack and open the gateway to excellence for yourself.

WHY TO SUBSCRIBE
- Rapid and intense course of study
- Covers important topics in concise yet complete form
- Most probable Qs which have large rate of incidence in exam
- If your foundation is good, then this is good pack to revise before the exam

BEST FOR
- Those who believe in doing extensive preparation for their Nursing competitive exams.
- The students who want to clear all of their last moment doubts.
- Working professionals who never want to compromise with their learnings for the competitive exams.

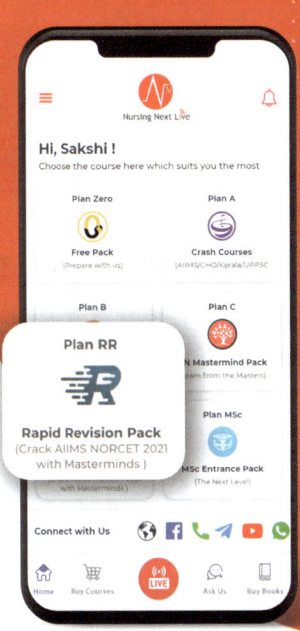

What all you will get

Plan RR

- **80-100 Hours of Rapid Revision Videos** covering Most Imp Topics for NORCET 2021 (Major Subjects including Nursing Management & Nursing Education)
- **2000+** Probable Qs with Rationale (MCQs + NCLEX Pattern)
- IBQ & VBQ Video Discussions by Master Mind Faculties (Relevant Subjects)
- **10 Special Mega Assessment Test** based on AIIMS NORCET Pattern
- Various Imp Tips/Trick & How to Prepare for NORCET 2021 Videos
- **15+** Imp Videos on COVID 19/Test & Discussion covering MCQ & NCLEX Pattern Qs
- COVID-19 Capsule (MCQs & Videos)
- Rapid Revision eBook in PDF format

MRP ₹2777/- | Validity: 2.5 Months

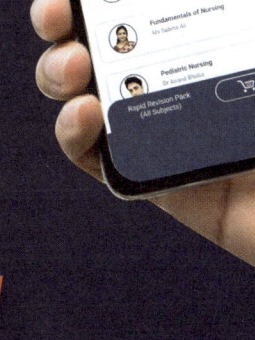

Plan RR+Mini TSP

Complete Ccontent of RR Pack + Mini TSP:
- **15k** Questions with Rationale
- **1000+** IBQs/VBQs with Rationale Subject-wise/System-wise approach
- **190+** Tests (Subject-wise/Grand Test)
- **1500** E-notes/Clinical Gems
- **400+** Hours of videos Lectures/Subject-wise Exam discussion/Skill Procedure Videos

MRP ₹7520/- | Validity: 3+1 Months

TESTIMONIALS

What our Subscribers say about our Rapid Revision Pack

GLORIFIED ACHIEVERS

With over 150+ AIIMS NORCET 2020/100+ CHO &

AIIMS NORCET 2020

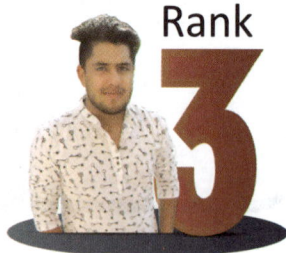
Rank 3
Rahul Dahiya
Roll No. 9016060

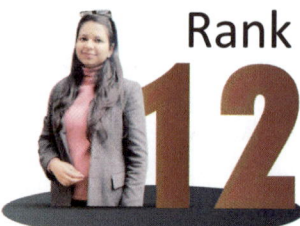
Rank 12
Nisha Singla
Roll No. 9101820

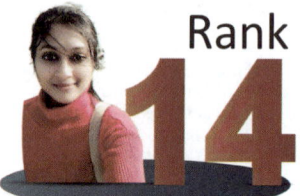
Rank 14
Arushi Mittal
Roll No. 9079646

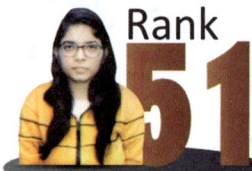
Rank 51
Komal Dhull
Roll No. 9024458

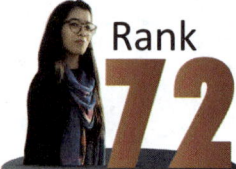
Rank 72
Shivani Bourai
Roll No. 9092877

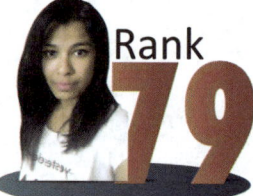
Rank 79
Nivedita Saini
Roll No. 9004587

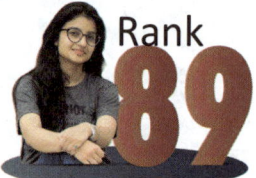
Rank 89
Rupali Garg
Roll No. 9054544

And many more

CHO 2020

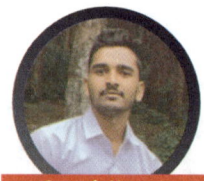
Suresh Kumsr
Rank- 1
Roll No. 12090
MP

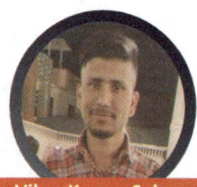
Vikas Kumar Sahu
Rank- 14
Roll No. 10011
MP

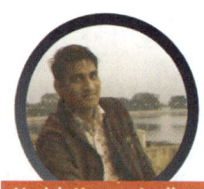
Harish Kumar Lodha
Rank- 18
Roll No. 7930
MP

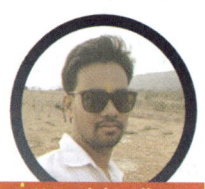
Heeralal Lodha
Rank- 33
Roll No. 10009
MP

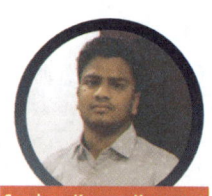
Sandeep Krumar Kumawat
Rank- 44
Roll No. 12585
MP

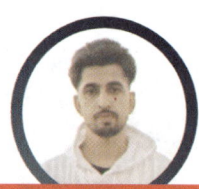
Mahadev Aanjan
Rank- 50
Roll No. 10130
MP

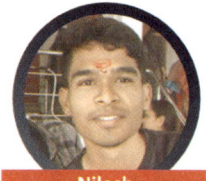
Nilesh
Rank- 81
Roll No. 10572
MP

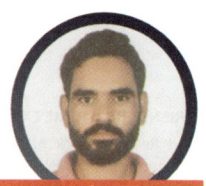
Balveer
Roll No. 619175
RAJASTHAN

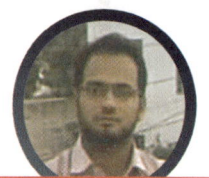
Mahendra Singh Gurjar
Roll No. 626167
RAJASTHAN

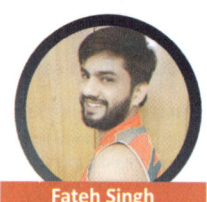
Fateh Singh
Roll No. 108169
RAJASTHAN

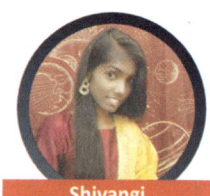
Shivangi
Roll No. 406105
RAJASTHAN

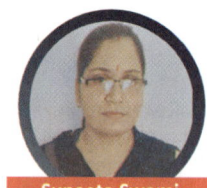
Suneeta Swami
Roll No. 619378
RAJASTHAN

And many more

OF NURSING NEXT LIVE

1200+ STUDENTS who cleared Various National/State Level Nursing Exams

BFUHS 2021

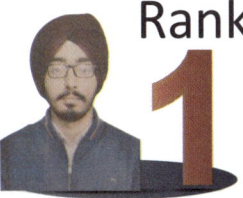

Rank 1
Harjeet Singh
Roll No- 472478

Rank 28
Kuljit Kaur
Roll No. 473956

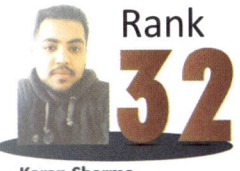

Rank 32
Karan Sharma
Roll No. 469134

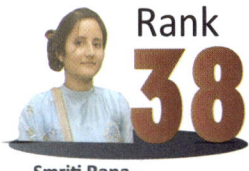

Rank 38
Smriti Rana
Roll No. 463342

Rank 107
Harpreet Kaur
Roll No. 474125

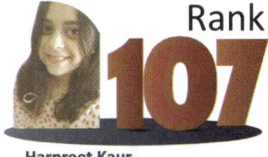

And many more

AIIMS MSc ENTRANCE EXAM 2021

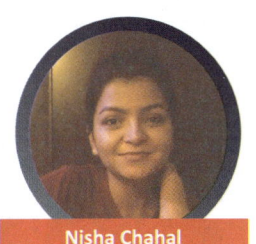

Nisha Chahal
AIIMS AIR-18

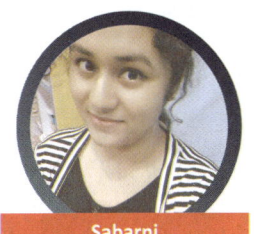

Sabarni
AIIMS AIR-21

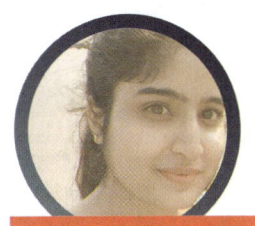

Ritika Rajpoot
AIIMS AIR-23

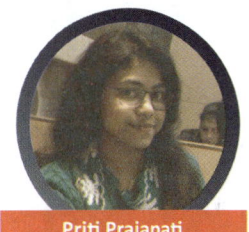

Priti Prajapati
AIIMS AIR-39

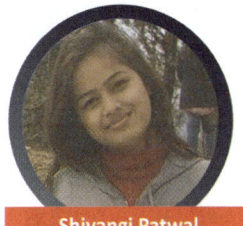

Shivangi Patwal
AIIMS AIR-64

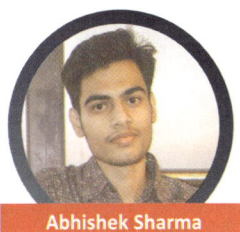

Abhishek Sharma
AIIMS AIR-97

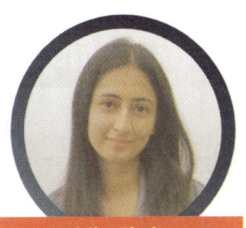

Pritika Thakur
AIIMS AIR-119

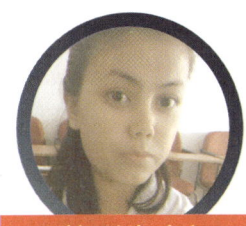

Shivani Shashni
AIIMS AIR-173

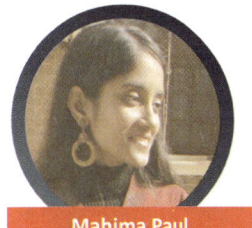

Mahima Paul
AIIMS AIR-175

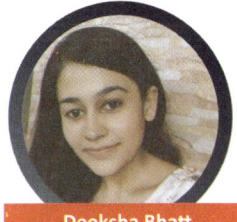

Deeksha Bhatt
AIIMS AIR-281

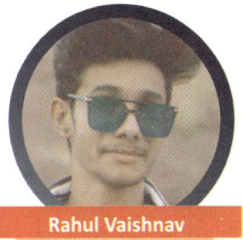

Rahul Vaishnav
AIIMS AIR-301

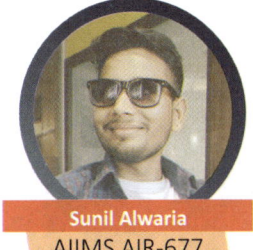

Chandan Sharma
AIIMS AIR-310

Sunil Alwaria
AIIMS AIR-677

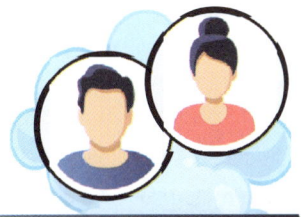

You Will Be The Next...

Scan the QR code to visit to our YouTube Channel to hear their success stories.

ONE PLACE FOR ALL! AN INVITATION FOR ALL THE NURSING FACULTY MEMBERS TO COME.

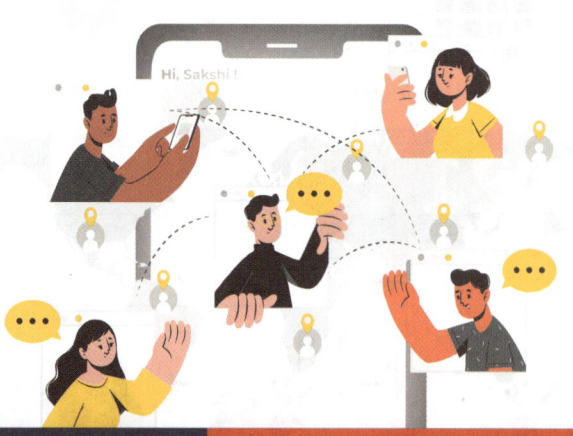

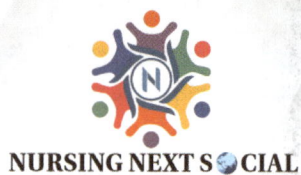

NURSING NEXT SOCIAL

Carrying on the legacy of being the best networking platform for the Nursing Segment!

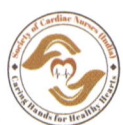 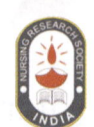 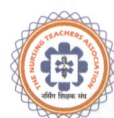 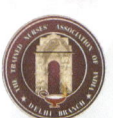

NOW DISTANCE WILL NOT BE A BARRIER

Knowledge is like money: to be of value, it must circulate, and in circulating it, it can increase in quantity!

Nursing Next Live always focuses on providing you with the best and beyond and nothing less than that. We aim to bring all the Nursing Faculties from across the nation closer and together on a single platform.
No social distancing can stop the circulation of learnings from the teachers to students now. With Nursing Next Social, all the faculties from every corner of the country can join at one platform without any barriers.
Nursing Next Social at your service!
ONE PLATFORM TO BECOME THE MENTORS AND MENTEE!

Rewards For You

• Get Acknowledgement & Appreciation Certificates • Get Sponsorships for Educational Programs • Get Credit hours for attending Webinars • Get Free Access to Nursing Next Live Content & CBS Nursing Books   • Get Latest Updates related to your subject • Get a chance to become Reviewer, Contributors in Nursing Next Live, Target High & in CBS Nursing Titles

BE THE MENTOR OR MENTEE

SHOWCASE YOUR ACHIEVEMENTS ➔ SHARE YOUR KNOWLEDGE ➔ ENHANCE YOUR KNOWLEDGE

Purposes
• Attend Webinars/ E- Workshops
• Connect with other Faculty Members
• Share Your Knowledge. Be the Mentor or Mentee
• Get Complimentary Books
• Latest Updates on State/National/International Conferences & Webniars

Special Features
• Create your profile
• Add your accomplishments to level up your portfolio
• Earn Reward Points & Redeem through various options
• Set your Professional GOALS with timelines
• Regular Updates on Upcoming Conferences, CNEs & webinars
• Become Mentor or Mentee
• Get a chance to become Reviewer, Contributor or Author
• Get Certificates with credit hours issued by renowned nursing societies

ARE YOU A NURSING FACULTY ?
BE THE PART OF NURSING NEXT LIVE SOCIAL!

PRE-REGISTER FOR NURSING NEXT SOCIAL
& Get 60 Days Free Subscription of **Nursing Next Live App**

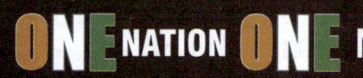

Scan the QR Code &
Fill the form to Pre-register

Or Use the below link to fill the form
http://nursingnextlive.com/NNSocial/

THE SMART DIGITAL LIBRARY

If Institutes Level Up, Students Level Up Automatically
GenNext

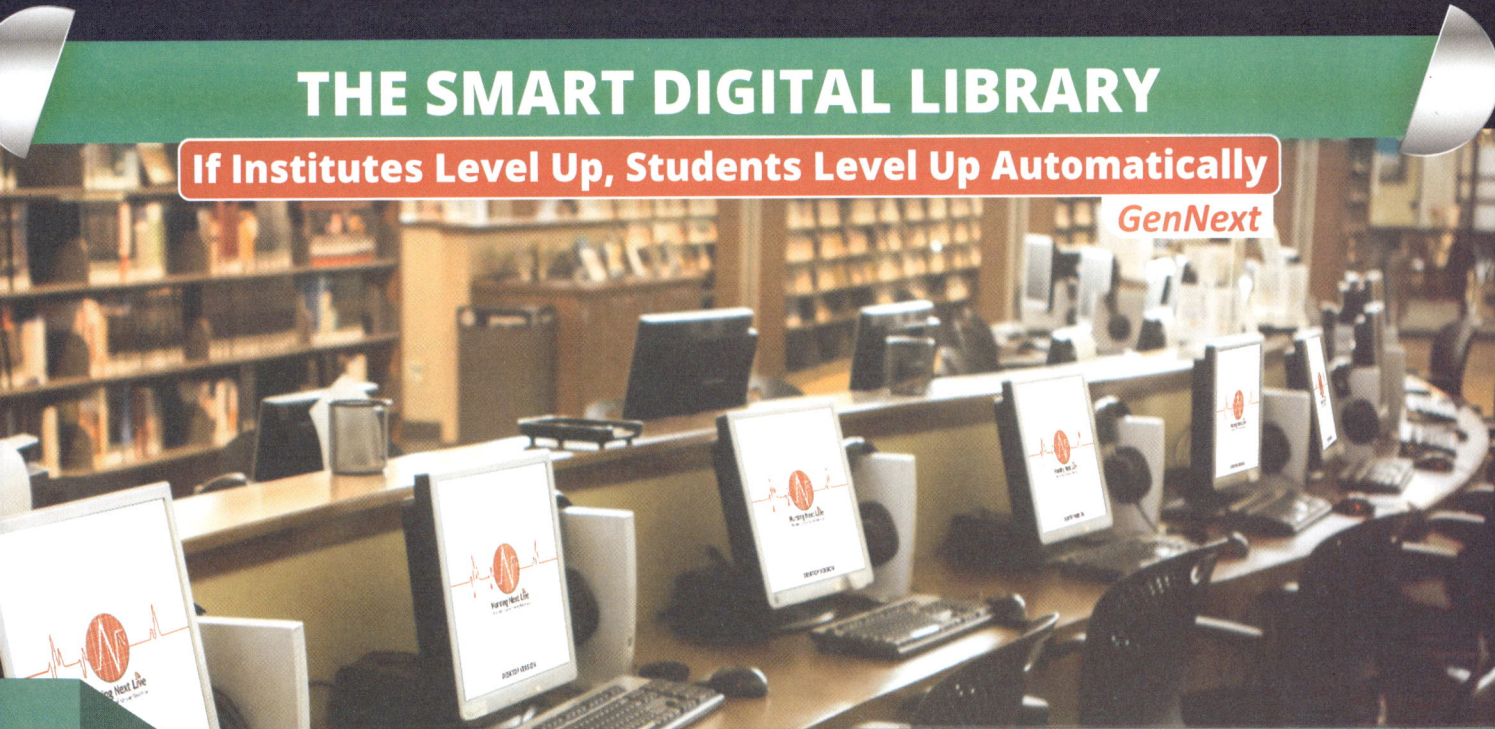

GET ACCESS TO A VARIETY OF CONTENT
Unlike the traditional library methods, we are here to provide you with the impeccable online learning resource where you avail yourself of diversified content to study from. Learn with a futuristic approach and make yourself ready for the in-trend competitions.

TAKE-ON FUTURISTIC STUDY PATTERN
The digital libraries store a wide range of content as per the trends in a virtual environment to give a complete in-vogue experience to the learners.

INCREASE YOUR INSTITUTION'S BRAND VALUE
Be the best Digit-ally to all the learners and increase your brand value. Enhance your traditional library methods by giving it high-tech touch and give your students and the institute the best learning e-learning resource.

COST & TIME-EFFECTIVE
Utilize your money where it needs to be utilized! Digital libraries cover a small space but give boundless information and content to study from. Moreover, if we look forward to our environment, it helps eliminate the paperwork and the time-consuming manual checking of papers.

NO OPENING OR CLOSING HOURS
To offer a sublime 24*7 study experience to your students the digital library works like a wonder. The students can get access and read the library content in digital format anytime and anywhere using their preferred devices. Many readers these days prefer digital libraries over conventional libraries to access the content at their own pace and convenience.

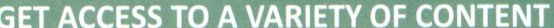

What all you will get

- Complete access to all the Content of all Courses (Crash Courses, Test Series Ver 2.0, Mastermind Pack) with Unlimited Watch Time & the option of re-attempting test.
- All Topics of All Subjects (as per INC syllabus) are covered in form of Video Lectures, MCQs with Rationales, E-Notes, Hand Written Notes (PDF form will be integrated in the app by Feb '21) & Subjective Qs along with IBQs, VBQs, Most Recent & Previous Year Papers, and Live Doubt Sessions per month with Faculties.
- New Content will be added every month. Therefore, the Quantity of your Content will increase gradually throughout your subscription period.

- Regular Online Training Sessions for Best Guidance & Support on "How to Prepare for Nursing Competitive Exams" from the Top experts.
- Get a Dashboard to monitor your Students Progress Chart and Total Usage. *(Forthcoming)*
- Smart Digital Library is available in 2 versions 1) Tablet Version 2) Desktop Application Version.
- Avail Best Discounts & Special Offers on Smart Digital Library. The Institutional Subscription starts with a minimum of 20 subscriptions

For Business Proposal-related enquiries, contact:

Bhupesh Arora
(Project Director)
+91-9555590180
bhupesharora@nursingnextlive.in

Plan-wise Comparison Chart

Compare and Choose the Best Suited to You

	Plan Zero	Crash Course	Test Series	Rapid Revision	Mastermind Plan C	Mastermind Plan C Plus
Videos						
1. All Subjects /Topics Videos	—	—	—	—	✓	✓
2. Video Lectures of Imp Topics	✓	—	✓	✓	—	✓
3. Exam Discussion Videos	—	—	—	—	—	✓
4. Procedure Videos	—	—	—	✓	—	✓
5. Rapid Revision Videos	—	—	—	✓	—	✓
6. IBQ/VBQ/Clinical Qs Discussion	—	—	—	—	—	✓
7. Live Doubt Sessions	—	—	✓	—	✓	✓
8. Student-faculty Meet	—	—	—	—	✓	✓
9. Zoom Sessions/Webinar	—	—	—	—	✓	✓
10. Youtube Videos	✓	—	✓	✓	✓	✓
Tests						
11. Special Mega Assessment Tests	—	✓	✓	✓	✓	✓
12. Grand Tests	✓	✓	✓	—	—	✓
13. Subject-wise Tests	✓	✓	✓	—	—	✓
14. Mini Tests	✓	—	✓	—	—	✓
15. IBQs/VBQs	✓	✓	✓	—	—	✓
16. Most Recent Papers	—	✓	✓	—	—	✓
17. Previous Years Papers	—	✓	✓	—	—	✓
18. Kerala Psc Crash Course	—	✓	✓	—	—	✓
19. CHO Exams Crash Course	—	✓	✓	—	—	✓
20. AIIMS NORCET 2020 Crash Course	—	—	✓	—	—	✓
21. UPPSC Crash Course	—	✓	✓	—	—	✓
22. Most Probable Qs	✓	—	✓	✓	✓	✓
23. National Scholarship Test	—	—	—	✓	✓	✓
24. Subject-wise Qs of All Topics	—	—	—	—	✓	✓
Notes						
25. Handwritten Notes Integrated With Lectures	—	—	—	—	—	✓
26. Last-minute Revision Notes	✓	✓	✓	—	✓	✓
27. Notes Integrated With Rapid Revision Videos	✓	—	—	✓	✓	✓
28. Printed Booklets(*Forthcoming*)	—	—	—	—	✓	✓
Features						
29. Desktop Version	✓	—	—	✓	✓	✓
30. Any Doubt Ask Us	✓	✓	✓	✓	✓	✓
31. Report A Query	✓	✓	✓	✓	✓	✓
32. National Level Ranking	✓	✓	✓	✓	✓	✓
33. Blogs	✓	✓	✓	✓	✓	✓
34. Daily Dose Of Knowledge	✓	✓	✓	✓	✓	✓
35. Forums Get Latest Info	✓	✓	✓	✓	✓	✓
36. Resume Learning	✓	✓	✓	✓	✓	✓
37. Buy Books	—	—	—	—	✓	✓
Supports						
38. Guidance & Counseling	—	—	—	✓	✓	✓
39. Faculty Telegram Channel	—	—	—	✓	✓	✓
40. Faculty Facebook Page	—	—	—	✓	✓	✓

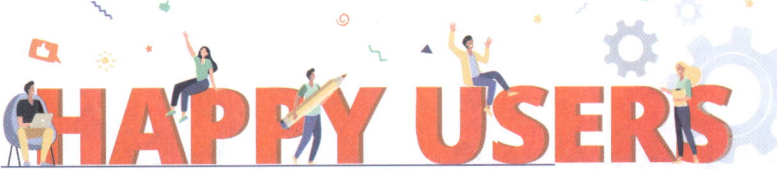

HAPPY USERS

Anisha Manna
★★★★★

DIVERSIFIED SPECIAL FEATURES TO BRACE YOU UP!

"The app is highly recommended for all nursing aspirants. The app has numerous special features with thorough information and is the best Nursing preparation option during these Pandemic times. Used for just 1 year and cleared my M.Sc. with excellent results."

Abhishek Kushwaha
★★★★★

RESULTED TO BE THE BEST NURSING PREPARATION APP!

"Hands down, it is the best Nursing app I have come across. All the tests, study content, CHO Crash Course will not let your expectations down but will prove to be really impressive. If you are a Nursing student/aspirant, then don't think just go for it."

Swatilekha Das
★★★★★

BECOME AN ACHIEVER FROM JUST AN USER WITH NURSING NEXT LIVE

"It has proved to be the best platform for me. If any student is looking for the perfect platform for Nursing Preparations, this is it. To become an achiever from just a dreamer, install this app and study from the plans now."

Nursing Guide Hindi
★★★★★

BEST PLAN FOR THE 1ST YEAR NURSING STUDENT

"The question bank, video lectures are amazing. Extremely helpful for any Nursing Aspirant. It is more preferable if you are in 1st year of Nursing. Do use this app if you want to make your knowledge vaster and achieve all your Nursing goals."

Harshit Upadhyay
★★★★★

IT HAS PROVED TO BE THE BEST NURSING PREPARATION ALLY!

"All the faculties especially Dr Sakshi, Dr Mukhmohit, Dr Rohan, Ms Sabina, all are excellent. The only drawback is that Dr Dharmendra needs to be a bit quick to make the notes and data. Else, it is an excellent prepping platform."

Naga Venkat
★★★★★

GET THE REAL-TIME TEST EXPERIENCE BY USING THE NNLIVE APP

"It is an excellent platform for learning and practicing for Nursing Competitive Exams. It consists of topic-wise explanations and helps us hold command of all. After attempting the real-time tests, I was able to progress gradually."

Sarangi Patel
★★★★★

THE ONE-STOP SOLUTION AS IT SAYS!

"I am grateful to the Nursing Next Live team for making great efforts towards providing us with the best and beyond preparation experience. The video lectures, e-notes, MCQs, and so on will suffice all your preparation needs and take it to the next level. "

Deepak Kumar
★★★★★

10/10 RECOMMENDATION FOR THE NN LIVE APP!

"This app is best for all Nursing students as it has the best quality content to study and learn from."

Shafat Maqbool
★★★★★

CLEAR ALL YOUR DOUBTS-101!

"The video lectures, study content is highly informative and the topics are understood effectively. Clear all your doubts with NNL in no time"

Video Testimonials

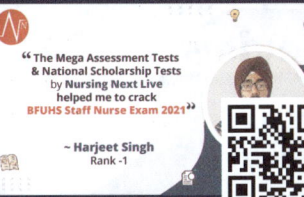

"The Mega Assessment Tests & National Scholarship Tests by Nursing Next Live helped me to crack BFUHS Staff Nurse Exam 2021"

~ Harjeet Singh
Rank -1

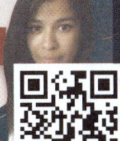

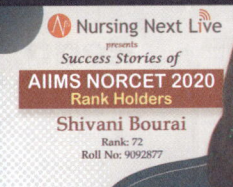

Nursing Next Live presents
Success Stories of
AIIMS NORCET 2020
Rank Holders
Shivani Bourai
Rank: 72
Roll No: 9092877

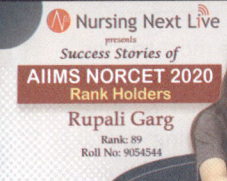

Nursing Next Live presents
Success Stories of
AIIMS NORCET 2020
Rank Holders
Rupali Garg
Rank: 89
Roll No: 9054544

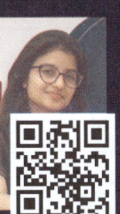

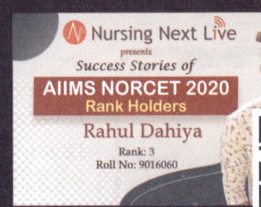

Nursing Next Live presents
Success Stories of
AIIMS NORCET 2020
Rank Holders
Rahul Dahiya
Rank: 3
Roll No: 9016060

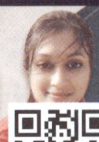

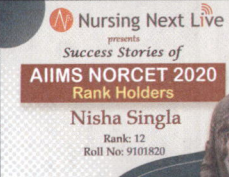

Nursing Next Live presents
Success Stories of
AIIMS NORCET 2020
Rank Holders
Nivedita Saini
Rank: 79
Roll No: 9004587

Nursing Next Live presents
Success Stories of
AIIMS NORCET 2020
Rank Holders
Nisha Singla
Rank: 12
Roll No: 9101820

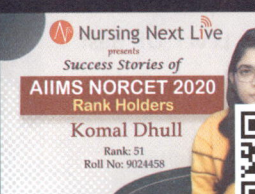

Nursing Next Live presents
Success Stories of
AIIMS NORCET 2020
Rank Holders
Komal Dhull
Rank: 51
Roll No: 9024458

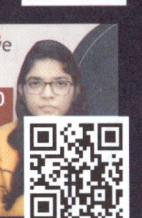

Nursing Next Live presents
Success Stories of
AIIMS NORCET 2020
Rank Holders
Arushi Mittal
Rank: 14
Roll No: 9079646

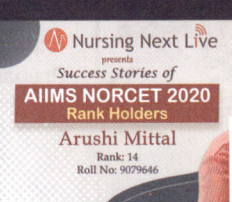

Scan the QR Codes to watch the videos on our YouTube Channel.

We Are Here 24X7

24×7 Guidance & Support

We provide personalized guidance and counseling to all our Subscribers, to ensure that their preparation is in the right direction, that is, toward success. That's why we have an active support service, handled especially by our:`

Nursing Counselors/Academic Counselors – To suggest you what to refer as per your need and want
Relationship Managers – To guide you throughout your learning journey and help you on every step
Guidance & Counselor – To teach you what to study and how to study
Scientific Team – To clear your Scientific Doubts within 24-48 Hours

How to connect with us?
Any Doubt, Ask Us : (In App Support 24x7)
Helpline and WhatsApp No : 9999117411 (Mon-Sat 9:00 am to 8:00 pm, Sunday 9:00 am to 2:00 pm)
Email : feedback@nursingnextlive.in
Web : www.nursingnextlive.com

Follow Us
(Scan the QR Code to Visit to Our Social Media Pages)

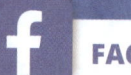 **FACEBOOK**
- Latest Updates & Discount Offers
- Read students feedbacks & Testimonials
- Fun & Learn Activities- Participate and win exciting prizes & free subscription

 INSTAGRAM
- Latest updates of upcoming events
- Participate in giveaways, contests, and quizzes
- See what's latest

 YOUTUBE
- Watch Success Stories, Tips & Tricks for easy preparation, from the top rank holders
- Videos of all Subjects/Important Topics by the mastermind faculty
- Various Last-minute revisions, motivational, and chanting videos
- Live Doubt Sessions every month for paid subscribers

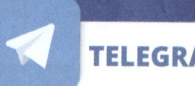 **LINKEDIN**
- Behind-the-scenes of Nursing Next Live
- Significant days of the staff members
- Get insights into the insides of NNLive

TELEGRAM
- Exclusive content for both paid and free subscribers
- Get Daily MCQs/IBQs, E-Notes, Video Teasers
- Latest updates, Daily dosage of learning, Quiz, Special discounts & Offers

Introducing TARGET HIGH DIGITAL
Now Read & Practice Together

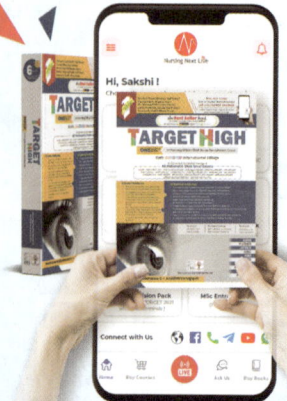

India's No. 1 and the most trusted book with exclusive & complete coverage of all National & State Level Exams is now going digital with no restrictions & additional content.

Explore The Next Level Of Best Preparation, Now!

 COMING SOON

Buy Best-Selling CBS Nursing Books

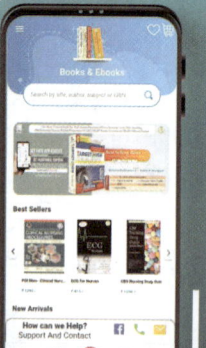

Read, Review & Buy

Now, buying CBS Nursing Books is extra convenient with Nursing Next Live App!

Get a Glimpse of **Sample Pages and TOC** before you proceed to buy the books.

Best Discounts & Special Offers on all the Books.

Textbook of
Pharmacology

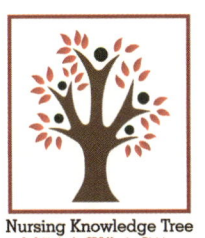

Nursing Knowledge Tree
An Initiative by CBS Nursing Division

For BSc Nursing Students

As per the syllabus of Kerala University of Health Sciences

Joginder Singh Pathania MBBS, MD (Pharmacology and Medicine)

Senior Medical Officer

(Government Hospital Shimla, HP)
Former Assistant Professor (Pharmacology)
IGMC Shimla (HP), India

Rupendra Kumar Bharti MD (Pharmacology)

Assistant Professor

Department of Pharmacology, Raipur Institute of Medical Sciences
Raipur, Chhattisgarh, India

Vikas Sood MSc, PhD

Lecturer

Shivalik Institute of Nursing and Shimla Nursing College
Shimla (HP), India

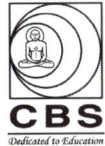

CBS
Dedicated to Education

CBS Publishers & Distributors Pvt Ltd

• New Delhi • Bengaluru • Chennai • Kochi • Kolkata • Lucknow
• Mumbai • Hyderabad • Nagpur • Patna • Pune • Vijayawada

Textbook of
Pharmacology

For BSc Nursing Students

As per the syllabus of Kerala University of Health Sciences

ISBN: 978-93-90619-28-3

First Edition: 2022

Published by **Satish Kumar Jain** and produced by **Varun Jain** for

CBS Publishers & Distributors Pvt Ltd

4819/XI Prahlad Street, 24 Ansari Road, Daryaganj, New Delhi 110 002, India.

Ph: +91-11-23289259, 23266861, 23266867   Website: www.cbspd.com

Fax: 011-23243014

e-mail: delhi@cbspd.com; cbspubs@airtelmail.in.

Corporate Office: 204 FIE, Industrial Area, Patparganj, Delhi 110 092

 Ph: +91-11-4934 4934   Fax: 4934 4935

e-mail: feedback@cbspd.com; bhupesharora@cbspd.com

Branches

- **Bengaluru:** Seema House 2975, 17th Cross, K.R. Road, Banasankari 2nd Stage, Bengaluru 560 070, Karnataka
  Ph: +91-80-26771678/79   Fax: +91-80-26771680   e-mail: bangalore@cbspd.com

- **Chennai:** 7, Subbaraya Street, Shenoy Nagar, Chennai 600 030, Tamil Nadu
  Ph: +91-44-26680620, 26681266   Fax: +91-44-42032115   e-mail: chennai@cbspd.com

- **Kochi:** 68/1534, 35, 36-Power House Road, Opp. KSEB, Cochin-682018, Kochi, Kerala
  Ph: +91-484-4059061-65   Fax: +91-484-4059065   e-mail: kochi@cbspd.com

- **Kolkata:** 6/B, Ground Floor, Rameswar Shaw Road, Kolkata-700 014, West Bengal
  Ph: +91-33-22891126, 22891127, 22891128   e-mail: kolkata@cbspd.com

- **Lucknow:** Basement, Khushnuma Complex, 7-Meerabai Ma Rg, (Behind Jawahar Bhawan), Lucknow-226001, Uttar Pradesh
  Ph: +0522-4000032   e-mail: tiwari.lucknow@cbspd.com

- **Mumbai:** PWD Shed, Gala No. 25/26, Ramchandra Bhatt Marg, Next to J.J. Hospital Gate No. 2, Opp. Union Bank of India, Noor Baug, Mumbai-400009
  Ph: +91-22-66661880/89   Fax: +91-22-24902342   e-mail: mumbai@cbspd.com

Representatives

- **Hyderabad**   +91-9885175004
- **Pune**   +91-9623451994
- **Patna**   +91-9334159340
- **Vijayawada**   +91-9000660880

Printed at: Goyal Offset Works Pvt. Ltd.

ॐ सर्वे भवन्तु सुखिनः सर्वे सन्तु निरामयाः।

सर्वे भद्राणिपश्यन्तु मा कश्चिद्दुःख भाग भवेत्॥

LIST OF REVIEWERS

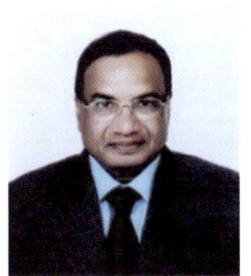

Dr AK Sahai MBBS, MD, PhD, MBA
Professor and HOD
Department of Pharmacology
IGMC, Shimla (HP), India

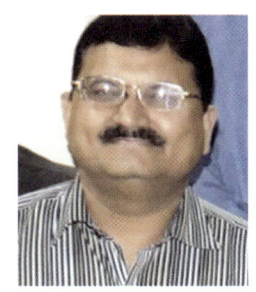

Dr PK Kaundal MBBS, MD
Professor
Department of Pharmacology
Dr YSP Medical College
Nahan, (HP), India

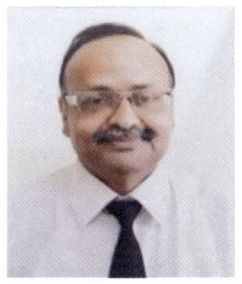

Dr DK Kansal MBBS, MD
Professor and HOD
Department of Pharmacology
RPGMC, Tanda (HP), India

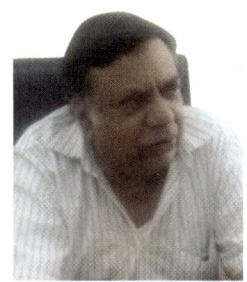

Dr PML Khanna MBBS, MD
Professor and HOD
Department of Pharmacology
Gian Sagar Medical College and
Hospitals,
Banur, Punjab, India

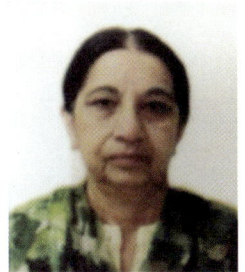

Dr Rani Walia MBBS, MD
Professor and HOD
Department of Pharmacology
MMIMSR, Mullana, Haryana, India

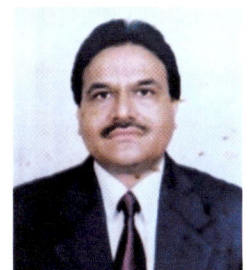

Dr Vijay K Sehgal
Associate Professor
Department of Pharmacology
Government Medical College
Patiala, Punjab, India

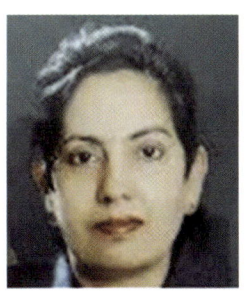

Dr Navpreet Kaur MBBS, MD
Professor and HOD
Department of Pharmacology
MM Medical College and Hospital
Kumarhatti, Solan (HP), India

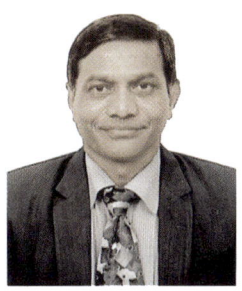

Dr Vijay M Motghare
Professor and HOD
Department of Pharmacology
GMC, Nagpur, India

PREFACE

Pharmacology is one of the basics as well as applied medical sciences that deals with the study of various drugs, their mode of action, pharmacological effects, side effects and drug-drug interactions. This subject is the backbone of all the drug treatments whatsoever are being used in medical practice as each and every medical specialty has to use drugs for the treatment of its patients. As, no treatment is complete without the use of drugs, appropriate knowledge of drugs is mandatory for all medical personnel involved in the use of drugs.

As we have been teaching Pharmacology to the nursing students since long, we have seen the dilemma in the minds of these students about the appropriate book to follow. A teacher sows the seeds of knowledge in the minds of students, but it is the book that provides water and manure to these seeds for sprouting and blooming into the flowers of knowledge. We could not find any suitable book of Pharmacology written strictly according to the syllabus prescribed by Kerala University of Health Sciences (KUHS). Hence, we conceived the idea of writing a Pharmacology book. This edition of the book is meant for the students of BSc Nursing as well as the nurses who are already in the medical practice. As this book has been written and organized strictly according to the syllabus, it will be of immense help to the nursing students all over India.

This book provides the basic concepts of Pharmacology in simple language with clinical correlations and adequate knowledge of the subject. The unnecessary theoretical details have been ignored. This book includes the recent drugs and latest concepts, which have been specially highlighted. It has been designed to provide a comprehensive, authoritative, simplified and precise knowledge of the subject. Most of the illustrations have been made in the easily understandable tabular forms, figures and highlighted forms for the ease of the students.

As we all are the lucky persons chosen by "The Almighty God" to work in the field of medicine, we will be dealing with the drugs till our last breath. This book is going to be useful not only for examination point of view, but also as a ready-reckoner to consult about the doses of drugs in different treatments.

Every care has been taken to keep the book free from errors, but absolute perfection is usually unattainable and there is always a scope for improvement. Hence, the readers are requested to communicate the errors and suggestions to us. The valuable suggestions from the readers and students will receive a warm welcome. The most suitable suggestions will be implemented and the suggestion makers will be suitably acknowledged in the coming editions.

We hope this book will make the learning of Pharmacology a pleasurable experience for the students.

Joginder Singh Pathania
joginderpathania30@gmail.com

Rupendra Kumar Bharti
rbharti000@gmail.com

Vikas Sood
vikas_env@yahoo.co.in

ACKNOWLEDGMENTS

Thanks to **The Almighty God** who provided us the strength and determination to accomplish the work of writing this book.

It is our proud privilege to express deep sense of gratitude and indebtness to **Dr AK Sahai** (Professor and Head), **Dr DD Gupta** (Professor) and **Dr PK Kaundal** (Professor) Department of Pharmacology IGMC, Shimla, for their encouragement, constant supervision and able guidance.

We are sincerely thankful to **Dr Ritu Shitak** (Associate Professor), **Dr Anamika Thakur** (Assistant Professor) Department of Pharmacology and **Dr Yogesh Diwan** (Assistant Professor) and **Dr Kunal Chawla** (Assistant Professor) Department of Anatomy for their positive attitude and valuable suggestions during this project.

We are thankful to the Senior Residents (**Dr Ramesh, Dr Meenakshi, Dr Aanchal**) and Junior Residents (**Dr Navdha Sharma, Dr Sandeep Kaushik, Dr Vivek Thakur, Dr Sushma Sharma**) Department of Pharmacology for their support and sincere cooperation for completion of this book.

We cannot forget the cooperation we got from **Mr Rajan Bhimta**, **Mr Vijay Thakur**, **Ms Aditi**, **Ms Nalini** and all other staff members of the department of Pharmacology, IGMC, Shimla.

We are sincerely thankful to **Ms Sampatti** for her sincere cooperation, constant encouragement and able guidance during the work.

I, **Dr JS Pathania**, express my profound gratitude to my parents, my wife **Dr Neelam Pathania**, my loving son **Siddharth Pathania** and all family members for their patience, unfailing support and cooperation throughout this endeavor. Without their support and encouragement, this book could not have seen the light of the day.

I, **Dr RK Bharti**, express my profound gratitude to my mother **Smt Bangla Bai**, father **Shri Jagdish Bharti** and all family members, for their showers of blessings, inspiration and encouragement at every stage of my life and career.

I, **Dr Vikas Sood**, express my profound gratitude to my parents, my wife **Mrs Babita Sood**, daughter **Ms Vasvi Sood**, son **Suryansh Sood** and all my family members for their patience, unfailing support and cooperation throughout this endeavor.

We all express our profound gratitude from the core of our heart to our families for their constant support and encouragement as they were the source of inspiration for us to accomplish this project.

Last but not the least, we extend our special thanks to **Mr Satish Kumar Jain** (Chairman) and **Mr Varun Jain** (Managing Director), M/s CBS Publishers and Distributors Pvt Ltd for their wholehearted support in publication of this book. We have no words to describe the role, efforts, inputs and initiatives undertaken by **Mr Bhupesh Aarora** [Sr. Vice President – Health Science Division (Publishing & Marketing)] for helping and motivating us.

We sincerely thank the entire CBS team for bringing out the book with utmost care and attractive presentation. We would like to thank Ms Nitasha Arora (Publishing Head & Content Strategist – PGMEE & Nursing), and Dr Anju Dhir (Product Manager cum Commissioning Editor – Medical) for their editorial support. We would also extend our thanks to Mr Shivendu Bhushan Pandey (Sr. Manager & Team Lead), Mr Manoj K Yadav (Production Manager), Mr Ashutosh Pathak (Sr. Proofreader cum Team Coordinator) and all the production team members for devoting laborious hours in designing and typesetting the book.

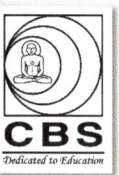

CBS Nursing Knowledge Tree

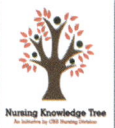

Extends its Tribute to

Florence Nightingale

For glorifying the role of women as nurses,
For holding the title of " The Lady with the Lamp,"
For working tirelessly for humanity—
Florence Nightingale will always be
remembered for her
selfless and memorable services to the
human race.

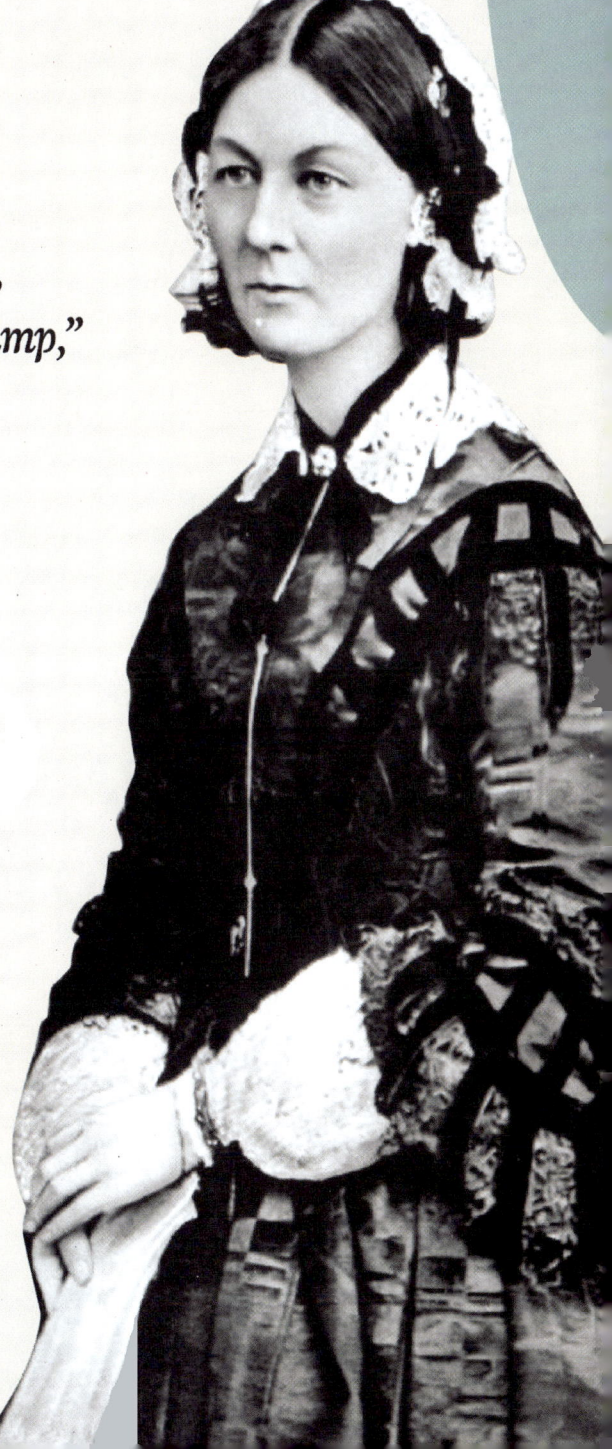

Florence Nightingale
(May 1820 – August 1910)

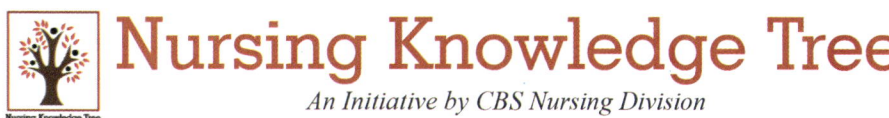

Nursing Knowledge Tree
An Initiative by CBS Nursing Division

"Coming together is a beginning. Keeping together is progress. Working together is success."

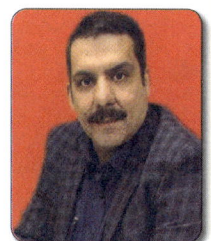

It gives us immense pleasure to share with you that the Nursing Knowledge Tree—An Initiative by CBS Nursing Division, has successfully established itself in the field of nursing as we have been able to stand as a strong contender by sharing approximately 50% of the market share. This growth could not have been possible without your invaluable contribution as our reader, author, reviewer, contributor and recommender, and your outstanding support for the growth of our titles as a whole. You people are the pillars of our series and we are so glad that you all have strengthened our basic foundation.

Nursing Knowledge Tree has been a pioneer and specialist in publishing best quality books for nursing education. Keeping in mind the changing trends in nursing education, we, at Nursing Knowledge Tree, have taken up a mission to bring student-friendly and syllabus-based books written by Subject Experts PAN India.

Our Noteworthy Achievements:
- Our nationally-acclaimed titles
  - *PGIMER NINE Clinical Nursing Procedures*—**Sandhya Ghai**
  - *Target High Staff Nurse Entrance Examination*—**Muthuvenkatachalam S, Ambili M Venugopal**
  - *CBS Nursing Drug Guide*—**Yogesh Gulati/Rakesh Sharma**
  - *Textbook of Nursing Foundations*—**Harindarjeet Goyal**
  - *Essentials of Biochemistry*—**Harbans Lal**
  - *Textbook of Nursing Education*—**Ratna Prakash**
  - *Nursing Research in 21st Century*—**Sukhpal Kaur and Amarjeet Singh**
  - *Essentials of Applied Microbiology*—**D R Arora and Brij Bala Arora**
  - *Textbook of Pediatric Nursing*—**Meharban Singh and Raman Kalia**
- Liaised with the topmost institutes of the country, like **AIIMS, NIMHANS, PGIMER NINE, CMC-Vellore, Manipal University, JIPMER, RAK-Delhi**, etc.
- Published **100+ Quality Nursing Books** and more than **50 New Books** on various subjects for Nursing Undergraduates, Postgraduates and Nursing superspecialty are under process and will be releasing in 2021.
- Increased our social presence by participating in more than **200+ National Conferences, CME's, College Exhibitions & Webinars** in previous years.
- We have come out with **Nursing Next Live**, an EdTech platform, the Next Level of Nursing Education, where we bring learning to people, instead of people going for learning. Through NNL App we are providing various study modules/plans covering All Subjects/All Topics, Video Lectures, Question Banks, E-notes and a Variety of Tests. Students can choose the plan according to their needs and requirements.
- We are excited to announce that we are coming out with our new initiative—**Nursing Next Live Social**, where nursing faculties can share as well as gain knowledge, with the aim to revolutionize the way the nursing segment connects. It's going to be India's first networking platform for Nursing Segment.

Our Journey towards providing Quality Nursing Education is Incomplete without YOU ! Join Us Now !

We specialize in publishing nursing books of superior quality, going ahead we see us publishing more and more quality content and it will only be possible when intellectuals from across the nation come together. Keeping pace with the advancements, we want to strengthen the nursing sector, which was long neglected, and establish a strong foundation when it comes to quality content for the segment.

We are determined to bring about changes in the Nursing Education system and with your support and contributions, we will do it for sure. We will be delighted if you join hands with us in the form of Author, Contributor or Reviewer and take the vision of quality education for nursing students ahead.

Let's join hands together and share our ideas and knowledge. Be the part of this Revolution. We are looking forward to your cooperation in future as well. Share your CVs at **bhupesharora@nursingnextlive.in** or scan the given QR code and fill the form or you can talk to me directly at +9555353330.

With Best Wishes
Mr Bhupesh Aarora
Sr. Vice President – Health Science Division
(Publishing & Marketing)

HOW TO MAKE MOST OUT OF THIS BOOK?

This book has been written after a thorough research about the requirements of nursing students in both theoretical as well as practical levels of knowledge in the subject of Pharmacology. While writing this book, we have studied a lot of Pharmacology books and we have tried to present the matter in a most simplified way keeping the sanctity of each topic.

As the way of presentation of different chapters is unique, the students are advised to go through the following general principles of study to extract most of the crux of the topics.

- Each chapter starts with the chapter outline to guide the students about the important topics of study in the whole chapter. The students should pay attention to this part.
- The **tables and figures** have been presented in a quite simplified way. Memorizing these will definitely sharpen the knowledge levels.
- The topics which are important from clinical point of view, have been highlighted in **separate pointer boxes** for the special attention of the students. These include the latest concepts, recent drugs and important management steps of different diseases.
- The important **Drug Interactions** have been specially highlighted and should be studied and memorized to avoid the errors in prescription and administration of drugs.
- **Nursing Implications** guide about the role of nurses in patient care and the practical aspects of use of various drugs.
- **Questions and MCQs** have been placed at the end of each chapter. The students can assess themselves better by trying to answer these questions themselves.

We hope, the students and other readers will find this book as a useful tool to enhance their knowledge of Pharmacology.

SPECIAL FEATURES OF THE BOOK

Chapter Outline enlist what the students will learn after studying the entire chapter

CHAPTER OUTLINE

- Diuretics and Antidiuretic Drugs
  - Renal physiology
  - Diuretics
  - Indications
  - Antidiuretics
  - Thiazide Diuretics, Amiloride

Important information that needs attention has been highlighted in these **pointer boxes**

Drotaverine
- It is an effective *non-anticholinergic spasmolytic drug*. It causes smooth muscle relaxation by inhibiting phosphodi-esterase-4 (PDE-4) enzyme.
- It is used both orally and parenterally for intestinal, biliary and renal colics, irritable bowel syndrome, uterine spasms, etc.

Remember boxes have been given covering important guidelines and concepts

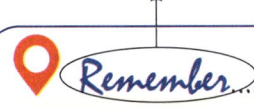
Remember

The common treatment guidelines for any poisoning are as follows:
- Resuscitation and maintenance of vital functions (*ABCD*)
  A- Airway, B- Blood pressure, C- Cardiac care, D- Uses of drugs.
- Termination of further exposure.
- To prevent the further absorption of poison.
- To promote elimination of drugs.
- Use of specific antidotes.

Drug-to-drug interactions have been given separately to help the nurses during their practice

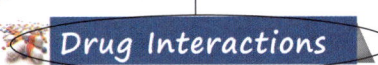
Drug Interactions

- Loop diuretics and spironolactone enhance the digitalis toxicity by causing hypokalemia.
- The levels of lithium are raised by loop diuretics. Hence, the combinations should be avoided.
- Thiazides or high ceiling diuretics are intentionally given in combination with anti-hypertensive to obtain synergistic effects.
- The combinations of high ceiling diuretics and aminoglycoside antibiotics should be avoided as both are ototoxic and nephrotoxic in nature.

Nursing implications enlist the various measures required by nurses while administering the drugs of every class

Nursing Implications

- Assess for contraindications or any known allergies to any vaccines or to the components.
- Nurse should keep a check during vaccination that the child is not suffering from active viral/bacterial infection. Do not administer if the patient exhibits signs of acute infection or immune deficiency because the vaccine can cause a mild infection and can exacerbate acute infections.
- Arrange for proper preparation and administration of the vaccine; check on the timing and dose of each injection because dose, preparation, and timing vary with individual vaccines.

Must know facts are covered under **Let's know boxes**

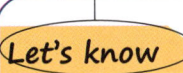
Let's know

Plasma Half-Life
The plasma half-life (t½) of a drug is the time taken for its plasma concentration to be reduced to half of its original value.
- After 1st t½–50% drug is eliminated.
- After 2nd t½–75% (50 + 25) drug is eliminated.
- After 3rd t½– 87.5% (50 + 25 + 12.5) drug is eliminated.
- After 4th t½–93.75% (50 + 25 + 12.5 + 6.25) drug is eliminated.

Thus, nearly complete drug elimination occurs in 4–5 half lives.

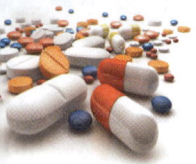

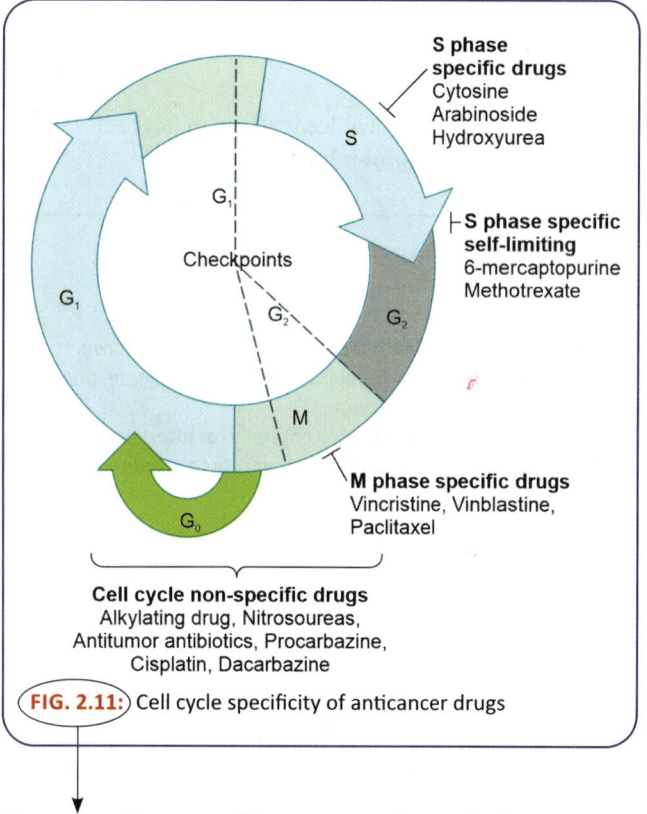

S phase specific drugs
Cytosine
Arabinoside
Hydroxyurea

⊢ **S phase specific self-limiting**
6-mercaptopurine
Methotrexate

Checkpoints

M phase specific drugs
Vincristine, Vinblastine,
Paclitaxel

Cell cycle non-specific drugs
Alkylating drug, Nitrosoureas,
Antitumor antibiotics, Procarbazine,
Cisplatin, Dacarbazine

FIG. 2.11: Cell cycle specificity of anticancer drugs

Numerous **Figures and image** are used to make learning easy for students

Numerous **Tables** are used to help students grasp the concepts quickly

Table 6.1: Classification according to efficacy of diuretics

High efficacy diuretics	Medium efficacy diuretics	Weak or adjunctive diuretics
Na+ K+2Cl⁻ cotransport Inhibitors	**Na+Cl⁻symport Inhibitors**	• Inhibitors of carbonic anhydrase enzyme: Acetazolamide

• Furosemide
• Torasemide
• Bumetanide
• Indacrinone
• Ethacrynic acid
	Thiazides diuretics:
	• Hydrochlorothiazide
	• Chlorthiazide
	• Benzthiazide,
	• Hydroflumethiazide, Bendroflumethiazide
	Thiazide-like diuretics:
	• Chlorthalidone
	• Indapamide
	• Xipamide
	• Metolazone
	• Quinethazone
		• **Potassium sparing diuretics:**
		  ▪ Aldosterone receptor antagonist
		  ▪ Spironolactone
		  ▪ Eplerenone
		• **Na+ channel inhibitors (at collecting duct):**
		  ▪ Triamterene
		  ▪ Amiloride
		• **Osmotic diuretics:**
		  ▪ Mannitol
		  ▪ Glycerol
		  ▪ Isosorbide

Important questions of the chapter are enlisted under **Assess Yourself boxes** to help students assess their learning

MCQs have been added to acquaint the students with probable questions for various examinations

Assess Yourself

Long and Short Answer Questions

1. What are diuretic agents? Classify them, describe loop diuretics.
2. Describe the complications of diuretic therapy.
3. What is the rational of combination of potassium sparing diuretic with loop diuretics?
4. Write short notes on:
   a. Urinary antiseptics   b. Bethanechol
   c. Alkalinizers   d. Furosemide
   e. Spironolactone

Multiple Choice Questions

1. The site of action of the loop diuretic furosemide is
   a. Thick ascending limb of loop of Henle
   b. Descending limb of loop of Henle
   c. Proximal tubule
   d. Distal tubule
2. Thiazides can cause:
   a. Hyperkalemic paralysis   b. Hypouricemia
   c. Hypolipidemia   d. Impotence

Answer Key

1.   (a)   2.   (d)

PHARMACOLOGY

Placement: II Year
Time: Theory 60 hours

Course description: This course is designed to enable students to acquire understanding of pharmacodynamics, pharmacokinetics, principles of therapeutics and nursing implications.

Unit	Time (hrs)	Learning objectives	Content	Teaching learning activities	Assessment methods
I	5	Describe pharmacodynamics, pharmacokinetics, classification and the principles of drug administration	**Introduction to Pharmacology** • Definitions • Sources • Terminology used • Types: Classification • Pharmacodynamics: Actions: therapeutic, adverse, toxic • Pharmacokinetics: Absorption, distribution, metabolism, interaction, excretion • Review: Routes and principles of administration of drugs • Indian pharmacopoeia: Legal issues • Rational use of drugs • Principles of therapeutics	• Lecture • Discussion	• Short answer • Very short answers
II	10	Explain chemotherapy of specific infections and infestations and nurse's responsibilities	**Chemotherapy** • Pharmacology of commonly used antibiotics ▪ Penicillin ▪ Cephalosporins ▪ Aminoglycosides ▪ Macrolide and broad spectrum antibiotics ▪ Sulfonamides ▪ Quinolones ▪ Antiamoebic ▪ Antimalarials ▪ Anthelmintic ▪ Antiscabies Agents ▪ Antiviral and anti fungal agents ▪ Antitubercular drugs ▪ Anti leprosy drugs • Anticancer drugs • Immunosuppressants • Composition, action, dosage, route, indications, contraindications, drug interactions, side effects, adverse effects, toxicity and role of nurse.	• Lecture • Discussion	• Essay • Short answers • Very short answers

Contd…

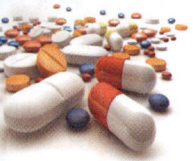

Textbook of Pharmacology for BSc Nursing Students for KUHS

Unit	Time (hrs)	Learning objectives	Content	Teaching learning activities	Assessment methods
III	2	Describe antiseptics, disinfectants, insecticides and nurse's responsibilities	**Pharmacology of Commonly Used Antiseptics, Disinfectants and Insecticides** • Antiseptics • Disinfectants • Insecticides • Composition, action, dosage, route, indications, contraindications, drug interactions, side effects, adverse effects, toxicity and role of nurse	• Lecture • Discussion	• Essay • Short answers • Very short answers
IV	4	Describe drugs acting on Gastrointestinal system and nurse's responsibilities	**Drugs Acting on GI System** • Pharmacology of commonly used: ▪ Antiemetics ▪ Emetics ▪ Purgatives ▪ Antacids ▪ Cholinergic ▪ Anticholinergics • Fluid and electrolyte therapy • Anti diarrhoeals • Histamines • Composition, action, dosage, route, indications, contraindications, drug interactions, side effects, adverse effects, toxicity and role of nurse	• Lecture • Discussion	• Essay • Short answers • Very short answers
V	3	Describe drugs used on respiratory system and nurse's responsibilities	**Drugs Used on Respiratory System** • Pharmacology of commonly used drugs: ▪ Anti asthmatics ▪ Mucolytics ▪ Decongestants ▪ Expectorants ▪ Antitussives ▪ Bronchodilators ▪ Bronchoconstrictors ▪ Antihistamines • Composition, action, dosage, route, indications, contraindications, drug interactions, side effects, adverse effects, toxicity and role of nurse	• Lecture • Discussion	• Essay • Short answers • Very short answers
VI	2	Describe drugs used on urinary system and nurse's responsibilities	**Drugs Used on Urinary System** • Pharmacology of commonly used: ▪ Diuretics and antidiuretics ▪ Urinary antiseptics ▪ Cholinergic and anticholinergics ▪ Acidifiers and alkalanizers • Composition, action, dosage, route, indications, contraindications, drug interactions, side effects, adverse effects, toxicity and role of nurse	• Lecture • Discussion	• Essay • Short answers • Very short answers

Contd...

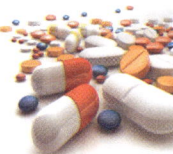

Unit	Time (hrs)	Learning objectives	Content	Teaching learning activities	Assessment methods
VII	4	Describe drugs used in de-addiction, emergency, deficiency of vitamins and minerals, poisoning, immunization and immunosuppression and nurse's responsibilities	**Miscellaneous Drugs** • Drugs used in de-addiction • Drugs used in CPR and emergency • Vitamins and minerals • Immunosuppressants • Antidotes • Antivenom • Vaccines and sera	• Lecture • Discussion	• Essay • Short answers • Very short answers
VIII	2	Describe drugs used on skin and mucous membranes and nurse's responsibilities	**Drugs Used on Skin and Mucous Membranes** • Topical applications for skin, eye, ear, nose and buccal cavity • Antipruritics • Composition, action, dosage, route, indications, contraindications, drug interactions, side effects, adverse effects, toxicity and role of nurse	• Lecture • Discussion	• Essay • Short answers • Very short answers
IX	10	Describe drugs used on nervous system and role of nurse	**Drugs Acting on Nervous System** • Basic and applied pharmacology of commonly used: ▪ Analgesics and anesthetics ▪ Analgesics ▪ Nonsteroidal anti-inflammatory (NSAID) drugs ▪ Antipyretics ▪ Hypnotics and sedatives ▪ Opioids ▪ Nonopioids ▪ Tranquilizers • General and local anesthetics—Gases: Oxygen, nitrous oxide carbon dioxide • Cholinergic and anticholinergics: ▪ Muscle relaxants ▪ Major tranquilizers ▪ Anti-psychotics ▪ Antidepressants ▪ Anticonvulsants ▪ Adrenergics ▪ Noradregenics' ▪ Mood stabilizers ▪ Acetylcholine ▪ Stimulants • Composition, action, dosage, route, indications, contraindications, drug interactions, side effects, adverse effects, toxicity and role of nurse	• Lecture • Discussion	• Essay • Short answers • Very short answers

Contd…

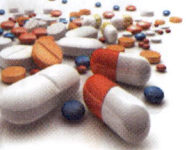

Textbook of Pharmacology for BSc Nursing Students for KUHS

Unit	Time (hrs)	Learning objectives	Content	Teaching learning activities	Assessment methods
X	6	Describe drugs used on cardiovascular system and nurse's responsibilities	**Cardiovascular Drugs** • Hematinics • Cardiotonics • Anti-anginals • Anti-hypertensives and vasodilators • Anti-arrhythmics • Plasma expanders • Coagulants and anticoagulants • Antiplatelets and thrombolytics • Hypolipidemics • Composition, action, dosage, route, indications, contraindications, drug interactions, side effects, adverse effects, toxicity and role of nurse	• Lecture • Discussion	• Essay • Short answers • Very short answers
XI	6	Describe drugs used for hormonal disorders and supplementation contraception and medical termination of pregnancy and nurse's responsibilities	**Drugs Used for Hormonal Disorders/ Supplementation Contraception and Medical Termination of Pregnancy** • Insulins and oral hypoglycemics • Thyroid supplements and suppressants • Steroids, anabolics • Uterine stimulants and relaxants • Oral contraceptives • Other estrogen progesterone preparations • Corticotrophine and gonadotropines • Adrenaline • Prostaglandins • Calcitonins • Calcium salts • Calcium regulators • Composition, action, dosage, route, indications, contraindications, drug interactions, side effects, adverse effects, toxicity and role of nurse	• Lecture • Discussion	• Essay • Short answers • Very short answers
XII	6	Demonstrate awareness of the common drugs used in alternative system of medicine	**Introduction to drugs Used in Alternative Systems of Medicine** • Ayurveda • Homeopathy • Unani • Siddha, etc.	• Lecture • Discussion	• Essay • Short answers • Very short answers

CONTENTS

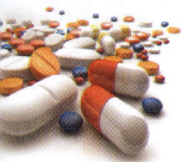

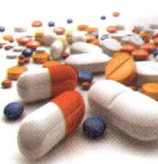

Contents

xxiii

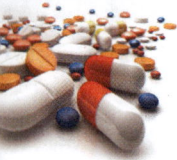

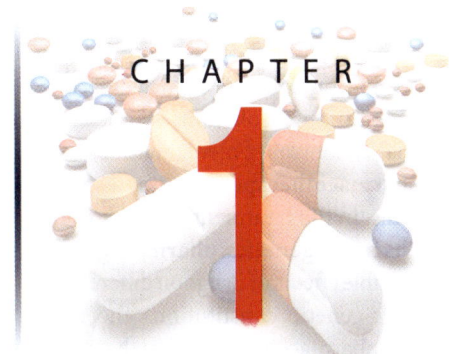

Introduction to Pharmacology

Pharmacology is one of the basic medical sciences, which deals with the detailed study of various drugs, such as their chemical structure, mode of action, pharmacological effects on various systems, side effects and interactions when two or more drugs are given together.

This subject is the backbone of all the drug treatments that are being used in medical practice.

The first institute of pharmacology was founded in 1847 in Germany by Rudolf Buchheim. Oswald Schmiedeberg, is regarded as the 'Father of Pharmacology', due to his extensive contribution in propounding the fundamental concepts in pharmacology.

DEFINITIONS

- **Pharmacology:** It is derived from the Greek word '*Pharmacon*' which means '*drugs*' and '*logos*' which means *study or knowledge*. It deals with the detailed knowledge about drugs including their history, sources, physical, chemical properties and their effects on the various body systems specially in relation to their effective and safe use for medicinal purpose.

- **Chemotherapy:** The therapeutic treatment of various local or systemic infections/malignancies, by using various drugs or chemicals (natural/synthetic/semisynthetic drugs) is called chemotherapy.

- **Drug:** Any substance, which is synthetic, semisynthetic, natural, or biotechnological used for diagnosis, prevention, treatment or cure of a disease or disorder is known as drug.

  According to WHO's definition "Drug is any substance or product that is used or is intended to be used to modify or explore physiological systems or pathological states for the benefit of the recipient". This term is derived from a French Word *drogue* meaning a *dry herb.*

- **Pharmacodynamics:** *(What the drug does to the body)*
  It is a branch of pharmacology, which deals with the effects of drugs on the different body systems and includes mechanism of action of drugs at the molecular, cellular and organ level.

- **Pharmacokinetics:** (*What the body does to the drug*)
  It is a branch of pharmacology, which deals with the journey or movements of drug *in, through and out* from the body. In other words, its deals with the scientific study of the administration, absorption, distribution, biotransformation (metabolism), and excretion (AADME) of drugs.

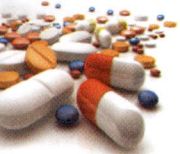

- **Pharmacy:** It is a branch of medical science, which deals with compounding and dispensing of drugs. It also includes preparing suitable dosage forms for administration of drugs to man or animals. It includes collection, identification, purification, isolation, synthesis, standardization and quality control of medicinal substances.
- **Pharmacotherapeutics:** It is a study of appropriate use of drugs in the treatment of various illnesses.
- **Pharmacogenetics/pharmacogenomics:** It is the study of variable effects of drugs on different individuals based upon their genetic constitution. The terms pharmacogenetics and pharmacogenomics can be used interchangeably.
- **Pharmacovigilance:** It deals with the detection, assessment, understanding and prevention of various drug-related problems.
- **Tachyphylaxis:** (*Tachy*: rapid; *Phylaxis*- Protection): When a drug is given repeatedly at shorter intervals, the effect of drug decreases due to development of tolerance. This is called tachyphylaxis. Example: Benzodiazepines, opioids analgesics.
- **Toxicology:** It is a study which deals with the toxic effects of various drugs. The drugs behave as poison if used in higher dosage than prescribed.
- **Teratogenicity:** It is the ability of a drug to produce harmful effect of various drugs on fetus when given in pregnancy.

SOURCES OF DRUGS

The drugs are obtained from various sources such as:
- **Natural sources:**
  - **Plants:** The drugs can be obtained from all part of a plant such as roots, stem, leaves and fruits. Examples: 1. Dhatura—a source of Atropine. 2. Cinchona Bark—a source of Quinine.
  - **Animals and humans:** The drugs can be obtained from animals and human beings also. Examples: Heparin-liver, insulin from the pancreas of cows and pigs, serum from animal source (horse) and human gonadotropin hormone from pregnant women.
  - **Microorganisms:** The bacteria and fungi are also the sources of various drugs, such as penicillin and streptomycin.
  - **Heavy metals, minerals and mineral oils:** Aluminium, fluoride, iron, gold and liquids paraffin are also used to treat various conditions (Table 1.1).
- **Synthetic and semi-synthetic sources:**
  - The drugs synthesized from various chemical substances are called synthetic drugs. Examples: paracetamol, aspirin, diclofenac sodium sulphonamides, calcium channel blockers.

TABLE 1.1: Medicinal uses of elements

Elements	Medicinal uses
Iron	Treatment of iron deficiency anemia
Calcium	Treatment of diseases due to calcium deficiencies, such as rickets in children and osteoporosis in adults
Aluminum and magnesium	As a part of various antacid combinations
Fluorine	Prevention of dental cavities, prevention of osteoporosis
Iodine	Radioactive iodine for diagnosis and treatment of various thyroid disorders
Gold	Treatment of rheumatoid arthritis

- The drugs obtained by changing the structure of naturally obtained substances are called semi-synthetic drugs. Examples: penicillin, ampicillin, amoxicillin dicloxacillin, etc.
- **Engineered sources:** Some drugs are obtained by using modern technology methods, such as human insulin by recombinant DNA technology, monoclonal antibodies and various vaccines for rabies and hepatitis, etc.

TERMINOLOGY

- **Addiction:** The physical and psychological dependence caused by drugs is called addiction.
- **Anaphylaxis:** It is a hypersensitive reaction, which occurs due to ingestion of drugs or any foreign protein material.
- **Antagonist:** The drug which opposes the action of other drugs, when given together or in combination is called antagonist. The net response obtained by the combination of these drugs is always on the lesser side.
- **Antidote:** The drug or chemical which counteracts the harmful effects of other drug or chemical is called antidote.
- **Aqueous solution:** The solution obtained by dissolving one or more drugs in water is called aqueous solution.
- **Brand name:** It is the name given by the manufacturer or pharmaceutical companies to a particular drug and is the trademark or property of that particular company.
- **Capsule:** Solid form of drugs or liquids composed in gelatin cover.
- **Chemical name:** It is the name assigned by the manufacturer to a formula before getting an approved name. It is based on chemical formula of drugs. This is not used in prescriptions.
- **Contraindication:** Any condition or factor, which prevents or withholds the use of medicines/drugs.
- **Dose:** The amount of drug to be administered or given is called dose of that drug. It is usually calculated and written in milligrams. Example, like Azithromycin 500 mg once

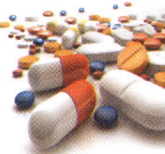

a day, or Amoxicillin with clavulanic acid (Augmentin) 625 mg thrice a day.

- **Emulsion:** It is the mixture of two immiscible liquids in which droplets of one liquid are dispersed throughout the body of second liquid. Example: Castor oil emulsion.
- **Enema:** This is a liquid preparation, which is administered rectally, for evacuation of the bowel. Example: Soap water enema.
- **Generic name:** It is the name by which the drug is known commonly. It is same throughout the world. It is based upon the salt name of a particular drug.
- **Half-life:** It is the time taken for the amount of drug in body to decrease to one half its peak level.
- **Iatrogenic:** The condition or disease, which is physician induced and is due to functional disturbances caused by the drug during treatment and persists even after the offending drug has been withdrawn. Example: Peptic ulcer by NSAIDs.
- **Idiosyncrasy:** It is genetically determined abnormal reactivity to a drug. Every drug has a potential to cause idiosyncratic reaction in the genetically susceptible individuals.
- **Inhalation:** Administering a drug invapor or gaseous form, through the nose.
- **Loading dose:** Administering drug at a dose higher than the routinely used dose is called loading dose. It is given to achieve the required peak levels in blood.
- **Lotion:** This is usually aqueous solution or suspension intended for local administration. Example: Calamine lotion.
- **Oral administration:** Giving drugs by mouth.
- **Ointment:** This is a semi-solid preparation for external application. Example: Betadine ointment.
- **Parenteral administration:** Drugs, which are given by injection into veins or muscles in various parts in body.
- **Poisoning:** Overdose of a drug that causes damage to multiple body systems and has the potential for fatal reactions.
- **Powder:** It is a dosage form, when a solid drug is given in finely divided powdered state. A simple powder contains one ingredient and a compound powder contains more than one ingredient.
- **Receptor:** It is a macromolecule, which is present on the cell surface or inside the cell and is a site for the drugs to act.
- **Rectal administration:** Route of administering drug via colon or rectum.
- **Response:** It is the effect seen after administering drugs causing improvement of health or decrease in sign and symptoms.
- **Schedule:** It is timing or frequency of administering the drugs to the patients.

- **Side effects:** Any undesirable actions which occur to the patient after administering the therapeutic dose levels.
- **Sublingual administration:** Route of administering the drug below the tongue.
- **Suspension:** According to **International Union of Pure and Applied Chemistry**, a suspension is dispersion of solid particles in a liquid.
- **Syrup:** This is a concentrated solution composed of sugar and various drugs to treat various conditions. Example: Cough syrup, B-complex syrup.
- **Tablet:** This is a solid disc-shaped form of medication prepared either by molding or compression in a special machine.
- **Tolerance:** The progressive decrease in the effectiveness of a drug, due to its repeated use.
- **Vitamin:** These are found in food and it is essential for growth and good health.

Commonly used Abbreviations in Prescriptions

- **R$_x$:** The symbol R is an abbreviation for the Latin word RECIPE, which means take thou or you take. The line on the foot of R is set to designate an invocation to Jupiter, the God of knowledge, learning and healing.
- **Tab:** Tablet
- **Cap:** Capsule
- **Inj:** Injection
- **IM:** Intramuscular
- **IV:** intra venous
- **SC:** Subcutaneous
- **I/D:** Intradermal
- **OD:** Once in a day
- **BD/bid:** (Bis in dic): Twice a day
- **TDS** (ter in dte sumendum): To be taken thrice a day
- **TID** (ter in die): Three times a day
- **QID** (Quarter in die): Four times a day
- **HS** (hora somni): At bed time
- **STAT** (staim): Immediately
- **Rept:** (Repitatur) Repeat
- **Non rept** (non reptatur): Non repeat
- **AC** (anti-cibum): Before meals
- **PC** (post cibum): After meals
- **NPO** (nil per orally): Nothing to taken by mouth
- **BBF:** Before breakfast
- **AD:** After dinner
- **SOS:** As and when required

DRUGS' CLASSIFICATION

The drugs can be classified into the following categories:

Prescription or Legend Drugs

The drugs, which can be sold to a patient in retail only against a prescription issued by a registered medical practitioner

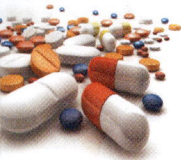

are called 'prescription drugs'. They have been placed in the *schedule H* of the Drugs and Cosmetic Rules (1945) in India.

Nonprescription or Over-the-counter (OTC) Drugs

The drugs, which can be purchased by anybody from the medical store. Such drugs are considered to be relatively safe. Few drugs like vitamins, paracetamol, aspirin, antacids, laxatives, etc. These drugs can be sold even by grocery stores.

Investigational Drugs

The drugs, which are still in the process of investigation regarding use in human subjects. These drugs are already proven to be effective in animals.

Illicit or Street Drugs

The drugs which cannot be sold legally in any country (e.g., heroin). Illicit drugs usually are used for non-medicinal purposes, generally to alter mood or feeling.

Orphan Drugs

The drugs or biological products, which are meant for diagnosis, treatment or prevention of a rare disease or condition. From the sale of these drugs, pharmaceutical companies may or may not be able to recover the cost of developing and marketing of these drugs. Examples: Liothyronine (T3), liposomal amphotericin B, miltefosine, rifabutin, somatropin, etc.

Essential Drugs

According to the WHO, essential drugs are defined as "those drugs that satisfy the basic healthcare need of the majority of the population". These drugs should be available at the affordable price, in adequate amounts and at all the times.

India prepared its first National Essential Drugs List in 1996 and the latest is 17th list prepared in 2011 titled as National List of Essential Medicines. It includes 348 medicines.

PHARMACODYNAMICS

(What the drug does to the body?)

Pharmacodynamics deals with the effects of drugs on the body and includes mechanism of action of drug at the molecular, cellular and organ level. It gives us a detailed view of the dose response relationship of various drugs and also helps us to understand how the action of drugs is modified, when two or more drugs are given together. Under pharmacodynamics we study:
- **The broad principles of drug action**
- **Therapeutic effects of drugs and their modifications**

Principles of Drug Action

The drugs, which are given to the patients, alter the basic physiological processes of the body. Broadly the drugs can control/alter the various body processes by following principles.
- **Stimulation:** The drugs play a role in increasing the level of activity of specialized cells. Example: Salivary glands are stimulated by pilocarpine, adrenaline stimulates heart, and metoclopramide increases GI motility causing diarrhea.
- **Depression:** The drugs play a role in decreasing the level of activity of specialized cells. Example: Decreased gastric acid secretion by omeprazole, codeine causes constipation due to depression in peristaltic movements.
- **Replacement:** Some diseases are caused by the deficiencies of certain hormones or some metabolites in the body, which are treated by replacing the deficient enzyme/hormones/metabolites. Example: Thyroid hormone in hypothyroidism, iron in iron deficiency anemia and insulin in diabetes mellitus.
- **Irritation:** Irritating effect of certain drugs are also helpful in therapeutics, such as irritant purgatives increase peristalsis. The various liniments act by irritation/counter irritation mechanisms, thus relieving pain. The decrease or loss of function can be achieved by strong irritation provided by certain drugs resulting in inflammation and morphological damage to the tissues. Examples: Necrosis of hemorrhoids with the help of local injections of almond oil and alcohol.
- **Antimicrobial action:** Some drugs act by killing or inhibiting the growth of microorganisms by interfering with various metabolic activities of microbes without affecting the host cell. Example: Ampicillin, azithromycin, acyclovir, etc.
- **By altering the immune system:** The drugs may modulate the immune system by increasing or decreasing the immune status. Example: BCG vaccination, hepatitis vaccination and polio vaccination.

Mechanism of Action of Drugs

The mechanism of action of drugs can be divided into following types:
- **Physical:** The drug actions are based upon its physical properties.
  - Laxative effect of agar, ispaghula, or psyllium seeds due to their mass effect
  - Diuretic effect of mannitol due to its osmotic properties
  - Soothing effect of pectin due to its demulcent property
  - Antifoaming effect of dimethicone
- **Chemical:** The drug actions are based upon its chemical properties. Examples:
  - Oxidizing effect of potassium permanganate

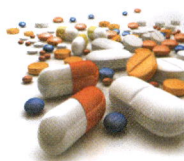

- Chelation by Dimercaprol
- Antacid having properties to decrease acid secretion into the stomach, used in peptic ulcer disease
- **Cellular:** The drugs act at the level of cell and its organelles, such as:

Enzymes

In the living system, almost all catalytic actions are carried out with the help of enzymes. The drugs may act by stimulation or inhibition of different enzymes depending upon the target cell (Table 1.2).

The inhibition of enzymes may be competitive or noncompetitive in nature.

Differences between the competitive and non-competitive enzyme inhibition are given in Table 1.3.

TABLE 1.2: Enzymatic receptors and their associated substances

Enzymatic receptor	Associated substance
Tyrosine kinase receptor	Insulin, endodermal growth factor, nerve growth factor, platelets derived growth factor, vascular endothelial growth factor, fibroblast growth factor
Tyrosine kinase associated receptor; tyrosine phosphatase receptor	Prolactin, interleukin -2, cytokines, T-cell, B-cell antigen receptor for depolarization of protein
Serine threonine kinase receptor	Phosphorylation of serine threonine residue
Guanyl cyclase receptor	Phosphorylation of atrial natriuretic peptide

TABLE 1.3: Differences between competitive and noncompetitive inhibition

Competitive inhibition	Noncompetitive inhibition
Antagonist binds with the same receptor	Binds to another site of receptor
Antagonist resembles chemically with the agonist	Does not resemble
The same maximal response can be attained by increasing dose of agonist (surmountable antagonism)	Maximal response is suppressed (unsurmountable antagonism)
Intensity of response depends on the concentration of both agonist and antagonist	Maximal response depends only on the concentration of antagonist
Examples: ACh—Atropine, Morphine—Naloxone	Diazepam—Bicuculline

TABLE 1.4: Action of various drugs on ion channels

Drugs	Action	Ion channel
Nifedipine	Blocks	L-type voltage sensitive calcium channel
Sulfonylurea	Inhibits	Pancreatic ATP sensitive K+ channels
Amioderone	Blocks	Myocardial sodium, potassium and calcium channels
Phenytoin	Modulates	Voltage sensitive Na+ channel
Quinidine	Blocks	Myocardial sodium channel
Mimantine	Blocks	Potassium and magnesium channel post-synaptically

Ions Channels

There are various ions channel located on the cell membrane, which participate in transmembrane signaling process. Example: Sodium channels, potassium channels calcium channels, etc. The drugs may act by stimulation or inhibition of different ions channels depending upon the target cell (Table 1.4).

Receptors

These are macromolecules, mostly protein in nature stimulation or inhibition of which causes biological/physiological effects. These are present on cell membrane or intracellularly (Table 1.5).

- The drugs may act by stimulation or inhibition of different receptors depending upon the target cell.
- The drug acts only, if it is having affinity for the receptor. As every lock has its own key to open it, similarly every drug acts through a particular receptor.
- Drug receptor combination is responsible for the activity through receptor.
  - **Agonist:** The drug having both affinity and intrinsic activity is called an agonist.

TABLE 1.5: Receptors acting on cell membrane and intracellular receptors

Receptors acting on cell membrane	Intracellular receptors

• Serpentine/seven pass/ G protein coupled receptor
• Ions channels
• Enzyme linked receptor
	• Divided into intracytoplasmic and intranuclear
	  ▪ **Intracytoplasmic:** Glucocorticoids, mineralocorticoids, liothyronine (T3), thyroxin (T4), vitamin-D or cholecalciferol
	  ▪ **Intranuclear:** Retinoid, some nucleus of T3 and T4
	• **Intracytoplasmic with intranuclear:** Progesterone, estrogen

5

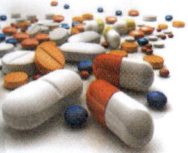

TABLE 1.6: Metabolites and transporters

Metabolites	Transporters	Drugs
Serotonin	Serotonin transporter neuron	Selective serotonin reuptake inhibitor
Dopamine	Dopamine transporter neuron	Amphetamine
Acetylcholine	Choline uptake neuron	Hemicholinium
GABA	GABA transporter GTA1	Tigabine
Noradrenaline	Norepinephrine transporter neuron	Cocaine

GABA, Gamma aminobutyric acid

- **Antagonist:** An agent which does not have any effect of its own, but prevents the action of an agonist on a receptor.
- **Inverse agonist:** An agent which activates a receptor to produce opposite effect to that of an agonist.
- **Partial agonist:** An agent which activates a receptor to produce submaximal effect.

Transporters

These are specific carriers present on the cell membrane, which serve the purpose of transporting the substrate across cell membrane in concentration gradient or against the concentration gradient using metabolic energy (Table 1.6).

Others

- **Counterfeit/false incorporation mechanisms:** The artificial analogues of natural substrates which have no effect on enzymes, ions, receptors or transporters, but are incorporated into specific macromolecules of the cell. It leads to alter the biological activity of cell causing destruction.
  Example: 5-flourouracil increases the mutation rate and chromosomal disturbances- (antineoplastic),
  Sulfa drugs: Nonfunctional folic acid- (bacteriostatic).
- **Protoplasmic poisons:** These drugs act as poison for the bacteria at their protoplasmic level. Examples: Germicides and antiseptics: phenol, formaldehyde
- **Formation of antibodies:**
  Active immunity: Vaccines induce antibody formation and stimulate defense mechanisms against the disease. Example: BCG, measles, DPT, hepatitis vaccination.
  Passive immunity: Readymade antibodies (antisera) are injected in the patients for immediate action. Example: Antisera against tetanus and diphtheria

- **Placebo:** Placebo (Latin word) means *I Shall Please.*
  - It is inert and harmless substance, which physically resembles the actual medicine.
  - These are pseudo drugs made by cellulose.
  - It works at psychological level and not at the pharmacodynamic level.
  - Patient may sometimes feel good on taking these placebo medicines.
  - These agents cause release of endorphins in brain and help to relieve subjective symptoms psychologically.
  - These are used in psychosomatic disorders and in clinical trials.

THERAPEUTIC EFFECT OF DRUGS AND THEIR MODIFICATIONS

Whenever drugs are administered to a patient, therapeutic effects are seen. The response is different with different dosages of a drug. A definite dose-response relationship is seen, which has two components:

1. **Dose: Plasma concentration relationship:** Dose is the appropriate amount of a drug required to produce a certain degree of response in a given patient. Dose of a drug is governed by its concentration at which it should be present at its target site.

   The recommended dose of a drug is based on population data and caters to an average patient. There are different types of dosages required to produce different level of plasma concentration, such as:

   The dose which is same and appropriate for most of the patients is called '**standard dose**'. The drugs given as standard dosages have a wide safety of margin. The effects of a drug differ with the different plasma concentrations.

   It is the dose which differentiate a drug from a poison.

   The plasma concentration of a drug may remain constant or keep on increasing as we go on increasing the dose. It depends upon the kinetics of elimination followed by a particular drug.

2. **Plasma concentration: Response relationship:** Optimum therapeutic response in every disease is obtained by maintaining a particular plasma concentration of a drug for the treatment of a particular disease.

   In other words, the therapeutic response changes with the change in plasma concentration of the drugs. The dose of a drug cannot be exceeded from the prescribed limit as it may lead to intolerable adverse effects. Sometimes a compromise has to be made between submaximal therapeutic effect and the tolerable side effects. Example: Anticancer drugs, corticosteroids.

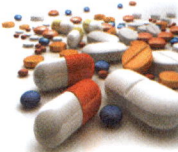

DRUG POTENCY AND EFFICACY

Drug Potency

It refers to the amount of drug needed to produce a certain response. Relative potency is a more meaningful term, in which we compare the dose of two similar drugs at which they produce the same response.

Example: 10 mg of morphine produces equal analgesic effect as produced by 100 mg of pethidine. It means that morphine is 10 times more potent than pethidine. Drug potency helps us to decide the dose of a drug.

Drug Efficacy

It refers to the maximum response, which can be elicited by a particular drug.

Example: Aspirin can never achieve the level analgesic effect, which can be achieved by morphine. This means that morphine is more efficacious than aspirin.

Therapeutic Efficacy

It refers to the degree of relief provided by the drug in the recommended dose range. It is a comparable term between two drugs having similar action.

Example: In case of mixed dyslipidemia, combination of drugs like statins with fenofibrate is much more beneficial than statins alone. It means that the therapeutic efficacy is higher in combination therapy than monotherapy of statins.

Therapeutic Index (TI)

It is also called safety margin of a drug. It refers to the ratio of *'the dose of drug that causes adverse effects'* to that which causes *'effective therapeutic effect'*.

The therapeutic index is calculated as follows:

$$TI = LD50/ED50$$

where TI: Therapeutic Index

LD_{50}: The amount of drug, which is lethal to 50% of general population.

ED_{50}: The amount of drug, which is beneficial to 50% of general population.

For the drugs with narrow therapeutic index

- The slight deviation from the prescribed dosage can be harmful for the patients.
- The plasma levels monitoring is advocated.

For the drugs with wide therapeutic index

- The deviation from the prescribed dosage may not be harmful for the patients.
- The plasma levels monitoring is not advocated.

The examples of drugs having narrow and wide therapeutic index are given in Table 1.7.

TABLE 1.7: Range of therapeutic indices of some drugs

Very narrow therapeutic index	Narrow therapeutic index	Wide therapeutic index
Vancomycin	Warfarin	Almost all
Amphotericin B	Levothyroxine	Antibiotics
Polymyxin	Carbamazepine	NSAIDS
	Lithium Carbonate	Hypnotics/
	DigoxinPhenytoin	Sedatives
	Theophylline	Beta- blockers
	Morphine	Benzodiazepines

COMBINED EFFECTS OF DRUGS

Most of the times, patients are prescribed two or more drugs simultaneously. This may affect the action of one drug by either increasing or decreasing the effect of other drug. When two or more drugs are given together or one after another, they may exhibit either synergism or antagonism. This is due to interactions at Pharmacokinetic or Pharmacodynamic level.

Synergism

(Greek: Syn—together; ergon—work)

When the action of one drug is potentiated or increased by the other, they are said to be synergistic.

Synergism can be:

- **Additive:** The effect of the two drugs is in the same direction and simply adds up. **(1 + 1 = 2)**
  Effect of drugs X + Y = effect of drug X + effect of drug Y

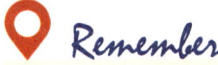

Additive Drug Combinations

- Aspirin + paracetamol as analgesic/antipyretic
- Amlodipine + atenolol as antihypertensive
- Glibenclamide + metformin as hypolycemic
- Ephedrine + theophylline as bronchodilator

- **Supraadditive (potentiation):** The effect of combination is greater than the individual effects of the components. **(1 + 1 = 11)**
  Effect of drugs X + Y > effect of drug X + effect of drug Y

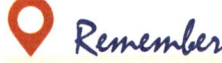

Supraadditive Drug Combinations

- Levodopa + carbidopa: Inhibition of peripheral metabolism
- Sulfamethoxazole + trimethoprim: Sequential blockade
- Telmisartan+ hydrochlorothiazide: Tackling two contributory factors in the management of hypertension.

Antagonism

(Greek: *Anta—opposite; ergon—work*)

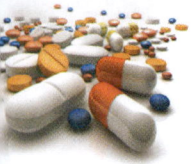

When one drug decreases or abolishes the action of another drug, they are said to be antagonistic.

Effect of drugs X + Y< effect of drug X + effect of drug

Depending on the mechanism involved, antagonism may be:

- **Physical antagonism:** Antagonism due to physical property of the drugs.
  Example: Adsorption-charcoal adsorbs alkaloids, so used in alkaloidal poisonings.
- **Chemical antagonism:** Antagonism due to the chemical property of the drugs. The two drugs react chemically and the product formed is inactive.
  Examples: Such as titration of acid with base.
  - Chelating agents (BAL, Cal. Disodium edetate) complex toxic metals (Arsenic and lead).
  - Potassium permanganate oxidizes alkaloids—used for gastric lavage in poisoning.
  - Nitrites form methemoglobin which reacts with cyanide radicals.
  - Two drugs should not be mixed in the same syringe or infusion bottle as they may react with each other. Example: Thiopentone sod. + Succinylcholine chloride, Heparin + penicillin.
- **Physiological/functional antagonism:** The two drugs may have pharmacological effects in opposite direction due to their overt effects on the same physiological function. The drugs act at different receptors and follow different mechanisms.
  - Glucagon and insulin on blood sugar level.
  - Histamine and adrenaline on bronchial muscles and BP.
- **Receptor antagonism:** Here, one drug (antagonist) blocks the receptor action of the other (agonist).
  Example: Acetylcholine- Atropine, calcium-iron

DRUG EFFECTS

Drugs are always given for the benefit of patients, but sometimes in addition to the desired effects, some undesirable events are seen in some patients, which may be trivial, serious or even fatal in nature. These undesirable events are called adverse drug effects.

Adverse effect is defined as 'any undesirable or unintended consequence of drug administration in normally used dosages and requires treatment or decrease in dose or indicates precaution in the future use of the same drug'.

Nature and severity of adverse drug effect differs with the route of administration employed.

Adverse Effects

- **Predictable (Type A or Augmented) reactions:** These are also called mechanism based adverse drug reactions.

These are dose related, preventable and usually reversible. These include the side effects of particular drug.

- **Unpredictable (Type B or Bizarre) reactions:** These are not based on drug's known actions but depend upon the different behavior of the patient's body system (genetic basis) to a particular drug. They are not dose related, less common, and generally more serious and mostly require withdrawal of the drug. It includes allergy and idiosyncrasy.

Severity of adverse drug reactions *can be graded as:*

- **Minor:** No treatment, antidote or prolongation of hospitalization is required.
- **Moderate:** Change in drug treatment may be required. Specific treatment is needed for treatment of reaction and hospital stay may be prolonged.
- **Severe:** The reaction is life-threatening, may cause permanent damage and requires intensive medical treatment. Example: Stevens-Johnson syndrome
- **Lethal:** It contributes to death of the patient directly or indirectly. Example: Anaphylactic shock

Side Effects

- These are unavoidable and unwanted pharmacodynamic effects of drug, which occur at routinely prescribed therapeutic doses.
- Generally, these are not serious in nature.
- By reducing the dose, symptoms usually improve.
- These are based on the same action as the therapeutic effect.
  Examples:
  - Glyceryl trinitrate relieves angina pectoris by dilating peripheral vasculature and this dilatation is the cause for postural hypotension and throbbing headache, which is seen as a side effect of this drug.
  - Atropine is used in preanesthetic medication for its antisecretory action. The same action produces dryness of mouth as a side effect.

Toxic Effects

- When some drug is used for prolonged period or in over dosage, excessive pharmacological action of the drug is seen. Which is termed as toxic effect of that drug.
- The symptoms are predictable and dose related.
  Examples:
  - Morphine (opioid analgesic) causes respiratory failure in overdosage.
  - Streptomycin (aminoglycoside) causes vestibular damage on prolonged use.

Poisoning

Poison is 'any substance which puts the life in danger by severely affecting one or more vital functions of the body'. The drugs,

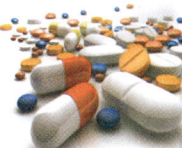
household and industrial chemicals, insecticides, etc. are frequently involved in poisoning. Every drug can behave as a poison, if administered in large dosages. Poisoning causes various harmful and deleterious effects on the human body, which can endanger life if not treated promptly. Example: Wild mushroom poisoning, organophosphorus poisoning.

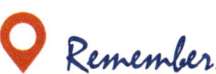 *Remember* ....

The common treatment guidelines for any poisoning are as follows:

- Resuscitation and maintenance of vital functions (*ABCD*) **A- Airway, B- Blood pressure, C- Cardiac care, D- Uses of drugs.**
- Termination of further exposure.
- To prevent the further absorption of poison.
- To promote elimination of drugs.
- Use of specific antidotes.

Idiosyncrasy

It is abnormal reactivity to a drug, which is genetically determined. This feature is not found in majority of patients and is a rare but important reaction. Every drug has a potential to cause idiosyncratic reaction in the genetically susceptible individuals.

Examples:

- In some individuals, barbiturates can cause excitement and mental confusion.
- In some individuals, quinine/quinidine can cause cramps, diarrhea, purpura, asthma and vascular collapse.
- Wheat (gluten) hypersensitivity.

Drug Allergy

- It is an abnormal individual immunologic response to a drug.
- It is not related to the pharmacodynamic behavior of the drug.
- It can occur even with very small doses of the drug.
- This is also called *drug hypersensitivity.*
- In drug allergy the skin, airways, gastrointestinal tract, blood and blood vessels are the major organs which are affected.
- Patients are advised to remember the drugs or food items to which they are allergic.
- These drugs or food items should be avoided in future.

TYPES OF ALLERGIC REACTIONS

Different types of allergic reactions are given in Table 1.8

TABLE 1.8: Types of allergic reactions

Humoral	Cell mediated
Immediate hypersensitivity reaction	Delayed hypersensitivity reaction
It includes: • Hypersensitivity reaction- I • IgE mediated Example: Wheal and flare reaction, anaphylaxis, atopic dermatitis, etc.	It includes: • Hypersensitivity reaction- IV • T cell mediated Example: Contact dermatitis, montoux test, multiple sclerosis, etc.

Photosensitivity

It is a cutaneous reaction on sun exposure, resulting due to drug induced sensitization of the skinto UV radiation. Example: Sulphonamide, thiazide, chloroquine, fluoroquinolone.

Drug Addiction

An individual likes to take the drug again and againto get the pleasurable effects of the drug. If not taken again, the person feels withdrawal symptoms which force him/her to take the drug again. Example: Alcohol, nicotine.

Physical Dependence

The drug seeking behavior develops in the individual, which is a strong impetus for continued drug use. Example: Amphetamines, cocaine, cannabis, LSD are drugs which produce addiction but little/no physical dependence.

There are specialized de-addiction centers which are helpful in de-addicting the patients.

Teratogenicity

The capacity of a drug to cause various abnormalities in fetus, when given during pregnancy, is called teratogenicity. The placenta behaves as an incomplete barrier, and any drug can cross it to a lesser or greater extent if given for a prolonged duration. The drug effects on the fetus are often irreversible and cause various malformations. Examples: The thalidomide disaster (1958–61) resulting in thousands of babies born with phocomelia (seal-like limbs).

Drugs can affect the fetus at three crucial periods of pregnancy:

1. **Fertilization and implantation:** Conception to 17 days, it causes failure of pregnancy or abortions, which often goes unnoticed.
2. **Organogenesis:** 18–55 days of gestation; it is the most vulnerable period and various deformities occur in the fetus, if exposed to any teratogenic drugs.
3. **Growth and development:** 56 days onwards—Various developmental and functional abnormalities can occur, e.g., NSAIDs may induce premature closure of ductus arteriosus, lithium cause fetal goiter and angiotensin

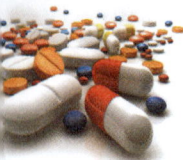

TABLE 1.9: Safe versus contraindicated drugs in pregnancy

Safe drugs (drugs which do not cross placenta)	Contraindicated drugs (Drugs which cross placenta or teratogenic drugs)
Heparin	Lithium
Insulin	Ciprofloxacin
Desmopressin	Tetracycline
Chloroquine	Aminoglycosides
Isoniazid, Rifampicin, Ethambutol	Angiotensin converting enzyme inhibitors
Methyldopa, Hydralazine	Atropine
Acyclovir	Metronidazole
Penicillin	Theophylline
Macrolides, most Cephalosporins	Chloramphenicol
Quinine	Diazepam, Corticosteroids,
Warfarin (can be given in 2nd trimester)	Phenytoin, Valproate
Prophylthiouracil	Retinoid, Temoxifen, Busulfan

TABLE 1.10: Safe versus contraindicated drugs during breast feeding

Safe drugs	Contraindicated drugs
Prophylthiouracil	Antithyroid drugs and radioiodine
Insulin	Lithium
Erythromycin, Cephalosporin	Tetracycline
Warfarin	Phenindione
Digoxin	Ergotamine, gold salt
Antacids	Anticancer/cytotoxic drugs, e.g., methotrexate, cyclophosphamide

converting enzyme (ACE) inhibitors can cause hypoplasia of organs, especially of lungs and kidneys. Drugs that are safe and contraindicated in pregnancy and drugs contraindicated in lactation are given in Tables 1.9 and 1.10, respectively.

PHARMACOKINETICS

(What the body does to the drug)

It is a branch of pharmacology, which deals with the journey or movement of the drug '**in, through and out from the body**'. In other words, it deals with the scientific study of the **absorption, distribution, metabolism (biotransformation), and excretion** (ADME) of drugs (Fig. 1.1).

- The transfer of drug from its sites of administration to the blood is called absorption.

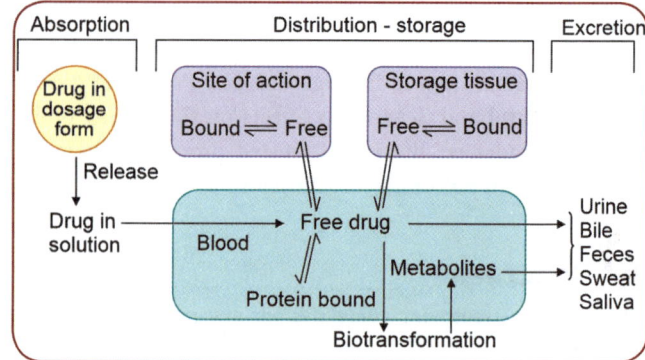

FIG. 1.1: Diagrammatic presentation of pharmacokinetics of a drug

- Its transfer from blood to tissues is called distribution. The drug attains its effective concentration at the site of action and produces its effects.
- Then the drug is metabolized, which is called metabolism or biotransformation.
- After the drug has done its work, it is to be thrown out of the body. This process is called excretion.

Absorption

Absorption is the process by which a drug passes from its site of administration into the blood stream or circulation of the body. From here, the drug moves to its site(s) of action. When given by oral route, absorption is the first step in the passage of a drug through the body. Whereas, it is introduced directly into the bloodstream when given by intravenous administration. Absorption of the drug is 100% when given by intravenous route and always less than 100% when given by intramuscular, subcutaneous or oral route.

Factors Affecting Absorption

- **Drug factors:**
  - **Aqueous solubility:** The drugs are absorbed in liquid form only. So the oral drug needs to be converted into liquid form before absorption. Drugs in liquid form are absorbed better. The dissolution and disintegration of a drug are the two important factors, which decide the rate and extent of absorption. Example: Dispersible tablets are absorbed and act faster (Fig. 1.2).
  - **Dose of drug:** The higher the dose, faster will be the absorption due to the concentration gradient and diffusion thereby.
- **Presence of food:** The presence of food may interfere with the dissolution and absorption of certain drugs, as well as delay the transit time of a drug from the stomach to the small intestine. Some food constituents may form absorbable complexes with the drugs which decrease absorption process. So most of the drugs are absorbed better if taken empty stomach, **until or unless contraindicated**.

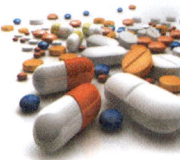

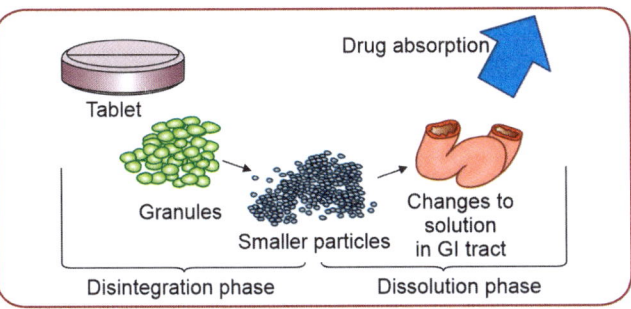

FIG. 1.2: Phases of solid drug absorption

- **Body factors:**
  - **Area of absorbing surface:** Absorption of the drug is faster, if area of the absorbing surface is more.
  - **Vascularity of the absorbing surface:** Increased blood flow at the site of absorption increases the rate of absorption, similarly as the wet clothes dry faster on exposure to the fast wind.
- **Route of administration:**
  - **Oral:** The barrier in absorption from this route is the epithelial lining (biological membrane) of GIT. The drugs have to cross the biological membrane, which is a lipid bilayer and allows the more lipid soluble drugs to be absorbed faster.
  - **Subcutaneous:** The drugs are deposited in the vicinity of capillaries and absorption occurs through the large paracellular spaces around the capillaries. The large molecules of drugs, which cannot be absorbed through capillaries, are absorbed via lymphatics. The absorption is slightly slower than the intramuscular route.
  - **Intramuscular:** The absorption is faster than subcutaneous and more consistent. The muscular exercise and application of heat at the site increases the rate of absorption.
  - **Intravenous:** Here the drug is directly put into the circulation and within no time the drug circulates throughout the body.

Bioavailability

- It is a measure or fraction of administered dose of a drug that reaches the systemic circulation in the unchanged or active form.
- Bioavailability of the drug injected intravenously is 100%.
- It is generally lower after oral ingestion because the drug may be incompletely absorbed or undergo first pass metabolism in the intestinal wall and liver.
- Bioavailability after subcutaneous or intramuscular injection is also less than 100% due to the local binding of drugs.
- Bioavailability variation have practical significance for drugs with low safety margin (digoxin) and also where

dosage needs fine control (oral hypoglycemic, oral anti-coagulants).
- It is also responsible for success or failure of an anti-microbial regimen.

Target Concentration of Drug

It is the minimum level of plasma concentration of drug which is necessary to get the desired therapeutic effect.

To achieve this target concentration, we need to administer the drug in loading or maintenance dose at right interval of time depending upon the type of drugs and disease the patient is suffering from.

Loading Dose

To attain the target concentration rapidly, sometimes a large single dose or few quickly repeated doses need to be given in the beginning, this is called the loading dose of a drug. Example: Digoxin, chloroquine, doxycycline, etc.

Maintenance Dose

To maintain the target concentration, the dose which is required to be given at specified intervals is called *maintenance dose*. This is always on the lower side than the loading dose. Example: Digoxin, chloroquine, doxycycline, etc.

Distribution

Drug distribution is the process by which a drug is carried from its site of absorption to its site of action. When a drug enters the bloodstream, it is carried most rapidly to the organs having rich blood supply, such as the heart, liver, kidneys, and brain. Areas with less blood supply receive the drug slowly, example: Muscle, skin, and adipose tissue.

- The drug remains in the body in bound and unbound (free) form.
- There is always equilibrium between bound and unbound form of the drug.
- The unbound form is the active form of the drug and while in the bound state, the drug is incapable of eliciting a pharmacological effect.
- When a plasma concentration of the unbound drug diminishes, the bound drug is released from its binding sites.
- The acidic drugs preferably bind to albumin and the basic drugs to alfa-acid glycoprotein.
- This protein-binding act as a temporary store house for drugs and also prolongs the drug action and acts like *sustained release technology*.

The distribution of drug depends upon following factors:
- Lipid solubility and lipid water partition coefficient

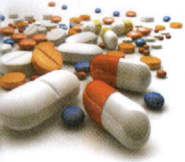

TABLE 1.11: Deposition of drugs in various tissues/organs

Tissue	Drugs
Bone and teeth	Tetracycline, heavy metals (bound to mucopolysaccharides of connective tissue)
Retina	Chloroquine (bound to nucleoproteins)
Liver	Chloroquine, tetracycline, emetinec, digoxin
Thyroid	Iodine
Kidney	Digoxin, chloroquine, emetine
Skeletal muscle, heart	Digoxin, emetine (bound to muscle proteins)

- Ionization at physiological pH
- Extent of binding to plasma and tissue proteins
- Differences in regional blood flow
- Diseases like renal failure, liver failure, heart failure and cirrhosis of liver

Some drugs have selective preference for the deposition in the various body tissues, which are important for the clinical as well as toxicological point of view and are given in Table 1.11.

Metabolism (Biotransformation)

It is also called the biotransformation of the drug. It is necessary for the elimination of a drug from the body through various excretory routes. To be eliminated from the body by way of the kidneys, a compound must be fairly soluble in water. Because many drugs are not very water soluble, they must first undergo drug metabolism or biotransformation to convert them to a more water-soluble form. In other words, it converts the drug in another form which is excretable.

- Metabolism permits the body to inactivate a potent drug before it accumulates and produces toxic effects.
- Metabolism permits the body to activate the prodrug into its active form.
- Most biotransformation reactions occur in the liver, but they also can occur in the gastrointestinal tract, lungs, kidneys, and skin.

Sites of Metabolism

The primary site is liver. The other sites are kidney, intestine, lungs and blood circulation.

Effects of Metabolism

Metabolism leads to:
- **Inactivation of the active drugs:** Drugs are made inactive or less active. Examples, paracetamol, ibuprofen, propranolol, etc.
- **Activation of the inactive drug:** Some drugs need conversion in the body to active form and are inactive as such. Such a drug is called prodrug (Table 1.12).

TABLE 1.12: Active forms of prodrugs

Prodrug	Active form
Acyclovir	Acyclovir triphosphate
Fluorouracil	Fluorouridine monophosphate
Bacampicillin	Ampicillin
Prednisone	Prednisolone
Sulindac	Sulfide metabolite
Enalapril	Enalaprilat
Alfa-methyldopa	α-methyl norepinephrine
Fosphenytoin	Phenytoin

- **Active metabolites formation from an active drug:** Some drugs are active even after their conversion to their metabolites. These metabolites can also act as the original drug. These are called active metabolites. The effect on the patients is sum total of the effect of drug and its active metabolites.

Types of Metabolism Reactions

- **Non-synthetic/phase I reactions:** A functional group is generated or exposed—metabolite may be active or inactive. The non-synthetic reactions involve oxidation, reduction, hydrolysis, cyclization and decyclization processes.
- **Synthetic/phase II reactions:** *Here the drug or its* phase I metabolites are conjugated with an endogenously derived substrate to form an easily excretable substance. This reaction requires energy. The synthetic reactions involve glucoronide conjugation, acetylation, methylation, sulphate/glycine/glutathione conjugation, etc.

The phase 1 and phase 2 reactions are given in (Table 1.13).

Microsomal and Non-microsomal Enzymes

The microsomal and non-microsomal enzymes that take part in metabolism are discussed as follows:

Microsomal enzymes

- These are located on smooth endoplasmic reticulum.
- Present primarily in liver, kidney, intestinal mucosa and lungs.

TABLE 1.13: Differences between Phase 1 and Phase 2 reactions

Phase I reaction	Phase II reaction
It changes functional group of drug molecule and uses cytochrome P450 monooxygenase	It attaches a conjugate to the drug molecule
Reactions are: • Oxidation (most common) • Reduction • Hydrolysis • Decyclization • Cyclization	Reactions are: • Glucuronide conjugation (most common) • Acetylation • Methylation • Sulfate conjugation • Glycine conjugation • Glutathione conjugation

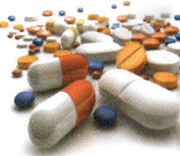

TABLE 1.14: Microsomal enzyme inducers and inhibitors

Microsomal Enzyme Inducer (GARIMAS)	Microsomal Enzyme Inhibitor
• G—Griseofulvin • A—Anti Epileptics (Phenobarbitone, Phenytoin and carbamazepine) • R—Rifampin • I—Isoniazid • M—Meat • A—Alcohol • S—Smoking • O—Other (Omeprazole, DDT, phenylbutazone,)	• Ketoconazole • Itraconazole • Metronidazole • Valproate • Verapamil • Protease Inhibitor (M/C Ritonavir) • Selective Serotonin Reuptake Inhibitor • Ciprofloxacin • Clarithromycin • Oral contraceptive pills • Cimetidine • Chloramphenicol • Allopurinol • Amiodarone • Erythromycin

- They catalyze the oxidation, reduction, hydrolysis and glucuronide conjugation.
- These are inducible by drugs, diet and other chemicals.
- Example: Monooxygenases, cytochrome P450, etc.
- Microsomal enzyme induces and inhibitors are given in Table 1.14.

Properties of microsomal enzymes

- All anti-fungal drugs are microsomal enzyme inhibitors except Griseofulvin.
- All anti-epileptic drugs are microsomal enzyme inhibitors except Valproate.
- Acute alcoholism is a microsomal enzyme inhibitor, while Chronic alcoholism is microsomal enzyme inducer.

Non-microsomal enzymes

- These are located in cytoplasm and mitochondria.
- Present primarily in liver and plasma.
- They catalyze some oxidation, reduction, many hydrolysis and all conjugations except glucuronide conjugation.
- These are not inducible by drugs, diet and other chemicals.
- Example: Esterases, Amidases, Flavoprotein oxidases and Conjugases.

  Some enzymes metabolize specific drugs such as alcohol by dehydrogenase, allopurinol by xanthine oxidase, succinylcholine and procaine by plasma cholinesterase, adrenaline by monoamine oxidase. Sometimes, the same enzyme can metabolize many drugs also.

Hofmann Elimination

This is the inactivation of drug in the body, where no enzyme is involved in the inactivation of the drug, but spontaneous molecular rearrangement occurs. Example: Atracurium, cistracurium.

First Pass Metabolism

It is the metabolism of a drug at the site of absorption during its passage from the site of absorption into the systemic circulation. All orally administered drugs are exposed to drug metabolizing enzymes in the intestinal wall and liver. This is called presystemic metabolism as it occurs before the drug reaches the systemic circulation. It can be avoided by administering the drug through sublingual, transdermal or parenteral routes because the portal circulation is bypassed. The extent of first pass metabolism differs for different drugs and is an important determinant of oral bioavailability. The first pass metabolism is highest, when the drug is given by oral route.

Due to this fact:

- Oral dose is always higher than sublingual or parenteral dose.
- Due to differences in the extent of first pass metabolism, the oral dose differs for individual patients.
- In patients with severe liver disease, the oral bioavailability is slightly increased.

Excretion

Excretion is the process of removing a drug or its metabolites from the body. Drugs and their metabolites may be eliminated from the body in several different ways, such as:

Urine or Renal Excretion

The substances which are made water soluble after biotransformation can be easily excreted through this route. The nephron is a basic renal unit. Three mechanisms of renal excretion operate simultaneously at the nephron level. These mechanisms are:

- **Glomerular filtration:** The drug/metabolites/substances, which are smaller in size than the glomerular capillary pores are easily filtered through the glomerulus and reach the proximal tubules. The protein bound drug and bigger molecules cannot be filtered through the glomerulus. Hence, excretion depends upon glomerular filtration rate.
- **Tubular reabsorption (selective):** The highly lipid soluble drugs are reabsorbed from the proximal tubules. The ionization of a drug also affects this process.
- **Tubular secretion:** Certain drugs and natural metabolites are actively secreted in the tubule for the purpose of excretion.

We can say that:

Net Renal excretion = (glomerular filtration + tubular secretion) - tubular reabsorption

Feces

Both the unabsorbed fraction of a drug and the drugs excreted through bile, are excreted in feces. Example: Erythromycin, OCPs, Ampicillin etc.

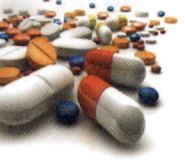

Exhaled Air

The volatile liquids and gases are excreted through this route. Example: Alcohol and anesthetic gases.

Saliva, Sweat and Tears

Lithium and some heavy metals are excreted through this route.

Breast Milk

More lipid soluble and less protein bound drugs are excreted through this route. Example: Tetracycline, Methotrexate, Indomethacin, etc.

Kinetics of Elimination

Kinetics of elimination are tabulated in Table 1.15.

Let's know

Plasma Half Life

The plasma half-life (t½) of a drug is the time taken for its plasma concentration to be reduced to half of its original value.
- After 1st t½–50% drug is eliminated.
- After 2nd t½–75% (50 + 25) drug is eliminated.
- After 3rd t½ – 87.5% (50 + 25 + 12.5) drug is eliminated.
- After 4th t½–93.75% (50 + 25 + 12.5 + 6.25) drug is eliminated.
Thus, nearly complete drug elimination occurs in 4–5 half lives.

Half-life of some drugs
- Aspirin   4 hr
- Digoxin   40 hr
- Azithromycin   >50 hr
- Digitoxin   7 days
- Doxycycline   20 hr
- Phenobarbitone   90 hr

Clinical implications of plasma half-life

Knowledge about the plasma half-life is an important factor which guides us to:
- Determine the frequency of drug administration
- Duration of drug action
- Time of excretion

TABLE 1.15: Kinetics of elimination

First order kinetics	Zero order kinetics
Rate of elimination of a drug is directly proportional to its plasma concentration	Rate of elimination is constant irrespective of its plasma concentration
Accumulation of drug does not occur	Accumulation of drug occurs
Level of drug remains constant, in spite of increase in dose	Toxicity can occur if dose of the drug is increased
Drug follows first order kinetics till the saturation of various elimination mechanisms	Drug follows zero order kinetics after the saturation of various elimination mechanisms
Example: Most of the drugs	Example: Phenytoin, Warfarin, Theophylline, Tolbutamide

DRUG INTERACTIONS

When two drugs are given together, a drug interaction occurs. The pharmacological effects of one drug are potentiated or diminished by another drug. This is due to the interaction at pharmacokinetic or pharmacodynamic level.

If the administration of two or more drugs produces a pharmacological response that is greater than that which would be expected by the individual effects of each drug together, the drugs are said to be acting synergistically. If one drug diminishes the action of another, it is said to act antagonistically.

- Drug interaction may be synergistic or antagonistic (explained earlier along with synergism/antagonism).
- Drug interactions may be beneficial or harmful:
  - **Beneficial:** For example, the use of a CNS stimulant such as caffeine with an antihistamine that may cause drowsiness as one of its side effects may be a useful drug interaction; the caffeine acts only to counteract the unwanted side effect (drowsiness) of the antihistamine without altering its intended pharmacological action.
  - **Harmful:** The use of an antacid with the antibiotic tetracycline would be likely to result in an undesirable drug interaction. Antacid forms a chemical complex with the tetracycline, thereby rendering it incapable of being absorbed into the bloodstream.
- Drug interactions may occur at any step in the passage of a drug through the body during its administration, absorption, distribution, metabolism, or excretion.
- Interactions may also take place at the receptor site of a drug.
- Drugs may interact with foods, laboratory test substances and environmental pollutants.

ROUTES AND PRINCIPLES OF ADMINISTRATION OF DRUGS

There are various routes available through which the drugs can be administered in the body, for their appropriate action. A detailed knowledge of exact route of drug administration is must for prescribing physician and nurses as well. The responsibility of administering various drugs lies on the shoulders of nurses, when the patient has been admitted indoor, day care centers or as an advisor to the outdoor patients.

The decision about the choice of route in a particular patient lies largely on the patient's requirement, condition as well as the drug preparation available.

The routes of drug administration can be divided into local and systemic routes.

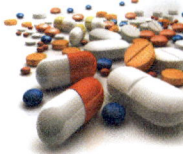

Local Routes

These routes are used where only the local action is desired keeping in view the patient's conditions, requirements, convenience and tolerability to systemic drugs. The following are the commonly used local routes for drug administration:

- *Topical:* Here the drug is applied topically/externally on skin and mucous membranes to get the local effects only. The various preparations to be applied on skin and mucous membrane are: creams, gel, ointments, lotion, liniments, paints, jellies, paste, pessaries, suppositories, drops, sprays, etc.
- *Local injections:* When we don't want to expose whole of the body to a particular medication. This is unnecessary when the patient is suffering from local disease only. We prefer local injection at a particular site as the drug remains confined to that particular diseased tissue. For example, intra-articular corticosteroid injection in arthritis, intramedullary anti-cancerous drugs in some bone cancers, intrafemoral or intrabrachial anticancerous drug infusion in some limb malignancies.

Systemic Routes

These routes are used, when the systemic action is desired keeping in view the patient's conditions, requirements, convenience and tolerability to systemic drugs. The drug administered by systemic routes reaches the blood circulation and it is distributed all over the body tissues including site of its action. The following are the commonly used systemic routes for drug administration.

Oral

- It is also called enteral route.
- It is the oldest, commonest and considered to be safest route of drug administration.
- Administering drug through this route does not need any assistance for adults. Pediatric and geriatric patients may need assistance.
- The oral formulations are usually cheaper than other formulations.
- The following forms of drugs can be given by oral route: tablets, capsules, spansules, caplets, powders, drops, syrup, gel, mixtures, suspensions, emulsions, elixirs, GITS (gastrointestinal therapeutic system), etc.

Gastrointestinal

There are some special preparations made for convenient dosing such as slow/sustained/extended/delayed/controlled/continuous release form of capsules or tablets. This is done to delay the absorption of the drug, so that frequency of dosing can be reduced. The enteric coated tablets protect the tablet from the acidic pH(HCl) of the stomach and the drug can safely pass into small intestine for better absorption.

Only scored tablets can be broken into the pieces. The unscored tablets should never be broken before administration. **This route is not suitable when,**

- The patient is noncooperative, unconscious and vomiting constantly.
- The patient has been brought in emergency.
- The drugs are irritant and nonpalatable. Example: Chloramphenicol
- The drugs are destroyed by gastric juice or enzyme. Example: Trypsin, chymotrypsin
- The drugs are having high first pass metabolism in liver. Example: Nitroglycerine (GTN)
- The drugs cannot be absorbed. Example: Streptomycin

Sublingual (S/L)

- The tablet or pellet containing the drug is placed under the tongue or crushed in the mouth to be spread over the buccal mucosa for absorption.
- Absorption is relatively rapid action that can be produced in minutes.
- The drug can be spit out once the desired effect has been obtained.
- Drugs given sublingually are: GTN, buprenorphine, desamino-oxytocin.
- This route is generally employed in emergencies. Example: GTN in myocardial infarction patients.

Rectal

- This route is used when the patient is having recurrent vomiting or is unconscious.
- The irritant and unpleasant drugs can be put into the rectum as suppositories or retention enemas for systemic effects.
- The absorption is slow and irregular by this route and the effect is unpredictable.
- Examples: Rectal diazepam for treating epilepsy in children; indomethacin, paracetamol, etc.

Cutaneous

- When slow and prolonged absorption of a drug is required for its systemic action, this route is preferred.
- The drug has to be highly lipid soluble.
- These drugs are presented in various forms like skin patches, etc.

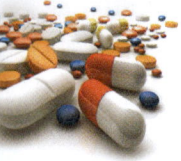
✔

Transdermal Therapeutic Systems (TTS)

These are devices in the form of adhesive patches of various shapes and sizes (5–20 cm²), which deliver the contained drug at a constant rate into systemic circulation via the stratum corneum layer of skin. The patch is to be peeled off just before application. The drug is delivered at the skin surface by diffusion for percutaneous absorption into the circulation. The usual sites for applying patches are chest, abdomen, upper arm, lower back, buttock and mastoid regions. Transdermal patches of GTN, fentanyl, nicotine, etoricoxib and estradiol are available in India. TTS have been designed to last for 1–3 days. Local irritation and erythema can occur in some patients, but is generally mild. This can be minimized by changing the site of application each time by rotation (Fig. 1.3).

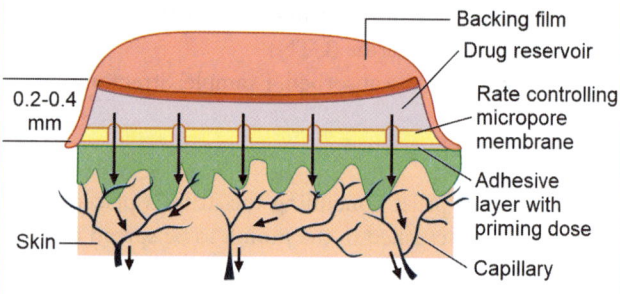

FIG. 1.3: Illustration of a transdermal drug delivery system

Inhalational

- Drugs given by this route are absorbed through respiratory tract.
- The drugs are either volatile liquids, aerosol form or gases that used to produce general anesthesia.
- This route is also used for the treatment for some local lung diseases.
- Drugs are presented in the form of inhalers, rotahalers and nebulizers.

Parenteral (Par—beyond, Enteral—intestinal) Routes

- It refers to administration of drug by injection.
- The action of the drug is faster and useful in emergency.
- This route is employed in unconscious, uncooperative or patients having vomiting.
- The preparation is costlier and has to be sterilized.
- The technique is painful as it is invasive.

The various parenteral routes are follows:

Intravenous (IV)

The drugs are directly injected into the superficial veins in the form of injection or infusion.

Advantages:

- The drug reaches directly into the blood stream.
- The onset of action is fastest.

- Effects are produced immediately.
- Very useful in emergency.
- The bioavailability is 100%.
- Response is accurately measurable.
- Highly irritant drugs can be injected by this route *as the intima of veins is insensitive to pain and the drug gets diluted with blood.*
- Titration of the dose with the response is possible.

Disadvantages:

- The technique is invasive and painful.
- The formulations are usually costlier.
- Strict aseptic measures need to be followed.
- Self-administration is usually not possible.
- Once the drug is injected, it cannot be withdrawn.
- Sometimes, thrombophlebitis of the injected vein and necrosis of adjoining tissues can occur if extravasation of the drug occurs. This can be minimized by diluting the drug or injecting it into a running IV line.
- Chances of causing air embolism is another risk.
- The vital organs like heart, brain, etc., get exposed to high concentrations of the drug, so it can prove to be a risky route also.

Precautions to be taken are:

- Drug sensitivity test should be performed before administration (where indicated).
- Make sure that needle is in the vein by withdrawal methods.
- Drug should be injected slowly.
- Oil-based preparations should not be injected by this route.

Intramuscular (IM)

- The site of injection of drug is one of the large skeletal muscles like, gluteus maximus, deltoid, triceps, rectus femoris, etc.
- The drug is deposited in the muscles mass and from there it is absorbed gradually into the systemic circulation taking some time.
- The time taken for action of drug is slightly more than the time taken by the IV route.

Advantages:

- Muscles are more vascular and absorption of drugs is faster than oral.
- Even the mild irritant drugs can be injected as muscles are less richly supplied with sensory nerves.
- The vital organs like heart, brain, etc., are not exposed to very high concentrations of the drug.
- Chances of causing air embolism are not there.

Disadvantages:

- It can produce local hematoma in patients with blood coagulation disorders.
- Self-injection impracticable.
- Assistance is required in case of children.

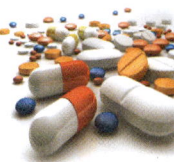

- Chances of local abscess formations are there, if strict aseptic measures are not followed.
- Inaccurate administration can lead to nerve injury sometimes (sciatic nerve injury).

Subcutaneous (SC)

- This route is used where, very prolonged action is required.
- The drug is deposited in the loose subcutaneous area.
- Self-injection is possible because deep penetration is not needed.

Disadvantages:
- The absorption is slower than intramuscular route as the subcutaneous area is less vascular.
- Irritant drugs cannot be injected as it is richly supplied by nerves.
- Only small volume of the drug can be injected.
- It is not a preferred route in shock patients as the absorption is delayed due to vasoconstriction.
- Preparations are expensive.

Intradermal (ID)

- The drug is injected under the epidermis raising a bleb.
- This route is employed for specific purposes only.
- Used for sensitivity testing of various drugs such as penicillin testing, montoux test.
- Used for BCG vaccination.

The comparative features of different routes of drug administration are discussed in Table 1.16.

Other Routes

- **Intraarterial:** Direct injection in arteries
- **Intracardiac:** Direct injection in chamber of heart
- **Intrathecal:** Direct injection in sub arachnoid space
- **Intraperitoneal:** Direct injection in peritoneal cavity
- **Epidural:** Direct injection in epidural space

Principles of Medication Administration

Principles include three Checks and ten rights:
Three checks are:
1. Check when obtaining the container of medicine.
2. Check when removing the medicine from the container.
3. Check when replacing the container.

Ten rights of medication administration are:

Medication errors can be detrimental to patients. To prevent these errors, these guidelines are the rights used in drug administration.

1. **Right patient:** Correct identification of the client cannot be over emphasized. This can be done by asking the client to mention his/her full name which should be compared with that on the identification bracelet or the patient's folder and medication/treatment chart for confirmation.
2. **Right medication:** Beware of same and similar first names and surnames to prevent the error of administering one person's medication to another and vice versa. Before administering any medicine, compare name on medication chart/medication order with that on the medication at least three times—checking medication label when removing it from storage unit, compare medication label with that on treatment chart and medication label and name on treatment chart with patient's name tag.
3. **Right time:** Drug timing is very special with some drugs like antibiotics, antimalarial drugs, etc., to achieve cure and prevent resistance. Some drugs must be given on empty stomach, e.g., antituberculosis drugs; and some

TABLE 1.16: Comparative features of different routes of drug administration

Route	Absorption pattern	Special utility	Limitations and precautions
Intravenous	Absorption circumvented; Potentially immediate effects; Suitable for large volumes and for irritating substances, or complex mixtures, when diluted	Valuable for emergency use; Permits titration of dosage; Usually required for high-molecular-weight protein and peptide drugs	Increased risk of adverse effects; Must inject solutions *slowly* as a rule; Not suitable for oily solutions or poorly soluble substances
Subcutaneous	Prompt, from aqueous solution; Slow and sustained, from repository preparations	Suitable for some poorly soluble suspensions and for instillation of slow-release implants	Not suitable for large volumes; Possible pain or necrosis from irritating substances
Intramuscular	Prompt, from aqueous solution; Slow and sustained, from repository preparations	Suitable for moderate volumes, oily vehicles, and some irritating substances; Appropriate for self-administration (e.g., insulin)	Precluded during anticoagulant therapy; May interfere with interpretation of certain diagnostic tests (e.g., creatine kinase)
Oral ingestion	Variable, depends on many factors	Most convenient and economical; usually safer	Requires patient compliance; Bioavailability potentially erratic and incomplete

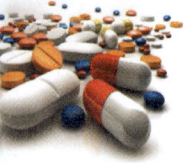

after meals, e.g., NSAIDS - these must be noted and adhered to. The interval of administration of drugs should also be adhered to because it is important for many drugs that the blood concentration is not allowed to fall below a given level and for others two successive doses closer than prescribed might increase blood concentration to a dangerous level that can harm the patient.

4. **Right dose:** This becomes very important when medications at hand are in a larger volume or strength than the prescribed order given or when the unit of measurement in the order is different from that supplied from the pharmacy. Careful and correct calculation is important to prevent over or under dosage of the medication.

5. **Right route:** An acceptable medication order must specify the route of medication. If this is unclear, the prescriber should be contacted to clarify or specify it. The nurse should never decide on a route without consulting the prescriber.

6. **Right to information on drug/client education:** The patient has the right to know the drug he/she is taking, desired and adverse effects and all there is to know about the medication. The charter on patient's right made this clear.

7. **Right to refuse medication:** The patient has the right to refuse any medication. However, the nurse is obliged to explainto patients why the drug is prescribed and the consequences of refusing medication.

8. **Right assessment:** Some medications require specific assessment before their administration, e.g., checking of vital signs. Before a medication like Digoxin is administered, the pulse must be checked. Some medication orders may contain specific assessments to be done prior to medication.

9. **Right documentation:** Documentation should be done after medication and not before.

10. **Right Evaluation:** Conduct assessment to ascertain drug action and side effect.

MEDICATION ORDER

The drug order, written by the physician, should have seven essential parts for administration of drugs safely.
1. Patients full name
2. Date and time
3. Drug name
4. Dosage
5. Route of administration
6. Time and frequency of administration
7. Signature of physician

Types of Medication Orders

Four types of medication orders are commonly used:
1. **Stat order:** A stat order indicates that the medication is to be given immediately and only once, e.g., morphine sulfate 10 mg IV stat.
2. **Single order:** The single order or one-time order indicates that the medication is to be given once at a specified time, e.g., Seconal 100 mg at bedtime.
3. **Standing order:** Standing order is written in advance carried out under specific circumstances. (e.g., amox twice daily × 2 days).
4. **PRN order:** "PRN" is a Latin term that stands for "pro re nata," which means "as the thing is needed." A PRN order or as-needed order, permits the nurse to give a medication when the client requires it. (e.g., Amphojel 15 mL PRN).

Special Drug Delivery System

Dermojet

In this method no needle is used. A high velocity jet of drug solution is projected through a micro-fine orifice using a gun like device. The solution gets deposited in the subcutaneous tissue. It is painless method.

Pellet Implantation

The drug is presented in the form of solid pellet. It is introduced surgically with the help of trochar and cannula. The drug keeps on releasing for weeks and month. Example. DOCA, testosterone

Implants

Crystalline drug packed in tube and capsule made of suitable material are implanted under the skin. Uniform and slow release of drug occurs for months together.

Liposomes

These are minute vesicles made of phospholipids into which the drug is incorporated. Used for targeted drug delivery. Example: Some anticancer drug and Amphotericin B.

Monoclonal Antibodies

These are antibodies which selectively react with specific antigen. These are produced using biotechnology and cell culture methods. This type is used for targeted drug delivery. Example: Rituximab, Cetuximab, etc.

INDIAN PHARMACOPEIA

Pharmacopeia (*Pharmacon—Drug, Poeia—is to make*) is the official publication, which contains all details about the established drugs, being in use in a particular country. It is

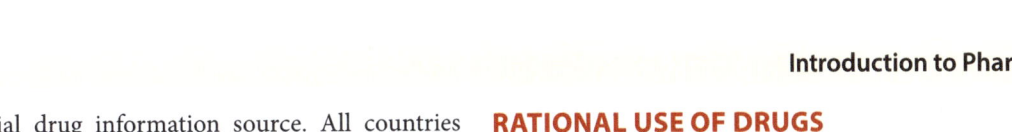

one of the official drug information source. All countries have their own Pharmacopeias such as Indian Pharmacopeia (IP), British Pharmacopeia (BP), United States Pharmacopeia (USP).

The Pharmacopeia includes various information such as:

- Description of chemical structure of drugs
- Physical and chemical characteristics of drugs
- Solubility, identification and assay methods
- Tests for their purity and potency
- Storage conditions
- Dosages, precautions and various indications for use

First Indian Pharmacopeia was published in 1868, but could not be followed for long under the British rule. After independence in 1947, a committee, which included experts from pharmaceutical industries, drug control laboratories and medical teaching institutions prepared a fresh Pharmacopeia and released it in 1955. The pharmacopeias are revised at regular intervals for adding the new research molecules (drugs) and deleting the harmful and un-useful drugs (proven by evidence based medicine).

LEGAL ISSUES

Preparation, dispensing and administration of medications are all covered by laws in every country. Dangerous Drug Act – 1930 and The Narcotic Drugs and Psychotropic Substances Act - 1985: These are the acts that govern the procurement and use of some drugs especially the narcotics, e.g., morphine, pethidine, cocaine, etc. These drugs are prescription only drugs, hence cannot be bought or administered without prescription.

Dangerous drugs are always kept under lock and key in the Dangerous Drug Cupboard under the care of trusted senior nurses.

It is worth knowing that nurses are responsible for their own actions regardless of the presence of a written order. If a nurse gives an overdose of a drug because it is written by a doctor, the error is accounted to the nurse and not the doctor.

The nurse should bear in mind that ALL substances are poisons: There is none that is not a poison. The right dose differentiates a poison from a remedy.

- The drug manufacturers have to strictly follow the Pharmacopeia of a particular country, wherever the manufacturing plant is established. If a particular formula from some other Pharmacopeia has been followed, they have to mention it on the strips.
- The regulatory authorities check the drug manufacturing units on the basis of Pharmacopeia.
- The prescribing physicians hardly require Pharmacopeia for their practical use but they can use it only for the reference purpose.

RATIONAL USE OF DRUGS

As per the World Health Organization (WHO)—'rational use of medicines requires that the patients receive medication appropriate to their clinical needs in doses that meet their own individual requirements for an adequate period of time, and at the lowest cost to them and to their community'.

Rational use of medicines requires to closely see every step in the supply-use chain of drugs, i.e., selection, procurement, storage, prescribing, dispensing, monitoring and feedback. For practical purpose, the rational prescribing needs to be studied in detail.

In simpler terms the rational prescribing is:

- Choosing an appropriate drug
- For an appropriate indication
- In appropriate dose, route and duration
- In an appropriate patient
- With correct dispensing
- Adequate monitoring

The following irrationalities should be avoided:

- Use of drug when not needed; example, antibiotics for viral fevers and nonspecific diarrheas.
- Use of drugs, which are not related to the diagnosis, example, chloroquine/ciprofloxacin for any fever, proton pump inhibitors for any abdominal symptom.
- Selection of the drug is wrong. Example: Tetracycline/ciprofloxacin for pharyngitis, β blocker as antihypertensive for asthmatic patient.
- Unnecessary prescription of vitamins/tonics should not be there.
- Doubtful efficacy drugs should not be prescribed. Example: Memory enhancers, cough mixtures, etc.
- Incorrect route of administration; injection when the drug can be given orally.
- Underdosing or overdosing should be avoided.
- Unnecessary prolongation of treatment should be avoided, example, prolonged postsurgical use of antibiotics or stoppage of antibiotics as soon as relief is obtained, such as in tuberculosis.
- Unnecessary and compulsive use of drug combinations, example, ciprofloxacin + tinidazole for diarrhea; ampicillin + cloxacillin for staphylococcal infection; ibuprofen + paracetamol as analgesic.
- Economical drugs with good efficacy should be preferred as they are equally effective.
- There should not be a craze for latest drugs, example, routine use of newer antibiotics.

Rational use of Drugs by Nurses

The nurses can add a lot to the rational use of drug (Fig. 14) by keeping a vigil on the drug in use, such as:

- Generic or brand name as prescribed

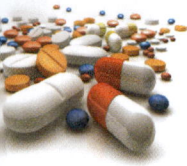

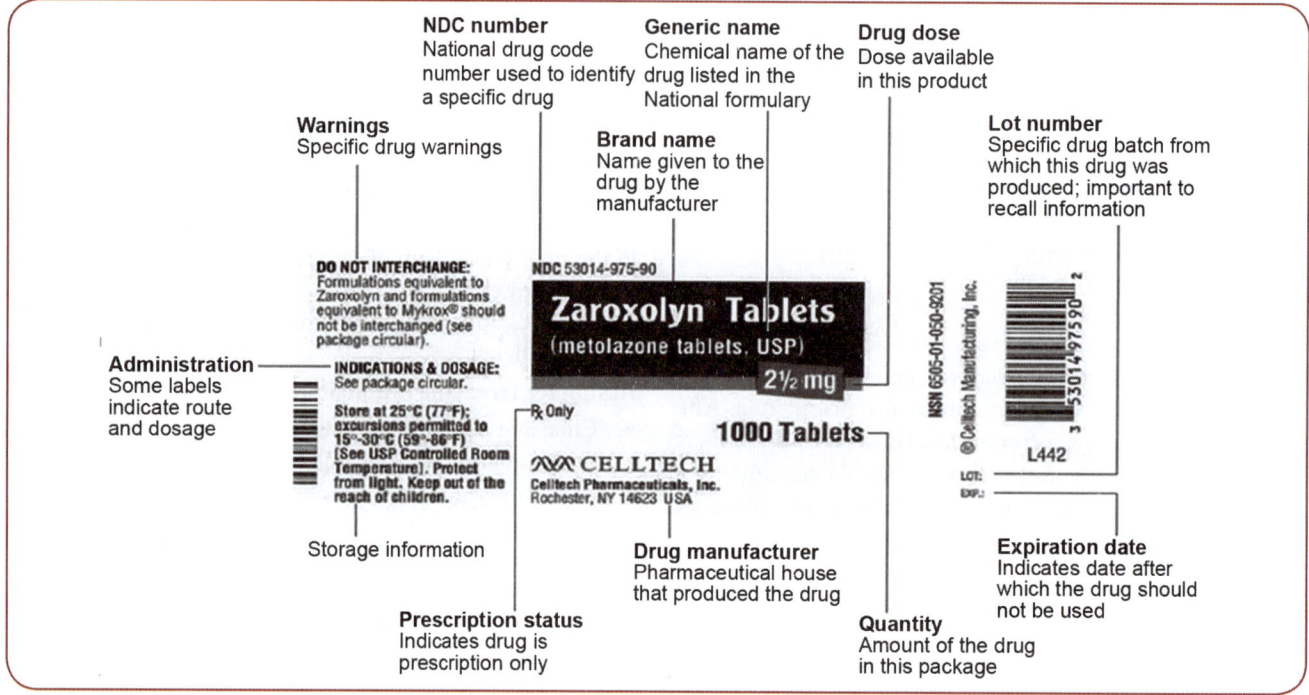

FIG. 1.4: Points to be taken care of by a nurse during rational use of drugs

- Drug manufacturer
- Date of manufacture
- Expiry date
- Indication
- Drug dose
- Route of administration
- Storage information
- Warning (if any written)

Points to be taken care of during rational use of drugs by a nurse is given in Figure 1.4

Advantages of Rational use of Drugs

- Timely relief and cure of disease
- Minimum adverse drug effects
- Minimum hospitalization
- Decreased morbidity and mortality
- Helpful in preventing microbial resistance
- Minimizing financial loss to the patient/community
- Gain of patient's confidence in the health system
- Strengthening of health standards of patients/community

PRINCIPLES OF THERAPEUTICS

The following principles should be followed for good therapeutic outcomes:

- Proper diagnosis should be made and therapeutic problem(s) should be identified. Example, pain, infection, etc.
- We should define the goals to be achieved by treatment. Example, symptom relief, cure, prevention of complications, etc.
- Selection of the drug capable of achieving each goal should be appropriate.
- It should be based on safety, efficacy and suitability of drug.
- The economical and best suitable drug should be chosen, keeping cost factor also in mind, as the paying capacity differs from patient to patient.
- The route, dose and duration of treatment should be decided, keeping the patient's condition in mind.
- The patient should be informed and instructed about the medication properly.
- Adherence/compliance to the medication should be monitored properly.
- Monitor the extent to which therapeutic goal is achieved, example, BP lowering, peptic ulcer healing, etc.
- The treatment should be reviewed promptly for any change required, keeping in view the latest clinical condition of the patients and therapy should be modified if needed.
- Monitor adverse drug events, if any, regularly.
- We should try to treat the patient as a whole not the symptoms only.
- The palliative therapy/care should not be denied, if the disease is incurable.
- Morale of the patient should be boosted by regular counseling and psychotherapy.

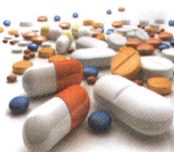

 ## Nursing Implications

- The different categories of drugs should be stored in different compartments. For example: Tablets, liquids, powders, etc.
- The drugs for external use and that for internal use should be kept separately.
- The containers should be arranged alphabetically, so that it is easy to find the required drug.
- All poisonous drugs should be marked "poison" in red ink.
- Emergency drugs should be kept in a place from where they can be obtained readily for emergency use.
- The physician's orders should be read carefully regarding the patients name, drugs to be given and the dose, route and frequency by which these are to be administered.
- Nurse should also be familiar with the trade names of the drugs and in case of any doubt, she should not hesitate to consult seniors, physicians or medical books.
- Nurse should know all the abbreviations and symbols, as these are frequently used in prescriptions.
- The medicines should be given before or after meals as per the prescription/orders.
- Nurse should stay with the patient until he/she has taken the medication.
- Any error, if occurs during the administration of drug, should be immediately brought in the notice of senior or physicians.
- Do not use the medicine with altered color, odor, consistency or taste and also guide the patients about the same.
- Always observe the five rights:
  - a. Right patients
  - b. Right medicine
  - c. Right dose
  - d. Right time
  - e. Right method of administration.
- Always give the drugs one-by-one.
- The notes about medicine should always be put soon after it has been administered and never before administering it.
- Nurse should be aware of his/her legal responsibilities.

Assess Yourself

Long and Short Answer Questions

1. What is a drug? Describe the various sources of drugs.
2. Describe the various routes of drug administration.
3. Describe the factors affecting drug absorption.
4. Describe the role of nurses in drug administration.
5. Discuss the advantages and disadvantages of oral route of drug administration.
6. Discuss the advantages and disadvantages of parenteral route of drug administration.
7. Describe the factors affecting the drug action.
8. Write short notes on:
   - a. Pharmacokinetics
   - b. Pharmacodynamics
   - c. First pass metabolism
   - d. Therapeutic Index
   - e. Competitive antagonism
   - f. Synergism
   - g. Idiosyncrasy
   - h. Loading dose
   - i. Prodrug
   - j. Teratogenicity
9. Write a short note on kinetics of elimination.
10. What is a placebo?
11. Write a short note on the types of allergic reactions.

Multiple Choice Questions

1. **Bioavailability of a drug is nearly 100% when given by route:**
   - a. Oral
   - b. IV
   - c. Transdermal
   - d. Inhalation

2. **Tick the prodrug:**
   - a. Enalapril
   - b. Dopamine
   - c. Nitroglycerin
   - d. Aspirin

3. **Major route of drug elimination is:**
   - a. Biliary
   - b. Alveolar
   - c. Renal
   - d. Dermal

4. **Solid drug preparation meant for rectal administration is:**
   - a. Suppository
   - b. Emulsion
   - c. Pessary
   - d. Tablet

21

Contd...

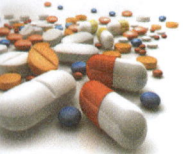
5. Maintenance dose is calculated by using value of:
   a. Clearance
   b. Volume of distribution
   c. Oral bioavailability
   d. Daily dosage

6. About rectal route true is:
   a. Used for irritant and unpleasant drugs
   b. Cannot be used in unconscious patient
   c. There is predictable absorption of drug
   d. Diazepam cannot be given via rectal route of administration

7. Drug administered by intranasal route is:
   a. Adrenaline
   b. Desmopressin
   c. Ganirelix
   d. Insulin

8. Major mechanism of transport of drugs across biological membranes is by:
   a. Passive diffusion
   b. Facilitated diffusion
   c. Active transport
   d. Endocytosis

Answer Key

1. b.	2. a.	3. c.	4. a.	5. a.	6. a.	7. b.
8. a.						

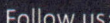

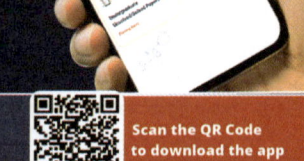

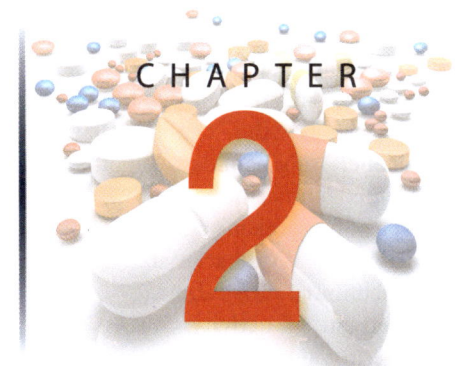

Chemotherapy

INTRODUCTION TO CHEMOTHERAPY

- **Chemotherapy:** Chemotherapy is defined as the 'treatment of systemic infections or malignancies with specific drugs that selectively suppress the infecting microorganisms or the malignant cells with minimal or no untoward effects on the host cells.
- **History of chemotherapy:**
  - In 1935, Domagk demonstrated the therapeutic effect of Prontosil, a sulfonamide dye, in pyogenic infections.
  - In 1941, penicillin was used as antibiotic, which was the beginning of *Golden Era* of antibiotics.
  - In the last 75 years, several new antibiotics and their semi-synthetic derivatives have been produced.
- **Chemotherapeutic agents:** These are the drugs or substances used in chemotherapy.

ANTIBIOTICS OR ANTIMICROBIAL AGENTS

- **Antibiotics:** These are the substances produced by microorganisms (fungi, bacteria, actinomycetes, etc.,) which selectively suppress the growth of or kill other microorganisms at very low concentrations.
  - **Antimicrobial agents (AMAs)** is more appropriate term as it includes most of the synthetic, semi-synthetic and naturally obtained drugs which attenuate microorganisms.

- The different AMAs have different modes of action. The AMAs may have action on the component of microbe or the metabolic processes occurring inside the microbial cell.
- **Types of antimicrobial agents:** They are either bactericidal or bacteriostatic as follows:

- **Bactericidal agents:** These are the antimicrobial agents, which irreversibly damage and kill the microorganisms. These drugs act better on the fast multiplying microorganisms. Examples: Cephalosporins, aminoglycosides and penicillin, etc.
- **Bacteriostatic agents:** These are the antimicrobial agents which do not kill the microorganisms but inhibit only the growth and multiplication of susceptible microorganisms. This inhibition is reversible in nature. Examples: Tetracyclines, sulfonamides, etc.

Modes of Action of Antimicrobial Agents

The different mechanisms of action are:
- **Cell wall synthesis inhibition:** Penicillins, cephalosporins, cycloserine, vancomycin, bacitracin, etc.
- **Causing damage to cell membranes:** *Polypeptides (polymyxins, colistin, bacitracin)*, polyenes (*amphotericin B, nystatin, hamycin*), etc.

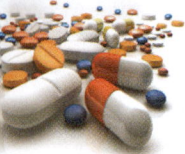

- **Protein synthesis inhibition:** Tetracyclines, chloramphenicol, erythromycin, clindamycin, linezolid, etc.
- **Inhibition of DNA gyrase:** Fluoroquinolones, Ciprofloxacin and others.
- **Interfering the intermediary metabolism in micobe:** Sulfonamides, sulfones, PAS, trimethoprim, pyrimethamine, metronidazole, etc.
- **Types of organisms against which the AMAs are active primarily:** Antibacterial, antifungal, antiprotozoal, anthelmintic, antiviral, etc.
- **Spectrum of activity:** AMAs may be bactericidal or bacteriostatic in nature. **Examples:**
  - **Bacteriostatic:** Sulfonamides, erythromycin, tetracycline, clindamycin, chloramphenicol, linezolid, ethambutol, etc.
  - **Bactericidal:** Penicillin, cephalosporins, aminoglycosides, vancomycin, ciprofloxacin, rifampicin, metronidazole, isoniazid, cotrimoxazole, pyrazinamide, etc.

Sources of Antibiotics/Antimicrobial Agents

The antibiotics may be obtained from natural sources or they may be semi-synthetic or completely synthetic in nature. The natural sources of commonly used antibiotics are:

- **Fungi:** Penicillin, cephalosporin, etc.
- **Bacteria:** Bacitracin, Colistin, polymixin B, etc.
- **Actinomycetes:** Macrolides, tetracycline, aminoglycosides, etc.

 Remember ....

Common Precautions to be Employed During Prescription of AMAs

Before prescribing antimicrobials, it should be made sure that there is some clinical evidence of microbial infection. As there are large number of AMAs available, the choice of a particular AMA depends upon the patient particulars, the infecting organisms and the drugs available.

- *Patient-related considerations:* The factors which are taken into consideration while prescribing the drug are—age of the patient, sex, any history of drug allergy, pregnancy, renal/hepatic/host defense status, etc.
- *Organism-related considerations:* Ideally, antibiotic sensitivity test should be performed before prescribing any antibiotic for any infection. But, the bacteriological testing is expensive as well as time consuming. So, we have to institute empirical therapy based upon our clinical judgment of the likely pathogens responsible for a particular infection. The empirical therapy should cover all likely organisms responsible for the infection.
- *Drug-related considerations:* Specific properties of the AMAs guide us in choosing a specific drug from a long list of AMAs. The most important factor is the spectrum of the activity of the drug and the sensitivity of the organism towards that drug. The final guide for the choice of antibiotic should be the evidence-based medicine, which further depends upon the reliable clinical trials data. The cost of the drug should also be taken into consideration.

TREATMENT WITH COMBINATION OF ANTIMICROBIAL AGENTS

Sometimes we have to use combination of different AMAs to treat certain infections. This is done:

- To get the synergistic effect, example: Rifampicin + isoniazid in tuberculosis; trimethoprim + sulfamethoxazole; to get a bactericidal effect whereas both individual components are bacteriostatic in nature.
- To widen the spectrum of action of AMAs.
- To treat the mixed infections.
- To prevent the development of resistance.
- To reduce the incidence of side effects, as in combination, the dose of the individual drug is usually on the lower side.

CAUSES OF FAILURE OF ANTIMICROBIAL THERAPY

Sometimes, the antimicrobial therapy may fail to cure an infection due to following reasons:

- The selection of drug, dose, route or duration of treatment is not proper.
- Delay in the beginning of treatment.
- The wrong diagnosis such as trying to treat untreatable (viral) infections or other causes of fever (malignancy, collagen diseases).
- Failure to remove the source of infection, such as abscess or foreign body.

PENICILLINS

HISTORY

Penicillin was discovered by Sir Alexander Fleming in 1928. This was the first antibiotic which was used in clinical practice in 1941. This was originally obtained from the fungus *Penicillium notatum*, but the present source is a high yielding mutant of *P. chrysogenum*. In 1957, the semi-synthetic penicillins were developed. These antibiotics have a β-lactam ring in their structure (Fig. 2.1).

Chemically, the penicillins have β-lactam ring in their structure. Some other antibiotics having β-lactam ring in their structure are cephalosporins, monobactam and carbapenams.

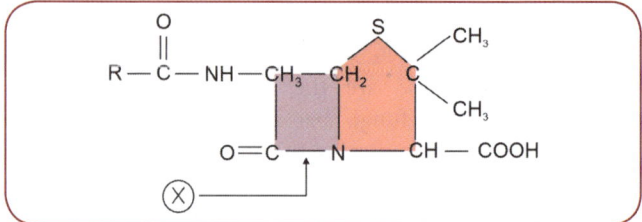

FIG. 2.1: Structure of penicillins
Thiazolidine ring 2. β-lactam ring 3. (X bond which is broken by penicillinase)

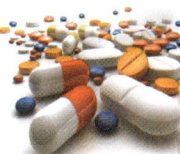

Collectively, all these above antibiotics are called β-lactam antibiotics.

MODE OF ACTION

All β-lactam antibiotics interfere with the synthesis of bacterial cell wall. The cell wall protects the bacteria and is essential for the survival of bacteria. The rigidity or strength to the bacterial cell wall is provided by peptidoglycans. The peptidoglycan is synthesized in the presence of an important enzyme called as transpeptidase (also known as penicillin binding proteins or PBPs). This transpeptidase is inhibited by the β-lactam antibiotics, thus inhibiting the formation of peptidoglycan and thus cell wall.

When susceptible bacteria divide in the presence of a β-lactam antibiotic, cell wall deficient forms are produced. Because the interior of the bacteria is hyperosmotic, the cell wall deficient forms swell burst. This causes bacterial cell lysis. This is how β-lactam antibiotics exert bactericidal action.

There is no cell wall in the human cells. Therefore, these β-lactam antibiotics are non-toxic to human cells. Blood, pus, and tissue fluids do not interfere with the antibacterial action of β-lactam antibiotics.

CLASSIFICATION

- **Acid-labile (natural) penicillin:** Penicillin G (PnG), procaine penicillin G, fortified penicillin G, benzathine Penicillin G.
- **Acid-resistant alternative to penicillin G:** Phenoxymethyl penicillin (penicillin V).
- **Penicillinase-resistant penicillins:** Methicillin, cloxacillin, dicloxacillin.
- **Extended spectrum penicillins:**
  - Aminopenicillins: Ampicillin, bacampicillin, amoxicillin.
  - Carboxypenicillins: Carbenicillin.
  - Ureidopenicillins: Piperacillin, mezlocillin.
- **β-lactamase inhibitors:** Clavulanic acid, sulbactam, tazobactam.

ACID LABILE (NATURAL) PENICILLIN: PENICILLIN G OR BENZYL PENICILLIN

- **Antibacterial spectrum:** PnG is a narrow spectrum antibiotic; activity is limited primarily to Gram-positive bacteria, few Gram negative ones and anaerobes.
- **Cocci:** *Streptococci, many Pneumococci, Staphylococcus. aureus* are highly sensitive *aureus, Neisseria gonorrheae* and *N. meningitidis,* although susceptible, but have developed partial resistance also.
- **Bacilli:** *Bacillus anthracis, Corynebacterium diphtheriae,* and practically all *Clostridia (tetani* and others), *Listeria, spirochetes, Treponema pallidum, Leptospira* are highly sensitive.

Mycobacterium tuberculosis, rickettsiae, chlamydiae, protozoa, fungi and *viruses* are totally insensitive to PnG.

Pharmacokinetics

- PnG is acid labile, therefore it is destroyed by gastric acid.
- Absorption of sod. Penicillin G from intramuscular site is rapid and complete; peak plasma level is attained in 30 min.
- It reaches most body fluids, but penetration in serous cavities and CSF is poor.
- However, in the presence of inflammation (synovitis, meningitis,etc.) adequate amounts may reach these sites.
- The plasma t½ of PnG in healthy adult is 30 min.
- It is excreted by the kidneys.
- Probenecid helps to prolong its duration of action by decreasing its excretion (the renal tubular secretion is decreased).
- Different penicillins available are given in Table 2.1.

TABLE 2.1: Different penicillins-dose, route and preparation

Drugs	Dose	Route	Available as and preparation
Sod. penicillin G (crystalline penicillin)	0.5–5 MU 6–12 hourly	IM/IV	Dry powder in vials to be dissolved in sterile water at the time of injection
Procaine penicillin G inj.	10.5–1 MU 12–24 hourly	IM	Dry powder in vials to be dissolved in sterile water at the time of injection
Fortified procaine penicillin G inj (3 lac U procaine penicillin + 1 lac U sod. penicillin G)	4 lac Unit Once daily	IM	Dry powder in vials to be dissolved in sterile water at the time of injection
Benzathine penicillin G (PENIDURE-LA)	0.6–2.4 MU every 2–4 weeks	IM	Dry powder in vials to be dissolved in sterile water at the time of injection

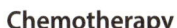

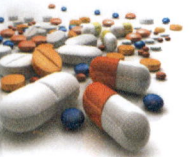

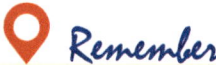 **Remember**...

Prior sensitivity testing is required before injecting penicillins in any patient. History of penicillin allergy must be elicited before injecting it. A scratch test or intradermal test (with 2–10 U) may be performed first. On occasions, it has caused fatal anaphylaxis. Testing with benzylpenicilloyl-polylysine is safer. However, a negative intradermal test does not rule out delayed hypersensitivity.

PnG is the most common drug implicated in drug allergy, because of which it has practically vanished from use in general practice.

In general practice, Benzathine penicillin is still used prophylactically in patients suffering from rheumatic fever, bacterial endocarditis and agranulocytosis.

Indications

PnG is the drug of choice for infections caused by organisms susceptible to it (unless the patient is allergic to it).

- **Respiratory tract infections:**
  - Streptococcal infections: Such as pharyngitis, otitis media, scarlet fever, rheumatic fever, etc.
  - Pneumococcal infections: Such as lobar pneumonia and meningitis.
  - Diphtheria infection.
- **Meningococcal infections:** Responsive with intravenous injection of high doses.
- **Gonorrhea and syphilis**
- **Tetanus and gas gangrene:** Antitoxin and other measures are more important; PnG 6–12 MU/day is used to kill the causative organism and has adjuvant value.
- **Leptospirosis:** PnG 1.5 MU injected IV 6 hourly for 7 days is curative.
- **Prophylactic uses:**
  - **Rheumatic fever:** Low concentrations of penicillin prevent colonization by streptococci that are indirectly responsible for rheumatic fever. Benzathine penicillin 1.2 MU every 4 weeks till 18 years of age or 5 years after an attack, whichever is more.
  - **Bacterial endocarditis:** Dental extractions, endoscopies, catheterization, etc., cause bacteremia in patients with valvular defects and can cause endocarditis. PnG can afford protection, but amoxicillin is preferred now.
  - **Agranulocytosis patients:** Penicillin has been used alone or in combination with streptomycin to prevent respiratory and other acute infections, but cephalosporins + an aminoglycoside or fluoroquinolone are preferred now.

Adverse Effects

- **Local:** Pain at the site of injection and thrombophlebitis of the injected vein can occur.

- **Hypersensitivity:** PnG is the most common drug implicated in drug allergy (with 1–10% incidence). Frequent manifestations of penicillin allergy are—rash, itching, urticaria and fever. Wheezing, angioneurotic edema, serum sickness and exfoliative dermatitis are less common. Anaphylaxis is rare (1–4 per 10,000 patients), but may be fatal.

  All forms of natural and semi-synthetic penicillins can cause allergy. Incidence is more common after parenteral than oral administration and is highest with procaine penicillin (*procaine itself is allergenic*). The course of penicillin hypersensitivity cannot be predicted, i.e., an individual who tolerated penicillin earlier may show allergy on subsequent administration and *vice versa*.

  If a patient is allergic to penicillin, it is best to use an alternative antibiotic. Hyposensitization by the injection of increasing amounts of penicillin intradermally at hourly intervals can be tried only if no other choice is available.

- **Direct toxicity to CNS:** It occurs only when large doses (>20 MU) are injected intravenously. The toxicity is manifested as mental confusion, muscular twitching, convulsions and coma.

Let's know

Jarisch-Herxheimer reaction: When penicillin is injected in a patient suffering from secondary syphilis, it may produce shivering, fever, myalgia, exacerbation of lesions and even vascular collapse. This is due to sudden release of spirochetal lytic products. These symptoms may last for 12–72 hours. It does not need interruption of therapy. Aspirin and sedation provide relief from symptoms.

Limitations of Penicillin G

- Poor oral efficacy.
- Susceptibility to penicillinases.
- Narrow spectrum of activity.
- Hypersensitivity reactions (this has not been overcome in any preparation).

Penicillinase

It is a β-lactamase enzyme which opens up the β-lactam ring of β-lactam antibiotics and inactivates them. Some of the bacteria which produce this enzyme are Staphylococci, Gonococci, *E. coli* and *H. influenza*, and are called Penicillinase producers. This production of Penicillinase is one of the primary mechanism of acquiring resistance in certain microorganisms.

ACID-RESISTANT ALTERNATIVE TO PENICILLIN G PHENOXYMETHYL PENICILLIN (PENICILLIN V)

It can be given orally as it is acid stable. The antibacterial spectrum is identical to PnG. It cannot be relied upon for

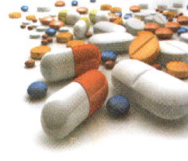
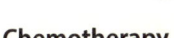

serious infections, but can be given for mild pharyngitis, sinusitis, otitis media and for prophylaxis of rheumatic fever.
Dose: Adults 250–500 mg, children 125–250 mg and infants 60 mg, given QID (250 mg = 4 lac U).

PENICILLINASE-RESISTANT PENICILLINS: METHICILLIN, CLOXACILLIN, DICLOXACILLIN

These drugs have side chain, which protects the β-lactam ring from attack by the penicillinase produced by some bacteria. These drugs are the drug of choice in the infections caused by Penicillinase producers.

Methicillin

It is not acid stable. Therefore, it has to be given parenterally. Methicillin resistant, staphylococcus aureus (MRSA) is resistant to it and are treated with vancomycin/linezolid.

Cloxacillin/Dicloxacillin

It can be given orally, as it is penicillinase as well as acid resistant drug. It should be given empty stomach for good absorption. The plasma t½ is about 1 hour.
Dose: 0.25–0.5 g orally every 6 hours; for severe infections 0.25–1 g may be injected IM or IV

Nafcillin

Its absorption from the gut is unreliable. Hence, it has to be given by parenteral route.

EXTENDED SPECTRUM PENICILLINS

These semisynthetic penicillins are active against a variety of Gram-negative bacilli as well. They can be grouped according to their spectrum of activity.

Aminopenicillins (Ampicillin, Bacampicillin, Amoxicillin)

This group is called aminopenicillins as the benzyl is substituted by the amino group in the side chain. Some are prodrugs and all have quite similar antibacterial spectra. No drug in this group is resistant to penicillinase or to other β-lactamases.

- **Antibacterial spectrum:** These are active against all organisms which are sensitive to PnG. In addition, many Gram-negative bacilli, e.g., *H. influenzae, E. coli, Proteus, Salmonella, Shigella* and *Helicobacter pylori* are also inhibited.

Ampicillin

- It is not degraded by gastric acid.
- Oral absorption is incomplete but adequate.
- Food interferes with absorption.

- Plasma t½ is 1 hour.
- Primary channel of excretion is kidney and partly excreted in bile and reabsorbed-enterohepatic circulation occurs.
Dose: 0.5–2 g oral/IM/IV depending on severity of infection, every 6 hourly; children 50–100 mg/kg/day.

Indications

- Respiratory tract infections; including bronchitis, sinusitis, otitis media, etc.
- Urinary tract infections
- Meningitis
- Gonorrhea
- Typhoid fever
- Bacillary dysentery
- Cholecystitis (It is a drug of choice because higher concentration is obtained in bile)
- Subacute bacterial endocarditis
- H. pylori infection
- Septicemias and mixed infections; injected ampicillin may be combined with gentamicin or one of the third generation cephalosporins.

[Ampicillin has been the drug of choice for most acute infections, but resistance has increased nowadays]

Adverse Effects

- Diarrhea is frequent after oral administration, due to its incomplete absorption and the unabsorbed drug irritates the lower intestines as well as causes marked alteration of bacterial flora.
- It produces a high incidence (up to 10%) of rashes, especially in patients with AIDS, EB virus infections and lymphatic leukemia.

Interactions

- Failure of oral contraception by inhibiting colonic flora, it may interfere with deconjugation and enterohepatic cycling of oral contraceptives.
- Hydrocortisone inactivates ampicillin if mixed together in the same IV solution.

Bacampicillin

It is an ester prodrug of ampicillin, which is nearly completely absorbed from the GIT. Hence, incidence of diarrhea is claimed to be lower and higher plasma levels are attained. It is given in a dose of 400–800 mg BD for 7–10 days.

Amoxicillin

- It is not a prodrug but close congener of ampicillin.
- It is similar to ampicillin in all aspects, except:
  - Oral absorption is better; food does not interfere with its absorption; higher and more sustained blood levels are produced.

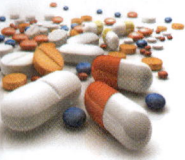

- Incidence of diarrhea is lower.
- It is more active against penicillin resistant *Streptococcus pneumoniae*.
- It is a component of triple drug *H. pylori* eradication regimens.
- It is given in a dose of 0.25–1 g TDS oral/IM; or slow IV injection, children 25–75 mg/kg/day.

Carboxypenicillins (Carbenicillin)

- The special feature of this penicillin congener is its activity against *Pseudomonas aeruginosa*, which is not inhibited by PnG or aminopenicillins.
- Carbenicillin is neither penicillinase-resistant nor acid resistant. It is inactive orally and is excreted rapidly in urine (t½ 1 hour).
- It is given in a dose of 1–2 g IM or 1–5 g IV every 4–6 hours.

(**Precaution**: *It is used as sodium salt. Hence at higher doses, enough sodium may be administered unknowingly to the patient. It may cause fluid retention and CHF in patients with borderline renal or cardiac functions*).

Indications

It is indicated in serious infections caused by *Pseudomonas* or *Proteus* such as:

- Burns
- Urinary tract infections
- Septicemia
- But, *Piperacillin is now mostly used for these serious infections.*

(**Precaution:** *Carbenicillin may be combined with gentamicin, but the two should not be mixed in the same syringe.*)

> **Carbenicillin indanyl:** It is an orally active ester of carbenicillin, used for treatment of UTIs caused by *Pseudomonas* and *Proteus*.

Ureidopenicillins (Piperacillin, Mezlocillin)

- **Piperacillin** is about 8 times more active than carbenicillin in its anti-pseudomonas activity.
- It is frequently used for treating serious Gram-negative infections in neutropenic, immunocompromised or burn patients.
- It has good activity against Klebsiella, many Enterobacteriaceae members and some Bacteroides.
- It can be combined with gentamicin or tobramycin in serious Gram-negative infections.
- Its elimination t½ is 1 hour.
- It is given in a dose of 100–150 mg/kg/day in three divided doses (max 16 g/day) IM or IV The IV route is preferred when >2 g is to be injected.

Mezlocillin is not available in India.

β-LACTAMASE INHIBITORS (CLAVULANIC ACID, SULBACTAM, TAZOBACTAM)

- β-lactamases are a family of enzymes produced by many Gram-positive and Gram-negative bacteria.
- These enzymes inactivate β-lactam antibiotics by opening the β-lactam ring.
- β-lactamase inhibitors bind irreversibly to the β-lactamases produced by the bacteria and inactivate them. This prevents the destruction of β-lactam antibiotics, thereby extending the spectrum of penicillins. β-lactamases are having very little intrinsic antibacterial activity.
- Three inhibitors of this enzyme clavulanic acid, sulbactam and tazobactam are available for clinical use.

Clavulanic Acid

- It is obtained from *Streptomyces clavuligerus*. It is a β-lactam molecule with little intrinsic antibacterial activity.
- It is called '**progressive inhibitor**' as the inhibition increases with time.
- It is also called a '**suicide inhibitor**' as it binds irreversibly to the β-lactamase and gets inactivated after binding to the enzyme.
- It inhibits the periplasmically located β-lactamase after permeating the outer layers of the cell wall of Gram-negative bacteria.
- It has good oral absorption and can also be given parenterally.
- Its elimination t½ is 1 hour.
- Its elimination t½ and tissue distribution matches with amoxicillin. So, it is usually combined with amoxicillin in both oral and parenteral preparations.
- Addition of clavulanic acid re-establishes the activity of amoxicillin against β-lactamase producing Gram-negative and positive bacteria.

Indications

- Skin and soft tissue infections.
- Intra abdominal and gynecological sepsis.
- Urinary, biliary and respiratory tract infections.
- Gonorrhea.

Dose

- **Orally:** Amoxicillin 250 mg + Clavulanic acid 125 mg TDS, also 500 mg + 125 mg TDS.
- **Parenterally:** Amoxicillin 1 g + Clavulanic acid 0.2 g single dose vial and 0.5 g + 0.1 g single dose vial; inject deep IM or IV 6–8 hourly for severe infections.
  It is more expensive than amoxicillin alone.

Sulbactam

- Its structure and activity is similar to clavulanic acid.
- It is preferably given by parenteral route as its oral absorption is inconsistent.

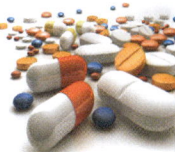

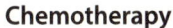

- Sulbactam has been combined with ampicillin, cefoperazone and ceftriaxone.

Indications

- Mixed aerobic-anaerobic infections.
- Intra-abdominal, gynecological, surgical, skin and soft tissue infections.
- It is *specially used in nosocomial infections.*

Dose

Ampicillin 1 g + sulbactam 0.5 g single dose vial; 1–2 vial deep IM or IV injection 6–8 hourly. Orally, 375 mg tab of Sultamicillin tosylate is given in 6–8 hourly doses.

Adverse Effects

Pain at the site of injection, thrombophlebitis of injected vein, rash and diarrhea are the main adverse effects.

Tazobactam

- It is similar to sulbactam.
- Its pharmacokinetics matches with piperacillin with which it has been combined for use in severe infections.
- The combination is not active against Pseudomonas as permeability to piperacillin is lost and resistance develops.
- Tazobactam can be combined with ceftriaxone also.
- Its main indications are serious pelvic, urinary, respiratory infections and Peritonitis.
- It is given in combination and in a dose of Piperacillin 4 g + 0.5 g tazobactam injected IV over 30 min TDS.

Drug Interactions

- ☞ Hydrocortisone should not be mixed with ampicillin in the same solution as ampicillin is inactivated by hydrocortisone.
- ☞ Ampicillin can cause failure of oral contraceptives due to inhibition of colonic flora and interference in enterohepatic circulation of oral contraceptives.
- ☞ Probenecid increases the blood levels of ampicillin by decreasing the renal excretion.

Nursing Implications

☞ **Penicillins**
  - ☞ The previous history of allergy to different penicillin must be taken carefully before administering penicillin injections.
  - ☞ If any sign of anaphylaxis is noticed after the injection, the treatment of the reaction should be started immediately and it should be informed immediately to senior and physician.
  - ☞ Intradermal sensitivity test should always be done before administering penicillin injections.
  - ☞ Emergency drug tray should always be ready for immediately handling of the reactions.
  - ☞ Patients should be informed beforehand that ampicillin can cause diarrhea.

- Cephalosporins are a group of semi-synthetic antibiotics derived from 'cephalosporin-C' which is obtained from a fungus *Cephalosporium.*
- The cephalosporins are chemically related to penicillins as they also have β-lactam ring in their structure.
- Cephalosporins have been conventionally divided into five generations based upon chronological sequence of development, potency and the overall antibacterial spectrum.

MECHANISM OF ACTION

- The mechanism of action is similar to penicillin.
- All cephalosporins are bactericidal in nature.
- They also inhibit the synthesis of bacterial cell wall.
- As they bind to different proteins than those which bind penicillins, no cross resistance is seen with penicillins and due to the same reason the spectrum and potency differs from penicillins.

Causes of Bacterial Resistance to Cephalosporins

The bacteria can acquire resistance to cephalosporins by various mechanisms. Some of the mechanisms are:
- Sometimes target proteins (PBPs) are altered which reduce affinity for the antibiotic.
- Sometimes impermeability to the antibiotic develops or its efflux increases, and the antibiotic can not reach its site of action.
- Production of cephalosporinases (β-lactamase) which destroy the cephalosporins specifically.

PHARMACOKINETICS

- These can be given both by oral or parenteral routes.
- Majority are given by parenteral route.
- Most of the cephalosporins are not metabolized in liver but, are excreted rapidly by the kidneys and have short elimination t½.
- Probenecid inhibits their tubular secretion and increases the t½.

CLASSIFICATION

Cephalosporins have been conventionally divided into five generations mentioned in Table 2.2.

(The potency and the overall antibacterial spectrum increases as we go to the higher generations).

The individual cephalosporins differ only in their:
- Antibacterial spectrum and relative potency against specific organisms.

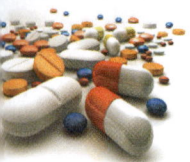

TABLE 2.2: Classification of cephalosporins

Generation	Oral	Parenteral
First generation	Cephalexin Cefadroxil	Cefazolin
Second generation	Cefaclor Cefprozil Cefuroxime axetil	Cefuroxime Cefoxitin
Third generation	Cefixime Cefpodoxime proxetil Cefdinir Ceftibuten Ceftamet pivoxil	Cefotaxime Ceftizoxime Ceftriaxone Ceftazidime Cefoperazone
Fourth generation	–	Cefepime Cefpirome
Fifth generation	–	Ceftobiprole Ceftaroline Ceftolozane

- Susceptibility to β-lactamases, and
- Pharmacokinetic properties-many have to be injected, some are oral.

First Generation Cephalosporins

- These were developed in the 1960s.
- These have high activity against Gram-positive but poor action against Gram-negative bacteria.
- No activity is seen against anaerobes (Table 2.3).

Second Generation Cephalosporins

- These were developed subsequent to the first generation compounds.
- These are more active against Gram-negative organisms *(but weaker than the first generation compounds against Gram-positive bacteria).*
- Some are active against anaerobes also, but none inhibits *P. aeruginosa.*
- Less preferred as compared to the third generation agents (Table 2.3).

Third Generation Cephalosporins

- These compounds were introduced in the 1980s.
- These are more active against Gram-negative organisms as compared to second generation agents.
- These are less active on Gram-positive cocci and anaerobes (Table 2.3).

Fourth Generation Cephalosporins

- These compounds were introduced in the 1990s.
- These have good activity against a variety of gram positive, Gram-negative and anaerobic organisms.
- These are resistant to β-lactamases.
- All agents of this group are administered parenterally (Table 2.3).

TABLE 2.3: Summary of different generations of cephalosporins

Drug	t½(Hr)	Route	Dose	Special features
First Generation Cephalosporins				
Cefazolin	2	IM or IV	Mild cases: 0.5 g 8 hourly Severe cases: 1 g 6 hourly Children: 25–50 mg/kg/day	• Active against most PnG sensitive organisms • Used for surgical prophylaxis
Cephalexin	1	Oral	Adult: 0.25–1 g 6–8 hourly Children: 25–100 mg/kg/day hourly	• Similar to cefazolin • Less active against penicillinase producing staphylococci and *H. influenzae*
Cefadroxil	2	Oral	0.5–1 g BD	• Has sustained action at the site of infection due to good tissue penetration
Second Generation Cephalosporins				
Cefuroxime	1	IM or IV	Adult: 0.75–1.5 g,8 hourly. Children: 30–100 mg/kg/day	• Resistant to gram-negative β-lactamases • Good activity on gram-positive cocci and certain anaerobes • Not active against *B. fragilis* • Attains higher CSF levels
Cefoxitin	1	IM or IV	1 gm 6–8 hourly	• Good activity against *B. fragilis* also
Cefuroxime axetil	1	Oral	Adults: 250–500 mg BD Children: 125–250 mg BD	• The activity depends on *in vivo* hydrolysis and release of cefuroxime

Contd...

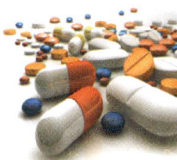

Cefaclor	1	Oral	0.25–1.0 g 8 hourly	• More active against *H. influenzae, E. coli, P. mirabilis* and some anaerobes
Cefprozil	1.3	Oral	Adults: 250–500 mg BD Children: 20 mg/kg/ day	• Active against *S. pyogenes, S. pneumoniae, S. aureus, H. influenzae, Moraxella* and *Klebsiella*
Third Generation Cephalosporins				
Cefotaxime	1	IM or IV	Adults: 1–2 g 6–12 hourly, Children: 50–100 mg/kg per day	• Attains high CSF levels • Indicated in meningitis by gram negative bacilli • Septicemias, immunocompromised patients
Ceftizoxime	1.5–2	IM or IV	0.5–2.0 g 8–12 hourly	• In addition to Cefotaxime, it inhibits B. fragilis also
Ceftriaxone	8	IM or IV	For skin/soft tissue/ urinary infections: 1–2 g IV/IM/ days Meningitis: 4g stat followed by 2 g IV (children 75–100 mg/kg) once daily for 7–10 days Typhoid: 2–4 g IV daily × 2 days followed by 2 g/day (children 75 mg/kg) till 2 days after fever subsides	• Attains high CSF levels • Longer duration of action • Indications: Meningitis, typhoid, complicated UTIs, septicemias and abdominal sepsis • To overcome resistance, it has been combined with sulbactam or tazobactam
Ceftazidime	2	IM or IV	0.5–2 g every 8 hourly	• Specially indicated for *P. aeruginosa* infections
Cefoperazone	2	IM or IV	1–3 g 8–12 hourly	• Good activity against *Pseudomonas, S. typhi* and *B. fragilis* • It may cause disulfiram-like reaction with alcohol
Cefixime	3	Oral	200–400 mg BD	• Highly active against Enterobacteriaceae, *H. influenzae, S. pyogenes* • Indicated in respiratory, urinary and biliary infections • Not active against S. aureus
Cefpodoxime proxetil	2	Oral	200–400 mg BD	• In addition to Cefixime, it has good activity against S. aureus also
Fourth generation cephalosporins				
Cefepime	2	IM/IV	1–2 g 8–12 hourly	• Has good activity against the bacteria, resistant to 1st, 2nd, and 3rd generation Cephalosporins • It is not active against MRSA • Indicated in serious nosocomial infections, septicemias and febrile neutropenia
Cefpirome	2.3	IM/IV	1–2 g 12 hourly	• Same as above

Fifth Generation Cephalosporins

- Ceftobiprole, Ceftaroline and Ceftolozane are fifth generation cephalosporins.
- These compounds were introduced in 2007 and after.
- These are not widely available in India.
- All agents of this group are used parenterally.
- In addition to the antimicrobial spectrum covered by all four generations, these agents have good activity against methicillin resistant S. aureus (MRSA) and vancomycin resistant S. aureus (VRSA) also, hence specifically indicated for complicated skin and skin structure infections (CSSSI) and community-acquired bacterial pneumonias.
- These agents have good activity against a wide variety of Gram-positive, Gram-negative and anaerobic organisms.

Antimicrobial Spectrum-Indications, Dose and Administration

Ceftobiprole has been approved for clinical use in the following conditions:

- CSSSI: 500 mg IV 12 hourly × 7–14 days. It should be given as infusion for 1 hour.
- For Gram-negative organism, infections in diabetic foot, community-acquired pneumonia, hospital-acquired pneumonia, and chemotherapy-induced neutropenia with fever: 500 mg IV 8 hourly × 7–14 days. It should be given as infusion for 2 hours.
- As 80% of drug is excreted in urine in an unchanged form, dose reduction is recommended keeping in view the renal status of patient (Table 2.4).

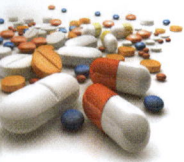

TABLE 2.4: Antimicrobial spectrum of fifth generation cephalosporins

Gram-positive	Gram-negative bacteria	Anaerobes
• Community acquired MRSA • VRSA • Penicillin, Macrolide and Fluoroquinolone resistant *S. pneumoniae* • Vancomycin resistant *Enterobacteriae foecalis*	• Similar to Ceftriaxone and Ceftazidime • β-lactamase producing and non-producing *H. influenzae* and *N. gonorrheae*	Mixed anaerobes

MRSA, methicillin resistant staphylococcus aureus; VRSA, vancomycin resistant staphylococcus aureus

Adverse Drug Reactions

- Dysguesia (taste changes).
- Nausea, vomiting.
- Both Ceftaroline and Ceftolozane have same spectrum of activity and indications as Ceftobiprole.
- Ceftolozane is sometimes combined with Tazobactam (a β-lactamase inhibitor), which prevents it from degradation and improves its activity in complicated UTIs and complicated intra-abdominal infections.

Common Adverse Effects of Cephalosporins

- **Pain** after IM injection occurs with some cephalosporins but most of these can be given by IV route.
- **Hypersensitivity reaction** is one of the most important adverse effect of cephalosporins. Rashes, angioedema and even anaphylaxis can occur. Ten percent patients allergic to penicillin show cross sensitivity to cephalosporins.
- **Diarrhea** can occur with oral cephalosporins due to the irritative effect of the orally given drug or due to alteration of gut flora.
- **Nephrotoxicity** can occur if given with an aminoglycoside or loop diuretic.
- **Neutropenia, thrombocytopenia** leading to *bleeding and a disulfiram-like interaction* with alcohol has been reported with some cephalosporins like cefoperazone.

Common uses of Cephalosporins

- Respiratory, urinary and soft tissue infections caused by Gram-negative organisms. Preferred agents for these infections are cefuroxime, cefotaxime and ceftriaxone.
- **Meningitis:** IV cefotaxime/ceftriaxone is generally combined with ampicillin or vancomycin or both (*For empirical therapy before bacterial diagnosis*).
- Septicemias caused by Gram-negative organisms.
- As an alternative to penicillins for ENT, upper respiratory and cutaneous infections.
- **Typhoid:** Currently, ceftriaxone and cefoperazone injected IV are the fastest acting and most reliable drugs for enteric fever.
- Mixed aerobic-anaerobic infections in cancer patients.

- **Surgical prophylaxis:** Cefazolin (IM or IV) is employed for most types of surgeries including those with surgical prosthesis such as artificial heart valves, artificial joints, etc. Also used for prophylaxis and treatment of infections in neutropenic patients: Ceftazidime or another third generation compound, alone or in combination with an aminoglycoside are used.
- Gonorrhea caused by penicillinase producing organisms: Ceftriaxone is the drug of choice for single dose therapy of gonorrhea. Cefuroxime and cefotaxime can also be used for this purpose.

MONOBACTAM

- Monobactams are β-lactam antibiotics having a single β-lactam ring (hence called as monobactam).
- Aztreonam is the only available monobactam.
- It is bactericidal in nature and acts by binding to specific protein binding proteins (PBP) and thereby inhibiting bacterial cell wall synthesis.
- It inhibits Gram-negative enteric bacilli and *H. influenzae* at a very low concentration and *Pseudomonas* at moderate concentration.
- It does not inhibit Gram-positive cocci or fecal anaerobes.
- There is no cross sensitivity with other β-lactam antibiotics except Ceftazidime.
- It is given parenterally in a dose of 0.5–2 g IM or IV 6–12 hourly.
- The elimination t½ is 1.8 hours.
- It is primarily given in hospital acquired infections originating from urinary, biliary, gastrointestinal and female genital tracts.

CARBAPENEMS

- Carbapenems contain a β-**lactam** ring fused with a five-membered penem ring.
- Members of this group have the widest spectrum of activity as compared to that of all currently available antimicrobials.
- Carbapenems have bactericidal action against Gram-positive and Gram-negative aerobic and anaerobic pathogenic bacteria.

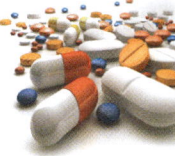

- These include **imipenem, meropenem, doripenem** and **ertapenem.**

Imipenem

- Imipenem is extremely potent and has a very wide spectrum of activity except MRSA.
- It is resistant to most of the β-**lactamases.**
- The t½ is 1 hour and it is inactivated rapidly by hydrolysis in the brush border of renal tubular cells with the help of an enzyme dehydropeptidase.
- The metabolic products are toxic to renal tubules.
- Dose of the drug is reduced when renal functions are impaired.
- *Imipenem has to be given in combination with Cilastatin.*
- *Combining Imipenem with cilastatin (a specific inhibitor of dehydropeptidase) prevents both inactivation of Imipenem and renal toxicity.*
- *It is given in a dose of Imipenem-cilastatin 0.5 g (250 + 250 mg) IV 6 hourly (max 4 g/day).*
- The imipenem and cilastatin are available in equivalent combined doses such as 125 +125 mg/250 + 250 mg/500 + 500 mg/1000 + 1000 mg.
- Adverse effects include GI upset, allergic reactions, confusion and convulsions.
- It is used commonly in septicemias, intra-abdominal infections and nosocomial pneumonia.
- It is used with aminoglycoside in pseudomonas infections.

Meropenem

- It is similar to imipenem, but is stable to renal dehydropeptidase and can therefore be given without Cilastatin.
- It penetrates into the CSF but is not associated with nausea and convulsions.
- It is given in a dose of 0.5–2.0 g (10–40 mg/kg) by slow IV injection at 8 hourly intervals.

Faropenem, doripenem and ertapenem are some other carbapenems.

Drug Interactions

- Patients on cefoperazone, cefotetan and cefamendol should avoid alcohol as a disulfiram-like reaction can occur.
- Concurrent use of cephalosporin, furosemide and aminoglycosides increases the risk of nephrotoxicity. Hence, the combination should be avoided.
- Probenecid prolongs the plasma half-life of cephalosporins by decreasing their tubular secretion.
- Antacids decrease the absorption of cefaclor and cefpodoxime. Hence, concurrent use should be avoided.

Nursing Implications

- **Cephalosporins**
  - Drug sensitivity test should be performed before administrating Cephalosporins.
  - If any sign of anaphylaxis is noticed after the injection, the treatment of the reaction should be started immediately and it should be informed immediately to senior and physician.
  - The renal functions should be regularly monitored.
  - Patients should be regularly enquired about any side effects.
  - The female patients should be especially enquired about vaginitis or any per-vaginal discharge.

AMINOGLYCOSIDES

- The aminoglycosides group includes streptomycin, gentamicin, amikacin, sisomicin, kanamycin, netilmicin, tobramycin, paromomycin, neomycin and framycetin.
- These are natural products or semi-synthetic derivatives of compounds produced by a variety of soil actinomycetes.
- Some compounds are isolated from stains of *Streptomyces griseus* (these end with –mycin in their spellings) whereas Gentamicin and Netilmicin are isolated from species of actinomycetes micromonospora (these end with—micin in their spellings).
- Chemically, these antibiotics have polybasic amino groups (hexose nucleus) linked to two or more amino sugar residues with glycosidic linkage.
- *Streptomycin* was the first member discovered in 1944 by *Waksman and his colleagues.*
- Aminoglycosides are bactericidal in nature.
- Aminoglycosides resemble one another in their mode of action, pharmacokinetics, therapeutic and toxic properties.

CLASSIFICATION

The classification of aminoglycosides is given in Table 2.5

TABLE 2.5: Classification of aminoglycosides

Systemic aminoglycosides	Topical aminoglycosides
• Streptomycin	• Neomycin
• Amikacin	• Framycetin
• Gentamicin	
• Sisomicin	
• Kanamycin	
• Netilmicin	
• Tobramycin	
• Paromomycin	

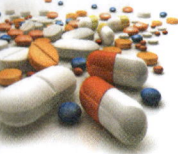

MECHANISM OF ACTION

- The aminoglycosides enter through the bacterial cell wall and cytoplasmic membrane through porin channels, which is a complex multistep process.
- After entering inside the bacterial cell, these agents bind to 30S ribosomes and lead to inhibition of protein synthesis. (*These proteins are essential for the bacterial replication*).
- The bactericidal effect of aminoglycosides is concentration dependent.
- The aminoglycosides show a unique phenomenon known as "*post antibiotic effect*" (bactericidal effect remains even after the plasma levels of aminoglycosides decrease). Therefore, single injection of the total daily dose of aminoglycoside may be more effective and possibly less toxic than its conventional division into 2–3 doses, despite having short half-life of 2–4 hours.

ANTIBACTERIAL SPECTRUM

- These drugs are highly effective against Gram-negative organisms including *E. coli, K. pneumoniae, Enterobacter, H. influenzae, Proteus, Serratia* and *P. aeruginosa.*
- Some Gram-positive bacteria are also susceptible, especially *Staph. aureus, Strep. faecalis* and some *Listeria, etc.*

PHARMACOKINETICS

- These are water soluble and do not readily cross cell membrane, so neither absorbed nor destroyed in the GIT.
- Absorption from injection site in muscles is rapid: peak plasma levels are attained in 30–60 minutes; they distribute mainly to the extracellular fluid only.
- They can cross placental barrier as well as higher concentrations are achieved in endolymph and renal cortex. This is responsible for ototoxicity and nephrotoxicity as side effects of these drugs.
- These are eliminated unchanged mainly by glomerular filtration.

COMMON PROPERTIES OF AMINOGLYCOSIDES

- They are bactericidal in nature and active against aerobic Gram-negative bacilli.
- They do not inhibit anaerobes.
- They are not absorbed orally.
- They are more active at alkaline pH.
- They are used as sulfate salts, which are highly water soluble; solutions are stable for months together.
- They have relatively narrow margin of safety.
- They exhibit ototoxicity and nephrotoxicity as their common adverse effects.

- There is only partial cross resistance amongst them. Common aminoglycosides and their special features are enlisted in Table 2.6.

COMMON ADVERSE EFFECTS OF AMINOGLYCOSIDES

Adverse effects of aminoglycoside occur when these drugs are given in a higher dose or for a longer duration. The risk increases when the renal clearance is inefficient (because of disease or age) or other potentially nephrotoxic drugs (loop diuretics, amphotericin-B) are co-administered or the patient is dehydrated.

- **Ototoxicity:** Both vestibular and auditory nerve damage may occur causing hearing loss, vertigo and tinnitus, which may be permanent. This is the most important dose and duration related adverse effect. Warning symptoms of auditory nerve damage is tinnitus and that of vestibular toxicity are motion related headache, dizziness or nausea. Serious ototoxicity can occur with ear drops when instilled in a patient with perforated tympanic membrane. Ototoxicity occurs due to attainment of higher concentration of these drugs in the labyrinthine fluid and local damage.
- **Nephrotoxicity:** The aminoglycosides attain high concentration in renal cortex (proximal tubules) and dose related changes (which are usually reversible) that occur in renal tubular cells. In the patients with normal renal functions, single daily dose is considered to be less nephrotoxic.
- **Neuromuscular blockade:** Aminoglycosides reduce acetylcholine release from the motor nerve endings and may impair neuromuscular transmission. This may aggravate myasthenia gravis or cause a transient mysthenic syndrome in patients whose neuromuscular transmission is normal. Dysfunction of optic nerve and perioral paraesthesia may be seen with *streptomycin.*
- **Other reactions:** *Rashes and hematological abnormalities, but are rare.

COMMON INDICATIONS OF AMINOGLYCOSIDES

- Gram-negative bacillary infections particularly septicemia, meningitis, UTIs, renal, pelvic and abdominal sepsis.
- Bacterial endocarditis: Usually gentamicin is preferred as a part of the regimen.
- Other infections such as tuberculosis (streptomycin preferred) tularemia, plague, brucellosis, etc.
- **Topical uses:** Neomycin, framycetin and sisomicin are used for various topical infections.

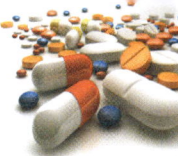

TABLE 2.6: Common aminoglycosides, their dose and special features

Drug	Dose	Special features
Gentamicin	3–5 mg/kg/day in 1–3 doses	• It is the most economical and 1st line aminoglycoside having narrow therapeutic index • Used in combination with piperacillin or 3rd generation cephalosporin for serious infections such as meningitis and SABE
Streptomycin	0.75–1 g IM OD/BD for 7–10 days	• It is the oldest aminoglycoside, having lowest nephrotoxicity • It is contraindicated during pregnancy due to fetal ototoxicity • Currently used in anti-tubercular regimen only
Amikacin	15 mg/kg/day in 1–3 doses	• It has widest spectrum of activity due to its resistance to bacterial aminoglycoside inactivating enzymes • It is a semi-synthetic derivative of kanamycin • In toxicity, hearing loss occurs more than vestibular disturbances
Tobramycin	3–5 mg/kg/day in 1–3 doses	• Similar to gentamicin except ototoxicity and nephrotoxicity, which is less than gentamicin. Hence, used as an alternative to gentamicin • It is given by inhalation for therapy of infective exacerbation of cystic fibrosis
Netilmicin	4–6 mg/kg/day in 1–3 doses	• It is effective against the strains of bacteria that resist gentamicin and tobramycin • It is less ototoxic and nephrotoxic than these drugs
Sisomicin	0.3% eye drops/ 0.1% cream	• It is more potent on pseudomonas infection
Kanamycin	15 mg/kg/day in 1–3 doses	• It is more toxic, both to the cochlea and vestibule. Rarely used these days
Neomycin	0.25–1 g QID oral, 0.3–0.5% skin and eye ointment	• Used topically, for infected wounds, ulcer, conjunctivitis and external ear infections • Used orally, for preparation of bowel before surgery and hepatic coma • Not used systemically due to high toxicity to internal ear and kidneys
Framycetin	1% skin cream and 0.5% eye drops and ointment	• Similar to neomycin
Paromomycin	25–30 mg/kg/day or 500 mg TDS	• It is chemically related to neomycin • Not absorbed from gut • Orally, it is used as an alternative to neomycin for hepatic encephalopathy • It has good activity against *E. histolytica*, *Giardia lamblia*, *Trichomonas vaginalis*, *Cryptosporidium* and *Leishmania*, in addition to many bacteria sensitive to neomycin • Parenterally, it is also used for visceral leishmaniasis

Current Role of Neomycin in Hepatic Coma

- Normally ammonia (NH_3) is produced by colonic bacteria. This is absorbed and converted to urea by liver. In severe hepatic failure, detoxification of ammonia does not occur and blood levels of ammonia rise which produce encephalopathy. Neomycin, by suppressing intestinal flora, diminishes ammonia production and lowers its blood level; clinical improvement is seen within 2–3 days.
  However, because of toxic potential, it is infrequently used for this purpose.
- *Paromomycin can be* used as an alternative to neomycin for hepatic encephalopathy.
- *Lactulose* is preferred agent these days because it reduces blood ammonia concentration by 25–50%. The ammonia produced by bacteria in colon is converted to ionised ammonium salts in the presence of breakdown products of lactulose which are acidic in nature. These ionised ammonium salts are not absorbed. For this purpose, lactulose 20 g TDS or more may be required.

Drug Interactions

- Aminoglycosides should not be given with other nephrotoxic drugs such as NSAIDs, vancomycin, amphotericin-B, etc.
- Aminoglycosides should not be given with other ototoxic drugs such as diuretics, vancomycin, minocycline, etc.
- Aminoglycosides potentiate the action of anaesthetics and muscles relaxants.
- These drugs should be used cautiously in patients above 60 years of age.

Nursing Implications

- **Aminoglycosides**
  - The renal functions should be regularly monitored.
  - Patients should be regularly enquired about any side effects.
  - Patients should be warned for not driving or operating the machinery.
  - Patient should be advised to take plenty of water during the course.
  - Monitor the signs and symptoms of hearing loss.

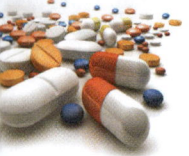

MACROLIDE ANTIBIOTICS

- Macrolide antibiotics contain a many membered lactone ring known as macrocyclic ring to which one or more deoxy-sugars are attached.
- Erythromycin, Clarithromycin, Roxithromycin and Azithromycin are macrolide antibiotics.
- *Erythromycin* is the first member of this group, and was isolated from a strain of *Streptomyces erythreus* in 1952.
- *Clarithromycin, Roxithromycin* and *Azithromycin* are semi-synthetic derivatives of erythromycin and these are also called *newer macrolides*.
- Some other macrolides are *dirithromycin, oleandomycin* and *troleandomycin*.

MECHANISM OF ACTION

- Macrolide antibiotics are bacteriostatic agents and inhibit the protein synthesis by binding reversibly to 50S ribosomal subunit of sensitive microorganism and interferes with 'translocation' step in the protein synthesis.
- The Gram-positive bacteria accumulate about 100 times more erythromycin than the Gram-negative bacteria, hence Gram-positive bacteria are more sensitive than the Gram-negative ones.
- Macrolides behave as bactericidal at very high concentrations.

ANTIMICROBIAL SPECTRUM

- These antibiotics are more active against Gram-positive cocci and inactive against most of the aerobic and enteric Gram-negative bacilli.

Some of the important drugs with their properties are given in Table 2.7.

Motilin Receptors

Erythromycin stimulates motilin receptors in the GIT which induces gastric contractions. This leads to early gastric emptying and increased intestinal motility without significantly affecting the colonic motility.

Due to this property, it is also used in diabetic gastroparesis and post operatively to promote the peristalsis in the cases of post-operative paralytic ileus.

TELITHROMYCIN

- It is a semi-synthetic derivative of erythromycin and also called as Ketolide, due to a keto group in its structure. Due to this changed structure, it is more active against the Macrolide resistant Gram-positive microorganisms.
- It is given orally as once daily dosage schedule in a dose of 400 mg OD.
- The half-life is 10 hours.
- Telithromycin is used as treatment of respiratory tract infections including acute exacerbation of chronic bronchitis, acute bacterial sinusitis and community-acquired pneumonia.
- The major side effects are: reversible hepatic dysfunction, prolongation of QTc interval and transient visual disturbances.

TABLE 2.7: Important macrolides and their properties

Drug properties	Erythromycin	Clarithromycin	Azithromycin	Roxithromycin
Dose	250–500 mg QID	250–500 mg BD	500 mg OD	150 mg BD
Route	Oral	Oral	Oral	Oral
Duration of treatment	7–14 days	7–14 days	3–5 days	7–14 days
Antibiotic spectrum	Narrow	Wide	Wide	Wide
Oral bioavailability	Low	Good	Good	Good
t½	1.5 hours	3–6 hours at low dose 3–9 hours at high dose	>50 hour	12 hours
Special properties	• Acid labile, given as enteric coated tablets. Poorly absorbed when given empty stomach • Has poor tissue penetration	• Acid stable, good absorption occurs when given empty stomach • Has good tissue penetration	• Acid stable, good absorption occurs when given empty stomach • Has good tissue penetration	• Acid stable, good absorption occurs when given empty stomach • Has good tissue penetration

Contd...

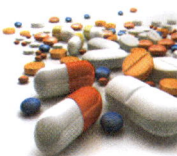

Drug properties	Erythromycin	Clarithromycin	Azithromycin	Roxithromycin
Indications	• As drug of choice in atypical pneumonia, whooping cough, and chancroid • As an alternative to Penicillin in Streptococcal pharyngitis, tonsillitis, mastoiditis, leptospirosis and prophylaxis of rheumatic fever SABE	• Upper and lower respiratory tract infections, sinusitis, otitis media, atypical pneumonia, skin and skin structure infections • As a component of triple drug regimen it eradicates *H. pylori* in 1–2 weeks • It is a first line drug in combination regimens for MAC infection in AIDS patients	• Pharyngitis, tonsillitis, sinusitis, otitis media, pneumonias, acute exacerbations of chronic bronchitis, skin and soft tissue infections • In the prophylaxis and treatment of MAC in AIDS patients • In multidrug resistant typhoid fever (patients allergic to cephalosporins) • Toxoplasmosis • As drug of choice: Legionnaires, *Chlamydia trachomatis*, Donovanosis and Chancroid	• It is an alternative to erythromycin for respiratory, ENT, skin and soft tissue and genital tract infections with similar efficacy
Side effects	• Epigastric distress causing nausea, vomiting and diarrhea • Allergic reaction such as fever and skin eruption • Cholestatic hepatitis (especially by erythromycin estolate) • Prolongation of QTc interval	• Side effects same as erythromycin but has better gastric tolerance • Reversible hearing loss at high doses	• Nausea, vomiting, diarrhea, and abdominal pain	• Nausea, vomiting, diarrhea, and abdominal pain

SPIRAMYCIN

- Spiramycin is also a macrolide antibiotic.
- It resembles erythromycin in spectrum of activity and properties.
- Its specific utility is for toxoplasmosis and recurrent abortions in pregnant women. It limits risk of transplacental transmission of *Toxoplasma gondii* infection.
- It is given in a dose of 3 million units (MU)BD/TDS for 3 weeks. (*Three week course is to be repeated after 2 weeks' gap till delivery*).
- Other indications are similar to erythromycin with a dose of 6 MU per day for 5 days.
- Common side effects are gastric irritation, nausea, diarrhea and rashes.

Drug Interactions

- ⚑ Erythromycin inhibits hepatic metabolism of many drugs (valproic acid, carbamazepine, warfarin, statins and ergotamine); increases the serum level of these drugs. This may cause toxicity symptoms. Hence, concurrent use of these agents should be avoided.
- ⚑ Macrolides block the degradation of digoxin by inhibiting intestinal flora causing increase in toxicity.
- ⚑ Linezolid (being inhibitor of MAO enzymes) causes cheese reaction. Hence, tyramine containing foods should be avoided by patients on linezolid therapy.

Nursing Implications

⚑ **Macrolide antibiotics**
- ☞ Azithromycin and clarithromycin should be given in empty stomach due to its acid stability and better absorption.
- ☞ These agents should be avoided during pregnancy as they cause cholestatic jaundice.
- ☞ The hepatic functions should be regularly monitored.
- ☞ Patients should be regularly enquired about any side effects.

LINCOSAMIDE ANTIBIOTICS

CLINDAMYCIN

- Clindamycin is a Lincosamide antibiotic.
- Its mechanism of action and spectrum of activity is similar to erythromycin.
- It also inhibits protein synthesis by binding to 50S ribosome.
- Clindamycin inhibits most Gram-positive cocci and many anaerobes.
- It is well absorbed orally.
- It attains good concentration in neutrophils, macrophages, skeletal and soft tissues.

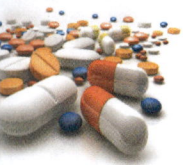

- It is metabolized in liver with a t½ of 3 hours and excreted in urine and bile.
- Side effects are rashes, urticaria, abdominal pain and diarrhea.
- Superinfection due to *Clostridium difficile* can occur. It causes pseudomembranous enterocolitis, which can be fatal if not treated timely. (*The treatment should be done by promptly stopping the drug and giving oral metronidazole (alternatively vancomycin).*)
- Clindamycin is indicated in anaerobic and mixed infections (abdominal, pelvic and lung abscess).
- Skin and soft tissue infections.
- Prophylaxis of subacute bacterial endocarditis (SABE) in penicillin allergic patients, who undergo dental procedures.
- Alternative to doxycycline for supplementing quinine/artesunate in treating multi-drug resistant malaria.
- Topically for infected acne vulgaris.
- **Dose:**
  - **Adults:** Oral dose is 150–300 mg QID, 200–600 mg IV 8 hourly
  - **Children:** Oral dose is 3–6 mg/kg QID.

LINCOMYCIN

Lincomycin has similar antibiotic and toxic properties to Clindamycin with higher incidence of diarrhea and fatal colitis. It was used extensively before the introduction of Clindamycin. It is rarely used nowadays.

GLYCOPEPTIDE ANTIBIOTICS

The glycopeptide antibiotics are vancomycin, and teicoplanin.

VANCOMYCIN

- It is a bactericidal drug which acts by inhibiting bacterial cell wall synthesis.
- It is not absorbed orally and has to be given by IV route.
- Its elimination t½ is 6 hours.
- As it is excreted unchanged by glomerular filtration, dose needs to be reduced in patients with poor renal functions.
- Vancomycin is indicated in:
  - Antibiotic-associated pseudomembranous enterocolitis by *C. difficile* or *Staphylococcus* is a second drug of choice as the drug of first choice is metronidazole.
  - Serious MRSA infections.
  - Enterococcal endocarditis in penicillin allergic patients.
  - As empirical therapy for bacterial meningitis (in combination with ceftriaxone/cefotaxime).

- Dose: Orally 125–500 mg QID, by IV route 500 mg QID or 1 g BD in the form of infusion.
- The common side effects are:
  - Higher doses of Vancomycin causes nerve deafness and renal damage.
  - IV injection can cause fall in BP and skin allergy.
  - Rapid IV injection can cause chills, fever, urticaria and intense flushing due to release of histamine by a direct action on the mast cells, this is called Red Men syndrome. (*It can be avoided by diluting Vancomycin and giving it in the form of IV infusion over a time period of 1–2 hours.*)

*Derivative of vancomycin, telavancin has better efficacy against Gram-positive organisms. It is given in a dose of 250–750 mg IV once a day.

TEICOPLANIN

- It is a newer glycopeptide with mechanism of action and spectrum of activity similar to vancomycin.
- It can be injected by IM route also.
- It has a long t½ of 3–4 days.
- It is less toxic than Vancomycin.
- Teicoplanin is indicated in:
  - Enterococcal endocarditis (along with gentamicin).
  - MRSA and penicillin-resistant streptococcal infections.
  - Osteomyelitis.
  - Surgical prophylaxis (as an alternative to Vancomycin).
- Dose: In moderate infections: 400 mg first day-then 200 mg daily IV or IM.

  In severe infections: 400 mg × 3 doses 12 hourly—then 400 mg daily.

*Some other newer derivatives of glycopeptides are Dalbavancin and Ramoplanin.

LINEZOLID

- Linezolid is the purely synthetic antimicrobial agent of oxazolidinones class.
- It acts by inhibiting bacterial protein synthesis by binding to the P site of the 50S ribosomal subunit and prevents the initiation of protein synthesis.
- It is very useful in the treatment of resistant Gram-positive aerobic, anaerobic and bacillary infections.
- It is well absorbed by oral route and the oral bioavailability approaches nearly 100%; hence oral and IV doses are equal.
- Linezolid is indicated in:
  - Community and hospital-acquired pneumonias.
  - Bacteremia.
  - Complicated skin and soft tissue infections such as MRSA, VRSA and VRE (vancomycin-resistant enterococci).

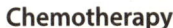

- It is given in a dose of 600 mg BD for 1–2 weeks.
- The common side effects are:
  - Mild abdominal pain, nausea, taste disturbance and diarrhea.
  - Rarely, optic neuropathy occurs if it is given for more than 4 weeks.

> **Linezolid** should be reserved as an alternative agent for the treatment of infections caused by multiple drug resistant strains and should never be used where other antimicrobial agents are likely to be effective. Indiscriminate use and overuse can lead to rapid development of resistant strains and eventual loss of effectiveness of this valuable new drug.

MISCELLANEOUS ANTIBIOTICS

Some important miscellaneous antibiotics are given in Table 2.8.

POLYPEPTIDE ANTIBIOTICS

- Polypeptide antibiotics are bactericidal in nature.
- These are used mainly by topical route and not systemically due to toxicity.
- All are produced by bacteria.
- Clinically useful polypeptides are: Polymyxin B, Colistin and Bacitracin.
- Some properties of these drugs are enlisted in Table 2.9.

TABLE 2.8: Some important miscellaneous antibiotics

Drugs	Special features
Spectinomycin	• Bacteriostatic, selectively inhibits protein synthesis in Gram-positive bacteria • It is given by IM route in a dose of 2 g single dose • Used only in drug resistant Gonorrhea
Quinupristin/Dalfopristin	• It is a synergistic combination inhibiting bacterial protein synthesis • It is bactericidal against Gram-positive organism such as MRSA and VRE • Used in serious nosocomial pneumonia • It is given by IV route only
Mupirocin	• It is a fermentation product of *Pseudomonas fluorescens* • It is used only as topical antibiotic in the form of 2% ointment in furunculosis, folliculitis, impetigo, infected insect bites and small wounds • Also used for eradication of *S. aureus* nasal carriage • It is bactericidal in higher concentrations
Fusidic acid	• It is used only as topical antibiotic in the form of 2% ointment in boils, folliculitis, sycosis barbae and other cutaneous infections • It is a narrow spectrum steroidal antibiotic, bactericidal and acts by inhibiting bacterial protein synthesis

MRSA, methicillin resistant staphylococcus aureus; VRE, vancomycin resistant enterococci

TABLE 2.9: Properties of polypeptide antibiotics

Properties of drugs	Polymyxin B and Colistin	Bacitracin
Source	*Bacillus polymyxa* and *B. colistinus*	Bacillus subtilis
Activity	Bactericidal against Gram-negative bacteria only	Bactericidal against Gram-positive organisms
Mode of action	Detergent-like action on the cell membrane	Inhibits cell wall synthesis
Route	Mainly topical, sometimes orally also	Topical only
Indications	• *Topically* used in combination with other antimicrobials for skin infections, burns, otitis externa, conjunctivitis, corneal ulcer • *Orally* used in Gram-negative bacillary infections	Used in infected wounds, ulcers, eye infections generally in combination with neomycin, polymyxin, etc.

Preparation and dose	• Polymyxin B: (1 mg = 10,000 U)
	  ▪ Neosporin powder: 5000 U with neomycin sulf. 3400 U and bacitracin 400 U/g
	  ▪ Neosporin eye drops: 5000 U with neomycin sulf. 1700 U and gramicidin 0.25 mg per mL
	  ▪ Neosporin-H ear drops: 10,000 U with neomycin sulf. 3400 U and hydrocortisone 10 mg/mL
	  ▪ Colistin sulfate: 25–100 mg TDS oral, 12.5 mg/5 mL and 25 mg/5 mL dry syrup
		NEBASUL: Bacitracin 250 U + neomycin 5 mg + sulfacetamide
		60 mg/g powder, skin ointment, eye ointment; in neosporin 400 U/g powder (1 U = 26 µg)

Adverse effects	No systemic side effects are seen as absorption does not occur from topical site	No systemic side effects are seen as absorption does not occur from topical site

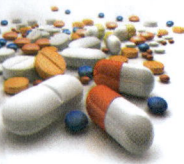

TETRACYCLINES

- Tetracyclines (*Tetra = four, cycline = rings*) are the antibiotics having a nucleus of four cyclic rings.
- The main tetracyclines in use are: Tetracycline, doxycycline, oxytetracycline, minocycline, demeclocycline and tigecycline (*Glycylcycline*).
- These were named as *broad spectrum antibiotics*, as tetracyclines were active against a wide range of microorganisms except fungi and viruses.

Mechanism of Action

- All are primarily bacteriostatic in nature.
- All have common mode of action and act by interfering with the protein synthesis by binding to the 30S ribosomes in the susceptible organism (Fig. 2.2).
- Their selective action in the organism is due to higher uptake by bacterial cells than by human cells.

Antimicrobial Spectrum

- Many Gram-positive and Gram-negative cocci were originally sensitive but now have become resistant to these drugs. These are still active against many Gram-positive and Gram-negative bacilli.
- *Spirochetes* (*T. pallidum*), all *rickettsiae* (typhus, etc.) and *Chlamydia* are highly sensitive. *Mycoplasma*, *Actinomyces*, Protozoa (*Entamoeba histolytica)* and *Plasmodia* are inhibited at higher concentration only.

Precautions

- Preparations should never be used beyond their expiry date (**A reversible Fanconi syndrome**—*like condition is produced by outdated tetracyclines. This is caused by degraded products—epitetracycline, anhydrotetracycline and epianhydrotetracycline, which damage proximal tubules*).
- Tetracyclines are contraindicated in pregnancy, lactation and children.
- They should be avoided in patients with renal or hepatic insufficiency.
- Injectable tetracyclines should never be mixed with penicillin as inactivation occurs.

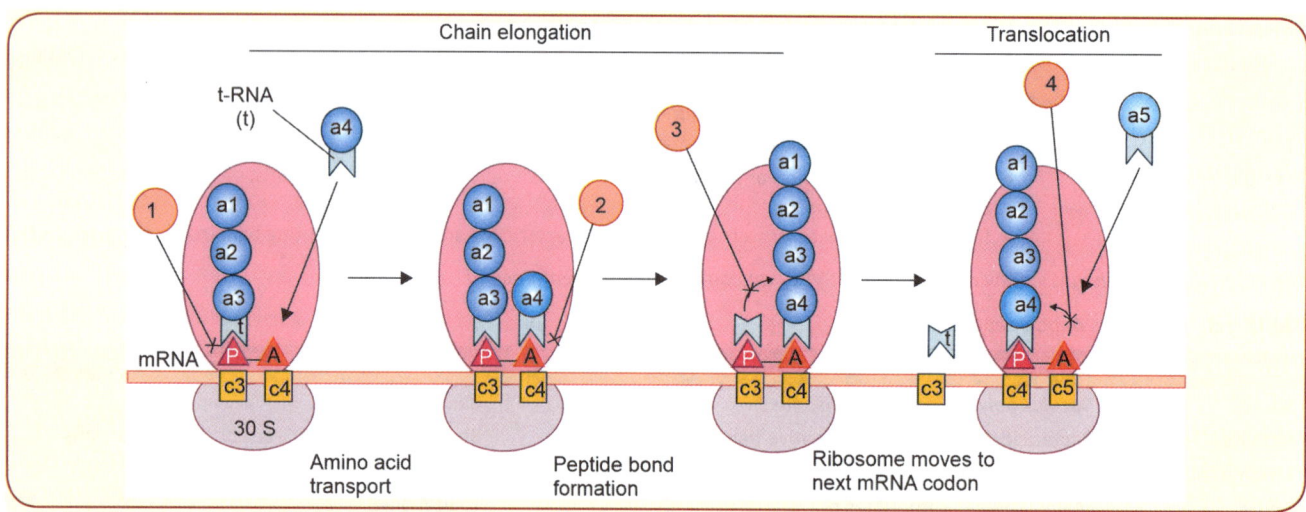

FIG. 2.2: Bacterial protein synthesis and the site of action of antibiotics

The messenger RNA (mRNA) attaches to the 30S ribosome. The initiation complex of mRNA starts protein synthesis and polysome formation. The nascent peptide chain is attached to the peptidyl (P) site of the 50S ribosome. The next amino acid (a) is transported to the acceptor (A) site of the ribosome by its specific tRNA which is complementary to the base sequence of the next mRNA codon (C). The nascent peptide chain is transferred to the newly attached amino acid by peptide bond formation. The elongated peptide chain is shifted back from 'A' to 'P' site and the ribosome moves along the mRNA to expose the next codon for amino acid attachment. Finally, the process is terminated by the termination complex and the protein is released.

Aminoglycosides bind to several sites at 30S and 50S subunits as well as to their interface—freeze initiation, interfere with polysome formation and cause misreading of mRNA code.

- Tetracyclines bind to 30S ribosome and inhibit aminoacyl tRNA attachment to the 'A' site.
- Chloramphenicol binds to 50S subunit—interferes with peptide bond formation and transfer of peptide chain from 'P' site.
- Erythromycin and clindamycin also bind to 50S ribosome and hinder translocation of the elongated peptide chain back from 'A' site to 'P' site and the ribosome does not move along the mRNA to expose the next codon. Peptide synthesis may be prematurely terminated.

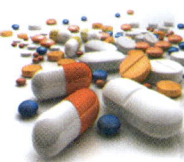

- Tetracycline should not be given with milk, iron preparations and antacid as chelation with calcium and other metals takes place leading to formation of unabsorbable complexes.

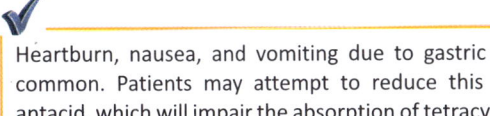

Heartburn, nausea, and vomiting due to gastric irritation are common. Patients may attempt to reduce this with milk or antacid, which will impair the absorption of tetracyclines. Hence, patients are especially advised to take this drug with plenty of water.

- Staining of teeth occurs in patients on tetracycline therapy.

Tetracyclines, due to their chelating property with calcium phosphate, selectively enter the teeth and growing bone of the fetus and children. This causes hypoplasia of dental enamel with pitting, cusp malformation, yellow/brown pigmentation and increased susceptibility to caries. The discoloration of permanent incisors and canines can be prevented by avoiding these drugs from the last two months of pregnancy to the age of four years and other teeth for the age of eight years. Even the short courses of these drugs can be damaging if given after the 14th week of pregnancy and in the first few months of life. Prolonged tetracycline therapy can also stain teeth at all ages.

Properties of various tetracyclines are given in Table 2.10.

Common Indications of Tetracyclines

These are used less commonly these days, due to availability of better, more efficacious and safer antimicrobial agents.
Tetracyclines are used as drugs of first choice in:

- **Rickettsial infections:** Typhus, rocky mountain spotted fever, Q fever, etc., respond dramatically. Chloramphenicol is an alternative.
- **Venereal diseases:**
  - Chlamydial non-specific urethritis/endocervicitis: 7 day doxycycline treatment is as effective as azithromycin single dose.
  - Lymphogranuloma venereum: 2–3 weeks course is required to resolve the infection.
  - Granuloma inguinale: 3 weeks treatment is required.
- **Cholera:** They reduce stool volume and limit the duration of diarrhea.
- **Atypical pneumonia:** Duration of illness is reduced.
- **Brucellosis:** Tetracyclines are highly efficacious; dose given is doxycycline 200 mg/day + Rifampicin 600 mg/day for 6 weeks.

Tetracyclines are used as drugs of second choice in:
- Tetanus, anthrax, actinomycosis and *Listeria* infections. (first choice is β-lactam antibiotics).
- Gonorrhea, especially for penicillin resistant non-PPNG (first choice is ceftriaxone, amoxicillin or azithromycin).
- Syphilis and chancroid (first choice is ceftriaxone, or azithromycin).
- Pneumonia due to *Chlamydia pneumoniae* (first choice is azithromycin).
- Leptospirosis 100 mg BD for 7 days is curative treatment (first choice is Penicillin).

Other Uses

- Acne vulgaris: Prolonged therapy with low doses may be used in severe cases (since *Propionibacterium acnes*

TABLE 2.10: Properties of various tetracyclines

Properties of drugs	Tetracycline and Oxytetracycline	Demeclocycline	Doxycycline & Minocycline
Source	Oxy T: *S. rimosus* T: semisynthetic (mutant)	S. aureofaciens	Doxy: semisynthetic Mino: semisynthetic
Potency	Low	Intermediate	High (Doxy < Mino)
Plasma protein binding	Oxy T: Low T: Moderate	High	High
Intestinal absorption	60–80%	60–80%	95–100% no interference by food
Plasma t½	6–10 hours	16–18 hours	18–24 hours
Dosage	250–500 mg QID or TDS	300 mg BD	200 mg initially, then 100–200 mg OD
Side effects	• Marked alteration of intestinal flora • Marked incidence of diarrhea • Low phototoxicity • Tetracycline causes discoloration of tooth if given in mid pregnancy	• Moderate alteration of intestinal flora • Moderate incidence of diarrhea • Highest phototoxicity • May cause diabetes insipidus by antagonising antidiuretic hormone (ADH) action	• Least alteration of intestinal flora • Least incidence of diarrhea • High phototoxicity • Minocycline is vastibulotoxic

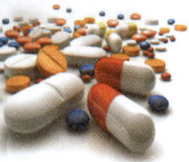

is sensitive to tetracyclines), but simpler treatments are preferred in most cases.

- Traveller's diarrhea.
- Protozoal infections such as chronic intestinal amoebiasis.
- Chloroquine resistant *P. falciparum* malaria (as adjuvant to artesunate or quinine).
- Urinary tract infections (UTIs) and pneumonia (if the causative organism is found sensitive).

TIGECYCLINE

- Tigecycline is the first of the glycylcyclines and is structurally and functionally similar to minocycline.
- No cross-resistance with other tetracyclines exists as tigecycline is unaffected by the two commonest tetracycline resistance mechanisms viz., ribosomal alteration and efflux pump.
- Tigecycline has useful bacteriostatic activity against a wide range of pathogens including streptococci and staphylococci (MRSA and VRE) and anaerobes.
- It is poorly absorbed from the oral route and is given by slow IV infusion only.
- Its elimination t½ is 37–67 hours.
- It is given in a dose of 100 mg loading dose, followed by 50 mg 12 hourly by IV infusion over 30–60 minutes, for 5–14 days.
- Tigecycline is indicated in:
  - Treatment of serious and hospital-acquired pneumonia.
  - Complicated skin and skin structure infections (except diabetic foot).
  - Complicated intra-abdominal infections.

It not suitable for UTIs as low concentration is achieved in urine.

- The most common side effects are epigastric distress, nausea, vomiting and superinfections.
- It should not be given in pregnancy and children.

CHLORAMPHENICOL

Chloramphenicol was initially obtained from *Streptomyces venezuelae* in 1947. The commercial product available is all synthetic and is intensely bitter in taste. It is used rarely these days due to its fatal side effect (bone marrow suppression).

Mechanism of Action

Chloramphenicol is primarily bacteriostatic and acts by inhibiting the bacterial protein synthesis by interfering with 'transfer' of the elongation of peptide chains. At high doses, it acts as bactericidal. It is effective against *S. typhi, H. influenzae* and *N. meningitidis.*

Pharmacokinetics

Chloramphenicol is rapidly and completely absorbed after oral ingestion. It freely penetrates serous cavities and crosses placental and blood-brain barrier. It is secreted in bile and milk. Plasma t½ is 3–5 hours. It is metabolized in liver and excreted mainly in urine.

Dose: It is given orally as follows:

- Adults: 250–500 mg 6 hourly (max. 100 mg/kg/day),
- Children: 25–50 mg/kg/day 6 hourly.

Adverse Effects

- **Bone marrow depression:** It causes aplastic anemia, leucopenia, agranulocytosis, thrombocytopenia or pancytopenia.
- **Hypersensitivity reactions:** It causes rashes and drug fever. Atrophic glossitis and angioedema are infrequent.
- **GIT effects:** Abdominal discomforts such as nausea, vomiting and diarrhea.
- **Superinfections:** On prolonged use, it causes superinfections (due to bone marrow supression and cidal effects on commensals).

Gray (Grey) Baby Syndrome

It occurs when neonates (especially premature) are exposed to high doses (~100 mg/kg). The baby stops feeding, vomits, becomes hypotonic, hypothermic, abdomen distends, respiration becomes irregular leading to cyanosis. Due to these ill effects, baby becomes ashen gray in color. If not treated timely, cardiovascular collapse and death can occur. It occurs due to inability of the newborn liver to metabolize and excrete chloramphenicol. *At higher doses, a similar "Gray syndrome" has been reported in adults also.*

Indications

Clinical use of chloramphenicol for systemic infections is now highly restricted due to fear of fatal toxicity (bone marrow suppression) and availability of safer alternatives. Some indications are as follows:

- **Pyogenic meningitis:** Chloramphenicol may be used as a second line drug for *H. influenzae* and meningococcal meningitis, especially in young children and cephalosporin allergic patients due to its better penetration into cerebrospinal fluid (CSF). Third generation cephalosporins (ceftriaxone) are presently the first line drugs for empirical therapy of bacterial meningitis.
- **Eye and ear infections:** Chloramphenicol attains high concentration in ocular fluid when given systemically. It is the preferred drug for endophthalmitis caused by sensitive bacteria. Eye aplicaps and eye/ear drops are available for topical use.

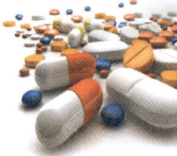

- **Enteric fever:** Earlier, chloramphenicol was the drug of choice for typhoid fever. Now, it has become resistant due to rampant and irrational use. The newer drugs like flouroquinolones and cephalosporins score over this because of their high effectiveness and BD dose compliance. These days, *S. typhi* has again found to be susceptible to chloramphenicol.

SULFONAMIDES

Sulfonamides were the first AMAs effective against pyogenic bacterial infections. It was used in the form of a dye (Prontosil Red) to treat streptococcal and staphylococcal infections. By 1937, it became clear that prontosil was broken down in the body to release sulfanilamide, which was found to be the active antibacterial agent.

CLASSIFICATION

The sulfonamides have been divided into following subtypes:

- **Systemically acting agents**
  - Short acting sulfadiazine (4–8 hours)
  - Intermediate acting sulfamethoxazole (8–12 hours)
  - Long acting Sulfadoxine, sulfamethopyrazine (~7 days)
- **Local acting agents**
  - Sulfacetamide sod., Mafenide, silver sulfadiazine.
- **Both systemic and local acting agents**
  - Sulfasalazine

MECHANISM OF ACTION

- Folic acid is essential for the synthesis of nucleic acid in bacteria and is required for the growth and multiplication of bacteria.
- Many bacteria synthesize their own folic acid from p-aminobenzoic acid (PABA) with the help of an enzyme called *folate synthase.*
- Sulfonamides are structurally similar to PABA and inhibit folic acid formation by inhibiting bacterial *folate synthase.*
- Human cells also require folic acid , but are unaffected by sulfonamides as they utilize folic acid supplied in diet.

PHARMACOKINETICS

- When given orally, these are rapidly and nearly completely absorbed.
- Sulfonamides are widely distributed in all body tissues and cross placental barrier.

- These are metabolized in liver and excreted in urine. The metabolism occurs by acetylation and the acetylated derivative is generally less soluble in acidic urine than the parent drug. It may precipitate and cause crystalluria.

COMMON ADVERSE EFFECTS OF SULFONAMIDES

The common side effects are:

- Anorexia, nausea, vomiting and epigastric pain.
- Crystalluria is dose related, but can be prevented by taking plenty of fluids and by alkalinizing the urine.
- Hypersensitivity reactions such as rashes, urticaria occur in 2–5% patients. Stevens-Johnson syndrome and exfoliative dermatitis are serious reactions reported with the long-acting agents.
- Photosensitivity reactions can be prevented by advising patients to avoid sun exposure.
- Hemolysis can occur in G6PD deficient individuals who are given high doses.
- Kernicterus may be precipitated in the newborn, especially in prematures, whose blood-brain barrier is more permeable by the displacement of bilirubin from plasma protein binding.

COMMON USES OF SULFONAMIDES

Systemic Uses

- Sulfamethoxazole is used in combination with trimethoprim (as cotrimoxazole) in many bacterial infections such as chronic urinary tract infection, streptococcal pharyngitis and gum infection (based upon culture sensitivity).
- Cotrimoxazole is the drug of choice in *Pneumocystis jiroveci* pneumonia in AIDS patients for prophylactic as well as therapeutic purpose.
- Along with pyrimethamine, certain sulfonamides are used for chloroquinine resistant malaria cases.
- Other uses of sulfonamides are in the treatment of nocardiosis, toxoplasmosis, ulcerative colitis and rhematoid arthritis (sulfasalazine).

Topical Uses

- Ocular sulfacetamide sod. (10–30%) is used in trachoma/inclusion conjunctivitis.
- Topical silver sulfadiazine is used for preventing infection on burn surfaces. It releases silver ions which are toxic to microorganisms. It is not effective in the presence of pus.
- Mefenide is active in the presence of pus and against *Pseudomonas, clostridia* alsom which are not inhibited by typical sulfonamides.

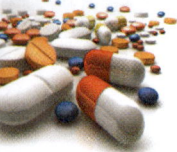

COTRIMOXAZOLE

- The fixed dose combination of sulfamethoxazole (sulfonamide) and trimethoprim (in a ratio of 5:1) is called *cotrimoxazole* and is the WHO approved combination.
- Both sulfonamide and trimethoprim are bacteriostatic, but the combination becomes cidal against many organisms.
- The combination prevents chances of resistance development.
- It is effective against both Gram-positive and Gram-negative bacteria such as—*S. typhi, Serratia, Klebsiella, Enterobacter, Yersinia enterocolitica, P. jiroveci* and many sulfonamide - resistant strains of *S. aureus, S. pyogenes, Shigella*, enteropathogenic *E. coli, H. influenzae*, gonococci and meningococci.

Mechanism of Action

It produces sequential blockade in bacterial folate production mechanism as shown below:

Sulfamethoxazole (sulfonamide) and trimethoprim act synergistically in two successive steps in the same metabolic pathway in folic acid synthesis. Sulfonamide inhibits folate synthase and trimethoprim inhibits dihydrofolate reductase and produces supra-additive effect (Fig. 2.3).

Pharmacokinetics

Cotrimoxazole is given orally and is rapidly and nearly completely absorbed. It is widely distributed in all body tissues and crosses placental barrier. It is metabolized in liver and excreted in urine.

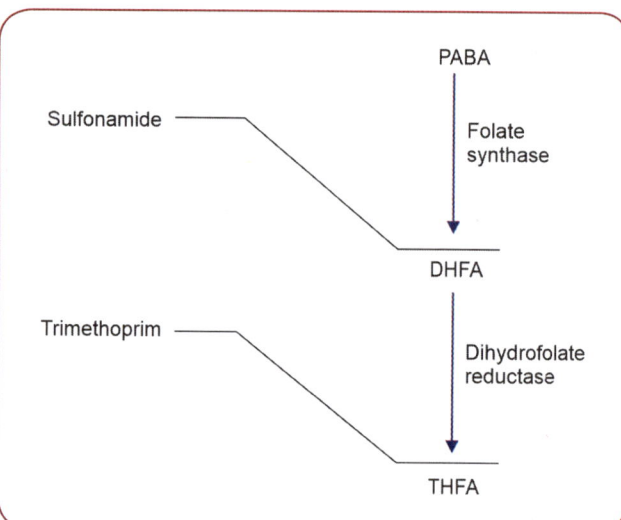

FIG. 2.3: Mechanism of action of cotrimoxazole

(PABA, Para aminobenzoic acid; DHFA, Dihydrofolic acid; THFA, Tetrahydrofolic acid)

Dose

Trimethoprim + Sulfamethoxazole

- 80 mg + 400 mg tab: 2 BD for 2 days then 1 BD for 5–7 days.
- 160 mg + 800 mg tab: Double strength (DS); 1 BD for 5–7 days.
- 20 mg + 100 mg pediatric tab. For 5–7 days.
- 40 mg + 200 mg per 5 mL suspension for 5–7 days.

Adverse Effects

The common side effects are:

- Anorexia, nausea, vomiting, epigastric pain, stomatitis and headache.
- Hypersensitivity reactions such as rashes, urticaria occur in 2–5% patients. Stevens-Johnson syndrome and exfoliative dermatitis are serious reactions.
- Photosensitivity reactions can be prevented by advising patients to avoid sun exposure.
- Hemolysis can occur in G6PD deficient individuals with high doses.
- Cotrimoxazole should not be given during pregnancy. Trimethoprim being an antifolate, there are chances of teratogenicity. Neonatal hemolysis and methemoglobinemia can occur.

COTRIMAZINE

- Cotrimazine is a combination of trimethoprim with sulfadiazine.
- Its usefulness is similar to that of cotrimoxazole.
- *Trimethoprim +Sulfadiazine (*90 mg + 410 mg). It is given in a dose of 2 tab BD for 2 days, then 1 BD.

Indications

- Urinary tract infections especially for chronic or recurrent cases or in prostatitis, because trimethoprim is concentrated in prostate
- Respiratory tract infections; both upper and lower respiratory tract infections
- Bacterial diarrheas and dysentery
- Chancroids
- *P. jiroveci* infections

P. jiroveci causes severe pneumonia in neutropenic and AIDS patients. Cotrimoxazole has prophylactic as well as therapeutic value, but higher doses are needed. One double strength (DS) tablet 4–6 times/day for 2–3 weeks is curative.

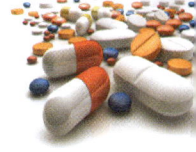

As better drugs with wide spectrum of activity and lesser side effects are available, the use of cotrimoxazole has decreased in the treatment of systemic infections.

Drug Interactions

↪ Sulfonamides increase the blood levels of warfarin, phenytoin, tolbutamide, sulfonylurea, methotrexate, etc., by inhibiting their hepatic metabolism and displacing them from their protein binding sites. The toxicity of these drugs can occur if given together.

Nursing Implications

↪ **Sulfonamides**
  ☞ Patients should be advised to take plenty of water during the course of these drugs to prevent crystalluria.
  ☞ These drugs should be avoided during pregnancy.
  ☞ The renal functions should be regularly monitored during co-trimoxazole therapy.
  ☞ Patients should be advised to avoid direct sun exposure.
  ☞ Patients should be regularly enquired about any side effects.
  ☞ Nurse should keep a vigil on the signs and symptoms of Stevens-Johnson syndrome.

QUINOLONES

- Quinolones are synthetic antimicrobials having a quinolone structure.
- These are active against most of the Gram-negative bacteria.
- The newer fluorinated quinolones also inhibit the Gram-positive bacteria.
- In 1960s, the first member of this group, *Nalidixic acid*, was introduced.
- The use of Nalidixic acid was limited to urinary and GIT infections. Therefore, resistance developed to this molecule. This problem was overcome in 1980s by development of fluoroquinolones.
- Fluoroquinolones have:
  ▪ High potency
  ▪ Expanded antimicrobial spectrum
  ▪ Better tissue penetration
  ▪ Good tolerability profile
  ▪ Very slow resistance development

Nalidixic Acid

- It was the first member in quinolones.
- It is active against Gram-negative bacteria.
- It acts by inhibiting bacterial DNA gyrase.

- It is bactericidal in nature.
- It is given orally.
- It attains high concentration (20–50 times that in plasma) in urine. Hence, most useful in UTIs. It is also called as *urinary antiseptic*.
- It attains good concentration in gut, lumen; hence useful in diarrhea caused by coliforms.
- Neurological toxicity presents as headache, drowsiness and vertigo. It is most commonly seen in children.
- It is contraindicated in infants and G6PD deficient patients.
- It is given in a dose of 0.5–1 g TDS or QID.

Drug Interactions

↪ Antacids decrease the absorption of fluroquinolones.
↪ Ciprofloxacin inhibits the metabolism of caffeine, theophylline and warfarin and lead to serious toxicity. Hence, the concurrent use should be avoided.
↪ Use of NSAIDs with fluroquinolones should be avoided as NSAIDs may potentiate CNS toxicity.
↪ Fluroquinolones should be used cautiously with antiarrhythmic drugs as they prolong the QT interval.

Nursing Implications

↪ **Quinolones**
  ☞ Patient should be advised to avoid direct sun exposure.
  ☞ Patient should be advised to take plenty of water during the course.
  ☞ Patient should be advised take medicine in empty stomach or with little meals for better absorption.
  ☞ Patients should be regularly enquired about any side effects.

FLUOROQUINOLONES

- Fluoroquinolones are quinolone antimicrobials having one or more fluorine substitutions at position 6 and introduction of piperazine substitution at position 7 in their structure.
- The first generation fluoroquinolones have one fluoro substitution and were developed in 1980s.
- The second generation fluoroquinolones have additional fluoro substitution, which extended the antimicrobial activity and were developed in 1990s.

Mechanism of Action

- The fluoroquinolones inhibit the enzyme DNA gyrase in Gram-negative microorganism and topoisomerase IV in Gram-positive microorganisms (*DNA gyrase and topoisomerase IV have role in formation of new bacterial*

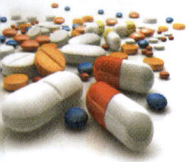

DNA by transcription in Gram-negative and Gram-positive bacteria respectively).

- The damaged DNA, thus produced is digested by the exonucleases. This leads to the bactericidal effect of fluoroquinolones.
- The mammalian cells possess an enzyme topoisomerase II in place of DNA gyrase or topoisomerase IV The toxicity of fluoroquinolones is very low as this topoisomerase II has very low affinity for fluoroquinolones.
- The resistance to fluoroquinolones develops when the bacteria produce a DNA gyrase or topoisomerase IV which have reduced affinity for fluoroquinolones, or the bacteria produce efflux pumps across bacterial membrane which shunt out the fluoroquinolones from the bacterial cell.

Classification of Fluoroquinolones

Fluoroquinolones have been divided into two generations. The first generation fluoroquinolones were developed in 1980s and have one fluoro substitution in the quinolones and the second generation fluoroquinolones were developed in 1990s and have additional fluoro substitution, which extended the antimicrobial spectrum as well as the metabolic stability (Table 2.11).

- **First generation Fluoroquinolones**: Norfloxacin, ofloxacin, ciprofloxacin, pefloxacin
- **Second generation Fluoroquinolones:** Levofloxacin, moxiflox-acin, lomefloxacin, gemifloxacin, sparfloxacin, prulifloxacin etc.

TABLE 2.11: Classification of fluoroquinolones

First Generation fluoroquinolones				
Drug	**t½ (Hr)**	**Route**	**Dose**	**Special features**
Ciprofloxacin	3–5	Oral, IV, topical	250–750 mg BD (oral) 100–200 mg BD (IV) 0.3% eye drops	• Most potent • Active against wide range of Gram-positive and Gram-negative bacteria • Bacteroides, clostridia and anaerobic cocci are resistant • First choice drug in Typhoid fever
Norfloxacin	4–6	Oral	400 mg BD	• Less potent than Ciprofloxacin • Attains good concentration in urine. Hence, useful in UTIs • Does not disturb anaerobic flora of the gut, hence useful in bacterial diarrhea
Ofloxacin	5–8	Oral, IV, topical	200–400 mg BD (oral) 200 mg BD (IV) 0.3% eye drops	• Food does not interfere in its absorption • It also inhibits *M. tuberculosis* and *M. leprae*, hence useful in drug resistant tuberculosis and leprosy
Pefloxacin	8–14	Oral or IV	400 mg BD (oral, IV)	• It is having 100% oral absorption • It attains good concentration in CSF, hence preferred for meningeal infections • Good alternative to ciprofloxacin in typhoid fever
Second Generation Fluoroquinolones				
Levofloxacin	8	Oral, IV, topical	500 mg OD (oral, IV) 0.5% eye drops	• It is a levo-isomer of ofloxacin • Good activity against Gram-positive, Gram-negative and anaerobes • Orally 100% bioavailable, hence oral and IV doses are equal
Lomefloxacin	8	Oral, topical	400 mg OD 0.3% eye drops	• Equal in activity to ciprofloxacin • Persists in tissues for a longer time • Prolongation of Q-T interval and phototoxicity are major side effects • Banned in USA but available in India
Sparfloxacin	16–30	Oral, topical	200–400 mg OD 0.3% eye drops	• Has good activity against Gram-positive, bacteroides, anaerobes and mycobacteria • Prolongation of Q-T interval and phototoxicity are major side effects • Banned in USA and India

Contd...

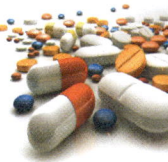

Drug	t½ (Hr)	Route	Dose	Special features
Moxifloxacin	10–15	Oral, IV, topical	400 mg OD (oral, IV) 0.5% eye drops	• Most potent fluoroquinolones against *M. tuberculosis* • Efficacy comparable to β-lactam antibiotics • Not good for UTIs • Can prolong Q-T interval but phototoxicity is rare
Gemifloxacin	7	Oral	320 mg OD	• Active against both Gram-positive and Gram-negative bacteria • Unchanged drug and its metabolites are excreted in urine, hence dose needs to be reduced in renal compromised patients • Prolongation of Q-T interval is major side effect
Prulifloxacin	10–12	Oral	600 mg OD	• It is prodrug of Ulifloxacin • Ulifloxacin attains good concentration in urine, hence useful in uncomplicated and complicated UTIs • Does not prolong Q-T interval
Gatifloxacin	7–14	Oral, topical	400 mg OD 0.5% eye drops	• It was useful in Gram-positive cocci (respiratory and ENT) infections • It has been banned in India since March 2011, due to prolongation of Q-T interval, arrhythmias, phototoxicity and unpredictable hypoglycemia

Pharmacokinetics

- These are given both by oral and intravenous route.
- These have good absorption, when given empty stomach and food delays the absorption.
- These have good tissue penetrability and attain good concentration in lungs, sputum, muscles, prostate and phagocytes.
- These are excreted in urine by glomerular filtration as well as tubular secretion.
- Urinary and biliary concentrations are 10–50 fold higher than plasma.

Common Features of Fluoroquinolones

- All fluoroquinolones are orally efficacious, tolerable, and bactericidal in nature.
- They have long post-antibiotic effect on Enterobacteriaceae, *Pseudomonas* and *Staphylococcus*.
- They are active against many β-lactam and aminoglycoside resistant bacteria.
- The intestinal commensals (streptococci and anaerobes) are not killed, hence diarrhea is rarely seen.
- Less active at acidic pH.

Common Adverse Effects of Fluoroquinolones

- **Gastrointestinal:** Nausea, vomiting, bad taste and anorexia.
- **CNS:** Headache, anxiety, insomnia, restlessness and impairment of concentration.
- **Skin:** Rash, pruritus, photosensitivity, urticaria, swelling of lips, etc.
- **Tendinitis and tendon rupture:** Risk of tendon damage is higher in patients above 60 years of age and in those receiving corticosteroids.
- Contraindicated in **pregnancy**.
- They should be used with caution in children as a few cases of joint pain and swelling have been reported and a risk of cartilage damage is suspected.

Indications

- **Bacterial gastroenteritis:** It is most commonly used drug for empirical therapy of diarrhea these days. Its use should be restricted for severe cases due to *EPEC, Shigella, Salmonella* and *C. jejuni* infections only.
- **Typhoid:** Ciprofloxacin (750 mg BD orally for 10 days or 200 mg IV 12 hourly) is recommended. Ciprofloxacin gives early relief from the symptoms and prevents the carrier state due to cidal action. It can also be used to treat typhoid carriers (750 mg BD for 4–8 weeks) as it attains good concentration in intestinal and biliary mucosa. Cephalosporins (ceftriaxone, cefotaxime/cefoperazone) are more commonly used these days due to their edge over fluoroquinolones.
- **Urinary tract infections:** In patients with UTIs, prostatitis and with indwelling catheters, high cure rates are achieved.
- **Gonorrhea:** Not used as a first line drug. These are used only if strain is sensitive.
- **Chancroid:** 500 mg BD for 3 days is a second line alternative drug to ceftriaxone/azithromycin.
- **Bone, soft tissue and gynecological infections:** Higher doses (750 mg BD) are required. Used along with clindamycin/metronidazole (to cover anaerobes) for diabetic foot.

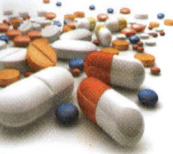

- **Respiratory infections:** Pneumonias and chronic bronchitis.
- **Tuberculosis:** As a second line drug and as a component of combination chemotherapy against multidrug resistant tuberculosis.
- **Gram-negative septicemias and Meningitis:** Parenteral ciprofloxacin may be combined with a third generation cephalosporin or an aminoglycoside.
- **Conjunctivitis:** Topical use only.

ANTIAMOEBIC DRUGS

Amoebiasis is an infectious protozoal disease and has a worldwide distribution. It is endemic in most parts of India and other developing countries. It is caused by Entamoeba histolytica and is acquired through ingestion of contaminated food and water.

The amoebic infection may present as:
- Asymptomatic cyst passers or mild intestinal amoebiasis.
- Acute amoebic dysentery.
- Chronic amoebiasis.
- Systemic amoebiasis in the form of amoebic abscesses in liver, lung, spleen, kidney, and brain.
  Presentation of amoebiasis is shown in Figure 2.4.

The drugs which are used in the treatment of any type of amoebiasis are called as antiamoebic drugs. These drugs are of following types:
- **For both intestinal and extra-intestinal amoebiasis:**
  - Nitroimidazoles: Metronidazole, tinidazole, secnidazole, ornidazole, satranidazole
  - Alkaloids: Emetine, Dehydroemetine
- **For extra-intestinal amoebiasis only:** Chloroquine
- **Luminal amoebicides:** Diloxanide furoate, nitazoxanide quiniodochlor, diiodohydroxyquin (iodoquinol) tetracyclines, paromomycin

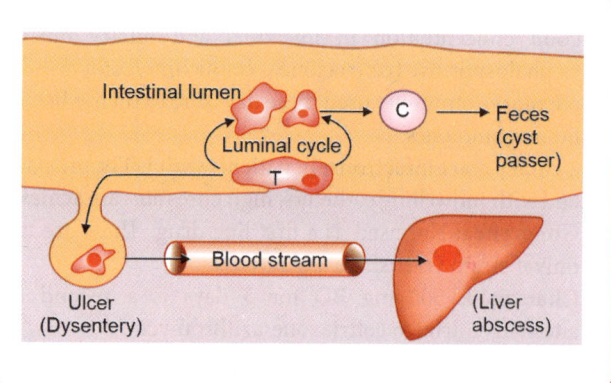

FIG. 2.4: Presentation of amoebiasis

METRONIDAZOLE

Metronidazole has a broad-spectrum cidal activity against amoebae, *Trichomonas* and *Giardia lamblia*. In addition, it is also having a good cidal activity against anaerobic protozoa and many anaerobic (and microaerophilic) bacteria. Metronidazole does not affect aerobic bacteria.

Mechanism of Action

It is selectively toxic to anaerobic and microaerophilic microorganisms. After entering the cell by diffusion, its nitro group is reduced to a *highly reactive nitro radical*. This reduction reaction is mediated by certain redox proteins which are operative only in anaerobic microbes. This *nitro radical* is cytotoxic to the microorganisms.

Pharmacokinetics

It is almost completely absorbed from the small intestines; little unabsorbed drug reaches the colon. It is widely distributed in the body and attains therapeutic concentration in vaginal secretions, semen, saliva and CSF. It is metabolized in liver and excretion occurs via renal route. Plasma t½ is 8 hours.

Adverse Effects

- Anorexia, nausea, metallic taste and abdominal cramps are the most common side effects. Sometimes, the stools become loose.
- Headache, glossitis, dryness of mouth and dizziness are also seen.
- Urticaria, flushing, heat, itching, rashes, and fixed drug eruptions occur in allergic subjects.
- Thrombophlebitis of the injected vein can occur if the solution is not well diluted.
- A disulfiram-like intolerance to alcohol occurs in some patients taking metronidazole.

Indications

Recommended dosage schedules in different indications are given in Table 2.12.

TINIDAZOLE

- Tinidazole is similar and equally efficacious to metronidazole in every respect with slight differences such as:
  - Metabolism is slower; t½ is ~12 hours; duration of action is longer; dosage schedules are simpler. Thus, it is more suited for single dose or once daily therapy.
  - It is better tolerated.
  - The incidence of side effects such as metallic taste and nausea is lower.
  - Recommended dosage schedules in different indications are given in Table 2.13.

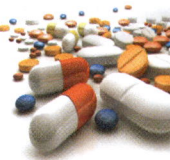

TABLE 2.12: Dose and duration of metronidazole in various indications

Indications	Dose and duration
• **Mild intestinal disease** • **Severe cases of amoebic dysentery or liver abscess** • **For invasive dysentery and liver abscess**	400 mg TDS for 5–7 days. 500 mg IV infusion slowly every 6–8 hours for 7–10 days or till oral therapy can be instituted. 800 mg TDS (children 30–50 mg/kg/day) for 7–10 days
Giardiasis	400 mg TDS for 7 days
Trichomonas vaginitis	400 mg TDS for 7 days or 2.0 g. Single dose
Anaerobic bacterial infections	15 mg/kg infused over 1 hour followed by 7.5 mg/kg every 6 hours till oral therapy can be instituted with 400–800 mg TDS
Pseudomembranous enterocolitis due to *C. difficile*	400–800 mg orally BD–TDS for 10–14 days
***H. pylori* gastritis/peptic ulcer**	400 mg TDS or tinidazole 500 mg BD are combined with amoxicillin/clarithromycin and a proton pump inhibitor in triple drug 2 week regimens
Acute necrotizing ulcerative gingivitis (ANUG)	200–400 mg TDS (15–30 mg/kg/day) is often combined with amoxicillin, tetracycline or erythromycin

TABLE 2.13: Dose and duration of tinidazole in various indications

Indications	Dose and duration
Intestinal amoebiasis	2 g OD for 3 days (children 30–50 mg/kg/day) or 0.6 g BD for 5–10 days
Amoebic liver abscess	2 g daily for 3–6 days
Trichomoniasis and giardiasis	2 g single dose or 0.6 g OD for 7 days
Anaerobic infections:	Prophylactic—2 g single dose before colorectal/biliary surgery. Therapeutic—2 g followed by 0.5 g BD for 5 days
***H. pylori* infection**	500 mg BD for 2 weeks in triple drug combination

SECNIDAZOLE

It is similar and equally efficacious to metronidazole in every respect with slight differences such as:

- Rapid and complete oral absorption.
- Metabolism is slower resulting in a plasma t½ of 17–29 hours.

TABLE 2.14: Dose and duration of senidazole in various indications

Indications	Dose and duration
• **Mild intestinal amoebiasis,** • **Giardiasis** • **Trichomonas vaginitis** • **Non-specific bacterial vaginosis**	2 g single dose (children 30 mg/kg) for 5 days
Acute amoebic dysentery	0.5 g TDS for 5 days

- In intestinal amoebiasis, a single 2 g dose has been found to yield high cure rates.
- Side effect profile is similar to metronidazole.
- Recommended dosage schedules are given in Table 2.14.

ORNIDAZOLE

Ornidazole is similar and equally efficacious to metronidazole in every respect with slight differences such as:

- Rapid and complete oral administration.
- A longer plasma t½ of 12–14 hours as the metabolism is slower.
- Side effect profile is similar to metronidazole.
- Recommended dosage schedules are given in Table 2.15.

SATRANIDAZOLE

Satranidazole is similar and equally efficacious to metronidazole in every respect with slight differences such as:

- Longer t½ (14 hours)
- Better tolerability
- Absence of nausea, vomiting or metallic taste, neurological disulfiram like reactions. Recommended dosage schedules are given in Table 2.16.

TABLE 2.15: Dose and duration of ornidazole in various indications

Indications	Dose and duration
• **Intestinal amoebiasis** • **Giardiasis** • **Trichomonas vaginitis** • **Non-specific bacterial vaginosis**	2 g single dose (children 30 mg/kg) for 5 days
In chronic intestinal amoebiasis and asymptomatic cyst passers	0.5 g twice daily for 5 to 7 days

TABLE 2.16: Dose and duration of satranidazole in various indications

Indications	Dose and duration
• **Amoebiasis**	300 mg BD for 3–5 days
• **Giardiasis and trichomoniasis**	600 mg single dose

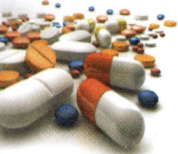

DILOXANIDE FUROATE

- Diloxanide furoate is a highly effective luminal amoebicide.
- It kills trophozoites, which are responsible for production of cysts.
- It has very little effect in invasive amoebic dysentery.
- It has no antibacterial action.
- This drug is very effective in mild intestinal amoebiasis and in asymptomatic cyst passers.
- The dose is 500 mg TDS for 5–10 days; children 20 mg/kg/day.
- It is used in combination with metronidazole or tinidazole for complete amoebiasis treatment.
- This drug is well tolerated.

NITAZOXANIDE

- Nitazoxanide is a prodrug which on absorption is converted to the active form *Tizoxanide*.
- Its mechanism of action is similar to metronidazole.
- It is also active against metronidazole resistant *Giardia*. **Besides protozoa, it is having good activity against helminthes (*Ascaris, H. nana*) also.**
- It is metabolized in liver and excreted in urine and bile.
- It is useful in giardiasis, amoebic dysentery (*as luminal amoebicide*) and diarrhea caused by *Cryptosporidium parvum* in children and AIDS patients.
- It is given in a dose of 500 mg BD × 3 days (children 7.5 mg/kg).
- The most common side effects are abdominal pain, headache, and vomiting.

QUINIODOCHLOR AND IODOQUINOL

- Both of these drugs had been used very frequently in the past and not used in routine these days.
- These drugs do not have tissue amoebicidal action, but kill the cyst forming amoebic trophozoites in the intestine, i.e., these have luminal amoebicidal action only.
- These are used in chronic intestinal amoebiasis and rated inferior to Diloxanide furoate.
- Both are orally absorbed, metabolized in liver, and excreted in urine.
- Some indications are giardiasis; local treatment of monilial and trichomonas vaginitis, fungal and bacterial skin infections.
- These drugs are economically affordable.

> Prolonged/repeated use of relatively high doses of quiniodochlor caused a neuropathic syndrome called 'subacute myelo-optic neuropathy' (SMON), in Japan in an epidemic form, affecting several thousand people in 1970. These drugs have been banned in Japan and few other countries, but in India, they are prohibited only for pediatric patients, because their use for chronic diarrheas in children has caused blindness.

- These are given in a dose of
  - Quiniodochlor: 250–500 mg TDS; (not to exceed 1.5 g/day for 14 days).
  - Iodoquinol: 650 mg TDS; (not to exceed 2.0 g/day for 14 days).

ANTI-AMOEBIC ANTIBIOTICS

Tetracyclines

- Tetracyclines have indirect anti-amoebic action.
- *Entamoeba* lives in symbiosis with bacterial commensals in gut.
- The tetracyclines kill these commensals and affect the proliferation of *Entamoebae*.
- These are used in combination with nitroimidazole + a luminal amoebicide in the treatment of amoebic dysentery.

Paromomycin

- Paromomycin is active against many protozoa like *Entamoeba, Giardia, Cryptosporidium, Trichomonas, Leishmania* and some tape worms.
- It is an aminoglycoside antibiotic.
- It binds to 30S ribosome and interferes with protein synthesis in protozoa.
- Given orally, it is neither absorbed nor degraded in the intestines, and acts only in the gut lumen.
- It does not have any systemic toxic effects.
- It is eliminated unchanged in the feces.
- Its major indications are:
  - As luminal amoebicide in asymptomatic cyst passers.
  - Chronic amoebic colitis.
  - As an alternative drug for giardiasis, especially during 1st trimester of pregnancy when metronidazole and other drugs are contraindicated.
  - In India and Africa, parenteral (IM) paromomycin is being used in resisting Kala azar.
  - Topically used in trichomonas vaginitis and dermal leishmaniasis.
- It is given in a dose 500 mg (children 10 mg/kg) TDS Orally, for 7 days for amoebiasis/giardiasis/cryptosporidiosis.
- The most common side effects are nausea, vomiting, diarrhea and abdominal cramps.

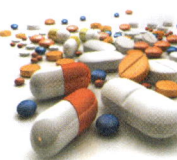

Drug Interactions

- Disulfiram-like reaction occurs with alcohol.
- The enzyme inducer drugs (phenobarbitone and rifampicin) reduce their therapeutic concentration.

Nursing Implications

- **Antiamoebic drugs**
  - ☞ Nurse should advise the patients to take these drugs with meals or immediately after meals to avoid gastric irritation.
  - ☞ Patients should be encouraged to take proper and hygienic meals, as they are malnourished.
  - ☞ Patients should be encouraged to take the full course of treatment.

ANTI-MALARIAL DRUGS

Antimalarial drugs are the drugs which are used for treatment, prophylaxis and prevention of relapses of malaria.

The treatment of malaria is available since 17th century. During those times, the bark of Cinchona tree was used in the crude form. Later in 1820, quinine (active principle) was isolated from this bark.

Since 1920, quinine and other drugs are commercially available in the market.

Malaria

- Malaria is an infectious disease of humans caused by parasitic protozoans (a group of unicellular microorganisms) belonging to the genus Plasmodium.
- Malaria is endemic in most parts of India and other tropical countries.
- As per WHO, malaria causes one death every minute globally and about 40,000 annual deaths in India.
- The disease is transmitted by the bite of an infected female Anopheles mosquito. Four species of protozoa *Plasmodium* cause malaria which are *P. falciparum*, *P. vivax*, *P. ovale*, and *P. malariae*.
- **Plasmodium falciparum** presents with most dangerous type of malaria, which can lead to death.
- **Plasmodium vivax** causes a milder form of the disease, which seldom results in death.
- **Plasmodium malariae** is endemic in many tropical countries and causes very mild signs and symptoms. It can cause more acute disease in travellers to endemic areas.
- **Plasmodium ovale** is rarely seen.

Life cycle of Plasmodium is given in Figs 2.5A and B.

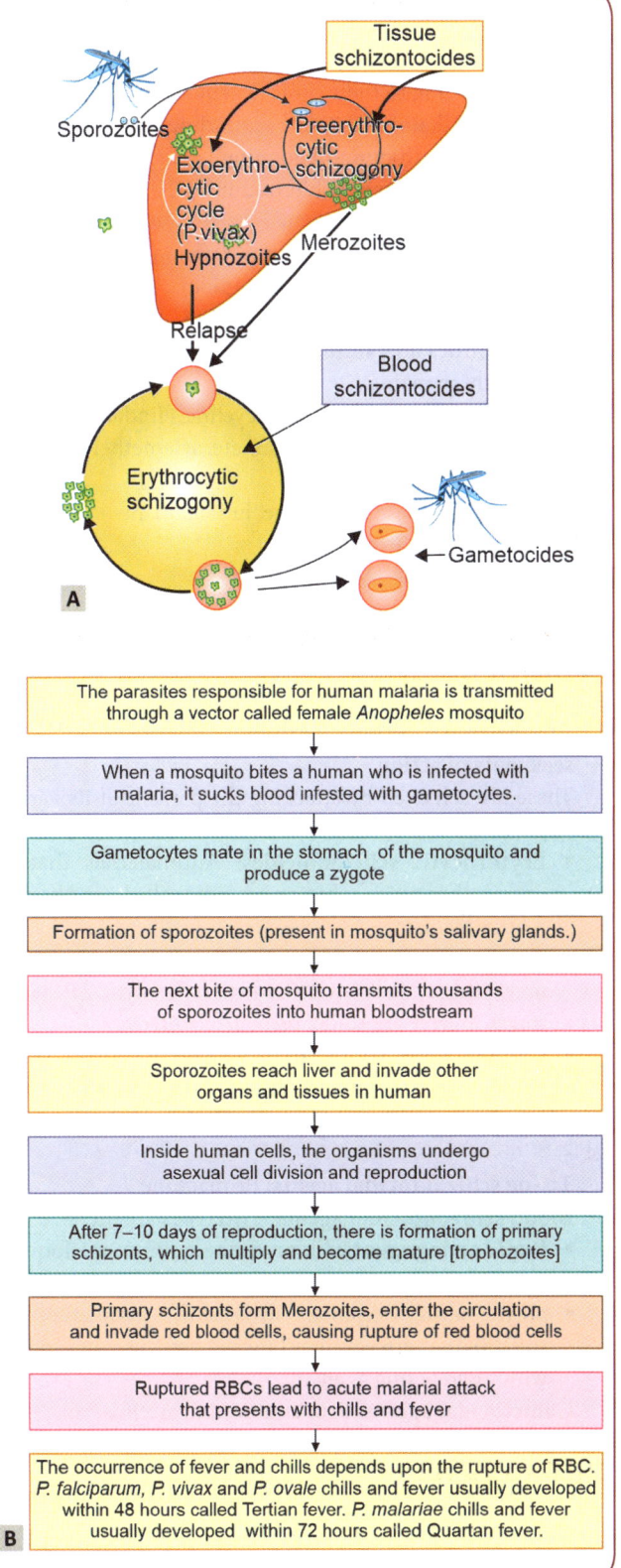

FIGS 2.5A and B: Life cycle of plasmodium

51

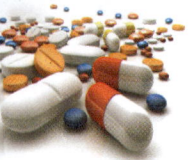

PHARMACOLOGICAL CLASSIFICATION

The various drugs used in the treatment of malaria can be classified according to their clinical structure as follows:

- **Cinchona alkaloid:** Quinine, quinidine.
- **Quinoline-methanol:** Mefloquine.
- **4-Aminoquinolines:** Chloroquine (CQ), amodiaquine (AQ), piperaquine.
- **8-Aminoquinoline:** Primaquine, tafenoquine.
- **Biguanide:** Proguanil (chloroguanide).
- **Diaminopyrimidine:** Pyrimethamine.
- **Sulfonamides and sulfone:** Sulfadoxine, Sulfamethopyrazine.
- **Antibiotics:** Tetracycline, doxycycline, clindamycin.
- **Sesquiterpine lactones:** Artesunate, artemether, arteether, arterolane.
- **Amino alcohols:** Halofantrine, lumefantrine.
- **Naphthyridine:** Pyronaridine.
- **Naphthoquinone:** Atovaquone.

CLINICAL CLASSIFICATION (*BASED UPON THE PARASITIC STAGE*)

- Antimalarial drugs exhibit considerable stage selectivity of action.
- These are achieved by attacking the parasite at its various stages of life cycle in the human host.
  - **Erythrocytic schizontocides:** Antimalarials that act on erythrocytic schizogony are called *erythrocytic schizontocides.*
  - **Tissue schizontocides:** Antimalarials that act on preerythrocytic as well as exoerythrocytic (*P. vivax*) stages in liver are called *tissue schizontocides.*
  - **Gametocides:** Antimalarials which kill gametocytes in blood are called *gametocides.*

Based on the parasitic stage, antimalarial can be classified as:

- **Tissue schizontocidal agents:** Primaquine
- **Blood schizontocidal agents:** Two types are there:
  - **Rapid acting agents:** Chloroquine, quinine, mefloquine, artemisinin derivative.
  - **Slow acting agents:** Proguanil, pyrimethamine, sulfadoxine, doxycycline (always used in combination with rapid acting agents)
- **Gametocidal agents:** Primaquine, and artemisinin

CHLOROQUINE

- Chloroquine acts as erythrocytic schizontocide against all species of plasmodia.
- The parasite disappears from peripheral blood in 1–3 days.
- It controls the clinical attacks of malaria within 1–2 days.

- It has no effect on pre and exo-erythrocytic phase of the parasite.
- It doesn't has any gametocidal activity.
- It is bitter in taste, so patient should be advised 'not to chew the tablet'.
- Chloroquine can be used for the treatment of malaria during pregnancy: No abortifacient or teratogenic effects have been reported.

Mechanism of Action

- Chloroquine gets concentrated in the infected RBCs and then is actively taken up by the susceptible plasmodia.
- *Normally hemoglobin (present in the RBCs) is degraded by parasitic lysosomes to Heme, which is toxic in nature for the parasite. This toxic heme is converted to non-toxic parasite pigment Hemozoin by polymerization process.*
- The Chloroquine binds to the heme and forms chloroquine heme complex.
- This complex inhibits the formation of hemozoin and also damages the *Plasmodium* membrane.
- The P. *falciparum* is resistant to Chloroquine, as the P. *falciparum* infected RBCs have low Chloroquine concentrating ability.

Pharmacokinetics

- It is well absorbed orally.
- 50% of the drug is plasma protein bound, gets concentrated in liver, spleen, kidney, lungs, skin and leukocytes.
- The plasma t½ is 3–10 days, whereas the terminal t½ is 1–2 months [due to tight tissue binding].
- On prolonged use, it gets accumulated selectively in the retina and causes ocular toxicity.
- It is partially metabolized in liver and slowly excreted in urine.

Adverse Effects

- Mild side effects like nausea, vomiting, anorexia, uncontrollable itching, epigastric pain, uneasiness are quite frequent.
- On prolonged use, it may lead to loss of vision and hearing, rashes, mental disturbances and graying of hair.

Indications

- It is the drug of choice for clinical cure of vivax, ovale and malariae malaria.
- P.falciparum is resistant to Chloroquine but it can still be used in the areas where *P. falciparum*:
- Extraintestinal amoebiasis
  - Lepra reaction
  - Rheumatoid arthritis and discoid lupus erythematosus
  - Infectious mononucleosis

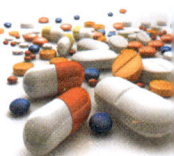

AMODIAQUINE

Amodiaquine is having similar properties to chloroquine except:

- It is fast acting and less bitter in taste.
- It is useful in uncomplicated falciparum malaria.
- In combination with artesunate (amodiaquine-artesunate combination), it is the first line treatment of falciparum malaria.
- Itching is less common with it, other side effects are same as that of chloroquine.
- It is given in a dose of 25–35 mg/kg over 3 days for the treatment of acute attack of malaria.

MEFLOQUINE

- Mefloquine is a fast acting erythrocytic schizontocide, but slower than Chloroquine.
- It is effective against Chloroquine sensitive as well as resistant *Plasmodium*.
- It has good activity against Chloroquine-resistant *P. falciparum*.
- It is bitter in taste, so patient should be advised '*not to chew the tablet*'.
- It can be safely given in pregnancy, but should be avoided in first trimester unless absolutely essential.

Mechanism of Action

- Similar to chloroquine, it accumulates in the infected RBCs (including those with Chloroquine-resistant *P.falciparum.*), binds to heme and this complex damages the cell membrane of parasite.

Pharmacokinetics

- It is given orally and is absorbed very slowly.
- It is highly plasma protein bound and gets concentrated in various organs such as liver, lungs and intestine.
- It is metabolized in liver and excreted in bile.
- It's t½ is long [2–3 weeks] due to its tissue binding and enterohepatic circulation.

Adverse Effects

- Mild side effects are: Nausea, vomiting, anorexia, and epigastric pain.
- Some patients may experience neuropsychiatric reactions (disturbed sense of balance, ataxia, errors in operating machinery, strange dreams, anxiety, hallucinations, rarely convulsions). These reactions subside after 2–3 weeks of discontinuation of treatment.

Indications

- Multidrug resistant *P. falciparum* malaria.
- In combination with artesunate as artemisinin based combination therapy for uncomplicated falciparum malaria, including Chloroquine-resistant and Chloroquine + sulfa-pyrimethamine (S/P) resistant cases.
- For the prophylaxis of malaria among travellers to areas with multidrug resistance; 5 mg/kg (adults 250 mg) per week is started preferably 1–2 weeks before travel. This is done to assess the side effects in the individuals.

QUININE

- Quinine is an erythrocytic schizontocide for all species of plasmodia.
- It is effective against Chloroquine and multidrug-resistant strains of *P. falciparum*.
- It is less effective and more toxic than Chloroquine.

Mechanism of Action

It is same as that of chloroquine.

Pharmacokinetics

- It is given orally and is absorbed rapidly and completely.
- It is 70% plasma protein bound.
- It is metabolized in liver and excreted in urine.
- It's t½ is 10–12 hours.

Adverse Effects

- The adverse effects are generally dose related.
- Mild side effects are: Nausea, vomiting, anorexia, and epigastric pain.
- At higher doses, it causes Cinchonism. Patient experiences nausea, vomiting, headache, tinnitus, vertigo, visual defects and mental confusion. Diarrhea, flushing and marked perspiration may also appear. This syndrome is reversible once the drug is stopped.
- At still higher doses, poisoning occurs in which the patient experiences the symptoms of cinchonism in an exaggerated form. In addition, delirium, fever, tachypnea followed by respiratory depression, pulmonary edema, hypoglycemia, marked weakness and prostration can occur. The patient may die due to hypotension and cardiac arrhythmias if the drug is injected rapidly by intravenous route.
- Quinine occasionally leads to hemolysis, especially in pregnant women and in patients of falciparum malaria, resulting in hemoglobinuria (black water fever) and kidney damage.

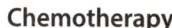

53

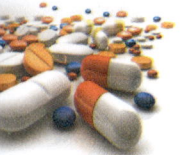

Indications

- Uncomplicated Chloroquine-resistant *P. falciparum* malaria [*drug is given by oral route*].
- Complicated and cerebral malaria [*drug is given by IV route*]
- Nocturnal muscles cramps [*mechanism not clear yet*]. 300 mg of quinine is given at bed time.
- Myotonia congenita.

PROGUANIL (CHLOROGUANIDE)

- It is pre-erythrocytic schizontocide for *P. falciparum* and erythrocytic schizontocide for both *P. falciparum* and *P. vivax*.
- It is a prodrug and the active metabolite is cycloguanil.

Mechanism of Action

It inhibits the plasmodial *dihydrofolate reductase-thymidylate synthase* in parasite, thereby exerting the cidal effect.

Pharmacokinetics

- It is given orally and having slow but complete absorption.
- It is metabolized in liver and excreted in urine.
- It's t½ is 16–20 hours.

Adverse Effects

It is well tolerated with mild abdominal discomfort. Rarely vomiting, stomatitis, hematuria, rashes and transient loss of hair may be seen.

Indications

It is used in prophylaxis and treatment of Chloroquine-resistant *P.falciparum* malaria (*in combination with atovaquone*).

PYRIMETHAMINE

- Pyrimethamine is a slow acting erythrocytic schizontocide for *P. falciparum*.
- It is a directly acting inhibitor of plasmoidal DHFRase.
- It has good but slow oral absorption.
- It is more potent and relatively safer than Proguanil.
- It is excreted slowly in urine.
- It is used in combination with sulfonamide for Chloroquine resistant *P. falciparum*.

PRIMAQUINE

- It is a poor erythrocytic schizontocide but more active against pre-erythrocytic (in liver) phase of *P. falciparum*.

- It differs from all other available antimalarials in having an additional effect on primary as well as secondary hepatic phases of the malarial parasite.
- It is also highly active against gametocytes and hypnozoites.

Mechanism of Action

Exact mechanism of action is not clearly known.

Pharmacokinetics

- It is given orally and has rapid and complete absorption.
- Metabolized in liver and excreted slowly in urine.
- Its t½ is 6–8 hours and excreted in urine within 24 hours.

Adverse Effects

- Mild side effects are: Nausea, vomiting, anorexia and epigastric pain.
- Dose dependent hemolysis, methemoglobinemia, tachypnea and cyanosis can also occur. *This is most commonly seen in glucose-6-phosphate dehydrogenase (G-6-PD) deficient persons. Spot tests are available for detecting G-6-PD deficiency. Passage of dark urine is an indication of hemolysis; primaquine should be promptly stopped if it occurs.*
- It should not be given in pregnancy, because the fetus is deficient in G-6-PD.

Indications

- Primaquine is indicated for radical cure of relapsing malaria caused by *P. ovale* and *P.vivax*. In India, 15 mg/day (children 0.25 mg/kg/day) for 2 weeks is given along with full curative dose of Chloroquine or another blood schizontocide to eliminate the erythrocytic phase.
- Falciparum malaria: A single 45 mg dose of primaquine is given with the curative dose of Chloroquine or artemisinin based combination therapy (ACT) to kill the gametes and cut down transmission to mosquito.

TETRACYCLINE, DOXYCYCLINE AND CLINDAMYCIN

- These antibiotics have slowly acting and weak erythrocytic schizontocidal action against all plasmodial species including Chloroquine, Mefloquine and S/P resistant *P. falciparum*.
- Tetracyclines are never used alone to treat malaria, but only in combination with quinine for the treatment of Chloroquine-resistant falciparum as well as vivax malaria.
- Doxycycline 100 mg/day is used as a 2nd line prophylactic drug for short-term travellers to Chloroquine-resistant *P. falciparum* areas.

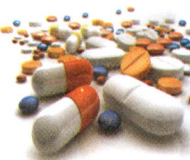

- Clindamycin is another bacteriostatic antibiotic that has slow acting erythrocytic schizontocidal property against all species of plasmodia including multidrug resistant strains of *P. falciparum*. It is always used in combination with quinine or artemisinin for better antimalarial activity.

ARTEMISININ DERIVATIVES

- Artemisinin is the active ingredient of the Chinese traditional medicine 'Quinghaosu' which is obtained from the plant *Artemisia annua*.
- Ms Tu Youyou was awarded half Noble prize in 2015 for the discovery of Artemisinin.
- Chemically, Artemisinin is sesquiterpene lactone endoperoxide.
- Its clinically used derivatives are:
  - Dihydroartemisinin
  - Artesunate
  - Artemether
  - α/β Arteether
  - Arterolane (totally synthetic oral compound)
  - All the above drugs are collectively known as 'Artemisinins'
- These derivatives are better tolerated, safer and highly efficacious.
- They are very potent and rapidly acting anti-malarial drugs.
- They produce high parasitic clearance than any other anti-malarial drug.
- They are effective in erythrocytic stage of all malarial parasites.
- They also have good gametocidal activity but do not affect hepatic forms.
- The dosing schedule of these derivatives is simple.

Mechanism of Action

Exact mechanism is unknown. Probably, the endoperoxide bridge in its molecule interacts with heme and releases a highly reactive free radical which binds to the membrane proteins of the parasite. This results in lipid peroxidation and damage to the endoplasmic reticulum; subsequently lysis of the parasite occurs.

Pharmacokinetics

- **Artesunate** is water-soluble and can be administered by oral, IM or IV routes.
- It is rapidly converted to the active metabolite dihydroartemisinin (DHA).
- **Artemether** is lipid-soluble and is administered by oral or IM but never by IV route. It is also converted to DHA.
- α/β **Arteether** has been developed in India and is available for IM. administration only.
- **Dihydroartemisinin and Arterolane** are available for oral use only.

Adverse Effects

Mild side effects are nausea, vomiting, abdominal pain, itching, drug fever, headache, tinnitus, dizziness, bleeding, and dark urine.

Indications

- Uncomplicated falciparum malaria
- Severe and complicated falciparum malaria

OBJECTIVES IN USE OF ANTIMALARIAL DRUGS

The antimalarial drugs are used with different objectives in mind. These are used both for prophylactic as well as therapeutic purpose.

The various objectives are:

- To prevent clinical attack of malaria (prophylactic).
- To treat clinical attack of malaria (clinical curative).
- To completely eradicate the parasite from the patient's body (radical curative).
- To cut down human-to-mosquito transmission (gametocidal).

Prophylactic Therapy (in India)

- Doxycycline 100 mg daily starting '*day before travelling to endemic area*' and taken '*till 4 weeks after returning from endemic area*' for chloroquine-resistant *P falciparum* (Chloroquine-resistant *P. falciparum* is prevalent in India).
- Mefloquine 250 mg started '*1–2 weeks before and taken weekly till 4 weeks after returning from endemic area*,' has been used for areas where chloroquine-resistant *P. falciparum* is prevalent.

  In India, use of mefloquine for prophylaxis is not allowed among Indian residents, but may be used by foreign travellers.

Clinical Curative Therapy

Treatment of uncomplicated malaria
A. Vivax (also ovale, malariae) malaria
• Chloroquine 600 mg (10 mg/kg) followed by 300 mg (5 mg/kg) after 8 hours and then for next 2 days. (Total 25 mg/kg over 3 days) + primaquine 15 mg (0.25 mg/kg) daily × 14 days   *In occasional case of chloroquine resistance*
• Quinine 600 mg (10 mg/kg) 8 hourly × 7 days + Doxycycline 100 mg daily × 7 days or + Clindamycin 600 mg 12 hourly × 7 days + Primaquine (15 mg (0.25 mg/kg) daily × 14 days)   or   Artemisinin-based combination therapy (see below) + primaquine (as above)

Contd...

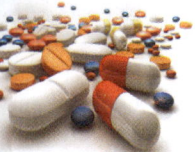

B. Chloroquine-sensitive falciparum malaria[£]

- Chloroquine (as above) + Primaquine 45 mg (0.75 mg/kg) single dose (as gametocidal)

C. Chloroquine-resistant falciparum malaria

- *Artesunate 100 mg BD (4 mg/kg/day) × 3 days + sulfadoxine[#] 1500 mg (25 mg/kg) + pyrimethamine 75 mg (1.25 mg/kg) single dose

or

- Artesunate 100 mg BD (4 mg/kg/day) × 3 days + mefloquine[#] 750 mg (15 mg/kg) on 2nd day and 500 mg (10 mg/kg) on 3rd day.

or

- Artemether 80 mg + lumefantrine 480 mg twice daily × 3 days (child 25–35 kg body weight (BW) ¾ dose; 15–25 kg BW ½ dose; 5–15 kg BW ¼ dose)

or

- Arterolane (as maleate) 150 mg + piperaquine 750 mg once daily × 3 days

or

- Quinine 600 mg (10 mg/kg) 8 hourly × 7 days + Doxycycline 100 mg daily × 7 days or + clindamycin 600 mg 12 hourly × 7 days

*First line artemisinin based combination therapy (ACT) under national vector borne disease control program (NVBDCP).

#Sulfadoxine-pyrimethamine (S/P) alone and mefloquine alone are also used, but should preferably be combined with artesunate.

£In India (including under NVBDCP) all *P. falciparum* cases, irrespective of Chloroquine-resistance status, are treated with artemisinin based combination therapy.

Treatment of severe and complicated falciparum malaria*

- Artesunate 2.4 mg/kg IV or IM, followed by 2.4 mg/kg after 12 and 24 hours, and then once daily for 7 days. Switchover to 3 day oral artemisinin based combination therapy in between whenever the patient can take and tolerate oral medication.

or

- Artemether 3.2 mg/kg IM on the 1st day, followed by 1.6 mg/kg daily for 7 days. Switchover to 3 days oral artemisinin based combination therapy in between whenever the patient is able to take oral medication.

or

- α/β Arteether 3.2 mg/kg IM on the 1st day, followed by 1.6 mg/kg daily for the next 4 days. Switchover to 3 days oral artemisinin based combination therapy in between whenever the patient is able to take oral medication.

or

- Quinine dihydrochloride 20 mg/kg (loading dose) diluted in 10 mL/kg 5% dextrose/dextrose-saline and infused IV over 4 hours, followed by 10 mg/kg (maintenance dose) IV infusion over 4 hours (in adults) or 2 hours (in children) every 8 hours, until patient can swallow. Switchover to oral quinine 10 mg/kg 8 hourly to complete the 7-day course.

α/β Arteether (IM) is slower acting than artesunate (IV), and appears to be less efficacious. It is used only in India.
- Volume of fluid for IV infusion of quinine should be reduced in patients with volume overload/pulmonary edema.

- If possible, oral quinine should be substituted by 3 days oral artemisinin based combination therapy, or doxycycline 100 mg daily should be combined with it.
- Chloroquine HCl IV to be used only if none of the above is available and only in adults.

*Adopted from Regional guidelines for the management of severe falciparum malaria in large hospitals (2006); WHO, Regional office for South-East Asia, New Delhi.

Radical Cure Therapy

- A radical cure is needed in relapsing malaria (*P. vivax* and *ovale* only).
- Drug of choice for radical cure of vivax and ovale malaria is: Primaquine 15 mg daily for 14 days.
- This treatment should be given concurrently with or immediately after chloroquine/other schizontocide only to individuals who test negative for G-6-PD.
- In case of falciparum malaria—no radical cure therapy is required as adequate treatment of clinical attack leaves no parasite in the body.

Gametocidal Therapy

- Primaquine 45 mg (0.75 mg/kg) is given as single dose.
- It is gametocidal to all species of plasmodia.
- This should be given even when an artemisinin is used for clinical cure because artemisinins do not kill all the gametes.
- Primaquine used for radical cure of vivax malaria eliminates *P.vivax* gametes as well.
- This therapy is of no benefit to the patient being treated, but reduces the transmission to mosquito.

Drug Interactions

- Mefloquine or amioadarone and chloroquine should not be given simultaneously, as QTc prolongation and cardiac arrest can occur.
- Concurrent use of metoclopramide with antimalarial therapy may precipitate extrapyramidal side effects.

Nursing Implications

- **Anti-malarial drugs**
  - Nurse should enquire the patients about unusual visual and auditory sensations.
  - Drug should be given with food to decrease the GI irritation.
  - Monitoring of urine output is mandatory during antimalarial therapy because it leads to renal damage.
  - Closely monitor the vital signs.
  - Closely monitor the blood glucose levels in patients receiving quinine therapy, as rapid IV injection can cause hypoglycemia.
  - Nurse should check that anti-malarial regimen is being followed properly.

Contd...

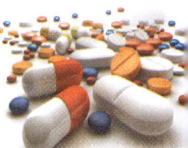

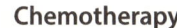

ANTHELMINTIC DRUGS

HELMINTHIASIS

The infection of an individual with helminths or parasitic worms is called Helminthiasis. It is a major cause of ill-health in the people living in the developing countries with poor personal and environmental hygiene. In the human body, these helminths are mostly present in the gastrointestinal tract. Some helminths (larva form) may migrate in tissues and different body organs.

Anthelmintics are drugs that either act locally to kill (vermicidal) or expel out (vermifuge) the infesting helminths from the gastrointestinal tract. They also include the drugs, which act systemically to eradicate adult helminths or developmental forms that invade organs or tissues.

Some of the important anthelmintic drugs are **mebendazole, albendazole, thiabendazole, pyrantel pamoate, piperazine, levamisole, tetramisole, diethylcarbamazine citrate (DEC), ivermectin, niclosamide, praziquantel, etc.**

MEBENDAZOLE

Mebendazole is a broad spectrum anthelmintic and produces nearly 100% cure rate in various helmintics infestations such as roundworm, hookworm, *Enterobius* and *Trichuris* infestations. In tapeworm infestation, up to 75% cure rate is obtained.

Mechanism of Action

- It acts on the microtubular protein 'β-tubulin' of the parasite and inhibits its polymerization.
- It blocks the glucose uptake in the parasite and also depletes its glycogen stores. Thus, the parasite dies due to starvation.

Pharmacokinetics

- It is given orally and absorbed poorly from the gastrointestinal tract. The unabsorbed drug (75–90%) remains in the gut and exerts its cidal effect on the worms.
- The absorbed fraction of the drug is excreted mainly as inactive metabolites in urine and feces.

Adverse Effects

- It is well tolerated and the systemic adverse effects are least due to poor absorption.
- Diarrhea, nausea, and abdominal pain may occur in patients having heavy worm infestation.
- It is contraindicated in pregnancy, lactation and children less than 1 year.

Indications and Dose

- **Roundworm, Hookworm, Whipworm infestation:** 100 mg BD for three consecutive days for >2 years of age and 50 mg BD for three consecutive days for 1–2 years of age group patients.
- **Pin worm** *(Enterobius):* 100 mg single dose, should be repeated after 2–3 weeks.
- **Trichinosis:** 200 mg BD for 4 days but is less effective than albendazole.
- **Hydatid disease:** 200–400 mg BD or TDS for 3–4 weeks, but is less effective than albendazole.

ALBENDAZOLE

It is a broad spectrum anthelmintic and produces nearly 100% cure rate in various helmintic infestations. It is the most preferred drug due to its advantage of single dose administration.

Mechanism of action: The mechanism of action is similar to Mebendazole.

Pharmacokinetics

- It is given orally and is well absorbed. The absorption increases when it is given with fatty meals. *Patient should be advised to chew the tablet properly for better absorption and efficacy.*
- It is metabolized in the liver and converted to an active metabolite known as albendazole sulfoxide. This active metabolite is widely distributed in the body tissues and also enters the brain. It is excreted in urine.

Adverse Effects

- Albendazole is well tolerated with mild gastrointestinal side effects in some patients.
- On prolonged use, as in hydatid cyst or in cysticercosis, it may cause headache, fever, alopecia, jaundice and neutropenia in some patients.
- It is contraindicated in pregnancy.

Dose

- In children above 2 years and adults: 400 mg single dose.
- In children 1–2 years of age: 200 mg single dose.

Indications

- Ascaris, hookworm, Enterobius and Trichuri: *400 mg daily for three days treatment is required in heavy infestation.*
- Tapeworms: *400 mg daily for three days.*
- Strongyloidosis
- Trichinosis
- Cutaneous larva migrans
- Neurocysticercosis
- Hydatid disease

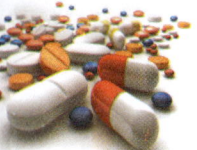

Neurocysticercosis

- Cysticercosis of various organs, including brain, occurs in *T. solium* infestation.
- It occurs due to migration of the larvae from the gut to various tissues via blood stream.
- The anthelmintic [albendazole] kills the larvae. It may precipitate the immunological reaction against the dead parasite, and results in meningeal irritation, rise in intracranial pressure, and seizures.
- The treatment is not required in the patients having inactive and calcified cysts.
- Albendazole is given in a dose of 400 mg BD [15 mg/kg/day] for 8–15 days. Treatment may need to be prolonged in patients having more number of cysts. Cysticercosis of other tissues (muscles, subcutaneous area) also responds simultaneously.
- Concurrent use of corticosteroids is also mandatory. Oral prednisolone in a 40–60 mg/day or dexamethasone in a dose of 8–12 mg/day is given.
- Corticosteroids must be started 2 days before and continued till 2 weeks after completing the anthelmintic course. This is necessary to suppress the inflammatory reaction to the products of killed larvae.
- Moreover, corticosteroids also enhance the absorption of albendazole.
- Most of the patients with neurocysticercosis present with seizures. Adequate anticonvulsant treatment should be given beforehand to control the fits. The most commonly used anti-convulsants are phenytoin and carbamazepine.

Hydatid Disease

- Hydatid disease occurs due to the human infection with Echinococcus granulosus and E. multilocularis.
- The human infections occur when the eggs passed in dog's feces are accidently swallowed. The liberated larvae penetrate the intestinal mucosa and enter the portal bloodstream. Then, these larvae [embryos] are carried to the liver where they become one or more hydatid cysts.
- Some larvae may reach the lung and develop into pulmonary hydatid cysts. Some other organs where hydatid cysts can form are brain, bones, skeletal muscles, kidneys, spleen, and some other tissues.
- Albendazole is the drug of choice in the treatment of hydatid disease. It is given in a dose of 400 mg BD for 4 weeks and repeated after 2 weeks (if required), up to 3 courses. It is the preferred treatment given before and after surgery as well as to inoperable cases.
- **Prevention:** In endemic areas, the prevention of this disease can be done by giving prophylactic treatment to pet dogs with 5 mg/kg of Praziquantel at monthly intervals to remove adult tape-worms and by health education of dog handlers.

THIABENDAZOLE

- Thiabendazole was the first poly anthelmintic drug introduced in 1961. It was effective against most of the nematodes.
- Given orally and well absorbed from the gastrointestinal tract.
- Due to good absorption, it causes various systemic side effects such as nausea, vomiting, abdominal pain, diarrhea, giddiness, impairment of alertness, itching, etc.
- Hence, it has gone out of use due to availability of better-tolerated mebendazole and albendazole.

PYRANTEL PAMOATE

It is highly effective drug in the treatment of pin worm, round worm and hook worm infestations.

Mechanism of Action

Pyrantel pamoate activates the nicotinic cholinergic receptors in the worms. It results in persistent depolarization, which in turn cause slowly developing contracture and spastic paralysis of worms. The paralyzed worms are then expelled out [vermifuge action].

Pharmacokinetics

It is given orally and 85–90% of the drug remains in intestines in unabsorbed form and then, this unabsorbed fraction is excreted in feces. The 10–15% absorbed drug is metabolized in liver and excreted in urine.

Adverse Effects

Occasionally gastrointestinal symptoms such as headache and dizziness may occur. It should not be prescribed to pregnant women and children less than 2 years of age.

Indications and Dose

- **Pin worm, round worm and hook worm** (*Ancylostoma duodenale*): Given in a single dose of 10 mg/kg of body weight.
- **Hook worm** (*Necator americanus*) **and Thread worm:** 10 mg/kg of for 3 days.

PIPERAZINE

Piperazine is a highly active drug against *Ascaris* and *Enterobius* with 90–100% cure rates. It is used less frequently due to availability of better tolerated drugs such as mebendazole and albendazole.

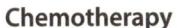

Mechanism of Action

- It causes flaccid paralysis in the worms by causing hyperpolarization of *Ascaris* muscles by a GABA agonistic action.
- It also opens the Cl⁻ channels which causes relaxation and decreased responsiveness of *Ascaris* muscle to contractile action of ACh.
- The worms are expelled alive due to the flaccid paralysis.

Pharmacokinetics

It is given orally and a considerable fraction of oral dose is absorbed, metabolized in liver and excreted in urine. It can be used during pregnancy while other drugs cannot be used.

Adverse Effects

- **At normal therapeutic doses:** Nausea, vomiting, abdominal discomfort and urticaria may occur in some patients.
- **At high doses:** Dizziness, excitement and convulsions may occur. It is contraindicated in patients with seizure disorders.

Indications and Dose

- **For roundworm infestation:** The curative dose is 4 g once a day for 2 consecutive days; children 0.75 g/year of age (maximum 4 g).
- **Pin worm:** 50 mg/kg (maximum 2 g) once a day for 7 days or 75 mg/kg (maximum 4 g) single dose, repeated after 3 weeks.

Combination of anthelmintic drugs with a purgative in the same formulation is banned in India (except piperazine).

LEVAMISOLE, TETRAMISOLE

- These drugs are used as a second line therapy in the treatment of ascariasis (round worm) and ancylostomiasis (hook worm).
- Tetramisole was developed in the late 1960s. Its racemic form (levo-isomer) levamisole is more effective and is preferred now.
- Both are active against many nematodes.

Mechanism of Action

The stimulation of ganglia in worms and interference with carbohydrate metabolism (inhibition of fumarate reductase) cause tonic paralysis and expulsion of live worms.

Pharmacokinetics

- It is given by oral route.
- It is effective in a single dose in most of the cases and is well tolerated.

Adverse Effects

- The incidence of side effects is very low. Rarely nausea, abdominal pain, and giddiness may occur.
- Severe reactions may be seen in patients who have to take the repeated doses for longer durations.

Indications and Dose

- **Ascariasis**—Adults: 150 mg single dose
  Children (20–39 kg): 100 mg single dose
  Infants (10–19 kg): 50 mg single dose
- **Ancylostomiasis**—150 mg BD for one day.
- Levamisole can be used as a disease modifying drug in rheumatoid arthritis and as an adjunct in cancer chemotherapy, aphthous ulcers , recurrent herpes and vitiligo. It acts as an immunomodulator and restores the depressed T cell function. (Rarely used these days)

DIETHYLCARBAMAZINE CITRATE (DEC)

DEC is the drug of choice for filariasis caused by the nematodes *Wuchereria bancrofti* (90% cases) and *Brugia malayi*. It is microfilaricidal.

Mechanism of Action

It promotes the cell death by altering the membranes of organelle of microfilaria and makes them more susceptible to the destruction by host defence mechanisms.

The adult worms are dislodged by alteration in the muscular activity.

Pharmacokinetics

It is given by oral route. After absorption, it is distributed all over the body, metabolized in liver and excreted in urine. Plasma t½ is 4–12 hours.

Adverse Effects

These may be drug or parasite induced.

- **Drug induced:** Mild headache, nausea, dizziness, anorexia and fatigue may be seen.
- **Parasite induced:** An allergic and febrile reaction occurs due to the antigens released by the dying parasite. It presents as rash, pruritus, enlargement of lymph nodes, bronchospasm and fall in BP. This reaction is treated by temporary drug withdrawal, and administering anti histaminic and/or corticosteroids. The drug can be started again but in a lower dose, 0.5 mg/kg.

Indications and Dose

- **Filariasis:** 2 mg/kg TDS for 3 weeks, eliminates microfilaria from the peripheral blood within 7 days. The slide

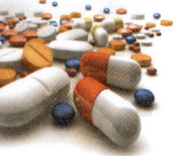

for peripheral blood smear to detect microfilariae is taken at night as the microfilariae. The adult worm remains alive in the lymphatics and may cause intermittent microfilariemia. It needs repeated courses to eliminate the adult worms with a gap of 3–4 weeks.

- Elephantiasis due to chronic lymphatic obstruction is not affected by DEC, because fibrosis of lymphatics is irreversible. In endemic areas, the transmission of filariasis is reduced by giving a combination of DEC (6 mg/kg) and albendazole (400 mg) in the form of a single dose on mass scale on yearly basis.
- **Tropical pulmonary eosinophilia:** DEC (2–4 mg/kg TDS) for 2–3 weeks.
- The associated cough mostly respond to inhaled corticosteroids.
- *Loa loa* and *O. volvulus* infections can also be treated with DEC, although Ivermectin is preferred.

IVERMECTIN

- Ivermectin is a potent semisynthetic drug obtained from *Streptomyces avermitilis.*
- It is effective against many nematodes, filariae and arthropods.

It is the only anthelmintic drug which is effective both in ectoparasitic and endoparasitic infestations.

Mechanism of Action

Ivermectin acts through a special type of glutamate gated Cl^- channels found only in invertebrates. In addition, it also enhances the GABA activity in the worm. These actions cause tonic paralysis and cidal effect on the worms.

Pharmacokinetics

- It is given orally, rapidly absorbed, widely distributed in the body, metabolized in the liver and excreted mainly in the feces.
- It has a long t½ of 48–60 hours.

Adverse Effects

The side effects are mild in the form of giddiness, nausea, pruritus, abdominal pain, constipation. Safety of ivermectin in pregnant women and young children is not established.

Indications and Dose

- Ivermectin is the drug of choice for onchocerciasis and strongyloidosis.
- Cutaneous larva migrans and ascariasis.
- Scabies and pediculosis.
- For above indications, ivermectin is given orally (0.2 mg/kg, single dose).

- **Filariasis:** A single 10–15 mg (0.2 mg/kg) oral dose of ivermectin, preferably with 400 mg albendazole is given annually for 5–6 years.

NICLOSAMIDE

- Niclosamide is a second drug of choice for *Taenia saginata, T. solium, Diphyllobothrium latum, Hymenolepis nana* and pin worm.
- It is given orally in the form of chewable tablets.
- It is poorly absorbed for gastrointestinal tract.
- It rapidly eliminates adult worms but not the ova.
- Niclosamide is safe during pregnancy and in patients with poor health.
- Not advised nowadays due to availability of better drugs.

PRAZIQUANTEL

Praziquantel has wide range of activity against Schistosomes, trematodes, cestodes and their larval forms but not nematodes.

Mechanism of Action

- The drug is rapidly taken up by susceptible worms and causes leakage of intracellular calcium from the membranes. This causes contracture and paralysis of worms.
- The worms loose grip of the intestinal mucosa and are expelled out.
- At relatively higher concentrations, it causes vacuolization of the tegument and release of the contents of tapeworms and flukes followed by their destruction by immune mechanisms of the host.

Pharmacokinetics

- It is given orally, rapidly absorbed, widely distributed in the body, metabolized in the liver and excreted mainly in the urine.
- It also crosses blood brain barrier.

Adverse Effects

- The side effects are mild in the form of giddiness, nausea, pruritus, abdominal pain, constipation, lethargy and myalgia.
- Destruction of cysticerci in the brain may produce neurological complications.

Indications and Dose

- *T. solium and T. saginata* (given orally in a single morning dose of 10 mg/kg).
- *H. nana and D. latum* (given orally in a single morning dose of 15–25 mg/kg).

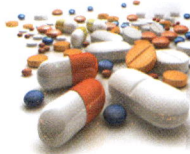

- *Schistosomiasis* (given orally in a single morning dose of 40–75 mg/kg or in divided doses).
- *Neurocysticercosis (second choice drug to albendazole), it is given in a dose of 50 mg/kg/day in three divided doses for 15–30 days.*

 ### Drug Interactions

↪ Pyrantel pamoate antagonizes the effect of piperazine.

Nursing Implications

↪ **Anti-helmintic drugs**
- ☞ Teach the patients proper hand washing technique.
- ☞ Patients should be encouraged to take the full course of treatment.
- ☞ Patients should be encouraged to take proper and hygienic meals, as they are malnourished.
- ☞ Nurse should educate the patients about getting all the members of family treated to avoid the recurrence of infections.
- ☞ Patients on DEC therapy should be monitored for any febrile reaction and nurse should be ready to manage it timely.

ANTI-SCABIES AGENTS

Scabies is an infestation caused by an ectoparasite *Sarcoptes scabiei* (arachnids).

It is highly contagious disease and mostly all family members get the infection.

The mite penetrate and burrows through the epidermis, laying eggs which form papules that itch intensely. Lesions start mainly in the fingers' webs and spread to forearms, trunk, genitals, and lower legs.

Pediculosis (lice infestation) is an infestation caused by an ectoparasite on head (*P. capitis*), body (*P. corporis*) or pubic region (*P. pubis*). The main presenting symptom is itching. They feed on host blood and transmit typhus and relapsing fever. The eggs are called *nits* and are found attached to the hair and clothing.

Anti-scabies agents are the drugs used to kill the ectoparasites like Mite (*Sarcoptes scabiei*) and Lice (*Pediculus sp.*).

The most common anti-scabies agents are:
- **Local agents:** Permethrin, Lindane (GBHC), Benzyl benzoate, Crotamiton.
- **Oral agents:** Ivermectin

LOCAL AGENTS

Permethrin

It is the first line and most efficacious drug in the treatment of both scabies and pediculosis. Complete cure rate is seen after even a single application.

For scabies: Patient is advised to apply 5% cream all over the body except face and head and take bath after 8–12 hours, preferably with 1% permethrin soap.

For head lice: Patient is advised to massage about 30 g of 1% cream or 1% lotion on the scalp and wash it off after 10 minutes.

Instructions

Other members of the patient's family should be treated concurrently; garments and bed linen should be washed in hot water and put in sun to prevent cross infection and re-infection.

Lindane (Gama Benzene Hexachloride, GBHC)

- GBHC is highly effective in the treatment of scabies and head lice, but lower in efficacy than permethrin.
- It penetrates through the chitinous cover of mites and lice, and causes paralysis as well as cidal effect.
- Being highly lipid soluble, it can be absorbed through skin and can produce systemic toxicity symptoms like CNS stimulation, vertigo, convulsions (in children) and arrhythmias. This occurs rarely if proper instructions for application are followed.
- It should be avoided in pregnancy.
- Patients should be instructed the method of application clearly to get the full benefit of treatment.
- **For scabies:** One percent lotion or 1% cream should be rubbed over the body below neck. It should be allowed to remain on the body for a minimum period of 12 hours to a maximum of 24 hours time. After this period, a good scrub bath should be taken. A single application is sufficient in most of the patients. If mites are still present, another application after one week may be required.
- **For pediculosis:** One percent lotion or 1% cream should be applied on the scalp and hair (protecting eyes). It should be allowed to remain as such for a period of 12–24 hours. After this period, it should be washed off. Shower cap should be used for long hair. If lice are still present, another application after one week may be required.

Benzyl Benzoate

Benzyl benzoate is a creamy white colored liquid (emulsion) with aromatic smell. It used to be a very popular drug before the advent of GBHC and Permethrin.

- **For scabies:** The patient is advised to take a good scrub bath in the morning (by rubbing, the pores of the burrows become exposed and the drug can enter easily inside the burrows for a good effect). The emulsion (25% lotion) is applied all over the body except face and neck, and is allowed to remain for 24 hours. A second coat is applied

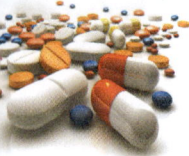

on next morning without taking a bath. It is allowed to remain for next 24 hours and should be washed off next morning. 76–100% cure rate is achieved if instructions are followed strictly. The systemic toxicity is very low, but should be avoided in children.

- **For pediculosis:** The emulsion (25% lotion) is applied to the scalp, taking care not to enter the eyes, and is washed off after 24 hours.

Crotamiton

- Crotamiton is a second choice drug for scabies and pediculosis treatment in children.
- It is an effective scabicide, pediculocide and antipruritic.
- Ten percent cream or lotion is applied all over the body below chin followed by a second application after 24 hours and a scrub bath 48 hours after last application.
- For the treatment of pruritis, massage gently into the affected areas 2–3 times daily.

ORAL AGENTS

Ivermectin

It is the only orally administered drug used for the treatment of ectoparasitosis.

- Although anthelmintic, this drug is highly effective both in scabies and pediculosis (head and body lice) as well.
- Scabies in AIDS patients also responds well.
- It is given as a single dose of 0.2 mg/kg (12 mg in adults).
- Ninety-one to hundred percent cure rate is seen with a single dose only.
- Not given to children <5 years, pregnant and lactating women.

Drug Interactions

- The concomitant use of antiviral agents with hepatic and renal toxic drugs should be avoided or closely monitored. For example, zidovudine with isoniazid, zidovudine with amphotericin-B.

Nursing Implications

- **Anti-scabies drugs**
  - ☞ Nurse should guide the patients about the proper application method of antiscabies agents.
  - ☞ Nurse should educate the patients about the maintenance of proper hygiene to prevent recurrence.
  - ☞ Nurse should educate the patients about the importance of treatment of whole family.
  - ☞ Patients should be regularly enquired about any local/systemic side effects.

ANTIVIRAL AGENTS

Viruses can replicate inside the host cell and utilize the host enzyme system for their food, growth, and multiplication.

Antiviral agents are the drugs which inhibit viral multiplication mainly by inhibiting the viral DNA/RNA replication. These drugs exert bad effects on host cells also. Therefore, selectively targeting the virus is very difficult.

Some antiviral agents are under-development, which are having cidal effect only on virus without affecting the host cell functions.

CLASSIFICATION

- **Anti-herpes virus agents:** Acyclovir, valacyclovir, ganciclovir, famciclovir, cidofovir, valganciclovir, foscarnet, fomivirsen, idoxuridine, docosanol and trifluridine.
- **Anti-influenza virus agents:** Oseltamivir, zanamivir, amantadine and rimantadine.
- **Anti-Hepatitis virus/Non-selective antiviral agents:**
  - **Primarily for hepatitis B**: Lamivudine, adefovir dipivoxil and tenofovir.
  - **Primarily for hepatitis C:** Ribavirin and interferon α.
- **Anti-retrovirus agents:**
  - **Nucleoside reverse transcriptase inhibitors (NRTIs):** Zidovudine (AZT), didanosine, abacavir, lamivudine stavudine, emtricitabine *and tenofovir (Nucleotide RTI)*
  - **Non nucleoside reverse transcriptase inhibitors (NNRTIs):** delavirdine nevirapine and efavirenz
  - **Protease inhibitors:** Indinavir, saquinavir, ritonavir, atazanavir, nelfinavir, amprenavir, and lopinavir.
  - **Entry (Fusion) inhibitors:** Enfuvirtide, sifuvirtide
  - **CD4 cell membrane receptor (CCR5 receptor) inhibitor:** Maraviroc
  - **Integrase inhibitor:** Raltegravir, elvitegravir, dolutegravir.

ANTI-HERPES VIRUS AGENTS

The drugs having activity against the Herpes group viruses are known as antiherpetic viral agents. The viruses included in this group are : *Herpes simplex virus-1* (HSV-1), *Herpes simplex virus-2* (HSV-2), *Cytomegalovirus* (CMV), *Varicella-Zoster virus* (VZV) and *Epstein- Barr virus* (EBV).

Acyclovir

- Acyclovir is mainly effective against HSV-1 and HSV-2 viral infections.
- It is less effective in VZV, EBV and ineffective against CMV infection.

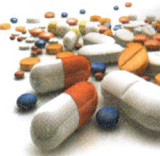

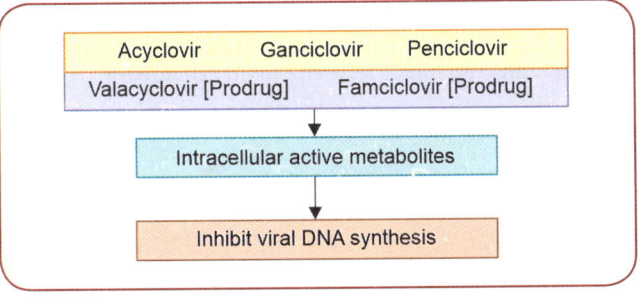

FIG. 2.6: Mechanism of action of acyclovir

- It is highly potent anti-herpes drug.
- It is less toxic to the host cell.

Mechanism of Action

The mechanism of action of acyclovir is shown in Figure 2.6.

Pharmacokinetics

- It can be given by oral, topical or intravenous route.
- Oral absorption is poor (20%).
- It is widely distributed with poor plasma protein binding.
- It crosses BBB and attains good CSF concentration (approximately 50%).
- It is metabolized in liver with a plasma t½ of 2–3 hours and excretion occurs via kidneys in an unchanged form.

Adverse Effects

- It is well tolerated.
- On topical application, it may cause mucosal irritation, itching, and transient burning when applied to genital lesions.
- Oral acyclovir has been associated infrequently with nausea, diarrhea, rash, or headache.
- On intravenous administration at therapeutic doses, it may cause headache, nausea, and diarrhea.
- At higher doses, it may precipitate nephrotoxicity, neurotoxicity, hallucinations and convulsions.
- In neonates, it has been associated with neutropenia.

Indications and Doses

- **Genital Herpes simplex (caused by HSV-2 virus):** It can be treated by topical, oral or parenteral acyclovir depending on stage and severity of disease.
  - **Primary disease:** Five percent ointment is applied locally after every 4 hours for a period of 10 days.
  - **Late and more severe cases:** Oral therapy 400 mg TDS for 10 days and concurrent use of topical application is also advised.
  - **Recurrent disease:** Five mg/kg IV infusion to be administered over 1 hour, repeated 8 hourly for 10 days.

Sequential oral therapy with 400 mg BD is helpful to prevent recurrences.
- **Mucocutaneous H. simplex (caused by HSV-1 virus):** The disease remains localized to lips, tongue, oral mucosa and gums. Five percent ointment is applied locally 6 times a day for 10 days.
- **H. simplex (type I) keratitis:** Eye ointment in a concentration of 3% should be applied 5–6 times/day.
- **H. simplex encephalitis (HSV-1 virus):** Acyclovir 10–20 mg/kg/8 hour IV for 10–14 days.
- **Herpes zoster (varicella-zoster virus):** It is less susceptible to acyclovir.
- *Chickenpox:* In adults and immunodeficient individuals, acyclovir is the drug of choice. It reduces the duration and severity of illness. In children, routine use of acyclovir is not recommended.

Valacyclovir

- It is a prodrug of acyclovir and is completely converted to acyclovir after first pass metabolism.
- The oral bioavailability is better (55–70%) than acyclovir (20%). Thus, higher plasma levels of acyclovir are obtained, which improves clinical efficacy.
- The metabolism occurs in liver with a plasma t½ is 3 hours and excretion occurs through kidneys.

Indications and Doses

- **For genital herpes simplex:** (Preferably both sexual partners should be treated)
  - First episode should be treated with 500–1000 mg twice a day for 10 days.
  - Recurrent episode should be treated with 500 mg twice a day for 3 days.
  - In suppressive treatment; it is given in a dose of 500 mg once daily for 6–12 months.
- **For orolabial herpes:** It is given in a dose of 2000 mg twice daily for 1 day and in immunocompromised individuals 1000 mg twice a day for 5 days.
- **For herpes zoster:** It is given in a dose of 1000 mg thrice a day for 7 days.

Ganciclovir

- Ganciclovir is an analogue of acyclovir.
- It works against all herpes viruses including *H. simplex, H. zoster,* and *EBV.*
- *It is most active against CMV* because the active metabolite attains much higher concentration inside CMV infected host cells.
- It has poor oral absorption.
- The plasma t½ is 2–4 hours, but in CMV infected host cell it is >24 hours.

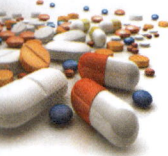

- It is highly toxic, and causes thrombocytopenia, granulocytopenia, bone marrow suppression, and neuropsychiatric disturbances.
- It is teratogenic and mutagenic in animals.
- It is indicated in serious CMV infection of retina in immunocompromised patients for both **prophylaxis** (10 mg/kg in two divided doses for 1–3 weeks, followed by 5 mg/kg/day) and **therapeutic treatment** (IV. infusion of ganciclovir 10 mg/kg/day)

Cidofovir

- It is a monophosphate nucleotide analogue of cytidine.
- It inhibits human herpes, papilloma, polyoma, pox, and adenoviruses.
- It is reserved drug for acyclovir and ganciclovir resistant cases.
- Plasma t½ is 2–3 hours.
- It is highly nephrotoxic and may also cause gastric disturbances, uveitis, neutropenia and hypersensitivity reactions.
- It is given in resistant cytomegalovirus (CMV) cases, in a dose of 5 mg/kg intravenously weekly, then after every 15 days.

Foscarnet

- Foscarnet inhibits viral DNA polymerase and reverse transcriptase enzyme.
- It works against *H. simplex,* CMV (even ganciclovir-resistant cases) in AIDS patients.
- The oral absorption of this drug is poor.
- Its t½ is 4–8 hours, and it is not metabolized.
- It is highly nephrotoxic, and also causes seizures, hallucinations, painful genital ulcerations, hypocalcemia, tremors and phlebitis.

Docosanol

- It is long-chain saturated alcohol.
- It is indicated in recurrent orolabial herpes.
- It is available as 10% cream for topical application.

Idoxuridine

- Idoxuridine (thymidine analogue) inhibits the replication of various DNA viruses, including herpes virus and poxvirus.
- It is not used systemically due to toxicity.
- Only topical preparation is available for treatment of *Herpes simplex* keratitis (0.1% eye drops to be instilled hourly, then 2 hourly and 4 hourly; apply 0.1% eye ointment at night).
- Edema involving the eyes or eyelids and photophobia are disturbing side effects, hence not preferred these days due to availability of better and safer drugs.

ANTI-INFLUENZA VIRUS AGENTS

(Amantadine, rimantadine, oseltamivir, zanamivir)

Amantadine and Rimantadine

- Both drugs work in a similar fashion.
- Rimantadine is a derivative of amantadine.
- Both inhibit an early step of uncoating and the late step of viral assembly in viral replication. They act by altering hemagglutinin processing.
- Both of these drugs are not effective against H1N1 (swine flu) and H5N1 (bird flu).
- These agents are effective against Influenza A virus strains.
- Rimantadine is more potent (4–10 times) and longer acting than amantadine.
- Amantadine releases dopamine from dopaminergic nerve endings, so it is also used in some cases of Parkinson's disease.
- Both drugs are well absorbed orally and have very large volumes of distribution. The plasma t½ of amantadine is 12–18 hours and rimantadine is 24–36 hours. Both are eliminated through urine.
- Both are given as follows:
  - Adults: 100 mg twice daily
  - Children: 5 mg/kg/day.
- The side effects are dose-related. Some common side effects are CNS and gastrointestinal disturbances which include nervousness, headache, confusion, insomnia, and loss of appetite.

Oseltamivir

- It is a sialic acid analogue, having broad spectrum activity covering influenza A, H1N1 (swine flu) H5N1 (bird flu) strains and influenza B.
- It acts by inhibiting influenza virus neuraminidase enzyme and thereby inhibits the multiplication of virus in the host cell.
- It is well absorbed from GIT, metabolized in liver to the active form *oseltamivir carboxylate.*
- The oral bioavailability is nearly 80% and it is excreted by the kidney with a t½ of 6–10 hours.
- It is indicated both for prophylaxis as well as treatment of influenza A, swine flu, bird flu and influenza B.
- It is given in a dose of 75 mg once daily for 5–10 days for prophylaxis and 75 mg oral twice daily for 5 days for therapeutic purpose.
- *It reduces the secondary complications (pneumonia) if started early.*
- The following side effects are seen with its use:
  - **GIT:** Abdominal pain, diarrhea, vomiting, nausea. (The drug should not be taken in empty stomach)

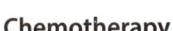

- **Respiratory system:** Cough.
- **CNS:** Insomnia, weakness, headache and mild depression.

Zanamivir

- Zanamavir is similar to oseltamivir in mechanism of action, efficacy and adverse reactions.
- It is given by inhalational route by special inhaler. It has low oral bioavailability with a t½ of 2–5 hours.
- It is given in a dose of 10 mg once daily for 7–10 days for prophylaxis and 10 mg oral twice daily for 5 days for therapeutic purpose through breath actuated inhaler.
- Inhalation of powder may lead to bronchospasm, therefore contraindicated in chronic obstructive pulmonary disease (COPD) and asthmatic individuals.

ANTI-HEPATITIS VIRUS OR NON-SELECTIVE ANTIVIRAL AGENTS

- The hepatitis presents clinically in a similar fashion irrespective of the causative agents. Hepatitis may occur due to viral infections, as a side effect of drug or due to toxic agents.
- The hepatitis causing viruses are:
  - Hepatitis A virus [HAV]
  - Hepatitis B virus [HBV[
  - Hepatitis C virus [HCV]
  - Hepatitis D virus also known as 'Delta agent' [HDV]
  - Hepatitis E virus [HEV]
  - Hepatitis G virus [HGV]

Hepatitis A and E are self-limiting infections and do not require any type of anti-viral drug treatment.

- HBV, like retroviruses can integrate into host chromosomal DNA to establish permanent infection. It is a DNA virus.
- HCV, does not integrate into chromosomal DNA but causes chronic hepatitis. It is a RNA virus.

Hepatitis B and hepatitis C require antiviral drug treatment and other supportive measures.

- The hepatitis D infection is always superimposed on hepatitis B infection.
- Hepatitis G is a flavivirus, transmitted by percutaneous route and does not cause any important liver disease, hence, does not require any active treatment.

ANTI-VIRAL DRUGS FOR HEPATITIS B AND C

- **Drugs for Hepatitis B:** Lamivudine, Adefovir dipivoxil, Tenofovir
- **Drugs for Hepatitis C:** Ribavirin, Interferon α

Lamivudine

- Lamivudine inhibits HBV DNA polymerase as well as human immunodeficiency virus (HIV) reverse transcriptase enzyme.
- It terminates the chain formation after getting incorporated into DNA.
- Its oral bioavailability is high and plasma t½ is 6–8 hours and intracellular t½ is longer (> 12 hours).
- It is mainly excreted unchanged in urine.
- For the treatment of chronic hepatitis B, lamivudine is the first drug of choice.
- It is also used along with other anti-HIV drugs for the treatment of HIV infection.
- It is given in a dose of 100 mg OD.
- It is well tolerated and has low toxicity. Hence, it is given priority in use.

Adefovir Dipivoxil

- Adefovir is active against HBV and some other DNA as well as RNA viruses. It is used only for hepatitis caused by HBV.
- On entering the host cells, it gets phosphorylated to the diphosphate form. Due to its high affinity to viral DNA polymerase no harm is caused to host cell.
- The plasma t½ is 7 hours and excretion occurs mainly through kidneys.
- It is indicated in chronic hepatitis B, including lamivudine-resistant cases and those having concurrent HIV infection.
- It is well tolerated in a daily dose of 10 mg.
- The minor side effects are headache, weakness, sore throat, abdominal pain and flu-like syndrome.
- It also exhibits dose dependent nephrotoxicity.

Tenofovir

- Tenofovir is active against HBV as well as HIV.
- It is incompletely but adequately absorbed after oral administration and excreted through kidneys. The plasma t½ is 14–16 hours.
- It is well tolerated with mild side effects such as nausea, flatulence, abdominal discomfort, loose motions and headache. The nephrotoxicity is rare.
- It is well tolerated in a daily dose of 300 mg.
- The major indication is chronic hepatitis B and is also preferred in lamivudine resistant hepatitis B infection.

Ribavirin

- Ribavirin is preferred in the treatment of chronic hepatitis C.
- It can also be given in combination with injectable peginterferon for 6–12 months in chronic hepatitis C infection.

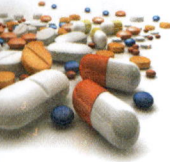

- Nebulized form of ribavirin is used for respiratory syncytial virus bronchiolitis in infants and children.
- The dose for patients is:
  - <75 kg is 200 mg four times a day
  - >75 kg is 400 mg thrice daily
  - Children: 15 mg/kg in 2–3 daily divided doses
- The prominent side effects are reversible anemia, hemolysis, bone marrow depression and insomnia.
- It is teratogenic and the nebulized form may cause conjuctival irritation, transient wheezing and reversible deterioration of pulmonary functions.

Interferon α

- Interferons (IFNs) are low molecular weight glycoprotein cytokines produced by host cells in response to viral infections, TNFα, IL-1 and some other inducers.
- They have non-specific antiviral effects with some complex effects on immunity and cell proliferation.
- Interferons are host specific and inhibit many RNA and DNA viruses.
- There are three types of human IFNs—α, β and γ. All three have antiviral activity.
- The clinically used interferons are only IFNα, 2A and IFNα 2B. These are produced by recombinant technology.
- These are administered by intramuscular/subcutaneous route. The pegylated forms are administered by SC route at weekly intervals.
- These are mainly used in chronic hepatitis B and C, condyloma and Kaposi's sarcoma associated with AIDS.
- The common adverse effects are flu-like symptoms, thyroid dysfunction, neurotoxicity and hypotension.

ANTI-RETROVIRAL DRUGS

The drugs which are effective against human immunodeficiency virus are called antiretroviral agents or antiretroviral drugs (ARVs).

HIV is a retrovirus.

Human Immunodeficiency Virus (HIV)

- Human immunodeficiency virus [HIV] is a retrovirus. HIV infection is a major global health problem and is a pandemic disease.
- In India, National AIDS Control Organization (NACO) distributes free antiretroviral therapy (ART) to all eligible registered patients.
- The anti-retroviral drugs do not cure the infection, but prolong life and also improve the quality of life. These drugs are helpful in postponing the complications of AIDS and AIDS related complex (ARC). After entering into the human body, the viral genome integrates with the host

DNA and directs the host DNA to produce multiple copies of HIV like genome. It multiplies at a rate of approximately 1010 copies/day.

- At such a high rate of replication, the virus often commits mistakes and results into mutants. This much high rate of mutation leads to development of multiple strains, threatens the development of drug resistance, and makes the treatment difficult.
- Once infected, the virus becomes an integral part of host cell and survives the full life span of infected host cell. Therefore, the eradication of the virus from the host cell appears impossible at present.
- The anti-retroviral drugs do not cure the infection. However, they prolong and improve the quality of life and are helpful in postponing the complications of acquired immunodeficiency syndrome (AIDS) or AIDS related complex (ARC). The first anti-retrovirus (ARV) drug zidovudine was made available for use in 1987.

Aim of Anti-retroviral Therapy

The anti-retroviral therapy (ART) is administered for suppressing the viral replication for a maximal period of time.

The ART drugs are always used in combination (at least three drugs) and the regimes are changed over time to avoid the problem of drug resistance. Therefore, lifelong therapy is required.

The site of actions of anti retroviral drugs are given in Figure 2.7.

Anti-retroviral Agents

- **Nucleoside reverse transcriptase inhibitors (NRTIs):** Zidovudine (AZT), Didanosine, Abacavir, Lamivudine Stavudine, Emtricitabine *and* Tenofovir *(Nucleotide RTI)*
- **Non nucleoside reverse transcriptase inhibitors (NNRTIs):** Delavirdine Nevirapine and Efavirenz
- **Protease inhibitors:** Indinavir, saquinavir, ritonavir, atazanavir, nelfinavir, amprenavir, and lopinavir.
- **Entry (Fusion) inhibitors:** Enfuvirtide, Sifuvirtide
- **CD4 Cell Membrane Receptor (CCR5 receptor) inhibitor:** Maraviroc
- **Integrase inhibitor:** Raltegravir, elvitegravir, dolutegravir.

Nucleoside Reverse Transcriptase Inhibitors (NRTIS)

Zidovudine [AZT]

- It is a thymidine analogue (azidothymidine, AZT) and effective against retroviruses only.
- AZT gets phosphorylated in the host cell and forms zidovudine triphosphate, which selectively inhibits viral reverse transcriptase. The affinity of zidovudine triphosphate towards viral reverse transcriptase is more than the cellular DNA polymerase (Fig. 2.8).

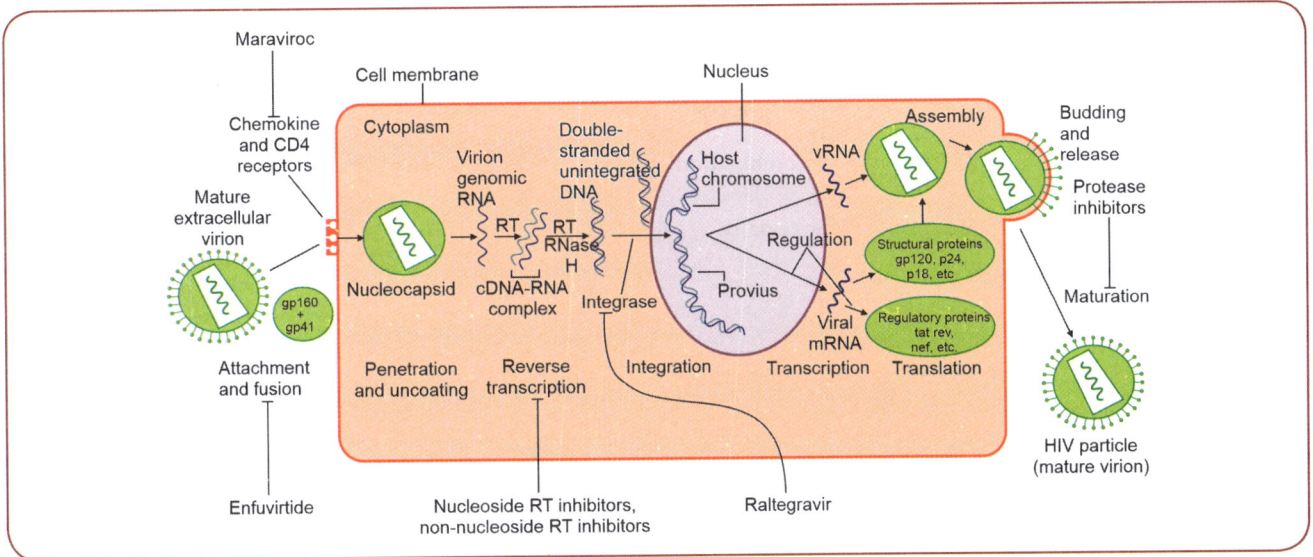

FIG. 2.7: Site of action of various antiretroviral drugs

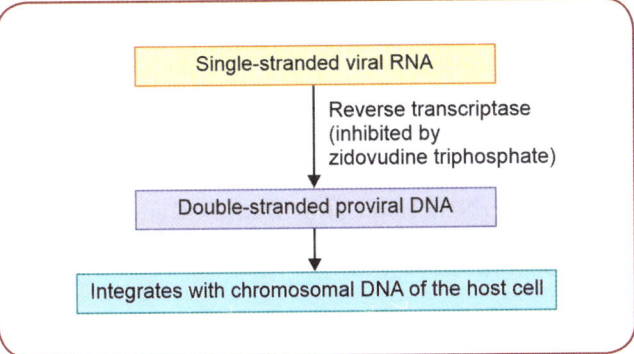

FIG. 2.8: Replication mechanism of HIV and role of zidovudine

- Zidovudine causes premature chain termination during proviral-DNA synthesis, therefore it prevents the formation of new pro-viral DNA and thus the infection of new cells by HIV. It has no effect on proviral DNA that has already integrated into the host chromosome.
- The oral absorption of AZT is rapid with bioavailability of 65%.
- The metabolism occurs in the liver and excretion via kidneys with t½ of 1 hour.
- AZT crosses placental and blood brain barrier and secreted in milk also.
- It is given in a dose of 300 mg BD to adults and 180 mg/m² (max 200 mg) in divided doses to children with plenty of water.
- Some of the dose-related side effects are anemia and neutropenia.
- Some other commonly seen adverse effects such as headache, anorexia, nausea, abdominal pain, loss of sleep

and muscular aches. These effects are common at the start of therapy, but diminish later.
- For HIV infected patients, AZT is used in combination with at least two other anti-retroviral drugs. For post-exposure prophylaxis and mother to offspring transmission of HIV, AZT is used along with two other antiretroviral drugs as a gold standard choice.

Didanosine (DDI)

- Antiretroviral activity of didanosine is equivalent to AZT and other NRTIs.
- The daily dose is 400 mg for the patients above 60 kg and 250 mg for the patients below 50 kg. Preferably the dose is given 1 hour before or 2 hours after meals.
- The major dose-related toxicity is irreversible peripheral neuropathy.
- The commonly seen adverse effects are nausea, dry mouth, diarrhea, and abdominal pain.
- It is not preferred due to higher toxicity than other NRTIs.

Stavudine (d4T)

- It is also a thymidine analogue which acts in the same way as AZT.
- It should not be given with AZT as it antagonizes the effect of stavudine.
- The anti-HIV efficacy of stavudine is equivalent to AZT.
- Stavudine is one of the optional components of first line regimen used by national AIDS control organization (NACO) in a fixed dose of 30 mg BD. (WHO and NACO guidelines 2007).

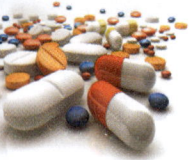

Lamivudine

- Lamivudine is an essential component of all first line triple drug NACO regimes for AIDS patients as it synergises with most other NRTIs for HIV.
- It is equally effective as AZT when used in combination with other anti-HIV drugs.
- The recommended dose is 300 mg once or twice daily.

Abacavir (ABC)

- This is a very potent guanosine analogue.
- Intracellularly, it gets converted to carbovir triphosphate and gets incorporated in proviral DNA and terminates chain elongation.
- Its oral bioavailability is 80% with a plasma t½ of 1–1.5 hour, but intracellular t½ of the active metabolite is >12 hours.
- The recommended dose is 600 mg once or twice daily.
- Common adverse effects include gastrointestinal disturbances, headache, and dizziness.
- Approximately 5% of patients exhibit the 'hypersensitivity reaction', which is usually characterized by drug fever with rash, gastrointestinal symptoms, malaise, and respiratory distress. Sensitized individuals should *never* be rechallenged because of rapidly appearing severe reactions that may lead to death.
- A genetic test (HLA-B*5701) is available to screen patients for the potential of this reaction.

Tenofovir

- This is a nucleotide (*not nucleoside*) analogue.
- In addition to HIV, it is also active against HBV.
- It is an inhibitor of HIV reverse transcriptase.
- It is given as a once daily regimen due its longer half-life.
- It has been included by NACO in the first line three drug regimen as an alternative when either zidovudine or nevirapine or efavirenz cannot be used.

Non-nucleoside Reverse Transcriptase Inhibitors (NNRTIs)

- These agents selectively inhibit the HIV-1 reverse transcriptase noncompetitively.
- They do not require intracellular phosphorylation for their activation, but directly inhibit HIV reverse transcriptase.
- They are more potent than AZT on HIV-1, but do not inhibit HIV-2.
- These are indicated in combination regimes for HIV. Either Nevirapine or Efavirenz is included in the first line triple drug regimen used by NACO.

TABLE 2.17: Features of NNRTIs

Drug	Dose	Special features and side-effects
Nevirapine	Initially 200 mg/day for 15 days, then 200 mg twice daily (because autoinduction reduces levels)	• The commonest side effects are rashes, nausea, headache, hepatotoxicity • In patients developing NVP toxicity, it should be replaced by EFV which has low hepatotoxicity
Efavirenz	600 mg OD on empty stomach	• Side effects are headache, rashes, dizziness, insomnia • These effects decrease over time • Contraindicated in pregnancy
Delavirdine	100 mg TDS	• Not recommended as a preferred or alternate NNRTI in the current HIV guidelines due to its inferior antiviral activity and thrice a day dosage schedule

- Some features of these drugs are given in Table 2.17:
- Some other NNRTIs are **Etravirine (ETR)** and **Rilpivirine.**

Protease Inhibitors (PIS)

- Protease inhibitors [PIs] are more effective viral inhibitors than AZT.
- They are effective in both newly as well as chronically infected cells as they act at a late step of viral cycle.
- They inhibit the functioning of protease enzyme.

Role of Protease Enzyme

A pro-viral DNA directed poly-protein is formed in the HIV infected cell. This poly-protein is cleaved into various structural and functional proteins by the protease enzyme. These cleavage products [enzymes] are necessary for the production of infective virions. The inhibition of protease enzyme prevents maturation of the viral particles and results in the production of non-infectious virions.

- The oral bioavailability of PIs is variable and the t½ of different PIs ranges from 2 hours to 8 hours.
- Nelfinavir, lopinavir and ritonavir induce their own metabolism.
- Combination of NRTIs with PIs is more effective than either drug given alone.

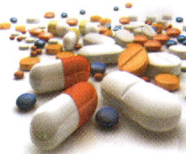

TABLE 2.18: Features of protease inhibitors

Drug	Dose	Special features and Side-Effects
Atazanavir (ATV)	• Given once daily 300 mg with 100 mg of ritonavir taken just before food.	• Administered with light meal improves its absorption. • S/E: Nausea, abdominal discomfort, skin rash, hyperbilirubinemia.
Indinavir (IDV)	• 800 mg TDS (BD if taken with 100 mg RTV)	• Should be taken before meals with plenty of fluids to avoid nephrolithiasis. At least >1.5 L daily. • S/E: Benign hyperbilirubinemia, nephrolithiasis.
Nelfinavir (NFV)	• 750 mg TDS	• Food increases its absorption. • S/E: Diarrhea, nausea, flatulence, rash.
Ritonavir (RTV)	• 600 mg twice daily • 100 mg BD to boost other PIs	• Capsules require refrigeration, tablets do not. • S/E: Diarrhea, nausea, taste alteration, vomiting, anemia.
Saquinavir (SQV)	• 1200 mg TDS on full stomach • 1000 mg BD (with RTV 100 mg).	• Should be taken with high-fat meal or within 2 hours of a full meal. • S/E: Diarrhea, nausea, abdominal discomfort, photosensitivity.
Lopinavir	• Given as twice daily at 400 mg + ritonavir 100 mg with food.	• S/E: Diarrhea, nausea, hyperlipidemia, insulin resistance.

- The triple drug regimen is more effective than double drug regimen.
- Commonly seen adverse effects are nausea, headache, dizziness, rashes, asthenia and GI disturbance.
- Lipodystrophy *(abdominal obesity, buffalo hump with wasting of limbs and face)* and dyslipidemia *(raised triglycerides and cholesterol)* may require hypolipidemic drugs. Diabetes may be exacerbated due to development of insulin resistance. Indinavir crystalizes in urine and increases risk of urinary calculi which can be avoided by taking plenty of fluids.
- Some other PIs are **fosamprenavir (FPV), darunavir** and **tipranavir (TPV).**
- Common features of inhibitors are given in Table 2.18.

Entry (Fusion) Inhibitors

Enfuvirtide

- *Enfuvirtide* is a fusion inhibitor.
- HIV fuses its membrane with that of the host cell to enter into the cell. This is accomplished by changes in the conformation of the viral transmembrane glycoprotein gp-41, which occurs when HIV binds to the host cell surface. *Enfuvirtide* is a polypeptide that binds to gp-41 and prevents the conformational change. This prevents fusion of the two membranes and entry of the virus into the cell.
- *Enfuvirtide* is not active against HIV-2 infection.
- It is administered by SC route twice daily.
- It is used less frequently due to its cost, pain on injection site and formation of local nodules.

CCR5 Receptor Inhibitor

Maraviroc

- Maraviroc is an entry inhibitor.
- It is an anti- HIV drug which targets the host cell CCR5 receptor and blocks it.

> **CCR5** is a chemokine receptor, which is present on the cell membrane of CD4 of host cell. The globular glycoprotein gp120 of the HIV attaches to CCR5 to gain entry into the host cell.

- Attachment of the virus and subsequent entry of viral genome into the cell is blocked.
- It is given orally and well tolerated.
- Since it blocks one of the human chemokine receptors, there is concern about impaired immune surveillance and increased risk of infection/malignancy.

Integrase Inhibitors

(Raltegravir, Elvitegravir and Dolutegravir)

Mechanism of action

CCR5 is a chemokine receptor, which is present on the cell membrane of CD4 of host cell. The globular glycoprotein gp120 of the HIV attaches to CCR5 to gain entry into the host cell Figure 2.9.

- The HIV-Integrase, integrates the proviral DNA with the DNA of host cell.
- This integration is must for the production of viral proteins.

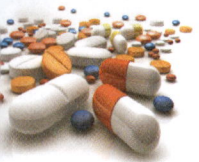

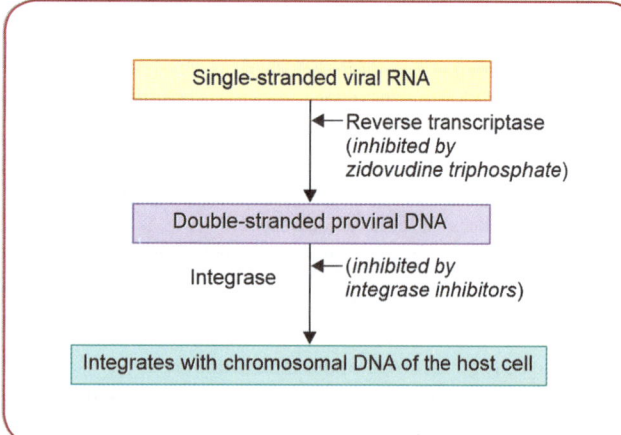

FIG. 2.9: Mechanism of action of integrase inhibitors

- Integrase inhibitors block this step by inhibiting the integrase enzyme.
- Raltegravir is an orally active drug and is effective against HIV-1 and HIV-2 infection.
- Along with two NRTIs, raltegravir is also a component of initial triple drug regimen. It is usually well tolerated with mild and non-specific myopathy in some patients.
- It is given in a dose of 200 mg twice daily.
- Some other integrase inhibitors are Elvitegravir and Dolutegravir.

HIV Treatment Principles and Guidelines

- The Monotherapy for HIV infection is strictly contraindicated.
- Whenever indicated, a combination of three or more anti-retroviral drugs [ARVs] is employed which is called 'Highly active antiretroviral therapy' (HAART).

When to Start Antiretroviral Therapy

- The best time to initiate anti- HIV therapy remains uncertain. Some guidelines are:
  - CD4 cell count is the major determinant of initiating therapy in asymptomatic cases.
  - ART should be started before the immune system is precariously damaged and the patient becomes ill or develops opportunistic infection.*
- Long-term clinical benefit has been demonstrated in asymptomatic cases with reasonable immune competence (CD4 cell count > 350/μL).
- Increased mortality occurs when treatment begins after CD4 count has fallen below 200/μL, and response to anti-HIV drugs is suboptimal.
- As per WHO guidelines, the optimum response to any regimen is reduction of plasma HIV-RNA to undetectable levels (<50 copies/μL) within 6 months.

The US Department of Health and Human Services Guidelines (2010)

It recommends instituting ART to:

- All symptomatic HIV disease patients.
- Asymptomatic patients when the CD4 cell count dips below 350/dL .
- All HIV patients co-infected with HBV/HCV requiring treatment.
- All pregnant HIV positive women.
- All patients with HIV-nephropathy.

In addition to above, the current NACO guidelines give priority in treatment to:

- All HIV-positive persons in WHO-clinical stage 3 and 4.
- All persons who tested HIV positive 6–8 years ago.
- Patients with history of pulmonary tuberculosis and/ or Herpes zoster.
- HIV infected partners of AIDS patients.
- All HIV positive children <15 years of age.

*In developed countries some authorities now recommend initiating ART in asymptomatic subjects at CD4 count < 500/ μL, and not wait till it falls below 350/μL.

Therapeutic Regimens

Whenever treatment is started, it should always be aggressive (HAART) with at least three anti-HIV drugs of different class.

First-line antiretroviral regimens as recommended by NACO are:

Preferred regimen

Lamivudine + Zidovudine + Nevirapine

Alternative regimens

- Lamivudine + Zidovudine + Efavirenz
- Lamivudine + Stavudine + Efavirenz
- Lamivudine + Stavudine + Nevirapine

Other options

- Lamivudine + Tenofovir + Nevirapine
- Lamivudine + Tenofovir + Efavirenz
- Lamivudine[3] + Zidovudine + Tenofovir

- Stavudine is substituted for Zidovudine if patient is anemic.
- Tenofovir is included when there is toxicity or other contraindication to both Zidovudine and Stavudine.
- NRTI regimen is only for patients unable to tolerate both Nevirapine and Efavirenz.

Prophylaxis of HIV Infection

Post-exposure Prophylaxis (PEP)

- **Aim of PEP:** The aim of PEP is to abort the infection before replication and dissemination of virus.

Contd...

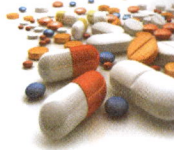

- **Whom to be given:**
  - Doctors, nurses, health care workers.
  - Any other individuals, who gets accidental exposure to HIV infection.
  - Whosoever gets accidentally exposed to the risk of HIV infection by needle-stick or other sharp injury *or* contact with blood/biological fluid of HIV patients *or* accidently HIV positive blood transfusion.
- **When to start:**
  - Ideally, PEP should be started as early as possible after the exposure.
  - Some guidelines suggest that, if the person reports late, it can also be started within 15 days of exposure.
- **When not to be given:** PEP is not necessary when the contact is only with intact skin, or with intact mucous membrane by only a few drops for short duration.
- **Regimens for Post Exposure Prophylaxis as recommended by NACO**

(Based upon magnitude of risk of HIV transmission)

Basic (2 drug) regimen (for low risk)*	
Zidovudine 300 mg Lamivudine 150 mg	Twice daily for 4 weeks

Expanded (3 drug) regimen (for high risk)**	
Zidovudine 300 mg ⎫ Lamivudine 150 mg ⎬ Indinavir 800 mg (or another PI)	Twice daily + All for 4 weeks Thrice daily

*Low risk:
- When the source is HIV positive, but asymptomatic with low HIV-RNA titer and high CD4 cell count.
- Exposure is through mucous membrane, or superficial scratch, or through thin and solid needle.

** High risk:
- When the source is symptomatic AIDS patient with high HIV-RNA titer or low CD4 count.
- Exposure is through major splash or large area of contact with mucous membrane or abraded skin for longer duration or puncture injury with blood stained needle.

Prophylaxis after Sexual Exposure

Though, there is no data to evaluate the value of prophylaxis after sexual exposure, the same regimen as for needle stick injury may be used.

Perinatal HIV Prophylaxis

HIV may be transmitted from the mother to the fetus/neonate through:
- The placenta
- During delivery [Maximum risk >66%]
- By breastfeeding.

As per current recommendations:
- All HIV positive women, who are not on ART, should be put on the standard three drug ART, which should be continued through delivery and into the postnatal period. The first line NACO regimen for pregnant women is: **Zidovudine + Lamivudine + Nevirapine.** This regimen prevents vertical transmission of HIV to the neonate as well as provides benefit to mother's own health.
- In HIV-positive women who are not taking ART, Zidovudine (300 mg BD) started during 2nd trimester and continued through delivery to postnatal period, with treatment of the neonate for 6 weeks has been found to reduce mother-to-child transmission by two-third.
- Even if not started earlier, AZT administered during labour and then to the infant is also substantially protective.
- Breastfeeding by HIV-positive mother is contraindicated, because it carries substantial risk of transmission to the infant.

Drug Interactions

- The concomitant use of antiviral agents with hepatic and renal toxic drugs should be avoided or closely monitored. For example, zidovudine with isoniazid, zidovudine with amphotericin-B.

Nursing Implications

- **Anti-viral agents**
  - Patients and their family members should be counselled and educated about the transmission modes and precautions of HIV/AIDS, various types of hepatitis, herpes and other viral diseases.
  - Hepatic and renal function should be monitored.
  - Nurse should adopt the 'universal precautionary measures' while taking care of the infected patients.
  - Biomedical waste of infected patients should be discarded properly.

ANTIFUNGAL DRUGS

The infections caused by the fungi are known as fungal infection or mycosis. The persons with normal immunological functions rarely get fungal infections. A variety of environmental and physiological conditions such as inhalation of fungal spores, diabetes, AIDS, over use of antibiotics and anti-cancer treatment can contribute to fungal infections. Fungal infections of the skin is the fourth most common skin disease.

The fungal infection can be classified as superficial and deep mycosis (Table 2.19).

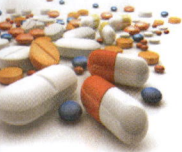

TABLE 2.19: Classified of fungal infections

Superficial mycosis	Deep [systemic] mycosis

• Dermatophytosis
  ▪ Epidermatophyton
  ▪ Trichophyton
  ▪ Microsporum
• Candidiasis
• *P. versicolor*
	• Candidiasis
	• Blastomycosis
	• Histoplasmosis
	• Cryptococcosis
	• Aspergillosis
	• Sporotrichosis
	• Coccidioidomycosis
	• Mucormycosis

CLASSIFICATION OF ANTIFUNGAL DRUGS

- *Antifungal Antibiotics*
  - **Polyenes:** Nystatin, Amphotericin B and Hamycin.
  - **Echinocandins:** Micafungin, Caspofungin and Anidulafungin.
  - **Heterocyclic benzofuran:** Griseofulvin.
- **Azoles**
  - **Imidazoles**
    Topical: Miconazole, Clotrimazole, Oxiconazole and Econazole.
    Systemic: Ketoconazole.
  - **Triazoles (systemic):** Fluconazole, Itraconazole, Luliconazole, Posaconazole and Voriconazole.
- **Allylamine:** Terbinafine and Butenafine, etc.
- **Other topical agents:** Butenafine, Tolnaftate, Benzoic acid, Quiniodochlor, Ciclopiroxolamine, Selenium sulfide, etc.

ANTIFUNGAL ANTIBIOTICS

Polyenes Antibiotics

Due to their highly double-bonded structure, these drugs have been named aspolyenes antibiotics.

All have common mechanism of action as given in Figure 2.10.

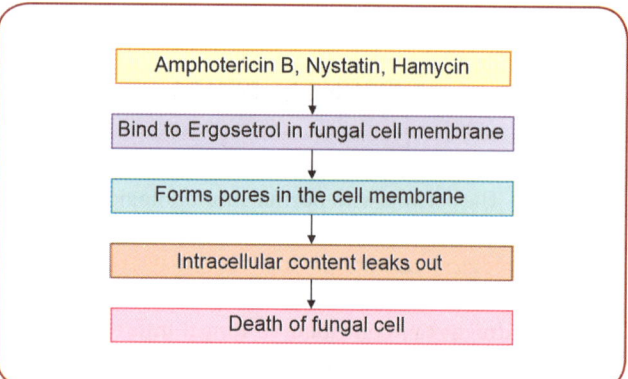

FIG. 2.10: Mechanism of action of polyenes antibiotics

Amphotericin B

It is obtained from the *Streptomyces nodosus*. It is a wide spectrum anti-mycotic drug and also effective against *leishmania* (protozoa).

Pharmacokinetics

- It is not absorbed orally. It is usually given by intravenous route.
- The volume of distribution is good with >90% of plasma protein binding.
- The metabolism occurs in the liver and excretion through liver and bile.
- The plasma t½ is 15 days.
- It does not penetrate blood brain barrier.
- Sometimes it is given orally for the treatment of intestinal candidiasis. There, it acts topically on the intestinal mucosa only as no absorption occurs.

Adverse effects

- It is most toxic of all antifungal agents [dose or formulation dependent].
- *Acute drug reaction* during infusion may occur. It consists of chills, fever, aches and pains. Premedication with IV paracetamol /hydrocortisone or both can be given to reduce the incidence of reactions.
- *Long-term toxicity* in the Nephrotoxicity is the most important long-term toxic effect.
- Thrombophlebitis of the injected vein can also occur.
- **Anemia:** Most patients develop reversible anemia, which is due to bone marrow depression.
- **CNS toxicity:** Occurs only on intrathecal injection—headache, vomiting, nerve palsies, etc.

Indications and dose

- Systemic mycoses such as mucormycosis, aspergillosis, cryptococcosis, spitotrichosis. It is highly effective intravenously used anti-fungal agent.
- Febrile neutropenia.

- Liposomal amphotericin B has been produced to improve tolerability of IV infusion of amphotericin B, reduce its toxicity and achieve targeted delivery. It consists of 10% amphotericin B incorporated in uniform-sized (60–80 nM) unilamellar liposomes made up of lecithin and other biodegradable phospholipids.
- The special features of this preparation are:
  - It produces milder acute reaction on IV infusion.
  - It can be used in patients not tolerating infusion of conventional amphotericin B formulation.

Contd...

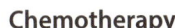

- It has lower nephrotoxicity.
- It causes minimal anemia.
- It delivers amphotericin B particularly to reticuloendo-thelial cells in liver and spleen—especially valuable for kala azar and in immunocompromised patients.
- The liposomal-amphotericin B produces equivalent blood levels, has similar clinical efficacy with less acute reaction and renal toxicity than conventional preparation.
- It can be infused at higher rates (3–5 mg/kg/day), but is many times costlier than conventional amphotericin B.

- Liposomal amphotericin B is specifically indicated for empirical therapy in antibiotics resistance febrile neutropenia, critically ill deep mycosis cases and in kala azar.

- Leishmaniasis.
- Topically used for oral, vaginal and cutaneous candidiasis and otomycosis.

  It is given orally in a dose of 50–100 mg QID for intestinal moniliasis and in infusion form in a dose of 0.3–0.5 mg/kg. The drug is dissolved in 5% dextrose and infused over four hours for other systemic fungal infections.

Nystatin

- It is obtained from *Streptomyces noursei.*
- Similar to amphotericin B in antifungal action and other properties.
- Only topically used as no absorption occurs from GIT when given orally.
- It is used to treat oral thrush, corneal, conjunctival, vaginal and cutaneous candidiasis in a dose of 1 Lac U tablet QID for 5–7 days.
- Utilizing its property of poor oral absorption, it can be given orally for monilial diarrhea and intestinal candidiasis for topical action in a dose of 5 Lac U TDS (1 mg = 2000 U). This does not cause systemic toxicity.
- Most common side effects are nausea and bad taste in mouth.

Hamycin

- It is similar to nystatin in all properties.
- It is used topically for oral thrush, cutaneous candidiasis, monilial, trichomonas vaginitis and otomycosis by *Aspergillus.*

Echinocandins

These are a new class of potent semi-synthetic antifungal antibiotics.

Caspofungin

- Caspofungin is the first and prototype member of the echinocandins class.
- It inhibits the synthesis of β-1, 3-glucan, due to which the fungal cell wall is weakened. Weakening of the cell wall by caspofungin leads to osmotic susceptibility of fungal cell.
- It is not absorbed orally, hence given by intravenous route only.
- The plasma t½ is 10 hours.
- It is used in deep and invasive candidiasis, esophageal candidiasis and salvage therapy of non-responsive invasive aspergillosis.
- It is given in intravenous infusion in a loading dose of 70 mg then 50 mg daily.
- *Micafungin* and *Anidulafungin* are the other echinocandins with similar properties.
- **Dose of Micafungin:**
  - Oesophageal candidiasis: 150 mg/ day,
  - Candidemia 100 mg/day and
  - For prophylaxis of fungal infection 50 mg/day.
- **Dose of Anidulafungin:**
  - Oesophageal candidiasis: Loading dose 100 mg IV, then 50 mg OD for 14 days,
  - Candidemia: Loading dose 200 mg IV, then 100 mg OD for 14 days.

Heterocyclic Benzofuran

Griseofulvin

- Griseofulvin is fungistatic for most dermatophytes.
- It is obtained from *Penicillium griseofulvum.*
- Griseofulvin interferes with mitosis due to which multinucleated and stunted fungal hyphae are produced. The drug gets deposited in the newly forming skin by binding to keratin and protects it from fungi.

Pharmacokinetics

- Griseofulvin is given orally and absorption is facilitated by taking it with fatty diet. The micronized/ultramicrofine forms are better absorbed.
- The metabolism occurs in liver and excretion through kidneys.
- The plasma t½ is 24 hours. It persists for weeks in skin and keratin.
- Griseofulvin gets concentrated in skin, hair and nails (in keratin forming cells).

Side effects

Commonly seen adverse effects are headache, gestrointestinal intolerance and gynecomastia.

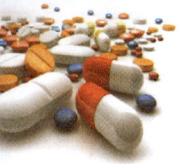

Dose

125–250 mg QID with fatty meals and the duration depends upon the site of infection.

- Scalp: 4 weeks
- Palm, soles: 6–8 weeks
- Finger nails: 6–8 months
- Toe nails:10–12 months

Indications

- Dermatophytosis.
- Onychomycosis.
- Athletes' foot.

AZOLES

- Azoles are the most extensively used antifungal agents.
- These have broad spectrum of activity with greater efficacy with least side effects.
- Imidazoles and Triazoles have similar mechanism of action.

Mechanism of Action

- These inhibit ergosterol synthesis and produce membrane abnormalities in the fungus.
- The cell growth of fungus is inhibited and finally it leads to fungal cell death.
- These have lower affinity for mammalian CYP450 enzymes and lesser propensity to inhibit mammalian sterol synthesis; hence, these are least toxic for human cells.

Common Drugs

Triazoles (Systemic)

Fluconazole, Itraconazole, luliconazole, posaconazole and voriconazole.

Imidazoles

- **Topical:** Miconazole, clotrimazole, oxiconazole and econazole.
- **Systemic:** Ketoconazole.

Clotrimazole

- It is used for oral, cutaneous and vaginal candidiasis, otomycosis and Athletes' foot.
- The effect of single application in vagina last for 7 days, hence, preferred in vaginitis.
- For oropharyngeal candidiasis, 10 mg troche of clotrimazole is allowed to dissolve in the mouth, given 3–4 times a day, or the lotion/gel is applied/swirled in the mouth for as long as possible.

- It has poor efficacy in tinea capitis (scalp) and tinea unguium (nails).
- Clotrimazole is well tolerated except local irritation with stinging and burning sensation occurs in some patients. No systemic toxicity occurs.
- Available as 1% lotion, mouth paint, cream, powder and 100 mg vaginal tab.

Econazole

- It is similar to clotrimazole in all respects with additional higher penetration in superficial layers of the skin.
- It is highly effective in dermatophytosis, otomycosis and oral thrush.
- It is inferior toclotrimazole in the treatment of vaginitis.
- It is available as ointment 1% and vaginal tablet 150 mg.

Miconazole

- Miconazole is more efficacious than clotrimazole for tinea, pityriasis versicolor, otomycosis, cutaneous/vulvovaginal candidiasis and onychomycosis.
- It has good penetrating power. Hence, even a single application on skin acts for a few days.
- No systemic adverse effects except slight irritation (*after cutaneous application*) are seen.
- In comparison to clotrimazole, a higher incidence of vaginal irritation is reported and even pelvic cramps can be experienced by some patients.
- It is available as 2% gel, 2% vaginal gel, 2% ointment and lotion, 2% powder and solution form, 1% ear drops and 100 mg vaginal ovules.

Oxiconazole

- Oxiconazole is effective in vaginal candidiasis, tinea and other dermatophytic infections.
- This is for topical application only and some patients may experience local irritation with its use.
- It is available as oxiconazole 1% with benzoic acid 0.25% cream/lotion for application once or twice daily.

Ketoconazole (KTZ)

- It is the first orally effective broad-spectrum antifungal drug.
- It is used both orally and by topical route. The oral absorption increases at lower pH.
- The metabolism occurs in liver and excretion via kidneys as well as feces.
- Its t½ varies from 1½–6 hours.
- It is given in a dose of 200 mg OD or BD in both dermatophytosis and deep mycosis. It is highly effective

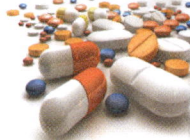

in seborrhea of scalp, dandruff, skin and vaginal fungal infections.

- It is available as 200 mg tablet 2% ointment, 2% shampoo (for dandruff), 2% cream and 2% lotion.
- KTZ is used in large doses in drug induced Cushing's syndrome as a therapeutic agent. (At large doses, it inhibits the biosynthesis of adrenal and gonadal steroidal hormones).
- When the drug is used for a few weeks, it decreases androgen production from testes, and displaces testosterone from protein binding sites. The major side effects which may appear are alopecia, gynecomastia, oligozoospermia and loss of libido.
- Due to suppression of estradiol synthesis in females, menstrual irregularities can occur in some patients.

Fluconazole

- Fluconazole is the most commonly used oral antifungal agent these days due to its higher efficacy, easy dosage schedule and minimal side effect profile.
- It has wide spectrum of activity as compared to ketoconazole.
- It is effective in normal and even immunocompromised patients.

Pharmacokinetics

- It is well absorbed orally and the oral bioavailability is nearly 94%.
- The absorption remains unaffected by food or gastric pH.
- Its fungicidal concentrations are achieved in nails, vagina and saliva.
- It attains good concentration in brain and CSF.
- The t½ is 25–30 hours and excretion occurs via kidneys.

Side Effects

- Dose and duration dependent adverse effects are headache, nausea, vomiting, abdominal pain and rash.
- It is not recommended in pregnancy and lactating mothers, as the safety has not been established yet .

Indications and Dose

- **Tinea infections and cutaneous candidiasis:** 150 mg weekly for 4 weeks.
- **Vaginal candidiasis:** 150 mg single dose [both partners]
- **Oropharyngeal and esophageal candidiasis:** 100 mg/day for 2–3 weeks.
- **Disseminated candidiasis, cryptococcal/coccidioidal. meningitis:** 200–400 mg/day for 4–12 weeks or longer.
- **Fungal keratitis:** 0.3% eye drops.

In AIDS patients with fungal meningitis, initial treatment is given with IV fluconazole/amphotericin B followed by long-term oral fluconazole maintenance therapy in a dose of 200–400 mg daily for 4–12 weeks durations or may be required for longer period.
Fluconazole is ineffective in aspergillosis and mucormycosis.

Itraconazole

Itraconazole has a broader spectrum of activities than KTZ or fluconazole. It is fungistatic, but effective in immunocompromised patients. It is preferred over KTZ as it does not affect the steroidal hormone synthesis.

Pharmacokinetics

- It is given both orally and intravenously.
- The absorption increases by food and low gastric pH. Fatty meals and drugs that reduce the gastric acidity [antacid/PPI/H_2 blockers] decrease the absorption.
- The metabolism occurs in liver and excretion occurs via feces.
- The plasma t½ varying from 30–64 hours.
- High concentration is attained in vaginal mucosa, skin and nails, but penetration into cerebrospinal fluid is poor.

Side Effects

- Commonly seen side effects are headache, dizziness and pruritus.
- Gastric intolerance may occur at doses >400 mg/day.
- Transient hepatitis and hypokalemia are some of the uncommon side effects.

Indications and Dose

- Vaginal candidiasis: 200 mg once daily, orally 3 days.
- Dermatophytosis: 100–200 mg OD for 7–15 days: more effective than griseofulvin, but less effective than fluconazole.
- Onychomycosis: 200 mg daily for 3 months.

In onychomycosis, an intermittent pulse regimen of 200 mg BD for 1 week each month for 3 months is equally effective. Relapses have occurred after Itraconazole therapy, though it remains in the nails for few months after completion of the course.

- Other uses are, histoplasmosis, blastomycosis, sporo-trichosis paracoccidioidomycosis, chromomycosis and aspergillosis in a dose of 200 mg daily for 3 months.
- In systemic aspergillosis, it may be used as a 'follow-on' therapy after the infection is controlled by amphotericin B preparation.

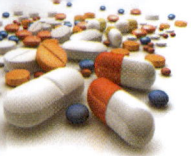

Voriconazole

- Voriconazole is a second generation broad pectrum triazole.
- It is given for difficult to treat fungal infections like invasive aspergillosis and fluconazole resistant candida induced disseminated infections.
- Serious cases are treated with sequential therapy of voriconazole, i.e., to start with parenteral and to continue with oral voriconazole.
- QTc prolongation and an acute reaction on IV injection are the significant adverse effects.
- It is given orally in a dose of 200 mg twice daily empty stomach or one hour after meals. Intravenously in a dose of 6 mg/kg, then 3–4 mg/kg twice daily.

Posaconazole

- Posaconazole is the only azole which has shown efficacy in mucormycosis.
- It is indicated for difficult to treat fungal infections. Because of its high cost and limited experience, it is reserved for non-responsive cases of aspergillosis and invasive candidiasis.
- It is given in a dose of 200 mg QID or 400 mg BD with fatty meals preferably.

Luliconazole

Luliconazole is used topically as 1% cream for the treatment of athletes' foot, tinea cruris (dhobi itch) and ringworm caused by dermatophytes.

Allylamine

Terbinafine

Terbinafine is a new synthetic allylamine. It is fungicidal and better than azoles which are fungistatic. It is active both orally and topically against dermatophytes and candida.

Mechanism of Action

- It inhibits 'squalene epoxidase' enzyme non-competitively.
- Accumulation of squalene within fungal cells is responsible for the fungicidal action.
- The mammalian squalene epoxidase enzyme is inhibited only by 1000-fold higher concentration of terbinafine.

squalene epoxidase is an early step enzyme in ergosterol biosynthesis by fungi.

Pharmacokinetics

- It is well absorbed by oral route, the oral bioavailability is 75%, while 5% or less is absorbed from unbroken skin.
- It strongly binds with the plasma proteins and widely distributed in tissues.

- It has high affinity for keratin. Therefore, it is concentrated in sebum, stratum corneum of skin and into the nail plates.
- The metabolism occurs in liver and excretion via kidneys.
- The plasma t½ is after a single dose of 11–16 hours but is prolonged to 10 days after repeated dosing.

Adverse Effects

- The mild side effects are gastric upset, rashes and taste disturbances.
- Topical terbinafine can cause erythema, itching, dryness, irritation, urticaria and rashes.

Indications and Dose

- **Localized tinea pedis/cruris/corporis and pityriasis versicolor:** Topical application of 1% cream given BD for 2-4 weeks.
- **Onychomycosis:** Oral 250 mg OD for 3–6 months.
- **Cutaneous and mucosal candidiasis:** Oral 250 mg OD for 2–4 weeks.

TOPICAL ANTIFUNGAL AGENTS

These drugs are used for Dermatophytosis. These drugs are summarized in Table 2.20.

Drug Interactions

- Aminoglycosides, vancomycin and other nephrotoxic drugs enhance the renal impairment caused by amphotericin-B and also increase the metabolism of warfarin.
- The antifungal decreases the effectiveness of oral contraceptives.
- Phenobarbitone may be a cause of failure of griseofulvin therapy.
- Griseofulvin may cause disulfiram-like reaction.
- The oral absorption of ketoconazole is reduced if given concomitantly with proton pump inhibitors H$_2$ blockers, and antacids.
- Rifampin, phenobarbitone, carbamazepine and phenytoin induce ketoconazole metabolism and reduce its efficacy.
- Fluconazole increases the plasma levels of phenytoin cyclosporine, zidovudine and sulfonylureas.

Nursing Implications

- **Anti-fungal drugs**
  - Patient should be encouraged to take the full course of treatment.
  - Nurse should educate the patient about the maintenance of proper hygiene to prevent recurrence of infections.
  - As the amphotericin-B is photosensitive, due precaution should be taken while administering the infusion.
  - Amphotericin-B infusion and infusion-line should be covered with some opaque material.

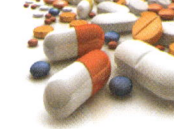

TABLE 2.20: Topical antifungal agents

Drug	Preparation	Special features
Tolnaftate	1% lotion, 1% cream	• Used for tinea cruris and tinea corporis for 1–3 weeks • Less effective in hyperkeratinized lesions • Used in combination with salicylic acid (keratolytic action) in hyperkeratinized lesions for better efficacy
Ciclopirox olamine	1% topical, 1% lotion, 1% cream	• Used for tinea infections, pityriasis versicolor and dermal candidiasis • Onychomycosis [as nail lacquer] • Vaginal candidiasis
Undecylenic acid	2.5% ointment Zinc undecenoate 8%	• Fungistatic and inferior to above two • Used for tinea pedis, nappy rash and tinea cruris
Benzoic acid	As a constituent of Whitfield's ointment (5% Benzoic acid with 3% salicylic acid)	• Used as Whitfield's ointment in hyperkeratotic lesions [salicylic acid acts as keratolytic agent]
Butenafine	1% cream	• Similar to terbinafine in mechanism of action but used only topically • Effective in tinea cruris/corporis/pedis
Quiniodochlor	3%, 4%, 8% cream	• Indicated in the treatment of furunculosis, pityriasis versicolor dermatophytosis, mycosis barbae, seborrheic dermatitis, infected eczema • Vaginal creams for monilial and trichomonas vaginitis • As luminal amebicide [by oral route]
Sodium thiosulfate	20% solution	• It is active against *Malassezia furfur* causing pityriasis versicolor
Selenium sulfide	2.5% suspension in shampoo based	• Used as anti-dandruff shampoo • It is active against *Malassezia furfur* causing pityriasis versicolor • *It is irritant to eye and unpleasant odor*

ANTI-TUBERCULAR THERAPY (ATT)

- Tuberculosis is a chronic granulomatous infectious disease.
- The causative organism is *Mycobacterium tuberculosis*, which is an acid-fast bacillus.
- In India, approximately 1000 people die from TB every day. In India, the control and treatment of TB is covered under a National programme called '*The Revised National Tuberculosis Control Programme* (RNTCP)', in which free and full course of treatment is provided to all TB cases.
- RNTCP was launched in 1997, and its treatment guidelines were further revised in 2010.
- Government of India has declared TB to be a notifiable disease in 2012, so that any clinician, who treats a TB patient, has to notify it to the Government.

According to their clinical utility, the anti-tubercular drugs have been classified as follows (Table 2.21):

- **First line anti-tubercular drugs:** These drugs are highly effective with low toxicity profile. These drugs are the first choice drugs and are used in routine. These drugs are always given in combinations for therapeutic purpose.
- **Second line anti-tubercular drugs:** These drugs have medium anti-tubercular efficacy. The toxic effects of these drugs appear due to the longer duration of anti-tubercular therapy. These drugs are used as reserve drugs and always given in different combinations with first line drugs.

ISONIAZID (ISONICOTINIC ACID HYDRAZIDE, H)

- **Isoniazid (INH)** is an essential component of all antitubercular regimens.
- It is primarily a tuberculocidal drug. It kills the fast multiplying organisms rapidly. The dormant organisms are inhibited only.

TABLE 2.21: Classification of anti-tubercular drugs

First line drugs		Second line drugs	
Rifampin (R)	Rifabutin	Fluoroquinolones	Injectable drugs
Isoniazid (H)	Thiacetazone	Moxifloxacin	Kanamycin
Ethambutol (E)	Ethionamide Prothionamide	Ciprofloxacin	Amikacin
Pyrazinamide (Z)	Cycloserine	Ofloxacin	Capreomycin
Streptomycin (S)	Para-aminosalicylic acid	Levofloxacin	

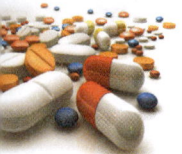

- It acts both on extracellular as well as intracellular TB (bacilli present within macrophages), and is equally active both in acidic and alkaline medium.

Mechanism of Action

- INH acts by inhibiting the synthesis of mycolic acids in the mycobacterial cell wall.
- The mycobacterial cell wall is composed as fatty acid known as mycolic acids.
- Inhibiting mycolic acid leads to a disruption in the mycobacterial cell wall and consequently cell death.
- INH has good resistance preventing action also.

Pharmacokinetics

- Isoniazid is readily absorbed after oral administration.
- Absorption is impaired if it is taken with food, particularly high-fatty meals.
- The drug diffuses into all body fluids, cells, and caseous material (*necrotic tissue resembling cheese that is produced in tuberculous lesions*).
- The cerebrospinal fluid concentration attained is equal to that in plasma.
- The metabolism occurs in liver and excretion occurs via kidneys.

Adverse Effects

- It is well tolerated.
- Peripheral neuritis and a variety of neurological manifestation (paresthesias, numbness, mental disturbances, rarely convulsions) are the most important dose-dependent toxic effects.

✔
- Pyridoxine given prophylactically (10 mg/day) prevents the neurotoxicity.
- Prophylactic pyridoxine must be given to diabetics, chronic alcoholics, malnourished, pregnant, lactating and HIV infected patients.
- INH neurotoxicity is treated by pyridoxine 100 mg/day.

- Hepatitis, a major adverse effect, is common in older people, but rare in children. It is due to dose-related damage to hepatocytes and is reversible on stopping the drug.
- Other side effects are lethargy, rashes, fever, acne and arthralgia.

RIFAMYCINS

(Rifampin (Rifampicin, R), Rifabutin, and Rifapentine)

- Rifampicin has broader antimicrobial activity than isoniazid and can be used as part of treatment for several different bacterial infections.

- Rifampicin is a semisynthetic derivative of *Rifamycin*.
- It has bactericidal action on *Mycobacterium tuberculosis* and all its subpopulations. *M. leprae* is also highly sensitive.
- *It is also acts similarly against a number of* Gram-positive and Gram-negative bacteria.
- It acts best on the slow/intermittent dividing bacilli (spurters).
- The cidal effect of rifampicin is similar to INH.
- It shows bactericidal effect on both extracellular and intracellular organisms.
- It has good sterilizing action (*making sputum AFB negative*) and the only drug, which shows cidal effect on persisters.
- It has good resistance preventing action also.

Mechanism of Action

- Rifampicin blocks mycobacterial DNA-dependent RNA polymerase enzyme, which inhibits RNA transcription and leads to bacterial cell death.
- This action is selective to mycobacterium only and not seen in human cells.

Pharmacokinetics

- It is well absorbed orally and the bioavailability is nearly 70%.
- Its absorption decreases when taken with food; hence, it should be taken empty stomach only.
- It is widely distributed in the body and penetrates intracellularly, enters tubercular cavities, caseous masses and placenta.
- It is converted to an active metabolite in liver, which is excreted mainly in bile and to lesser extend in the urine and undergoes enterohepatic circulation.
- It has variable plasma t½ ranging from 2–5 hours.

✔
[Note: Urine, feces, sweat, tears, saliva and other secretions become orange-red in color, so patients should be informed in advance that it is harmless. Tears may even stain soft contact lenses orange-red.]

Adverse Effects

These are similar to INH.
- Hepatitis, a major adverse effect, is dose-related and generally occurs in hepatic impaired patients. It is rarely seen with a dose less than 600 mg/day.
- Jaundice, if occurs, is reversible on discontinuation of the drug.
- Minor adverse reactions are nausea, vomiting, abdominal cramps, flu like syndrome and cutaneous syndrome in which patient presents as flushing, pruritus and rash.

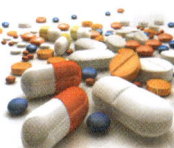

Other uses of Rifampicin

- Rifampicin is used in the treatment of Leprosy.
- It is used in prophylaxis of *Meningococcal* and *H. influenzae* meningitis and carrier state.
- Rifampicin + Doxycycline is the first line therapy of brucellosis.

> **Rifabutin**
> - Rifabutin is a derivative of rifampin, and is preferred for TB patients coinfected with the human immunodeficiency virus (HIV) who are receiving protease inhibitors (PIs) or non-nucleoside reverse transcriptase inhibitors (NNRTIs).

> - Rifabutin is a less potent inducer of cytochrome P450 enzymes as compared to rifampicin. Hence, drug interactions are less.
> - Rifabutin has adverse effects similar to those of rifampicin but can also cause uveitis, skin hyperpigmentation, and neutropenia.

PYRAZINAMIDE (Z)

- Pyrazinamide (Z) is chemically similar to INH.
- It is weakly tuberculocidal and more active in acidic medium.
- It is more lethal to intracellularly located bacilli and to those at sites showing an inflammatory response (pH is acidic at both these locations).
- It is highly effective during the first 2 months of therapy.
- By killing the residual intracellular bacilli it has good 'sterilizing' activity.

Mechanism of Action

- It is not well established, but like INH, it is also converted inside the mycobacterial cell into an active metabolite pyrazinoic acid by an enzyme pyrazinamidase.
- This metabolite gets accumulated in acidic medium and probably inhibits mycolic acid synthesis.

Pharmacokinetics

- Pyrazinamide is absorbed orally and widely distributed. It has good penetration in CSF due to which it is highly useful in meningeal tuberculosis.
- The metabolism occurs in liver and excretion via kidneys.
- The plasma t½ is 6–10 hours.

Adverse Effects

- The dose related side effect is hepatotoxicity.
- Other adverse effects are abdominal distress, hyperuricemia, arthralgia, flushing, rashes, fever and loss of diabetes control.

ETHAMBUTOL (E)

- Ethambutol is a tuberculostatic antitubercular drug.
- It is more active against fast multiplying bacilli.
- It helps the early conversion of sputum positive patients to sputum negative ones when added to the triple drug regimen of RHZ.
- Primarily, it is used to prevent development of drug resistance.

Mechanism of Action

- The exact mechanism of action of ethambutol is unknown.
- Probably, it interferes with the mycolic acid incorporation in mycobacterial cell wall.

Pharmacokinetics

- It is absorbed orally and is widely distributed in all compartments of body.
- It penetrates meninges in completely and is temporarily stored in RBCs.
- The excretion occurs via kidneys through glomerular filtration as well as tubular secretion.
- The plasma t½ is nearly 4 hours.

Adverse Effects

- It has very few side effects.
- The most important dose and duration dependent side effect is Optic neuritis. It causes *loss of visual acuity, color vision and field defects*.
- In color vision defect, there is loss of ability to differentiate between red and green color.
- Hyperuricemia may occur due to interference with urate excretion.

The adverse effects of first line anti-tubercular drugs and their management are given in Table 2.22.

STREPTOMYCIN (S)

- The pharmacology of streptomycin has been already described with aminoglycosides.
- It is the first clinically useful antitubercular drug.
- The tuberculocidal effect is less as compared to INH or Rifampicin.
- It exerts its effect on extracellular bacilli only (because of poor penetration into cells).
- It penetrates tubercular cavities, but does not cross the CSF, and has poor action in acidic medium.
- It has lower margin of safety.
- Ototoxicity and nephrotoxicity are the major side effects like other aminoglycosides.

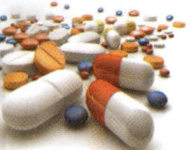

TABLE 2.22: Adverse effects of first line anti-tubercular drugs and their management

Drug	Adverse effects	Comments
Isoniazid	Hepatic enzyme elevation, hepatitis, peripheral neuropathy	Take baseline hepatic enzyme measurements; repeat if abnormal or patient is at risk or symptomatic. Clinically significant interaction with phenytoin and Carbamazepine.
Rifampicin	Hepatitis, GI upset, rash, flu-like syndrome, significant interaction with several drugs	Take baseline hepatic enzyme measurements and CBC; Repeat if abnormal or patient is at risk or symptomatic. Warn patient that urine and tears may turn red-orange in color.
Ethambutol	Optic neuritis with blurred vision, red-green color blindness	Establish baseline visual acuity and color vision; test monthly.
Pyrazinamide	Nausea, hepatitis, hyperuricemia, rash, arthralgia, gout (rare)	Take baseline hepatic enzymes and uric acid measurements; repeat if abnormal or patient is at risk or symptomatic.

- Streptomycin is used in addition to other anti-tubercular therapy (ATT) in directly observed treatment, short-course (DOTs) category-II for a period of two months.
- It is also labeled as a 'supplemental' first line drug.

SECOND LINE ANTI-TUBERCULAR DRUGS

Second line anti-tubercular drugs are more toxic and less efficacious as compared to first line anti-tubercular drugs. These are used when the tubercular bacilli show a resistance to the first line antitubercular drugs or when first line anti–tubercular drugs are not tolerated or contraindicated.

Kanamycin (Km), Amikacin (Am)

- These are tuberculocidal aminoglycosides and very much similar to streptomycin in antitubercular activity, pharmacokinetic properties and adverse effects.
- Many streptomycin resistant and multi-drug resistant strains of M. tuberculosis are sensitive to these drugs.
- During the intensive phase of MDR-TB treatment, one of these drugs is mostly included in the regimen.
- The RNTCP standardized regimen for MDR-TB includes kanamycin due to its lesser cost as compared to amikacin.
- It is administered intramuscularly in an OD dose of 0.75–1.0 g/day (10–15 mg/kg/day).

Capreomycin (Cm)

- It is chemically very different from aminoglycosides, but has similar bactericidal activity against Mycobacterium.
- It is administered by IM. route.
- It is used only as an alternative to Streptomycin and Amikacin resistant M. tuberculosis.
- It is administered intramuscularly in an OD dose of 0.75–1.0 g/day.

Fluoroquinolones

- The pharmacology of fluoroquinolones has been already described.
- The fluoroquinolones are potent oral bactericidal drugs for TB. The preferred ones are moxifloxacin and levofloxacin.
- They have an important place in the treatment of multidrug-resistant tuberculosis as they penetrate cells and kill mycobacteria lodged inside the macrophages.
- The antitubercular doses are:
  - Moxifloxacin–400 mg OD, levofloxacin–750 mg OD, ofloxacin–800 mg OD.

Ethionamide

- This is sulfur containing structural analog of isoniazid that also disrupts mycolic acid synthesis. It acts on both extracellular and intracellular bacilli.
- It is widely distributed in all compartments of the body, including the cerebrospinal fluid.
- The metabolism occurs in liver with plasma t½ of 2–3 hours.
- Adverse effects are anorexia nausea, sulfurous belching, vomiting, hepatotoxicity and peripheral neuritis. Pyridoxine (100 mg/day) can be used to treat the neurological adverse effects.
- Ethionamide is given in escalated dosage scheduled as follows: 250 mg/day, and increased every 5–6 days to reach 750 mg daily (10–15 mg/kg/day). This is done to improve tolerance.

Cycloserine

- This is an orally effective tuberculostatic drug.
- It disrupts d-alanine incorporation into the bacterial cell wall.
- It is well distributed in all compartments of the body, including the cerebrospinal fluid.

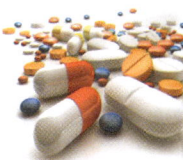

- The only 1/3 fraction in liver and the remaining part is excreted via kidneys in an unchanged form.
- Commonly seen side effects are CNS disturbances like lethargy, anxiety, and suicidal tendency. Therefore, in patients with history of seizure and other mental illness, it is contraindicated.
- Pyridoxine (100 mg/day) can be used to treat the neurological adverse effects.
- It is given in escalated dosage scheduled as follows: Start with 250 mg BD and increase to 750 mg/day, if tolerated.

Para-amino Salicylic acid (PAS)

- PAS acts by the same mechanism as sulfonamides.
- It is tuberculostatic and one of the least active drugs.
- It is absorbed completely by the oral route and distributed all over body except in cerebrospinal fluid.
- Some of the common side effects are anorexia, nausea, epigastric pain, rashes, fever, malaise, hypokalemia, goiter, liver dysfunction and rarely blood dyscrasias.
- PAS is used only in resistant tuberculosis when one of the tuberculocidal drugs or static drugs cannot be used.
- PAS is given in divided doses of 10–12 g daily.

TREATMENT OF TUBERCULOSIS

- In the previous days, the full treatment course for a tuberculosis patient used to be for 9–12 months.
- The therapy of tuberculosis has undergone remarkable changes now.
- The 'conventional' treatment has been replaced by more effective and less toxic 6 months (short course) treatment. Due to shortening of duration of treatment, the *treatment completion rate* has increased.

Short Course Chemotherapy (DOTS)

- After several years of trials, the WHO introduced 6–8 months multidrug 'short course' regimens in 1995 under DOTS program (*Directly Observed Treatment, Short course chemotherapy*).

- In DOTS program, the patients are treated in two phases.
- All regimens have an initial *intensive phase* with 4–5 drugs given for 2–3 months and a *continuation phase* with 2–3 drugs lasting 4–5 months.
- **The aims of intensive phase is:**
  - To kill the Mycobacterium rapidly
  - To bringing about rapid sputum conversion (*from sputum positive to sputum negative)*
  - To provide fast symptomatic relief.
- **The aim of continuation phase is:**
  - To eliminate the remaining bacilli so that relapse does not occur.
- Previously, there used to be three categories of tuberculosis patients for the purpose of treatment under DOTS. These were Category I, Category II and Category III.
- New guidelines with revised categorization of patients were brought out in 2010. According to these guidelines, the category III was merged with category I, and patients of TB are now classified as:
  - *'New cases' or category I patients*
  - *'Previously treated' or category II* patients
  - Drug resistant *MDR-TB patients*

Recommended doses of antitubercular drugs are given in Table 2.23.

New Patients (Category I Patients)

Category wise treatment regimens for tuberculosis are given in Table 2.24.
- The new smear positive TB patients who in the past have never been exposed to anti-TB drugs are called New patients or Category I patients.
- In these type of patients, the intensive phase treatment for two months is started with Four drugs (HRZE) which include three bactericidal drugs. This reduces the risk of bacilli becoming resistant.
- After the intensive phase, the continuation phase is started which includes two highly effective mycobactericidal drugs (HR). This phase is continued for four months, which is enough for effective cure as only few bacilli are left after the intensive phase.

TABLE 2.23: Recommended doses of antitubercular drugs

DRUG	Daily dose mg/kg	Maximum dose	3 times per week dose mg/kg	Daily maximum
Isoniazid (H)	5 (4–6)	300 mg	10 (8–12)	900 mg
Rifampin (R)	10 (8–12)	600 mg	10 (8–12)	600 mg
Pyrazinamide (Z)	25 (20–30)	—	35 (30–40)	—
Ethambutol (E)	15 (15–20)	—	30 (25–35)	—
Streptomycin (S)*	15 (12–18)	—	15 (12–18)	1000 mg

*Patients over 60 years age—10 mg/kg or 500–750 mg/day (IM).
[*Adopted from Treatment of Tuberculosis: Guidelines, 4th edition (2010), WHO, Geneva*]

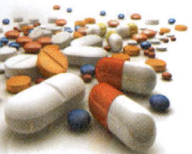

TABLE 2.24: Category wise treatment regimens for tuberculosis

Category	Intensive phase	Continuation phase	Duration (months)	Comment
I **New patient**	2* HRZE daily	4* HRE daily	6*	Optimal
	2 HRZE daily	4 HRE thrice weekly	6	Acceptable if DOT ensured
	2 HRZE thrice weekly	4 HRE thrice weekly	6	Acceptable if DOT ensured, and no HIV coinfection or its risk
II Previously treated patients pending DST result	2 HRZE daily + 1 HRZE daily	5 HRE daily	8	For patient with low/medium risk of MDR-TB (failure, default, etc.)
	Empirical** (Standardized) MDR-regimen	Empirical (Standardized) MDR-regimen	18–24 or till DST result	For patient with high risk of MDR-TB (failure, 2nd default, contact of MDR-TB.

DST—Drug sensitivity testing; DOT—Directly observed therapy
H, R, Z, E, S—Standard codes for isoniazid, rifampin, pyrazinamide, ethambutol and streptomycin, respectively.
*The numerals indicate duration of a phase/total duration in months.
**Empirical (Standardized) MDR regimen is country specific depending upon local data and situation *(adopted from WHO guidelines 2010)*

Previously Treated Patients (Category II Patients)

- The smear positive TB patients who in the past had been exposed to anti-TB drugs, but did not complete the course or took inadequate/irregular medication, or relapsed after responding, or failed to respond run a higher risk of harboring drug resistant (DR) bacilli. These type of patients are included in previously treated or Category II patients.
- In these type of patients, *the intensive phase treatment is started with Five drugs (HRZES)* which include four bactericidal drugs. The 1ˢᵗ line drugs hourZES (5 drugs) are given daily for 2 months and hourZE (4 drugs) for another one month.
- This is followed by the *continuation phase of 3 drugs* (HRE) for the next 5 months.

Multidrug-Resistant (MDR) Tuberculosis

- When the tuberculosis is due to the tubercular bacilli resistant to both INH and rifampicin and may be any number of other first line drug/drugs, it is called multidrug-resistant (MDR) tuberculosis.
- It has a more rapid course with worse outcomes.
- Its treatment requires complex multiple second line drug regimens, which are more expensive, more toxic, and has to be given for longer duration.

General Principles of MDR-TB Treatment

The regimen often includes 5–6 drugs, out of which at least four drugs should be certainly effective as efficacy of some drugs may be uncertain. RNTCP program has specified the regimen for treatment of TB (Table 2.25).

TABLE 2.25: RNTCP regimen for MDR-TB

Intensive phase (6–9 months)	Continuation phase (18 months)
Kanamycin (Km)	Ofloxacin or Levofloxacin
Ofloxacin or Levofloxacin	Ethionamide
Ethionamide (Eto)	Cycloserine
Cycloserine (Cs)	Ethambutol
Pyrazinamide (Z)	
Ethambutol (E)	
+ Pyridoxine 100 mg/day	

Extensively drug-resistant tuberculosis (XDR-TB)

- The MDR-TB cases, which are *also resistant to*
  - Fluroquinolones,
  - *One of the injectable second line drugs* and
  - *May be any number of other drugs*, are called as XDR-TB patients.
- The bacilli are resistant to at least four most effective mycobactericidal drugs, *viz.* H, R, FQs and one of Kanamycin or Amikacin or Capreomycin.
- The extensively drug-resistant tuberculosis (XDR-TB) patients are very difficult to treat.

- Bedaquiline fumarate, a newer anti-tubercular drug has been recently approved by US-food and drug administration (FDA) for multi-drug resistant tuberculosis.
- Pyridoxine 100 mg/day is given to all patients during the whole course of therapy to prevent neurotoxicity of the anti-TB drugs.

✔

Tuberculosis Treatment in Pregnant Women
- The standard 6 months (2HRZE +4HR) regimen can be given to pregnant women with TB *(The WHO and British Thoracic Society recommendations)*.

Contd...

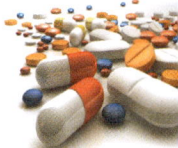

- Streptomycin is contraindicated because it is ototoxic to the fetus.
- Treatment of TB should not be withheld or delayed because of pregnancy.
- All pregnant women being treated with INH should also receive pyridoxine 10–25 mg/day.

Chemoprophylaxis of Tuberculosis

- The aim of chemoprophylaxis is to prevent progression of latent tubercular infection to active disease.
- The standard drug for chemoprophylaxis of TB is Isoniazid (H) 300 mg (10 mg/kg in children) daily for 6 months.

The Candidates for Chemoprophylaxis are as follows:

- Contacts of open cases that show recent Montoux conversion.
- Children with positive Montoux test and a TB patient in the family.
- Neonate of the tubercular mother.
- Patients of leukemia, diabetes, silicosis, or those who are HIV positive but are not anergic, or are on corticosteroid therapy who show a positive Montoux test.
- Patients with old inactive disease who are assessed to have received inadequate therapy.

Corticosteroid Therapy in Tuberculosis

Corticosteroids should not be used in routine in tubercular patients. However, they are used:

In miliary or severe pulmonary TB patients till the antitubercular drugs start acting.

- When patients show sensitivity to antitubercular drugs
- To reduce exudation and to prevent strictures formation in organ TB
- Corticosteroids are contraindicated in intestinal tuberculosis because perforation of intestines remains silent (painless and with poorly localized symptoms).

Precaution: Corticosteroids should always be tapered gradually when the general condition of the patient improves.

Tuberculosis Treatment in Aids Patients

- In case of *M. tuberculosis* infection in HIV patients, drugs used are the same as in non-HIV cases.
- Initial intensive phase therapy with daily hourZE for 2 months is started immediately on the diagnosis of TB.
- It is followed by a continuation phase of hour for 4–7 months (total 6–9 months).
- Thrice weekly regimen is not advised due to chances of relapse among HIV positive patients.
- In addition, the risk of acquiring resistance to Rifampicin is increased as compared to daily treatment.

Bedaquiline

- Bedaquiline fumarate, a newer anti-tubercular drug has been recently approved by US-FDA for multi-drug resistant tuberculosis.
- It is included in the WHO list of essential drugs.

Mechanism of Action

- It inhibits mycobacterial ATP (adenosine 5'-triphosphate) synthase, by binding to subunit c of the enzyme. This enzyme is essential for the production of energy [ATP] in *M. tuberculosis*.

Pharmacokinetics

- It is well absorbed orally with wide distribution in all compartments of body.
- The metabolism occurs in liver and excretion via feces.
- The plasma t½ is approximately 5.5 months.

Indications: Pulmonary MDR TB.

Dosage schedule:

- 400 mg once daily orally for initial two weeks then 200 mg thrice weekly up to 24th week.
- The total duration of treatment is up to 24th week only.

Adverse effects

- Commonly seen adverse effects are, nausea, headache, arthralgia.
- It also leads to QT prolongation and increases liver enzyme levels.

ANTILEPROTIC DRUGS

- Leprosy is also known as Hansen's disease and is caused by *Mycobacterium laprae*, which is related to *Mycobacterium tuberculosis*.
- It primarily affects skin, mucous membranes and nerves.
- It is more prevalent among the lowest socioeconomic population.
- It was considered incurable since ages.
- But now, the fact is that it is completely curable due to availability of highly effective antileprotic drugs.
- The antileprotic drugs (Table 2.26) can cure the disease but not the deformities or defects which have already incurred. The deformities can be corrected to some extent by surgery only.
- In India, Multi-Drug Therapy [MDT] was introduced for the treatment of leprosy as apart of National Leprosy Eradication Program (NLEP) in 1982.

TABLE 2.26: Antileprotic drugs

Drug Class	Drugs
Sulfone	Dapsone (DDS)
Phenazine derivatives	Clofazimine
Antitubercular drugs	Rifampicin and ethionamide
Other antibiotics	Ofloxacin, minocycline, moxifloxacin and clarithromycin

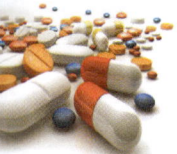

DAPSONE (DDS)

- Dapsone is the oldest, most active and most commonly used drug.
- At very low concentrations, it is leprostatic and at relatively higher concentrations, it is cidal to many other sulfonamide sensitive bacteria.
- Dapsone is active against certain protozoa and shows some anti-inflammatory activity also.

Mechanism of Action

Dapsone is chemically related to sulfonamides and has the same mechanism of action, i.e., inhibition of PABA incorporation into folic acid by folate synthase.

Pharmacokinetics

- It is well absorbed orally with a widely distribution in different body parts but, penetration in CSF is poor.
- It is concentrated in skin (especially lepromatous skin), muscles, liver and kidney. The plasma protein binding is 70%.
- The metabolism occurs in liver and excretion occurs in urine.
- The metabolites undergo *enterohepatic circulation*.
- The plasma t½ is more than 24 hours. Due to retention in tissues and enterohepatic circulation, the elimination may take 1–2 weeks or longer.

Adverse Effects

- Dapsone is generally well tolerated. Some dose related side effects like hemolytic anemia and gastric intolerance can occur in some patients.
- Patients with G-6-PD deficiency are more susceptible to hemolysis at doses >50 mg/day.
- It is contraindicated in severe anemia (Hb <7 g/dL), G-6-PD deficiency and in patients who are hypersensitive to dapsone.

✔
Sulfone Syndrome
This reaction develops 4–6 weeks after starting dapsone therapy. It appears with fever, malaise, lymphadenopathy, desquamation of skin, jaundice, and anemia. This reaction has become frequent after the introduction of MDT and mostly seen in malnourished patients. Some or all of the above symptoms may occur.
The treatment of this syndrome includes
- Stopping dapsone,
- Corticosteroid therapy and
- Supportive measures.

Indications

- Multibacillary and paucibacillary leprosy.
- Other than leprosy: Chloroquine resistant malaria, toxoplasmosis, and *P. jirovecii* infection (in combination with pyrimethamine).

CLOFAZIMINE (CLO)

Clofazimine is a dye with leprostatic and anti-inflammatory properties.

Mechanism of Action

In M. *leprae*, it inhibits the mycobacterial growth by interfering with the template function of DNA, altering the membrane structure and disrupting the mitochondrial electron transport chain.

Pharmacokinetics

- It is absorbed orally (40–70%) and accumulates in macrophages and gets deposited in many tissues including subcutaneous fat.
- The cerebrospinal fluids penetration is poor.
- The plasma t½ is 70 days.
- Dose: 50–100 mg once daily.

Indications

- Leprosy (as a component of multidrug therapy [MDT])
- Lepra reaction (due to its anti-inflammatory property)

Adverse Effects

- Commonly seen side effects are nausea, anorexia, abdominal pain, weight loss, and enteritis with intermittent loose stools.
- One major disadvantage with the use of clofazimine is photosensitivity in which reddish-black discoloration of skin (*specially exposed parts*) occurs. Discoloration of hair, conjunctiva and body secretions cause cosmetic problems. Dryness of skin and itching can also occur.
- Clofazimine should be avoided during early pregnancy and in patients with poor liver or kidney functions.

RIFAMPICIN (R)

The pharmacology of rifampicin has been already described with antitubercular drugs. In addition,
- It is the most potent cidal drug for *M.leprae*.
- The leprosy patients are made noncontagious within 3–7 days of starting therapy with rifampicin as 99.99% *M. leprae* are killed within this period.

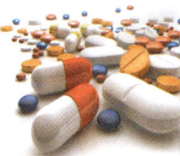

- It is not given alone but has been included in the MDT of leprosy whereby it shortens the duration of treatment and prevents the development of resistance.
- In MDT, rifampicin is given in a 600 mg monthly dose. It is effective and practically non-toxic.
- It should not be given during '*erythema nodosum leprosum*' (ENL) and '*reversal reaction*' in leprosy patients, because it can release large quantities of mycobacterial antigens by inducing rapid bacillary killing.
- It should be avoided in renal and hepatic compromised patients.

FLUOROQUINOLONES

- Many fluoroquinolones like ofloxacin and moxifloxacin are highly effective against *M. leprae*.
- The most commonly used FQ in leprosy is ofloxacin.
- It is cidal to *M. leprae*.
- It is used only when rifampicin is intolerable.
- Dose: 400 mg daily.

MINOCYCLINE

The pharmacology of Minocycline has been already described with tetracyclines. In addition,

- It has good anti leprotic activity, but lesser than rifampicin.
- It penetrates the *M. leprae* as well.
- It is a part of alternative MDT regimens.

TREATMENT OF LEPROSY

- Before starting anti-leprotic treatment, the lesions should be properly diagnosed, identified and classified.
- The most commonly used classification of leprosy was given by Ridley and Jopling in 1966 and leprosy was divided into:
  - Lepromatous (LL)
  - Borderline lepromatous (BL)
  - Borderline (BB)
  - Borderline tuberculoid (BT)
  - Tuberculoid (TT)
- The two extreme types are Tuberculoid (*mild form*) and Lepromatous (*severe form*) (Table 2.27).

For operational purposes, WHO has divided leprosy into:

- **Paucibacillary leprosy (PBL):** Patient has few bacilli and is noninfectious. It includes the TT and BT types.
- **Multibacillary leprosy (MBL):** Patient has large bacillary load and is infectious. It includes the LL, BL and BB types.

WHO reclassified leprosy in 1998 into:

- **Single lesion paucibacillary leprosy (SL PB):** With a solitary cutaneous lesion.

TABLE 2.27: Difference between tuberculoid and lepromatous leprosy

Tuberculoid leprosy (TT)	Lepromatous leprosy (LL)
Anaesthetic patch	Diffuse skin and mucous membrane infiltration, nodules
Cell mediated immunity (CMI) is normal	CMI is absent
Lepromin test—positive, Bacilli rarely found in biopsies	Lepromin test-negative, Skin and mucous membrane lesions teeming with bacilli
Prolonged remissions with periodic exacerbations	Progresses to anaesthesia of distal parts, atrophy, ulceration, absorption of digits, etc.

TABLE 2.28: Multidrug therapy (MDT) of leprosy

Drugs	Multibacillary Leprosy	Paucibacillary Leprosy
Rifampicin	600 mg once in a month (under supervision)	600 mg once in a month (under supervision)
Dapsone	100 mg daily self administered	100 mg daily self administered
Clofazimine	300 mg once a month supervised and 50 mg daily self administered	–
Duration	12 months	6 months

Doses should be reduced suitably for children.

- **Paucibacillary leprosy (PB):** With 2–5 skin lesions. Both SLPB and PB cases are skin smear negative for *M. leprae*.
- **Multibacillary leprosy (MB):** With >6 skin lesions, as well as all smear positive cases.

TABLE 2.29. Classification of leprosy

The classification being followed by NLEP since 2009	
Paucibacillary (PB)	**Multibacillary (MB)**
1-5 skin lesions	6 or more skin lesions
No nerve/only one nerve involvement, + 1–5 skin lesions	>1 nerve involved irrespective of number of skin lesions
Skin smear negative at all sites	Skin smear positive at any one site

Table 2.28 is depicting the multidrug therapy of leprosy. Both type of leprosy reaction are given in Table 2.29.

Alternative Regimens

The alternative regimens are used only in case of rifampin-resistance or when it is not possible to employ the standard MDT regimen.

Some of these regimens are:

- **Intermittent ROM:** <u>R</u>ifampin 600 mg + <u>O</u>floxacin 400 mg + <u>M</u>inocycline 100 mg are given once a month

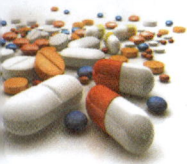

TABLE 2.29: Reactions in leprosy

	Lepra reaction (ENL)	Reversal reaction
Seen in	Lepromatous leprosy	Tuberculoid and borderline lepromatous leprosy
Time of Start	Coincides with institution of chemotherapy and/or any intercurrent infection	Occurs suddenly even after completion of therapy
Cause	Jarisch Herxheimer (Arthus) type of reaction due to release of antigens from the killed bacilli	A manifestation of delayed hypersensitivity to *M. leprae* antigens
Symptoms	Abrupt onset; existing lesions enlarge, become red swollen and painful; several new lesions may appear Malaise, fever and other constitutional symptoms generally accompany and may be marked	Cutaneous ulceration, multiple nerve involvement with swollen, painful and tender nerves, occurs suddenly
Severity	May be mild, severe or life-threatening, i.e., erythema nodosum leprosum (ENL)	Moderately severe form
Treatment	• Temporary discontinuation of dapsone • Clofazimine (200 mg daily) • Prednisolone (40–60 mg/day) • Thalidomide (100–300 mg OD) at bedtime as an alternative to Prednisolone	• Clofazimine (200 mg daily) • Prednisolone (40–60 mg/day) • Thalidomide is ineffective

for 3–6 months for PBL and for 12 or 24 months for MBL cases.

- **Single dose ROM:** A single dose of rifampin + ofloxacin + minocycline was given for single lesion PBL, but this has been discontinued now.
- **Intermittent RMMx:** Moxifloxacin 400 mg + Minocycline 200 mg + Rifampicin 600 mg is given once a month. Total six doses for PBL and 12 doses for MBL are given.

Reactions in Leprosy

- Two types of reactions can occur in the patients of leprosy.
- The reaction occuring on start of treatment is known as *Lepra reaction* and that on completion of therapy is known as *Reversal reaction*.

Drug Interactions

- Absorption of isoniazid is inhibited by aluminium hydroxide.
- Isoniazid is an inhibitor of hepatic enzymes. Hence, it decreases the metabolism of carbamazepine, phenytoin theophylline and warfarin and may increase their blood levels.
- PAS inhibits isoniazid metabolism and prolongs its plasma half-life.
- Rifampicin is a microsomal enzyme inducer. Hence, it decreases the levels of many drugs such as corticosteroids, HIV protease inhibitors, oral contraceptives, warfarin, sulfonylureas, non-nucleoside reverse transcriptase inhibitors, metoprolol, fluconazole, ketoconazole, phenytoin, etc.
- Rifampicin causes failure of oral contraceptives. Hence, patient should be advised to take alternative methods of contraception.

Nursing Implications

- **Anti-tubercular and Anti-leprosy drugs**
  - Educate the patients about taking all the drugs as advised.
  - Educate the patients and their family members about the adverse reactions and instruct them to report to physician if any reactions occur.
  - Patient is advised that discoloration of body secretions is a normal phenomenon with rifampicin.
  - Monitoring of hepatic and renal function test should be done in routine.
  - Patient should be advised to take balanced and protein rich diet.
  - Nurse should boost the morale of leprosy patients.
  - Nurse should be well aware about the treatment of lepra reaction and reversal reaction seen in the patient of leprosy on treatment.
  - Nurse should adopt the 'universal precautionary measures' while taking care of the open tuberculosis patients and the leprosy patients with open lesions.

ANTI-CANCER DRUGS

- Cancer is one of the leading causes of death in the world. In India too, cancer shows an ascending pattern.
- Cancer arises from a single abnormal cell that multiplies and grows progressively (Fig. 2.11). Over the time, these abnormal cells proliferate uncontrollably, invading and damaging surrounding healthy tissues. The host cells are devoid of energy and nutrients at the cost of purposeless proliferation of cancerous cells.

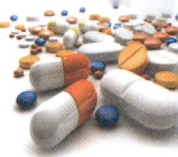

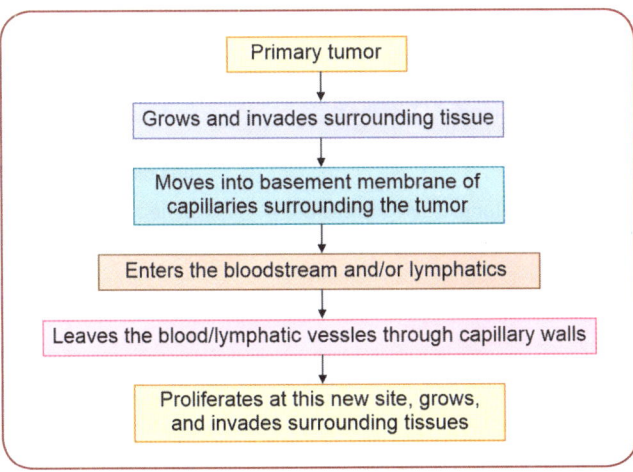

FIG. 2.11: Development of cancer

- In addition, the cancerous cells intrude the normal cells, leading to a loss of normal cellular function.
- Some of the cancer cells remain in a dormant phase. These cells are not sensitive to anti-cancer drugs and can become active at any time causing recurrence.

AIM OF ANTI-CANCER TREATMENT

The anti-cancer drugs have been classified in Table 2.30.

The aim and modalities of treatment of cancer depends on the stage at which the disease has been diagnosed. The different modalities of treatment can be anti-cancer drugs only, anti-cancer drugs in combination with surgery, radiotherapy or immunotherapy in the *combined modality approach.*

Different features of targeted anti-cancer drugs are given in Table 2.31

TABLE 2.30: Classification of anti-cancer drugs

Cytotoxic drugs	
Alkylating agents	Mechlorethamine, cyclophosphamide, ifosfamide, chlorambucil, melphalan, busulfan, carmustine, lomustine, dacarbazine, temozolomide, procarbazine
Platinum analogs	Cisplatin, carboplatin, oxaliplatin
Antimetabolites	• **Folate antagonist:** Methotrexate (Mtx), pemetrexed • **Purine antagonist:** 6-Mercaptopurine (6-MP), 6-Thioguanine (6-TG), azathioprine, fludarabine • **Pyrimidine antagonist:** 5-Fluorouracil (5-FU), capecitabine, cytarabine
Microtubule damaging agents	Vinca alkaloids: Vincristine, vinblastine, vinorelbine Taxanes: Paclitaxel, docetaxel
Topoisomerase-2 inhibitors	Etoposide, tenipocite
Topoisomerase-1 inhibitors	Topotecan, irinotecan
Antibiotics	Actinomycin D (Dactinomycin), doxorubicin, daunorubicin, epirubicin, mitoxantrone, bleomycins, Mitomycin C
Miscellaneous	Hydroxyurea, L-Asparaginase, tretinoin, arsenic trioxide
Targeted drugs	
Tyrosine protein- kinase inhibitors	Imatinib, nilotinib
Endothelial growth factor [EGF] receptor inhibitors	Gefitinib, erlotinib, cetuximab, panitumumab, sorafenib
Angiogenesis inhibitors	Bevacizumab, sunitinib
Proteasome inhibitor	Bortezomib
Unarmed monoclonal antibody	Rituximab, trastuzumab
Hormonal drugs	
Glucocorticoids	Prednisolone and others
Estrogens	Fosfestrol, ethinylestradiol
Selective estrogen receptor modulators	Tamoxifen, toremifene
Selective estrogen receptor down regulators	Fulvestrant
Aromatase inhibitors	Letrozole, anastrozole, exemestane
Antiandrogen	Flutamide, bicalutamide
5-α reductase inhibitor	Finasteride, dutasteride
GnRH analogs	Nafarelin, leuprorelin, triptorelin
Progestins	Hydroxyprogesterone acetate, etc.

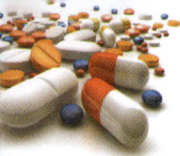

TABLE 2.31: Targeted anti-cancer drugs

Drug	Mechanism of action	Dose	Clinical applications	Acute toxicity	Delayed toxicity
Erlotinib	Inhibits EGFR tyrosine kinase leading to inhibition of EGFR signaling	150-mg tablet daily	Non-small cell lung cancer, pancreatic cancer	Diarrhea	Skin rash, diarrhea, anorexia, interstitial lung disease
Gefitinib	Same as erlotinib	250 mg OD, orally	Non-small cell lung cancer	Hypertension, diarrhea	Same as above
Imatinib	Inhibits Bcr-Abl tyrosine kinase and other receptor tyrosine kinases, including PDGFR, stem cell factor, and c-kit	400–600 mg/day, orally	CML, gastrointestinal stromal tumor (GIST), Philadelphia chromosome-positive ALL	Nausea and vomiting	Fluid retention at ankle and periorbital edema, diarrhea, myalgias, congestive heart failure
Cetuximab	Binds to EGFR and inhibits downstream EGFR signaling; enhances response to chemotherapy and radiotherapy	Single loading dose of 400 mg/m²IV, followed by weekly doses of 250 mg/m² IV for the duration of treatment	Colorectal cancer, head and neck cancer (used in combination with radiotherapy), non-small cell lung cancer	Infusion reaction	Skin rash, hypomagnesemia, fatigue, interstitial lung disease
Panitumumab	Binds to EGFR and inhibits downstream EGFR signaling; enhances response to chemotherapy and radiotherapy	6 mg/kg IV given once every 2 weeks	Colorectal cancer	Infusion reaction (rarely)	Skin rash, hypomagnesemia, fatigue, interstitial lung disease
Bevacizumab	Inhibits binding of VEGF to VEGFR leading to inhibition of VEGF signaling. Enhances tumor blood flow and drug delivery	5–15 mg/kg IV every 2–3 weeks	Non-small cell lung cancer, breast cancer, renal cell cancer	Infusion site reaction & hypertension	GI perforations, delay wound healing, thromboembolism, proteinuria
Sorafenib	Inhibits VEGF leading to inhibition of angiogenesis, invasion, and metastasis	Orally, 400 mg twice daily	Renal cell cancer, hepatocellular cancer	Nausea, hypertension	Skin rash, fatigue and asthenia, bleeding complications, hypophosphatemia
Sunitinib	Same as above	50 mg once daily for 4 weeks followed by 2 weeks off treatment	Renal cell cancer, GIST	Hypertension	Skin rash, fatigue and asthenia, bleeding complications, cardiac toxicity leading to congestive heart failure in rare cases

EGFR: Endothelial growth factor receptor, VGFR: vascular endothelial growth factor receptor, PDGFR: platelet-derived growth factor receptor.

The aim of treatment can be:

- **Cure or prolonged remission:** Chemotherapy is the primary treatment modality that can achieve cure or prolonged remission.
- **Palliation:** If the cancer is incurable, the aim of treatment is to improve the quality of life by controlling signs and symptoms with supportive measures only.

- **Adjuvant chemotherapy:** After surgery or radiotherapy, anti-cancer drugs are used in routine to kill any micro-metastatic cells or residual malignant cells. This is done to achieve apparent cure and prevent recurrence.

The anti-cancer drugs arrest the cell division by acting specifically at a particular stage of cell division or non specifically as shown Figure 2.12.

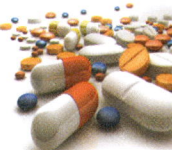

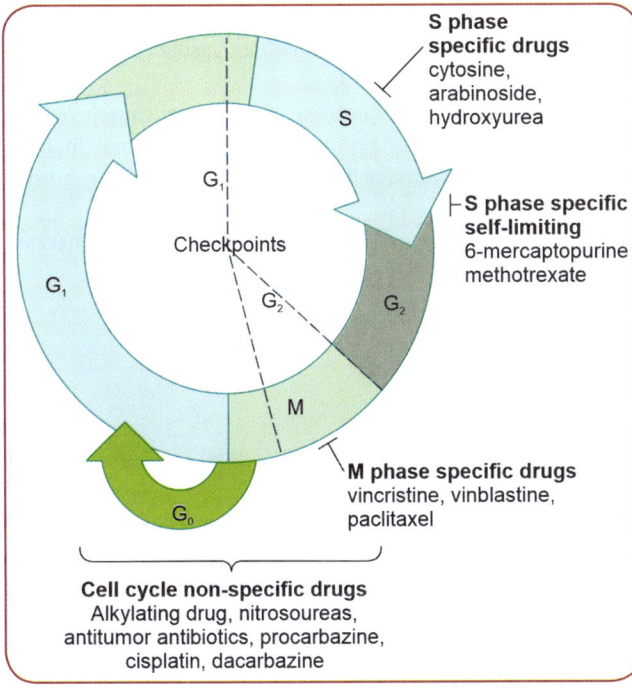

FIG. 2.12: Cell cycle specificity of anti-cancer drugs

✔
The dose of all chemotherapeutic agents varies from patient to patient.

The dose is calculated keeping in view the various factors such as age, sex, body surface area, stage of disease, organ involved, type of cancer, hepatic and renal status of the patient.

The product monograph inserted in the package should always be consulted before initiating the treatment.

ALKYLATING AGENTS

- All the alkylating agents cause alkylation of DNA, which leads to DNA damage and lethal effects to the tumor cells.
- Alkylating agents do not discriminate between cycling and resting cells, even though they are most toxic for rapidly dividing cells.
- They are used in combination with other agents to treat a wide variety of lymphatic and solid cancers.
- In addition to being cytotoxic, all are mutagenic and carcinogenic and can lead to secondary malignancies such as acute leukemia.
- These agents are used in soft tissue sarcoma, breast cancer, ovarian cancer, neuroblastoma, Hodgkin's and non-Hodgkin's lymphoma chronic lymphocytic leukemia, Wilms' tumor, and rhabdomyosarcoma.
- The immediate side effects of alkylating agents are nausea and vomiting and on prolonged treatment, bone marrow depression and alopecia are also seen.

- Cyclophosphamide causes hemorrhagic cystitis, which is associated with dysuria and hematuria. This can be prevented with adequate hydration and IV mesna (2-mercaptoethanesulphonate).
- Busulfan is specially associated with pulmonary fibrosis, adrenal insufficiency and skin pigmentation.
- Before administering these agents, the packaged inserts should always be referred for dosage and schedule.

PLATINUM ANALOGS

- These are all platinum-containing compound.
- They get converted to the active form to the cell, inhibit DNA synthesis and cause cytotoxicity like alkylating agents.
- Cytotoxicity can occur at any stage of the cell cycle, but cells are most vulnerable to the actions of these drugs in the G_1 and S-phases.
- These agents are used in testicular, ovarian, bladder, lung, colorectal, head and neck and prostate cancers.
- The immediate side effects are nausea and vomiting and on prolonged treatment, bone marrow depression, ototoxicity nephrotoxicity, and peripheral sensory neuropathy are also seen.
- Before administering these agents, the package inserted should always be referred for dosage and schedule.

ANTIMETABOLITES

Folate Antagonists

- These agents inhibit the dihydrofolate acid reductase enzyme, which is essential for the active folic acid formation (tetrahydrofolic acid).
- Methotrexate is one of the most common used anti-cancer agents. In addition to its anti-cancer activity, it also produces anti-inflammatory and immunosuppressant effect.
- These agents are used in choriocarcinoma, osteogenic sarcoma, mesothelioma, head and neck, bladder, breast, and non-small cell lung cancers.
- The immediate side effects are nausea, vomiting and diarrhea and on prolonged treatment, bone marrow depression, megaloblastic anemia, hepatic fibrosis and hand-foot syndrome are also seen.
- Leucovorin or folinic acid is used as antidote for methotrexate overdose.
- Before administering these agents, the package inserted should always be referred for dosage and schedule.

Purine and Pyrimidine Antagonists

- Purine and pyrimidine are required for RNA and DNA synthesis in the cells.

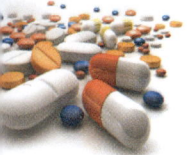

- After entering into the cells, these drugs get incorporated into their place of DNA and inhibits RNA and DNA synthesis.
- These agents are used in head and neck, bladder, breast, non-small cell lung, gastroesophageal, and colorectal cancers.
- The immediate side effects are nausea and vomiting and on prolonged treatment and bone marrow depression, immunosuppression are also seen.
- Before administering these agents, the package inserted should always be referred for dosage and schedule.

MICROTUBULE DAMAGING AGENTS

- These agents inhibit the cell division in metaphase by binding to microtubular protein, tubulin that forms mitotic spindles. Hence, mitosis is inhibited.
- These agents are cell cycle specific.
- The vinca alkaloids are obtained from periwinkle plants and taxanes from taxus baccata tree.
- These agents are used in Kaposi's sarcoma, rhabdomyosarcoma, Wilms' tumor, Hodgkin's and non-Hodgkin's lymphoma, breast, non-small cell lung, ovarian and germ cell cancers.
- The immediate side effects are nausea and vomiting and on prolonged treatment, bone marrow depression, syndrome of inappropriate secretion of antidiuretic hormone (SIADH), paralytic ileus, and peripheral neuropathy alopecia are also seen.
- Before administering these agents, the package inserted should always be referred for dosage and schedule.

TOPOISOMERASE-I AND II INHIBITORS

- These drugs cause DNA damage and cause cell death.
- These agents are used in small cell lung cancer, non-Hodgkin's lymphoma, gastroesophageal, gastric, colorectal and ovarian cancers.
- The immediate side effects are nausea, vomiting and hypotension and on prolonged treatment, bone marrow depression, neutropenia, and alopecia are also seen.
- Before administering these agents, the package inserted should always be referred for dosage and schedule.

ANTIBIOTICS

- These anti-cancer antibiotics produce oxygen free radicals, which bind to DNA and cause single- and double-stranded DNA breaks.
- These are cell cycle non-specific drugs.
- These agents are used in small cell lung cancer, anti-lymphocytic leukemia (ALL), acute myeloid leukemia

(AML), Hodgkin's and non-Hodgkin's lymphoma, head and neck cancer, superficial bladder, gastric, germ cell and ovarian cancers.
- The immediate side effects are nausea, vomiting, fever and hypotension and on prolonged treatment, bone marrow depression, pulmonary fibrosis, and cardiotoxicity are also seen.
- Before administering these agents, the package inserted should always be referred for dosage and schedule.

MISCELLANEOUS

L-Asparaginase

- It hydrolyzes circulating L-asparagine, resulting in rapid inhibition of protein synthesis.
- This agent is indicated in ALL.
- It is given in a dose of 6000-10,000 IU every third day for 3-4 weeks.
- The immediate side effects are nausea and vomiting and on prolonged treatment, bone marrow depression, hepato and renal toxicity are also seen.
- Before administering these agents, the package inserted should always be referred for dosage and schedule.

HORMONAL DRUGS

[Detailed Description is given in Chapter on Hormones]
- All hormonal drugs are used for palliative therapy.
- These drugs are not cytotoxic.
- They modify the growth of hormone-dependent tumors.

Glucocorticoids

- They have marked lympholytic action therefore they are primarily used in acute childhood leukemia and lymphomas.
- They are also helpful for the control of malignancy/chemotherapy associated complications like hypercalcemia, hemolysis, bleeding due to thrombocytopenia and increased intracranial tension.
- They potentiate the antiemetic action of ondansetron and metoclopramide.
- Most commonly used glucocorticoids for this purpose are prednisolone and dexamethasone.

Estrogens

Estrogens are mostly used in androgen-dependent tumors such as carcinoma prostate.

Fosfestrol, a phosphate derivative of stilbestrol, is specifically used in carcinoma prostate. It is given intravenously 600–1200 mg initially then as maintenance dose of 120–240 mg orally.

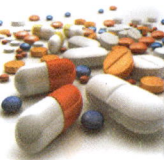

Selective Estrogen Receptor Modulators (SERMs)

Tamoxifen

- It acts as potent estrogen antagonist in breast carcinoma cells, blood cells.
- It is used in the treatment of breast carcinoma as adjuvant therapy.

Selective Estrogen Receptor down Regulators (SERDs)

Fulvestrant

- It is a fully estrogen antagonist, used in tamoxifen resistant breast cancer.
- It is given in a dose of 250 mg IM deep intragluteally.

Aromatase Inhibitors (Letrozole)

It inhibits the conversion of androgen to estrogen by inhibiting aromatase enzyme.

Androgen

↓ ← Aromatase enzyme

Estrogen *(Inhibited by Aromatase inhibitors)*

- It is used in early and advance breast cancer.

Antiandrogen (Flutamide and Bicalutamide)

- These are androgen antagonists used in the palliative therapy.
- These antagonize androgen action on prostate carcinoma and have palliative effects in advanced/metastatic cases.

5-α Reductase Inhibitors (Finasteride and Dutasteride)

- These drugs inhibit conversion of testosterone to dihydrotestosterone in prostate and other tissues.
- They have palliative effects in advanced carcinoma prostate.

GnRH Agonists (Leuprolide, Nafarelin, Goserelin, Busereline, Triptorelin)

- These drugs indirectly inhibit estrogen/androgen gland secretion by suppressing FSH and LH release from pituitary.
- They provide palliative effects in advanced estrogen/androgen dependent carcinoma breast/prostate.
- They are most commonly used in combination with anti-androgens or SERMs.

Progestins

- They provide palliative effects by giving temporary remission in some cases of advanced, recurrent and metastatic endometrial carcinoma.
- They are used in high doses after surgery and radiotherapy.

GENERAL TOXICITIES OF CYTOTOXIC DRUGS

- Majority of the cytotoxic drugs have lethal effect on rapidly multiplying cancer cells. They are also toxic/lethal to the normal host (proliferating) cells of the skin, mucous membrane, lymphoid organs and gonads.
- The toxicity of anti-cancer drugs is dose dependent and also depends upon individual susceptibility.
- The common adverse effects are:
  - **Bone marrow depression**: Pancytopenia, granulocytopenia, thrombocytopenia, aplastic anemia, leucopenia and anemia. The dose may need to be reduced.
  - **Suppression of proliferating cells:** Mucous lining is highly susceptible to cytotoxic drugs because of high epithelial cell turnover. This leads to stomatitis, bleeding gums, glossitis, esophagitis, gastritis, proctitis, GI ulcer and diarrhea.
  - **Skin:** Dermatitis and alopecia [damage to the cells in hair follicles]. The alopecia is reversible and do not require any medication.
  - **Gonads:**
    - **In males:** Oligozoospermia due to inhibition of gonadal cells.
    - **In females:** Amenorrhea due to inhibition of ovulation.
  - **Hyperuricemia:** It occurs due to massive cell destruction and may lead to acute renal failure, gout and urate stones in the urinary tract. Allopurinol can be used to inhibit hyperuricemia.
  - **Carcinogenicity:** Cytotoxic drugs, themselves may cause secondary cancers, due to depression of cell mediated and humoral immunity.
  - **Teratogenicity:** The cancer therapy is cytotoxic and inhibits the cell division or growth or both; therefore they are teratogenic and contraindicated in pregnancy but not at the cost of mother's life.
  - **Emetogenicity** [vomiting causing potential]: The different anti-cancer drugs cause emesis of different intensity. They are as given in Table 2.32.

TABLE 2.32: Emetogenic potential of cytotoxic drugs

High	Moderate	Mild
• Cisplatin	• Vinblastine	• Fluorouracil
• Actinomycin D	• Cytarabine	• Etoposide
• Mustine	• Carboplatin	• Bleomycin
• Dacarbazine	• Paclitaxel	• Busulfan
• Cyclophosphamide	• Ifosfamide	• Chlorambucil
• Lomustine	• Daunorubicin	• L-Asparaginase
	• Procarbazine	• Hydroxyurea
	• 6-Mercapto-purine	• Vincristine
		• Methotrexate

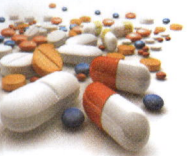

Drug Interactions

- Allopurinol prolongs the action of 6-marcaptopurine. Hence, dose of 6-marcaptopurine should be reduced inpatients taking allopurinol.
- Procarbazine causes disulfiram like reaction with alcohol. Hence, patients should be warned not to consume alcohol.
- Doxorubicin and daunorubicin shouldn't be administered to the patient suffering from cardiomyopathy.

Nursing Implications

- **Anti-cancer drugs**
  - Arrange for blood tests periodically before, during and for at least 3 weeks after therapy to monitor bone marrow function.
  - Administer medication according to scheduled protocol and in combination with other drugs as indicated to improve effectiveness.
  - Ensure that the patient is well hydrated to decrease risk of renal toxicity.
  - Protect the patient from exposure to infection; limit invasive procedures when bone marrow suppression limits the patient's immune/inflammatory responses.
  - Provide small, frequent meals, frequent mouth care, and dietary consultation as appropriate to maintain nutrition when GI effects are severe. Anticipate the need for antiemetic drugs if necessary.
  - Arrange for proper head covering at extremes of temperature if alopecia occurs; a wig, scarf, or hat is important for maintaining body temperature. If alopecia is an anticipated effect of drug therapy, advice the patient to obtain a wig or head covering before the condition occurs to promote self-esteem and a positive body image.
  - Monitor patient response to the drug (alleviation of cancer being treated, palliation of signs and symptoms of cancer).
  - Monitor for adverse effects (bone marrow suppression, GI toxicity, neurotoxicity, alopecia, renal or hepatic dysfunction).
  - Evaluate the effectiveness of the teaching plan (patient can name the drug, dosage, possible adverse effects to watch for, and specific measures to help avoid adverse effects).

IMMUNOSUPPRESSANT DRUGS

- Immunosuppressants are the drugs, which suppress the immunity by inhibiting cellular/humoral or both types of immune responses.
- The main therapeutic applications of immunosuppressants are in organ transplantation and autoimmune diseases.

TABLE 2.33: Sites of action of selected immunosuppressive agents on T-cell activation

Drug	Site of action
Cyclosporine	Calcineurin (inhibits the activity of phosphatase enzyme)
Tacrolimus	Calcineurin (inhibits the activity of phosphatase enzyme)
Sirolimus	Protein kinase involved in cell-cycle progression (mTOR) (inhibits activity)
Azathioprine	DNA (false nucleotide incorporation)
Mycophenolate mofetil	Inhibits the activity of Inosine monophosphate dehydrogenase enzyme
Glucocorticoids	Glucocorticoid response elements in DNA (regulate gene transcription)
Daclizumab, basiliximab	IL-2 receptor (block IL-2-mediated T-cell activation)
Muromonab-CD3	T-cell receptor complex (blocks antigen recognition)

Abbreviations: IL, interleukin; mTOR, mammalian target of rapamycin.

Classification of Immunosuppressant Drugs

- **Inhibitors of Calcineurin (Specific T-cell inhibitors):** Cyclosporine and Tacrolimus
- **Inhibitors of m-TORenzyme:** Sirolimus and Everolimus
- **Cytotoxic or Antiproliferative drugs:** Methotrexate, Cyclophosphamide, Azathioprine, Mycophenolate mofetil (MMF) & Chlorambucil
- **Glucocorticoids:** Prednisolone and other corticosteroids
- **Biological agents**
  - TNFα inhibitors: Etanercept, Infliximab, Adalimumab
  - Antagonist of IL-1 receptor: Anakinra
  - Antagonists of IL-2 receptor: Daclizumab, (anti CD-25 antibodies) Basiliximab
  - Anti CD-3 antibody: Muromonab CD3
  - Polyclonal antibodies: Antithymocyte antibody (ATG), Rho(D) immuneglobulin.

Sites of action of some immunosuppressive on T-cell activation are given in Table 2.33.

m-TOR INHIBITORS

Sirolimus

- Sirolimus is obtained from *Streptomyces hygroscopicus*, earlier named Rapamycin.
- It binds to immunophillin FKBP. FKBP complex inhibits another kinase called 'mammalian target of rapamycin' (m-TOR).
- It inhibits the proliferation and differentiation of T-cells activated by IL-2 and other cytokines.

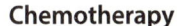

- The oral absorption is good, while fatty food decreases its absorption.
- The excretion occurs primarily via biliary system.
- The plasma t½ is 60 hours.
- It is used both for prophylaxis and therapy of graft rejection reaction.
- The recommended loading dose is 1 mg/m² daily, then has to be titrated to lower doses for maintenance.
- Some other indications for its use are psoriasis and choreoretinitis.
- Nowadays, drug eluting stents are incorporated with sirolimus. It inhibits local cell proliferation and thereby restenosis.

CALCINEURIN INHIBITORS

The common side effects are bone marrow suppression, thrombocytopenia hyperlipidemia, diarrhea, liver damage, and pneumonitis.

Different features of calcineurin inhibitors are given in Table 2.34.

Everolimus

- It is another m-TOR inhibitor, having profile very much similar to sirolimus.
- It is better absorbed orally with consistent bioavailability.
- The t½ is shorter (40 hours) and attains steady state levels earlier as compared to sirolimus.

ANTIPROLIFERATIVE DRUGS

Azathioprine

- It is a prodrug.
- 6-mercaptopurine (6-MP) is the active metabolite of azathioprine.
- It inhibits the *de novo* purine synthesis and damages the DNA. By affecting the differentiation and functioning of T-cells, it inhibits the functioning of cytolytic lymphocytes.
- It is given in renal and other grafts to prevent graft rejection.
- The effectiveness of azathioprine is less than cyclosporine. Therefore, usually azathioprine is given in combination with cyclosporine.
- It is given alone in patients developing cyclosporine toxicity.
- The other indications are:
  - Inflammatory bowel disease
  - Rheumatoid arthritis

Dose

- Therapeutic: 3-5 mg/kg daily
- Maintenance: 1–2 mg/kg daily.

Cyclophosphamide

- Cyclophosphamide acts better on 'B-cells' than 'T-cells', which means effects on humoral immunity are better than on cell mediated immunity (CMI).

TABLE 2.34: Calcineurin inhibitors

Drug	Mechanism of action	Dose & route	Indications	Special features
Cyclosporine [Obtained from Beauveria nivea fungi]	Inhibits the enzyme calcinuerin phosphates, this inhibits T-cell activation, IL-2 production and also suppress the proliferation cytotoxic-T cells.	**Initially:** Intravenously 3–5 mg/kg infusion, then 10–15 mg/kg daily (with milk or fruit juice) for 1–2 weeks after transplantation. **Maintenance dose:** 2–6 mg/kg daily	Organ transplantation and autoimmune disorders	It is most effective when administered before antigen exposure. Causes opportunistic Infections, hypertension, precipitation of diabetes, hyperkalemia, hyperuricemia, hirsutism.
Tacrolimus [Obtained from **Streptomyces tsukubaensis**]	Same as above In addition, also binds 'FK 506 binding protein (FKBP)'inhibit Helper-T cells.	**For renal transplant patients:** 0.05–0.1 mg/kg twice daily, orally. **For liver transplant:** 0.1–0.2 mg/kg twice daily. **Topically:** 0.03–0.1%	Organ transplantation, atopic dermatitis, vitiligo Crohn's disease	Requires blood level monitoring for dose adjustment. 100 times more potent than cyclosporine Causes gum hyperplasia, precipitate diabetes, cause neurotoxicity, alopecia and diarrhea

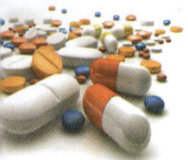

- It is used in a higher dosage for bone marrow transplantation for short duration only.
- It is also used in systemic lupus erythematosus, idiopathic thrombocytopenic purpura and pemphigus in a low dose formulation.

Methotrexate (MTx)

- Methotrexate inhibits dihydrofolate reductase [DHFR], thus inhibiting the formation of tetrahydrofolate synthesis (THF).
- The deficiency of THF results in inhibition of protein synthesis, affecting the rapidly multiplying cells the most.
- It also inhibits the cellular immunity and production of cytokines (anti-inflammatory action).
- It is primarily used in rheumatoid arthritis, pemphigus, uveitis, severe psoriasis and myasthenia gravis.

Chlorambucil

- Chlorambucil has weak immunosuppressant activity
- It is rarely used nowadays due to availability of better drugs.
- It is indicated in autoimmune diseases and maintenance therapy for organ transplantation.

Mycophenolate Mofetil (MMF)

- It is a prodrug and converted to mycophenolic acid.
- It inhibits formation of inosine monophosphate dehydrogenase, noncompetitively and thereby, inhibits the proliferation and function of lymphocytes.
- It is well absorbed orally and excretion occurs via kidneys.
- The plasma t½ is 16 hours.
- The recommended dose is 1.0 gm given twice daily.
- Commonly seen adverse effects are GI disturbance such as nausea, vomiting, diarrhea, and abdominal pain.
- It is indicated as an adjuvant with other immunosuppressant drugs to prevent organ transplant rejection.
- MMF + glucocorticoid + sirolimus is a preferred non-nephrotoxic combination.

GLUCOCORTICOIDS (DESCRIBED IN STEROIDS)

- Glucocorticoids are naturally secreted from the adrenal cortex.
- The glucocorticoids used pharmacologically are synthetic in nature.
- They possess potent immunosuppressant and antiinflammatory actions.
- They inhibit the proliferation of T-lymphocytes.
- They also inhibit interleukin and cytokines and possess anti-inflammatory action.
- They are the first pharmacologic agents to be used as immunosuppressants both in transplantation and in various autoimmune disorders.
- The most common agents in use are *prednisone* and *methylprednisolone*.

BIOLOGICAL AGENTS

These are biotechnologically produced recombinant proteins or monoclonal/polyclonal antibodies directed to cytokines or lymphocyte surface antigens which play a key role in immune response. They are important recent additions, mostly as supplementary/reserve drugs for severe and refractory cases of autoimmune diseases and graft versus host reaction.

TNF-α INHIBITORS (ETANERCEPT, INFLIXIMAB, ADALIMUMAB)

- Macrophages, T helper and CD 4 cells produce TNF-α, which plays a major role in pathogenesis of granulomatous conditions such as rheumatoid arthritis and Crohn's disease.
- TNF-α also amplifies immune inflammation by releasing other cytokines and enzymes which promote inflammatory response.
- TNF-α blocked by biological products (TNF-α inhibitors) has proved highly effective therapy against inflammatory and granulomatous diseases.
- Different TNF-α in inhibitors are given in Table 2.35.

TABLE 2.35: TNF-α inhibitors

Etanercept	Infliximab	Adalimumab
• It is a recombinant molecule and consists of TNF receptor coupled to Fc component of IgG-1	• It is chemical monoclonal antibody of IgG-1	• It is fully human monoclonal antibody of IgG-1 (less antigenic)
• It neutralizes TNF α and β	• Effective against TNF-α only	• Effective against TNF-α only
• It is used mostly in combination with MTx	• It is used mostly in combination with MTx	• It is used mostly in combination with MTx
• Dose: 25 mg SC twice weekly	• Dose: 3 mg/kg IV, every 4–8 weeks	• Dose: 40 mg SC, on alternate week
• Used in rheumatoid arthritis, psoriatic arthritis	• Used in rheumatoid arthritis, psoriatic arthritis, Crohn's disease	• Used in rheumatoid arthritis, psoriatic arthritis

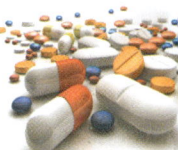

ANTAGONIST OF IL-1 RECEPTOR

- IL-1 amplifies immune inflammation by releasing other cytokines and enzymes, which promote inflammatory responses by activation of helper T cells.
- IL-1 receptor antagonist areproduced biotechnologically [human recombinant] for clinical use. They are variants of an endogenously isolated IL-1 receptor antagonist.

Anakinra

- It is an anti IL-1 monoclonal antibody.
- It prevents the binding of interlukin-1 to its receptors.
- It has been approved for use in rheumatoid arthritis not controlled by conventional DMARDs.
- The therapeutic efficacy of anakinra is lesser than TNF-α inhibitors.

ANTAGONISTS OF IL-2 RECEPTOR

Antagonists of IL-2 receptor are given in Table 2.36.

ANTI CD-3 ANTIBODY

Muromonab CD3

- It is a **murine** monoclonal antibody, which is against the CD3 molecule on the surface of human T cells.
- It is mainly used in steroid-resistant acute transplant rejection reaction cases.
- The recommended dose is 5 mg daily/intravenously given for 10–14 days.
- It is antigenic in nature and may cause anaphylaxis.

TABLE 2.36: Antagonists of IL-2 receptor

Daclizumab (anti CD-25 antibodies)	Basiliximab
• It is humanized murine chimeric IgG-1 monoclonal antibody. • It binds with IL-2 and inhibits lymphocytes production. • The t½ is 20 days.	• It is murine human chimeric IgG-1 monoclonal antibody. • It also binds with IL-2 and inhibits lymphocytes production. • The t½ is 7 days.

Common features
- These drugs are used in combination with glucocorticoids, azathioprine/MMF and/or calcineurin antagonists.
- They are used to prevent renal and other transplant rejection reaction.
- These drugs have no significant adverse effects, but in some cases anaphylactic reactions and opportunistic infections can occur.

✓ Cytokine Release Syndrome
- It is a major side effect of anti-CD3 therapy, which typically begins within 30 minutes after infusion (but can occur later also) and may persist for hours.
- This is due to release of TNF α, ILs and interferons.
- The most common presenting symptoms are fever, chills/rigor, nausea, vomiting, diarrhea, headache, tremors, myalgia and arthralgia.
- These symptoms usually are worst with the first dose. Tapering the dose causes remission of symptoms.
- Pretreatment administration of corticosteroids prevents the release of cytokines, hence reduces the first dose reaction. This procedure is used as a standard protocol for anti CD3 therapy.

POLYCLONAL ANTIBODIES

Antithymocyte Globulin (ATG)

- It is used as immunosuppressant used in steroid resistant allograft rejection patients.
- It is administered in a dose of 1.5 mg/kg intravenously, daily for 1–2 weeks.
- The most commonly presenting side effects are fever, chills, and hypotension.
- Serum sickness, glomerulonephritis, and anaphylaxis are rarely seen.

Anti-D Immunoglobulin (Rh$_o$ [D])

- Rh$_o$ (D) immunoglobulin is a concentrated solution of antibodies directed against the Rh$_o$ (D) antigen of the red cell.
- It prevents the formation of antibodies against Rh$_o$ (D) antigen in Rh$_o$ (D) negative individuals by binding to the Rh$_o$ (D) antigen.
- If Rh-negative mother is having Rh-positive fetus in the womb and certain complications like miscarriages or normal delivery occurs, then the fetal RBCs leak into the mother's bloodstream and cause sensitization of mother's immune system to D antigen present on fetal RBCs.
- In next pregnancy, hemolytic disease of the newborn (*erythroblastosis fetalis*) occurs in third trimester due to the destruction of fetal RBCs by the circulating maternal antibodies against Rh-positive cells.
- The treatment is advocated to Rh-negative mothers at 26–28 weeks, gestation with history of:
  - Miscarriages
  - Previous ectopic pregnancies, or
  - Previous abortions,
  - When the blood type of the previous fetus is unknown.

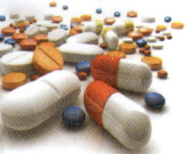

- The dose's schedule is as follows:
  - **Prophylaxis after delivery/abortion:** 300 mcg IM within 72 hours of the event.
  - Antepartum prophylaxis before 20 weeks of gestation: 250 IU, IM.
  - Antepartum prophylaxis after 20 weeks of gestation: 500 IU, IM.

- In case of transplacental hemorrhage: 1200 mcg, IM.

It is well tolerated with mild discomforts like pain at injection site and slight rise in body temperature.

Rh_o(D) immune globulin is injected to the mother and not to infant.

 ## Drug Interactions

✧ The nephrotoxic drugs such as aminoglycosides, vancomycin, amphotericin-B and NSAIDs increase the toxicity of cyclosporine. Hence, combination should be avoided.

✧ The enzyme inducer drugs like phenobarbitone, rifampicin, phenytoin, etc., decrease the effectiveness of cyclosporine and other immunosuppressant drugs.

✧ The enzyme inhibitors drugs like ketoconazole, erythromycin & related drugs, increase the blood levels of these drugs and can cause toxicity.

✧ Potassium sparing diuretics and K^+ supplements should not be given in the patient with cyclosporine therapy as fatal hyperkalemia can occur.

Nursing Implications

✧ **Immunosuppressant drugs**
  ☞ Arrange for blood tests periodically before, during and for at least 3 weeks after therapy to monitor bone marrow function.
  ☞ Administer medication according to scheduled protocol and in combination with other drugs as indicated to improve effectiveness.
  ☞ Protect the patient from exposure to infection; limit invasive procedures when bone marrow suppression limits the patient's immune/inflammatory responses.
  ☞ Monitor patient's response to the drug (alleviation of cancer being treated, palliation of signs and symptoms of cancer).
  ☞ Monitor for adverse effects (bone marrow suppression, GI toxicity, neurotoxicity, alopecia, renal or hepatic dysfunction).
  ☞ Evaluate the effectiveness of the teaching plan (patient can name the drug, dosage, possible adverse effects to watch for, and specific measures to help avoid adverse effects).

Assess Yourself

Long and Short Answer Questions

1. Define antimicrobial agents. Classify them according to their mechanism of action.
2. What are antitubercular drugs and describe mechanism of action and adverse effects of 1st line drugs.
3. What is the rational of using pyridoxine with INH?
4. Pharmacological management of leprosy.
5. What is Acyclovir? Describe its mode of action and enlist its uses.
6. Describe two anti-malarial drugs.
7. What are anti-retroviral agents? Classify them and describe zidovudine.
8. What is perinatal HIV prophylaxis?
9. What is DOTS? Describe the regimen used in category-I patients.
10. What are antihelmintic drugs? Describe albendazole.
11. What are antiamebic drugs? Describe metronidazole.
12. Write a short note on:
    a. Bactericidal & bacteriostatic drugs
    b. Chemoprophylaxis
    c. Sulfonamides
    d. Beta-lactam antibiotics
    e. Beta-lactamase inhibitors
    f. Quinolones
    g. Aminoglycosides
    h. Erythromycin
    i. Tetracycline
    j. Amphotericin-B
    k. Toxicity of cytotoxic drugs
    l. Treatment of scabies
    m. Uses of immunosuppressants

Contd...

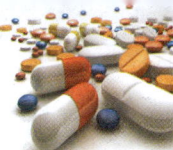

Multiple Choice Questions

1. One of the antitubercular drugs is contraindicated in children below 6 years of age, because they may be unable to appreciate and report visual field defects or changes in vision, which is a known side effect of that drug. Which among the following is that drug?
   a. Ethambutol
   b. INH
   c. Rifampicin
   d. Pyrazinamide

2. Which fluoroquinolone is highly active against mycobacterium leprae and is being used in alternative multidrug therapy regimens?
   a. Norfloxacin
   b. Ofloxacin
   c. Ciprofloxacin
   d. Lomefloxacin

3. Which of the following ATT is not hepatotoxic?
   a. Isoniazid
   b. Rifampicin
   c. Pyrazinamide
   d. Streptomycin

4. Mucormycosis, drug of choice is:
   a. Amphotericin B
   b. Itraconazole
   c. Voriconazole
   d. Griseofulvin

5. Voriconazole is not effective against:
   a. Candida albicans
   b. Mucormycosis
   c. Candida tropicalis
   d. Aspergillosis

6. Most effective drug in severe falciparum malaria:
   a. Quinine
   b. Cholorquine
   c. Artesunate
   d. Mefloquine

7. Not a drug recommended for *P. falciparum* is:
   a. Quinine
   b. Ciprofloxacin
   c. Artemether
   d. Doxycycline

8. Which of the following drugs is not used in scabies?
   a. Benzene haxachloride
   b. Permethrin
   c. Ciclopirox olamine
   d. Crotamiton

9. Wrong statement about albendazole is:
   a. Poor CSF penetration
   b. Contraindicated in pregnancy
   c. Useful in neurocysticercosis
   d. Can cause hepatotoxicity

10. Cyclophosphamide is:
    a. Alkylating agent
    b. Antitumor antibiotic
    c. Monoclonal antibody
    d. Antimetabolities

11. True about cyclophosphamide:
    a. Antimetabolites
    b. Alkylating agent
    c. Platinum compound
    d. Topoisomerase inhibitors

Answer Key

1.	a.	2.	b.	3.	d.	4.	a.	5.	b.	6.	c.	7.	b.
8.	c.	9.	a.	10.	a.	11.	b.						

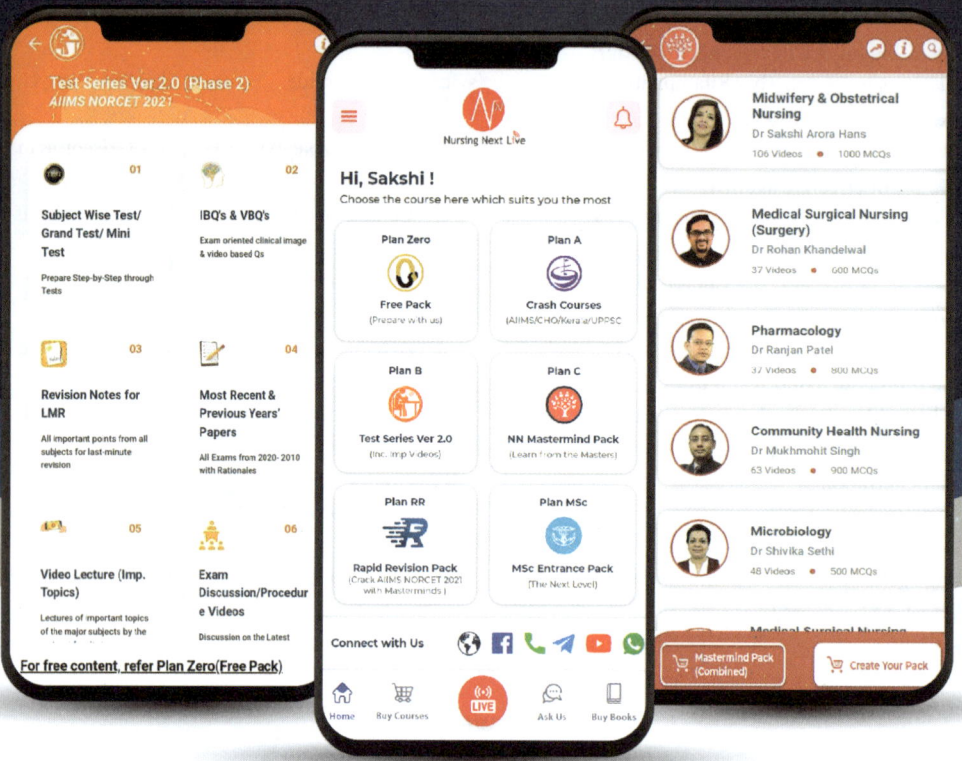 
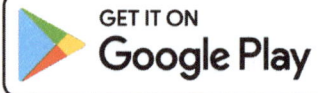

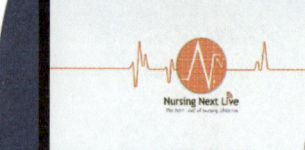
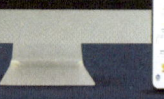

Pharmacology of Commonly used Antiseptics, Disinfectants and Insecticides

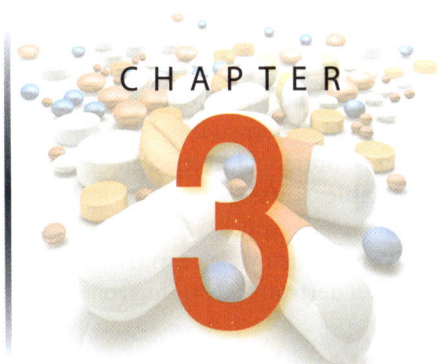

CHAPTER

3

ANTISEPTICS AND DISINFECTANTS

Antiseptics are the agents, which are used to inhibit or kill the microbes *on living tissue*. These agents are applied topically on skin, mucous membranes, or wounds. In concentrated form, some of the antiseptics can be used as disinfectants also.

Disinfectants are the chemical agents, which are used to inhibit or kill the microbes *on inanimate objects* such as surgical instruments/tables, floor, etc. These agents should never be applied on living tissue.

The common term used for both is *'Germicide'*.

Sterilizing agents are the chemical agents used to completely kill all forms of microorganisms (*vegetative and dormant forms*).

Properties of an Ideal Antiseptic/Disinfectant

- It should have cidal effect against all pathogens (bacteria, fungi, virus, protozoa).
- It should be sporicidal also.
- It should be chemically stable.
- It should be economical and affordable.
- It should be easily available at all times.
- It should be non-staining.

- It should be odorless or with tolerable odor.
- It should require brief time of exposure for its cidal effect and should have sustained protection.
- It should be able to spread through organic films and enter folds and crevices.
- It should be active even in the presence of blood, pus, exudates and excreta.
- It should be non-irritating to tissues, should not delay healing.
- It should be non-absorbable, and if absorbed, should produce minimum toxicity.
- It should be non-sensitizing or non-allergic type.
- It should be compatible with soaps and other detergents.

CLASSIFICATION OF ANTISEPTICS/DISINFECTANTS

- **Phenol derivatives:** Phenol, cresol, hexylresorcinol, chloroxylenol, hexachlorophene.
- **Oxidizing agents:** Potassium permanganate, hydrogen peroxide, benzoyl peroxide, ethylene oxide (ETO), Low temperature gas plasma, ozone sterilization.
- **Halogens:** Iodine, Iodophores, chlorine, chlorophores.
- **Biguanide:** Chlorhexidine.

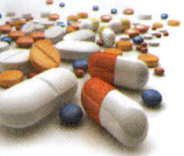

- **Quaternary ammonium (Cationic):** Cetrimide, benzalkonium chloride, dequalinium chloride.
- **Soaps:** Of sodium and potassium.
- **Alcohols:** Ethanol, isopropanol.
- **Aldehydes:** Formaldehyde, glutaraldehyde.
- **Acids:** Boric acid, acetic acid.
- **Metallic salts:** Silver nitrate, silversulfadiazine, zinc sulfate, zinc oxide.
- **Dyes:** Gentian violet, acriflavine, proflavine.
- **Furan derivative:** Nitrofurazone.

PHENOLS

Phenol (Carbolic Acid)

- It is one of the earliest and relatively weak antiseptic agents having poor action on bacterial spores.
- It is a general *protoplasmic poison* which damages both microbes and tissue cells alike.
- It can cause skin burns at higher concentrations.
- It acts by disrupting bacterial membranes and denaturing bacterial proteins.
- It is used to disinfect urine, feces, pus, and sputum of patients.
- It is static at 0.2% and microbicidal at >1% concentration.

Cresol

- It is a methyl derivative of phenol.
- It is three to ten times more active than phenol but less damaging to tissues.
- It is used for washing hands, disinfection of utensils and excreta.
- Lysol is a 50% soapy emulsion of cresol.

Hexylresorcinol

- It is a more potent derivative of the phenolic compound resorcinol.
- It is odorless and non-staining.
- It is used as mouthwash, lozenge and as antifungal.

Chloroxylenol

- It is non-irritating to intact skin, but efficacy is reduced in the presence of organic matter.
- It is poorly water soluble and loses activity if diluted with water and kept for a long time.
- Commonly, it is used for:
  - Washing hands (4.8% solution)
  - Skin cream and soap (0.8%)
  - Lubricating obstetric cream (1.4%)
  - Mouthwash

Hexachlorophene

- It inhibits bacterial enzymes and causes cell lysis at higher concentration.
- It is non-staining, non-irritating and odorless (rather good deodorant also).
- Its activity is reduced in presence of organic matter.
- It does not kill spores and Gram-negative bacteria.
- The degerming action is slow but persistent due to deposition on the skin as a fine film that is not removed by rinsing with water.
- It is commonly incorporated in soap and other cleansing antiseptics for surgical scrub.
- Not used in concentration >2% as some cases of premature neonatal brain damage have occurred in USA around 1970.

OXIDIZING AGENTS

Potassium Permanganate

- Potassium permanganate acts as an oxidizing antiseptic. Its crystals are purple in color and are readily soluble in water.
- When dissolved in water, it liberates nascent oxygen that oxidizes bacterial protoplasm.
- It is less popular as higher concentration can cause burns and blisters.
- It is mainly used as disinfectant in different dilutions. 1/20 dilution for hand wash, 1/5000 dilution for mouthwash and 1/10000–1/30000 dilution for urethral and vaginal lavage.
- It is also used to disinfect and deodorize the water of ponds and wells.
- It is used as an antidote for stomach wash in morphine poisoning in 0.1–0.3% concentration.
- It is not good for disinfection of surgical instruments as it promotes rusting.

Hydrogen Peroxide

- It is a colorless watery liquid and loses potency on keeping for a longer time.
- It liberates nascent oxygen on coming in contact with tissues, which oxidizes necrotic matter and bacteria. Catalase enzyme is present in tissues, which speeds up decomposition resulting in foaming and helps in loosening and removing slough, earwax, etc.
- It is used for cleaning dirty wounds and abscess cavities.
- It can also be used to disinfect contact lenses, plastic implants, surgical prosthesis, etc.
- It is sporicidal in a concentration of 10–20%.

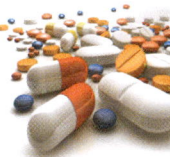

Benzoyl Peroxide

- It is specifically active against *P. acnes* and used on acne vulgaris.
- It should only be applied on the surface of acne, because it causes skin irritation, marked scaling, erythema, and contact sensitization.
- It should be applied in 5–10% conc. in a form of cream/gel/lotion.

Ethylene Oxide (ETO)

- It is the most common form of chemical sterilization.
- It has lethal effects on proteins and DNA of bacteria.
- It is also sporicidal and virucidal.
- It is highly inflammable. Therefore, it is generally mixed with carbon dioxide.
- It is used to sterilize heat sensitive plastics, petri dishes, catheterization equipment and plastic syringes, etc.

Low Temperature Gas Plasma

- It is an alternate to ETO.
- It is used with hydrogen peroxide (H_2O_2) for generation of free radicals, which kills microorganisms.

Ozone Sterilization

- It is a new technique of sterilization, recently approved by the US.
- In this technique, the oxygen is converted to atomic oxygen, which binds to another oxygen molecule and forms ozone.
- It destroys many pathogens and prions.
- It is used to treat foods such as meat, eggs, and poultry.
- It is also used to disinfectant water and sewage.

HALOGENS

Halogens are strong oxidizing agents; they include iodine, chlorine, and fluorine.

Iodine

- Iodine is an microbicidal agent and acts by iodinating and oxidizing microbial protoplasm.
- It acts very fast and a 1:20,000 solution kills most vegetative forms within 1 minute. Higher concentration and longer duration of contact kill the bacterial spores also.
- Germicidal action decreases in the presence of organic matter.
- It is used for degerming skin before surgery and on cuts.
- Some individuals are hypersensitive to iodine. Rashes can occur.
- Different preparations with different uses are:

- **Tincture iodine** (2% in alcohol) stings on abrasions (>5%) cause burning and blistering of skin.
- **Mandl's paint** (1.25% iodine is dissolved with the help of potassium iodide) is applied on sore throat.
- **Lugol's iodine** contains 5% iodine in 10% solution of potassium iodide and is used in thyrotoxicosis.

Iodophores

- These are non-irritating, non-toxic and non-staining forms of iodine. Hence, the treated areas can be bandaged or occluded without risk of blistering.
- These exert prolonged germicidal action.
- These are soluble complexes of iodine and serve as carriers of iodine, and release free iodine slowly.
- The most popular one is Povidone (Polyvinylpyrrolidone) iodine.
- It is used for surgical scrubbing, disinfection of endoscopes and instruments.
- It is also used on boils, furunculosis, burns, otitis externa, ulcers, tinea, monilial, trichomonal and non-specific vaginitis.
- Its different preparations are Povidone iodine 5% solution, 5% ointment, 7.5% scrub solution, 200 mg vaginal pessary, Piodin 10% solution, 10% cream,
- 1% mouthwash and 5% spray.

Chlorine

- Chlorine is a rapidly acting potent germicide which kills most pathogens.
- It is used to disinfect urban water supplies at 0.1–0.25 ppm concentration.
- *'Chlorine demand' of water:* The organic matter binds to chlorine and excess chlorine has to be added to obtain free chlorine concentration of 0.2–0.4 ppm (parts per million). The chlorine demand of water is measured by *Horrock's apparatus*.

Chlorophores

- Chlorine is a gas and difficult to provide as such for routine use, chlorophores are used instead.
- Chlorophores are compounds that slowly release hypochlorous acid (HOCl) and then liberate free chlorine for the action. These are used in preference to gaseous chlorine because of ease of handling.

Some of the important chlorophores are as follows:

Chlorinated Lime (Bleaching Powder)

- It is obtained by the action of chlorine on lime; resulting in a mixture of calcium chloride and calcium hypochlorite. On exposure, it decomposes releasing 30–35% W/W chlorine.

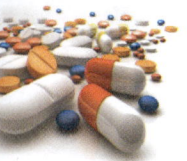

- It is used as disinfectant for drinking water, swimming pools and sanitizer for toilets, etc.

Sodium Hypochlorite Solution

- It is a powerful disinfectant and contains 4–6% sodium hypochlorite.
- It is used as disinfectant in dairies for milk cans and other equipment.

Fluoride

It mainly acts as anticaries agent, but studies show that it is germicidal also.

BIGUANIDE

Chlorhexidine

- It is a non-irritating and powerful antiseptic and more active against Gram-positive bacteria.
- It acts by disrupting bacterial cell membrane and by denaturing the microbial proteins.
- It is used for surgical scrubs, neonatal bath, obstetric and general skin antiseptic.
- It is the most commonly used antiseptic in dentistry to prevent or treat gingivitis.
- It is used as 0.12–0.2% oral rinse or 0.5–1% toothpaste.
- The only disadvantage is an unpleasant after taste and brownish discoloration of teeth on prolonged use.

QUATERNARY AMMONIUM OR CATIONIC ANTISEPTICS

Cetrimide

- Cetrimide is a soapy powder with a slight fishy odor.
- It acts as non-irritating detergent and is cidal to bacteria, fungi and viruses.
- It acts by altering permeability of cell membranes and denaturing the bacterial proteins.
- It is commonly used as hospital antiseptic sanitizer, and disinfectant for surgical instruments, and gloves, etc. but, does not have sterilizing action.
- It removes dirt, grease, tar and blood from wounds very efficiently due to its good cleansing action.
- It is used either alone or in combination with chlorhexidine.
- It is available in different forms as:
  - Concentrate solution (cetrimide 20%), as disinfectant.
  - Liquid antiseptic (chlorhexidine gluconate 1.5% + Cetrimide 3%).
  - Cream (chlorhexidine HCl 0.1% + cetrimide 0.5%),
  - Hospital concentrate (chlorhexidine gluconate 7.5% + cetrimide 15%).

Benzalkonium Chloride

A 1:1000 solution is used to sterile instruments and 1: 5000 to 1 :10,000 is used for douches, irrigation, etc.

Dequalinium Chloride

It is used in gum paints and lozenges.

SOAPS (ANIONIC ANTISEPTICS)

- Soaps are weak antiseptics and anionic in nature.
- They have detergent (cleansing) action and affect only Gram-positive bacteria.
- One of the most advocated and effective methods of preventing transmission of infection is by washing hands with soap and warm water.

ALCOHOLS

They act by denaturing bacterial proteins and precipitating them.

Ethanol or Ethyl Alcohol

- It acts as antiseptic and cleansing agent at 40–90% concentration.
- Up to concentration of 70%, the rapidity of action increases and then it decreases above 90%.
- When a cotton swab soaked in 70% ethanol is rubbed on the skin, 90% bacteria are killed in 2 minutes. Therefore, it is used before hypodermic injection and on minor cuts.
- It is an irritant and should not be applied to open wounds, mucous membranes or to delicate skin.
- It is not used to disinfect instruments as it promotes rusting and does not kill spores.
- Hand sanitizers contains 65–70% of ethyl alcohol.

Isopropanol or Isopropyl Alcohol

- It is more potent and less volatile than ethanol.
- It can be used to disinfect clinical thermometers.
- It is used in 60–70% concentration as an antiseptic.

ALDEHYDES

The aldehydes denature proteins and act as general protoplasmic poisons. The aldehydes are very good sterilizing agents.

Formaldehyde

- It is a pungent gas, broad-spectrum germicide and used for fumigation of operation theaters and wards.

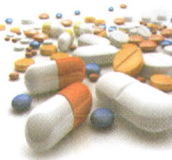

- A 37% aqueous solution of formaldehyde is called *Formalin*.
- A 4% diluted solution is used for hardening and preserving dead tissues.
- Formalin is also used to precipitate *toxoids* from toxins.
- It can cause allergic reactions.
- The urinary antiseptic methenamine also acts by releasing formaldehyde in acidic urine.

Glutaraldehyde

- A 2% solution is used to disinfect surgical instruments and endoscopes, but prolonged contact is needed.
- It is less pungent, less irritating and better sterilizing agent than formalin.

It needs to be activated by alkalinization of the solution.

- The alkalinized solution has a short shelf life (2 weeks) unless stablilizing agents are added.

Orthophthalaldehyde (OPA)

- It is a phenolic dialdehyde and has sterilizing effect also.
- It is rapidly acting bactericidal than other aldehydes.
- Disinfection can be achieved within 12 minutes with 0.55% OPA, whereas, 2.4% glutaraldehyde takes 45 minutes.

It does not require activation for its action.

- It is less irritant to mucous membranes and does not precipitate asthma.
- It has good materials-compatibility and an acceptable environmental safety profile.
- It is used for disinfection or sterilization of endoscopes, surgical instruments, rubber anesthetic tubes, and other medical devices.
- No resistance to OPA has been recorded yet.

ACIDS

Boric Acid

- It is non-irritating weak antiseptic and bacteriostatic in nature.
- It is available in different preparations.
  - **Solutions:** 4% saturated aqueous solutions are used for irrigating eyes, mouthwash, douche, etc.
  - **Paint:** In 30% conc. It is used for stomatitis and glossitis (Boroglycerine paint).
  - **Ointment:** A 10% ointment is used for cuts and abrasion.
  - Powders and ear drops: It is included in prickly heat powders and eardrops.
  - Systemic absorption causes vomiting, abdominal pain, diarrhea, visual disturbances and kidney damage. Hence, not recommended for use in infants.

Benzoic Acid

- It acts as antibacterial and antifungal.
- It is a constituent of Whitfield's ointment (6% benzoic acid + 3% salicylic acid) for ringworm infections.

FURAN DERIVATIVES

Nitrofurazone

- It is microbicidal to Gram-positive, Gram-negative, aerobic and anaerobic bacteria.
- It acts by inhibiting enzymes necessary for carbohydrate metabolism in bacteria.
- It is highly efficacious in burns and for skin grafting.
- It is available as furacin 0.2% cream, soluble ointment and powder.
- Nitrofurantoin and furazolidone are other furan derivatives used for urinary and intestinal infections respectively.

METALLIC SALTS

Silver Salts
Silver Nitrate

- It is used as an antiseptic and has astringent properties.
- It kills the microbes rapidly and performs sustained effect because of interaction between cellular protein and silver ions. It stains the tissue black in color due to this interaction.
- 1% solution is used to treat ophthalmia neonatorum and conjunctivitis.
- Silver nitrate swab is applied on oral ulcers and inflamed tonsils.

Silver Sulfadiazine

- 1% cream is used topically on burn wounds to prevent Pseudomonas infection, but it is not much effective once the infection has established.
- Pseudo-barrier layer of silver sulfadiazine (>2 mm thick) should be developed over the burn area to prevent the infection and activation of opportunistic pathogens.
- It is non-irritating, but the combination with chlorhexidine may cause burning sensation.

Nano-Silver Gel

- Nano-silver is fast acting, highly efficacious, non-poisonous, non-irritating gel containing nanoparticles silver measuring 25 nm.
- They have extremely large surface area which increases their contact with bacteria or fungi; thereby improving the bactericidal and fungicidal effects.

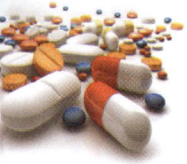

- The nano-silver adversely affects the cellular metabolism (respiration and basal metabolism) and inhibits the cell growth.
- Its major uses are dressing for burns, scalds, skin donor and recipient site, acne and cavity wounds.
- It is available as 0.002% in concentration.

Zinc Salts

Zinc Sulfate

- It has antiseptic and astringent properties.
- It is highly water-soluble.
- It is used in 0.1–1% preparation for washing eyes for the prevention of conjunctivitis.
- It decreases perspiration; thereby used as a component of deodorants.

Zinc Pyrithione (ZPTO)

- It is having antifungal action.
- It is an active ingredient of anti-dandruff shampoos.

Zinc Oxide

- Zinc oxide in combination with ferric oxide forms a flesh color lotion (Calamine). This lotion possesses antiseptic and astringent effects and used for nappy rash.
- In addition to being mildly antiseptic, the combination is popular dermal protective and adsorbant.

DYES

- Two groups of dyes aniline and acridine have been widely used as antiseptics.
- They are mainly bacteriostatic.

Aniline Dye

They include Malachite Green, Brilliant Green, and Crystal Violet (Gentian violet).

- They are non-irritating antiseptics.
- It is effective against Gram-positive bacteria and fungi.
- It is used in burns, infected eczema, furunculosis and oral and vaginal thrush.
- Its major disadvantage is that it is non-effective against Gram-negative bacteria and stains the tissue.

Acridine Dye

They include acriflavine, proflavine, aminacrine and euflavine.

- They are non-irritating antiseptics.
- It is effective against Gram-positive bacteria and gonococci.
- It is used in chronic ulcers and wounds.
- Also used to irrigate urinary bladder and vagina.
- It should be stored in amber color bottle as it degrades on exposure to sun light (Photosensitive).
- Non-effective against Gram-negative bacteria.

Methylene Blue

It acts as reducing agent and given intravenously to convert methemoglobin to hemoglobin.

Triple Dye Lotion

Contains Gentian violet 0.25% + brilliant green 0.25% + acriflavine/proflavine 0.1%. This dye is used in burn patients.

SUCRALFATE

Topical application of sucralfate is used in combination with antiseptics in burns, bedsores, diabetic/radiation ulcers, excoriated skin, etc. where it forms a protective layer.

DEBRIDEMENT AGENTS

- **Eusol solution:** It is freshly prepared solution of Boric acid 12.5 g + bleching powder 12.5 g desolved in 1 L of distal water. It liberates chlorine which inhibits the growth of microorganisms.
- **Tetracholrodecaoxide, Collagenase, Superoxide solutions, etc. are some other debridement agents.**

INSECTICIDES

Insecticides are the substances used to kill insects. They include ovicides and larvicides used against insect eggs and larvae, respectively. Insecticides are used in agriculture, medicine, industry and by consumers. All insecticides have significant potential to alter ecosystem. Many are toxic to humans; some concentrate along the food chain.

Insecticides can be classified into two major groups:

- Systemic insecticides, which have residual or long term activity.
- Contact insecticides, which have no residual activity.

Furthermore, based upon their nature, insecticides can be distinguished into three types:

- Natural insecticides, such as nicotine, pyrethrum and neem extracts, made by plants as defence against insects.
- Inorganic insecticides, which are metals.
- Organic insecticides, which are organic chemical compounds, mostly working by contact.

ORGANOCHLORIDES

The best known organochloride, DDT, was created by Swiss scientist Paul Muller. For this discovery, he was awarded the 1948 Nobel Prize for physiology or medicine. DDT was introduced in 1944. It functions by opening sodium channels in the insect's nerve cell. The rise of the chemical

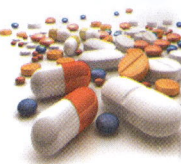

industry facilitated large-scale production of DDT and related chlorinated hydrocarbons. Use of these insecticides has been banned these days due to their non-biodegradable nature and adding to the depletion of the precious ozone layer.

ORGANOPHOSPHATES AND CARBAMATES

Organophosphates are another large class of contact insecticides. These also target the insect's nervous system. Organophosphates interfere with the enzyme acetylcholinesterase and other cholinesterase, disrupting nerve impulses and killing or disabling the insect. Organophosphate insecticides and chemical warfare nerve agents (*such as tabun, sarin, soman*) work in the same way. Organophosphates have a cumulative toxic effect to wildlife, so multiple exposures to the chemicals amplifies the toxicity. Carbamate insecticides have similar mechanisms to organophosphates, but have a much shorter duration of action and are somewhat less toxic.

There are many other insecticides which can harm human beings and behave as poisons.

Drug Interactions

- In most of the antifungal combinations, salicylic acid is added; both have synergistic effect as salicylic acid acts as keratolytic agents and helps in better penetration of antifungal agents.

Nursing Implications

- Hydrogen peroxide should be stored in the tightly closed dark containers and patient should be informed about the discomfort, which is going to occur on its application.
- The crystals of potassium permanganate should be completely dissolved before using it.
- Never apply alcohol to the abraded areas of the skin or open wounds.
- Nurse should ask about the history of allergy to any iodine preparation before applying any iodinated compound.
- Aseptic measures should be strictly followed.
- Universal precautions should be strictly followed.

Assess Yourself

Long and Short Answer Questions

1. What are the properties of ideal antiseptic/disinfectant?
2. Write short notes on:
   a. Halogen compounds
   b. Chlorhexidine
   c. Cetrimide
   d. Silver compounds
   e. Aldehydes

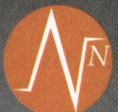
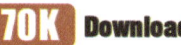 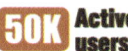 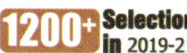 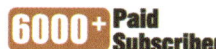 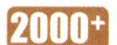 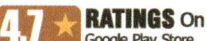
 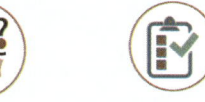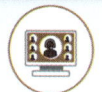
 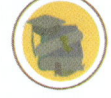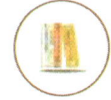

Drugs Acting on Gastrointestinal System

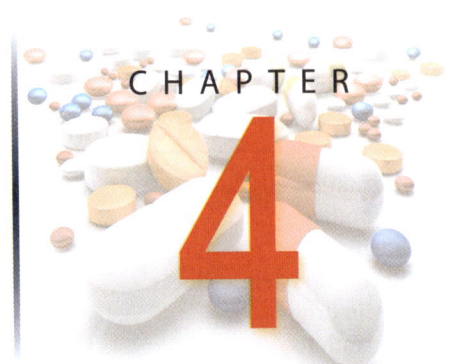

EMETICS AND ANTIEMETICS

('Emesis Means Vomiting')

Emesis (vomiting) is a protective reflex, which is induced by irritation of stomach (*peripheral stimuli*) or/and stimulation of vomiting center in the brain (*central stimuli*) whereas, nausea denotes the feeling of impending vomiting.

In case of ingestion of certaintoxic substances, vomiting may need to be induced for therapeutic purpose also.

MECHANISM OF VOMITING

- Vomiting occurs due to stimulation of the *emetic center and chemotherapy trigger zone* (CTZ) situated in the medulla oblongata.
- The CTZ is not protected by the blood-brain barrier; hence, many stimuli can stimulate it easily (Fig. 4.1).

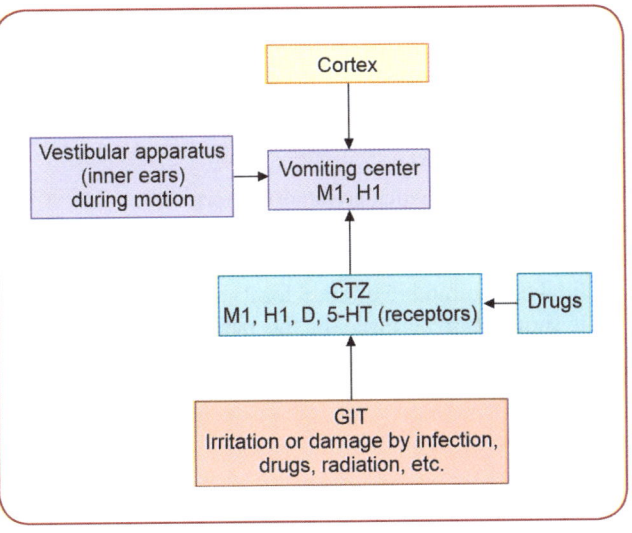

FIG. 4.1: Mechanism of vomiting

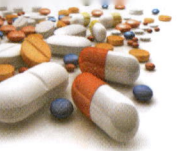

- The CTZ relays the stimulus to vomiting center also to initiate complex series of actions for a coordinated vomiting reflex.

CAUSES AND STIMULI OF VOMITING

- GI irritation
- Chemotherapy
- Radiations
- Infections/systemic illness
- Certain drugs
- Labyrinthitis
- Motion sickness during travelling
- Pregnancy (morning sickness)
- Severe vomiting during pregnancy (hyperemesis gravidarum).
- Painful stimuli
- Postoperative vomiting
- Metabolic and emotional disturbances
- Pseudotumor cerebri

Main Neurotransmitters Involved in Vomiting
- Acetylcholine
- Histamine
- 5-hydroxy tryptamine (5HT)
- Dopamine

EMETICS

- The drugs and other substances that cause emesis are called emetics. Common examples of emetics are: powdered mustard suspension, strong common salt solution, powdered ipecac and apomorphine.
- Mustard and common salt are commonly-used household emetics because they are easily available.
- They are indicated in case of poisonings.
- They act reflexly by irritating the stomach.

Apomorphine

- It is a semisynthetic derivative of morphine.
- It acts on CTZ.
- It is given in a dose of 6 mg by IM/SC route.
- It takes minimum 5 minutes for its action.
- It should not be given in the patients who are having respiratory distress as it also acts as a respiratory depressant.
- Its action is unpredictable when given by oral route.
- For induction of vomiting, very high dose is required, which is not safe.

Ipecacuanha

- It is obtained from dried root of Cephaelis ipecacuanha which contains an alkaloid called *Emetine*.

- It causes vomiting by irritating the gastric mucosa reflexly as well as by acting on CTZ.
- To induce vomiting, it is given orally in a dose of 15–30 mL in adults, 10–15 mL in children and 5 mL in infants.
- It takes minimum 15 minutes for its action.
- The syrup of ipecac is safer than apomorphine.

Conditions where Emetics are Contraindicated
- Kerosine poisoning (*aspiration may cause chemical pneumonia*).
- CNS stimulant drug poisoning (*emetics precipitate convulsions*).
- Morphine poisoning (*emetics do not work properly*).
- Corrosive poisoning (*it may lead to GI perforation/ esophageal erosions*).
- Unconscious patients (*increased chances of aspiration*).
- Paediatric patients. (*increased chances of aspiration*).

ANTIEMETICS

Drugs that are used to prevent or control the emesis are called antiemetics.

Although vomiting is a protective mechanism to eliminate the unwanted harmful material from the body, in some situations it may not serve a useful purpose, rather may only be troublesome. In such type of circumstances, vomiting needs to be suppressed with the help of antiemetic drugs.

Classification of Antiemetics

Refer to Table 4.1 for classification of antiemetics.

TABLE 4.1: Classification of antiemetics

Anticholinergics	Hyoscine, dicyclomine
H₁ antihistaminics	Promethazine, diphenhydramine, dimenhydrinate, doxylamine, meclozine (meclizine), cinnarizine.
Neuroleptics (D2 blockers)	Chlorpromazine, triflupromazine, prochlorperazine, haloperidol, etc.
Prokinetic drugs	Metoclopramide, domperidone, cisapride, mosapride, itopride, levosulpride.
5-HT3 antagonists	Ondansetron, granisetron, palonosetron, ramosetron
NK1 receptor antagonists	Aprepitant, fosaprepitant
Adjuvant antiemetics	Dexamethasone, benzodiazepines, cannabinoids

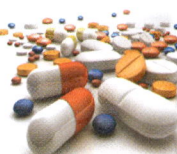

Cholinergics and anticholinergics are discussed separately (in chapter on cholinergic)

Antiemetic action is exerted by blocking conduction of nerve impulses from the vestibular apparatus to the vomiting center (which involves cholinergic link).

These drugs have poor efficacy in vomiting of other etiologies.

Hyoscine and Dicyclomine are the most commonly used anticholinergic drugs in GI system.

Hyoscine

It has shorter duration of action. It is given in a dose of 0.2–0.4 mg orally or IM. It is very effective for motion sickness. The most common adverse effects are dry mouth and sedation. Transdermal hyoscine patch is applied behind the pinna. It contains 1.5 mg of Hyoscine and delivers the drug for consecutive three days.

Dicyclomine

It is also used for motion sickness as a prophylaxis. It is given in a dose of 10–20 mg orally. It is used as an antispasmodic agent. The most common adverse effects are dry mouth and sedation.

H_1 Antihistaminics

- H_1 antihistaminic drugs have weak antiemetic property.
- The antiemetic action is due to antihistaminic, anticholinergic and weak antidopaminergic action.
- These drugs are useful to prevent motion sickness, morning sickness and postoperative vomiting.
- The main side effects are dry mouth, sedation, confusion, dizziness, and urinary retention. Commonly used H_1 antihistaminics with their dose, route and main uses are given in Table 4.2.

TABLE 4.2: H_1 antihistaminics

Drug	Dose and Route	Main uses
Promethazine	25 mg, oral and IV	Motion sickness, chemotherapy induce vomiting
Diphenhydramine	25–50 mg oral	
Dimenhydrinate	25–50 mg oral	
Doxylamine	10-20 mg oral	Morning sickness
Meclozine (Meclizine)	25–50 mg oral	Sea sickness
Cinnarizine	25–50 mg oral	Vertigo, labrynthitis

NEUROLEPTICS (D_2 BLOCKERS)

(Chlorpromazine, triflupromazine, prochlorperazine, haloperidol)
- The neuroleptics act as potent antiemetics also.
- They act by blocking D_2 receptors in CTZ.
- These are less effective in motion sickness as the vestibular pathway does not involve D_2 receptors.
- They are mainly used in:
  - Postoperative/drug induced/radiation sickness, nausea and vomiting
  - Vomiting due to uremia, liver disease, migraine, etc.
  - Malignancy associated and cancer chemotherapy (mildly emetogenic) induced vomiting.
- The major side effects are acute muscle dystonia and extrapyramidal side effects.

Prochlorperazine

A D_2 antagonist, given in a dose of 5–10 mg BD/TDS oral, and/or 12.5–25 mg by deep IM injection and it is indicated in vertigo and some cases of chemotherapy induced vomiting.

These drugs are least preferred as antiemetics due to availability of better and safer antiemetics.

Prokinetic Drugs

(Metoclopramide, domperidone, cisapride, mosapride, itopride, levosulpride)
The drugs, which promote gastric emptying by enhancing the coordinated propulsive motility of upper gastrointestinal tract are called prokinetic drugs.

Metoclopramide

- It is also called gastric hurrying agent. It has both peripheral and central actions.
  - **Peripherally:** Metoclopramide has more prominent effect on upper GIT; increases gastric peristalsis while relaxing the pyloric sphincter and the first part of duodenum. It also increases the tone of lower esophageal sphincter (LES).
  - **Centrally:** Metoclopramide blocks the D2 receptors in CTZ.

Pharmacokinetics

- It is rapidly absorbed orally. It acts in ½–1 hour when given orally, within 10 minutes after IM and 2 minutes after IV injection. Action lasts for 4–6 hours.
- It crosses the blood brain barrier and placental barrier.
- It is metabolized in liver and excreted in urine.

Dose

- Adults: 10 mg TDS oral or IM
- Children: 0.2–0.5 mg/kg TDS oral or IM

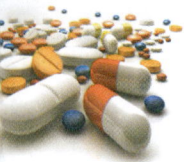

Indications

- Vomiting due to different reasons such as drug induced, disease associated, postoperative and radiation sickness, etc. It is not preferred in motion sickness due to poor effectiveness.
- It can be used for morning sickness only when other drugs fail.
- It is used as *Gastrokinetic agent* to accelerate gastric emptying in conditions such as: diabetic gastroparesis associated-gastric stasis and when in emergency general anesthesia has to be given and the patient has taken food in less than 4 hours before.
- Dyspepsia and persistent hiccups.

Adverse Effects

- The most common side effects are loose stools, sedation, dizziness and muscle dystonias (due to extrapyramidal side effects in children).
- Long-term use can cause galactorrhea, gynecomastia and parkinsonism.

Domperidone

- **Domperidone** is a D_2 receptor inhibitor.
- It acts as metoclopramide but has chemical structure like haloperidol.

Pharmacokinetics

- It is well-absorbed orally, but due to first pass metabolism, it has poor bioavailability (15%).
- It is metabolized in liver and excreted in urine.
- The plasma t½ is 7.5 hours.

Dose

- Adult: 10–40 mg TDS.
- Children: 0.3–0.6 mg/kg in three divided doses.

Indications

- These are same as metoclopramide but less effective as gastrokinetic agent.
- It is not useful in chemotherapy induced emesis.

Adverse Effects

- The side effects are less as compared to metoclopramide.
- The mild side effects are headache, loose stools and dry mouth.

Cisapride

- It is 5-HT$_4$ receptors agonist and promotes Ach release in the gut wall causing prokinetic activity.

- It is not an antiemetic as it does not act on D_2 receptors. Therefore, no extrapyramidal side effects are seen. The t½ is 10 hours.
- It was commonly indicated as prokinetic agent, particularly for gastroesophageal reflux disease and gastroparesis.
- Its clinical use has been banned in India since 2011 due to cardiac side effects like Q-T prolongation, etc.

Mosapride

- It is a congener of Cisapride. It is also a 5-HT$_4$ receptor agonist and has poor 5-HT$_3$ antagonistic action on myenteric plexus.
- Like cisapride, it does not act on D_2 receptors hence, hyperprolactinemia and extrapyramidal side effects are not seen.
- The common side effects are abdominal pain, diarrhea, headache, dizziness, and insomnia. It may also cause Q-T prolongation when co-prescribed with macrolides and azoles. So, it should be given carefully in cardiac patients.
- It is given in a dose of 5 mg (elderly 2.5 mg) TDS.
- It is indicated in diabetic gastroparesis, non-ulcer dyspepsia, GERD (as adjuvant to H$_2$ blockers/PPIs), and some cases of chronic constipation.

Itopride

- It is a safer prokinetic drug.
- It has D_2 antidopaminergic and anti-cholinesterase activity. Thus, it potentiates the Ach action on GIT causing prokinetic activity.
- No drug interactions are seen with macrolides and azoles. It can be given safely to cardiac patients as no Q-T prolongation has been recorded yet.
- The side effects are diarrhea, abdominal pain, headache. Galactorrhea and gynecomastia occur rarely. No extrapyramidal side effects are seen.
- It is given in a dose of 50 mg TDS before meals.

Levosulpiride

- It is a selective antagonist of dopamine D_2 receptor activity on both central and peripheral levels.
- It is typical neuroleptic and a prokinetic agent.
- It is used in a treatment of anxiety disorders, dyspepsia, irritable bowel syndrome (IBS), etc.
- It is metabolized in liver and excreted in urine with a t½ of 9.7 hours. When given orally and 4.3 hours by IV route.
- It is usually given in combination with PPI (rabeprazole) (rabeprazole 20 mg + levosulpiride 75 mg).
- It can be given safely to cardiac patients as no Q-T prolongation has been recorded yet.

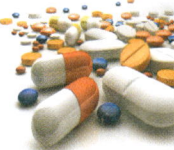

- The common side effects are diarrhea and constipation (dose dependent).
- It should not be used to stimulate the GI motility in presence of GI hemorrhage, obstruction and perforation.
- The patients should be advised to avoid driving or work on machinery as it causes dizziness and somnolence in some patients.

The newer prokinetic drugs are sultopride and tiapride.

5-HT₃ Antagonists

(Ondansetron, Granisetron, Palonosetron, Ramosetron)

- These antiemetic drugs were developed to control cancer chemotherapy or radiotherapy induced vomiting and proved their worth.
- They block the depolarizing action of 5-HT exerted through 5-HT receptors on vagal afferents in the GIT as well as in nucleus tractus solitarius (NTS) and CTZ.

Cytotoxic drugs/radiation produce nausea and vomiting by causing cellular damage → release of mediators including 5-HT from intestinal mucosa → activation of vagal afferents in the gut → emetogenic impulses to the NTS and CTZ → vomiting.

- They are highly effective in postoperative nausea and vomiting (PONV) and disease or drug-induced vomiting.
- They are not effective in apomorphine or motion sickness induced vomiting.
- Nowadays, these drugs are the most commonly used antiemetics.

Ondansetron

- It is given by both oral and IV route.
- It is metabolized in liver and excreted in urine and feces.
- The t½ 3–5 hours and duration of action is 8–12 hours, which may be longer at higher doses.

Indications and Dose

- **Cancer chemotherapy (highly emetogenic drugs) induced vomiting:** The dosage regimen is 8 mg IV by slow injection over 15 minutes to be given half hour before chemotherapeutic infusion, followed by 2 similar doses at 4 hours interval. Alternatively, single 24 mg IV dose on first day can also be used.
- **To prevent delayed emesis:** 8 mg oral is given twice a day for 3–5 days.
- **To prevent postoperative nausea and vomiting:** 4–8 mg IV given before induction of anesthesia and given 8 hourly postoperatively if required.
- **For radiotherapy and less emetogenic drugs:** 8 mg orally given 1–2 hours prior to the procedure and then at eight hourly interval till required.

Granisetron

- It is ten times more potent than ondansetron.
- It is more effective during the repeat cycle of chemotherapy.
- Its t½ is 8–12 hours therefore, given in BD doses.
- The side effects are similar to ondansetron.

Indications and Dose

- **Cancer chemotherapy (highly emetogenic drugs) induced vomiting:** 1–3 mg diluted in 20–50 mL saline and infused IV over 5 minutes before chemotherapy, repeated after 12 hours.
- **For radiotherapy and less emetogenic drugs:** 2 mg oral 1 hour before chemotherapy or 1 mg before and 1 mg 12 hours after it.
- **To prevent post-operative nausea and vomiting:** 1 mg diluted in 5 mL saline and injected IV over 30 sec before starting anesthesia or 1 mg orally every 12 hours.

Palonosetron

- It is the longest acting 5-HT₃ antagonist and given in a single dose only.
- It is more effective in suppressing delayed vomiting occurring between 2–5 days after chemotherapy.
- It is given by both oral and IV routes.
- It is metabolized in liver and excreted in urine.
- It has t½ of 40 hours.
- In addition to the common side effects of 5-HT₃ antagonists, it also causes Q-T prolongation, when co-administered with erythromycin, moxifloxacin, anti-psychotics, antidepressants, etc.
- It should always be given by slow IV infusion as rapid IV injection may cause blurring of vision.

Indications and Dose

- **Cancer chemotherapy (highly emetogenic drugs) induced vomiting:** 250 µg by slow IV injection 30 minutes before chemotherapy. Do not repeat before 7 days.
- **To prevent post-operative nausea and vomiting:** 75 µg IV as a single injection just before induction.

Ramosetron

- It is similar to ondansetron in general properties.
- It is also indicated for diarrhea predominant IBS as it has shown potential to normalize disturbed colonic function.

Indications and dose

- **Cancer chemotherapy (highly emetogenic drugs) induced vomiting:** 0.3 mg injected IV before chemo-therapy, and repeated once daily.

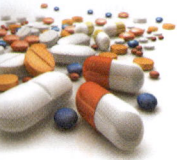

- **For low emetogenic chemotherapy:** It is given orally in a dose of 0.1 mg once daily.
- **To prevent post-operative nausea and vomiting:** Ramosetron 0.3 mg IV equally effective as ondansetron 8 mg IV.

NK1 Receptor Antagonists

(Aprepitant, Fosaprepitant)

- The substance-P released due to emetogenic chemotherapy activates neurokinin (NK1) receptors in CTZ and NTS and plays a role in the causation of vomiting.
- Aprepitant and Fosaprepitant antagonists block the NK1 receptors and act as antiemetics in chemotherapy-induced vomiting.

Aprepitant

- Aprepitant has high affinity to NK1 receptors.
- It is well absorbed orally. It penetrates blood-brain barrier and is metabolized in liver and excreted in feces and urine. Its $t\frac{1}{2}$ is 9–13 hours.
- It should not be given to the patients who have been already prescribed Q-T interval prolonging drugs.
- The main side effects are weakness, fatigue, flatulence and rarely rise in liver enzymes.

Indications and Dose

- **Cancer chemotherapy (highly emetogenic drugs) induced vomiting:** Oral aprepitant (125 mg + 80 mg + 80 mg over 3 days) combined with standard IV ondansetron/palonosetron + dexamethasone regimen significantly enhances the antiemetic efficacy against highly emetogenic cisplatin-based chemotherapy. It is highly useful in patients undergoing multiple cycles of chemotherapy.
- **To prevent post-operative nausea and vomiting:** A single (40 mg) oral dose of aprepitant is well effective in PONV.

Fosaprepitant

- It is a parenterally administered prodrug of aprepitant.
- It is given as 150 mg running IV infusion administered over 20-30 minutes.
- It is used in *Cancer, chemotherapy (highly emetogenic drugs) induced vomiting*. It is given in a dose of 150 mg in conjunction with standard IV ondansetron/palonosetron + dexamethasone regimen.

ADJUVANT ANTIEMETICS

(Corticosteroids, Benzodiazepines, Cannabinoids)

Corticosteroids

- Corticosteroids (dexamethasone, methylprednisolone) have antiemetic properties, but exact mechanism of action is unknown.
- These agents enhance the efficacy of 5-HT$_3$ receptor antagonists.
- The commonly used corticosteroid is dexamethasone, which is given in a dose of 8–20 mg intravenously before chemotherapy, followed by 8 mg/day orally for 2–4 days.

Benzodiazepines (BZDs)

- BZDs have sedative action and relieve the psychogenic component of vomiting; thereby used as adjuvant to antiemetics.
- They also suppress dystonic side effects of metoclopramide.
- The commonly used BZDs are diazepam, lorazepam (oral/IV), and alprazolam (oral only).

Cannabinoids

- They are obtained from *Cannabis indica,* and possess good antiemetic activity. Tetrahydrocannabinol (THC) is the active principle.
- They act by agonistic action on cannabinoid receptors (CB-1), which are located in vomiting center and CTZ.
- They are also good appetite stimulants.
- They are metabolized in liver and metabolites are excreted slowly over days to weeks in the feces and urine.
- They are not commonly used due to availability of better drugs.
- They are used only in those patients, who do not respond to other antiemetics.
- The common side effects are euphoria, dysphoria, sedation, hallucinations, and dry mouth.
  - **Dronabinol** is the purest form of THC and is usually given in a dose of 5 mg/m² just prior to chemotherapy and every 2–4 hours as needed.
  - **Nabilone**
    - It is a man-made cannabinoid, having antiemetic property.
    - It has been approved by US-food and drug administration (FDA) for its clinical use.
    - It is used only in those patients, who do not respond to other antiemetics.
    - It is given in a dose of 1–2 mg before 1–3 hours of chemotherapy; then every 8–12 hours during the course of chemotherapy and for 2 days following cessation of chemotherapy.

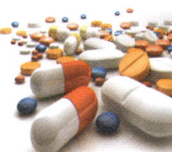

 Nursing Implications

⇨ **Emetics and antiemetics**
- ☞ Assess for possible contraindications or cautions: History of allergy to antiemetic to avoid hypersensitivity reactions.
- ☞ Assure that route of administration is appropriate for each patient to ensure therapeutic effects and decrease adverse effects.
- ☞ If used to prevent motion sickness, the antiemetic drug should be given 30 minutes before activity that involves motion.
- ☞ Monitor the patient response to the drug (relief of nausea and vomiting).
- ☞ In medicolegal cases, the vomitus should be preserved.
- ☞ Unconscious patient should be kept in lateral position to prevent aspiration.
- ☞ These patients should be given small, frequent, and light meals.
- ☞ Metoclopramide injection should be given slow IV and not very fast.

PURGATIVES AND LAXATIVES

- These drugs facilitate evacuation of stools from bowel.
- Laxatives facilitate evacuation of soft but formed stools.
- Purgatives facilitate evacuation of watery stools.
- *Laxatives have mild action than purgatives.*
- Some drugs act as laxatives in low dose and as purgatives in higher dose.

CLASSIFICATION

Refer to Table 4.3 for classification of purgatives and laxatives.

Bulk Purgatives

Dietary Fibers

- These are indigestible plant-based fibers and colloids such as bran, methylcellulose, lignins, gums, pectins, glycoproteins and polysaccharides.
- They absorb water, swell up and increase the bulk of stools.

TABLE 4.3: Classification of purgatives and laxatives

Class	Drugs
Bulk forming agents	Dietary fiber: Bran, psyllium, ispaghula, methylcellulose
Stool softeners	Docusates (DOSS), liquid paraffin
Stimulant purgatives	• *Diphenylmethanes*: Phenolphthalein, Bisacodyl, Sodium picosulfate • *Anthraquinones*: Senna, cascara sagrada • *5-HT4 agonist*: Prucalopride • Castor oil
Osmotic purgatives	• Magnesium sulfate, magnesium hydroxide • Sodium sulfate, sodium phosphate • Sodium potassium tartrate • Lactulose • Polyethylene glycol

- Some studies show that:
  - Fibers in the diet help in reducing the calorie intake as they remain longer in the gut and promote the satiety.
  - They promote the growth of colonic commensals, which help to improve bowel habits and even prevent diarrhea.
  - They improve the hepatic catabolism of cholesterol thereby; reducing the LDL-Cholesterol.
- A large amount of water should be taken with bulk forming laxatives to avoid intestinal obstruction.
- Increased intake of fiber helps in the prevention of functional constipation.
- They may cause flatulence.
- They should not be used in patients with gut ulcerations, stenosis, and obstruction.

Psyllium and Ispaghula

- They are plant fibers obtained from Psyllium and Ispaghula respectively.
- They should be freshly prepared by mixing with water or cold milk or fruit juice.
- The dose is 3–8 g OD/BD.
- They should not be swallowed dry.

Methylcellulose

It should be taken 4–6 g/day with large amount of fluids.

Stool Softeners

Liquid Paraffin

- It is a pharmacologically inert mineral oil that cannot be digested.
- It lubricates and softens the stools.
- It is taken in a dose of 15–30 mL OD.
- It is rarely used due to its unpalatable taste and oily consistency.
- It decreases the absorption of fat-soluble vitamins.
- It may leak out from the anus causing discomfort.

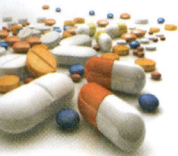

Docusates (Dioctyl Sodium Sulfosuccinate: DSS)

- It is an anionic detergent.
- It softens the stool by lowering surface tension, emulsifying the colonic contents and retaining the water content into the feces.
- It is bitter in taste and causes nausea; hence, capsule formulation is preferred.
- It is given orally in a dose of 100–400 mg/day and as enema 50–150 mg in 50–100 mL.
- Its prolonged use should be avoided as it may cause hepatotoxicity.

Stimulant Purgatives

- **Diphenylmethanes:** Phenolphthalein, bisacodyl, sodium picosulfate
- **Anthraquinones:** Senna, cascara sagrada
- **5-HT$_4$ agonist:** Prucalopride
- **Fixed oil:** Castor oil
- They promote water and electrolyte accumulation in the colon and stimulate evacuation of stool, increasing intestinal motility through stimulation of myenteric plexuses.
- Large and regular doses can cause colonic atony and electrolyte imbalance mainly hypokalemia.
- They cause uterine contractions; therefore contraindicated in pregnancy.
- They are also contraindicated in subacute and chronic intestinal obstruction.

Diphenylmethanes

Phenolphthalein

- A small proportion of phenolphthalein gets absorbed and resecreted into enterohepatic circulation. This is responsible for longer action and repeated purgation.
- After administration, it takes 6–8 hours to perform its action on colon and produces soft semi liquid stools.
- It should be given at bedtime.
- The common side effects are pink urine (if urine is alkaline), pink-colored skin and allergic eruptions. Hepatic damage may occur after repeated purgation.
- **Dose:** 60–130 mg HS.
- Nowadays, it is obsolete.

Bisacodyl

- It acts like phenolphthalein.
- It acts within 6–8 hours when given orally and 15–45 minutes when given in suppository form (bisacodyl + glycerin).

- It is relatively safe, but prolonged use may cause GI mucosal inflammation.
- Dose:
  - Orally: 5–15 mg.
  - Suppository- Children: 5 mg
  - Adults: 10 mg

Sodium Picosulfate

- It is similar to bisacodyl.
- After administration, it is hydrolyzed by colonic flora and converted to active form.
- The active form stimulates the myenteric plexus and increases colonic motility.
- It acts within 6–12 hours when given orally.
- Dose: 5–10 mg HS.
- Nowadays, it is used for investigative procedures (colonoscopy) and colonic surgery.
- The common side effects are skin rashes. Rarely Stevens-Johnson syndrome may be seen.

Anthraquinones

Senna and Cascara Sagrada

Ethnobotany confirms that Senna is traditional Indian therapy for constipation.

- These are natural products obtained from the plants. Senna from *Cassia sp.* (Amaltas) and *Cascara sagrada* from buck-thorn tree (powdered bark of the tree).
- After administration, colonic flora converts them to the active form *anthrol*, which acts locally and enters into enterohepatic circulation; therefore takes 6–8 hours to produce its action.
- The common side effect is skin rashes. Prolonged use causes mucosal pigmentation and colonic atony.
- These are contraindicated in lactating mothers as they secreted in milk.
- Dose: 10–20 mg HS.

The WHO Essential Drug List includes only Senna as laxative, whereas National Essential Drug List also includes Bisacodyl and Isapgol along with Senna.

5-HT$_4$ Agonist

Prucalopride

- It is a specific 5-HT$_4$-receptor agonist that facilitates cholinergic neurotransmission.
- It increases oro-cecal transit and colonic transit without affecting gastric emptying.
- It improves colonic transit and stool frequency in patients with chronic idiopathic constipation.

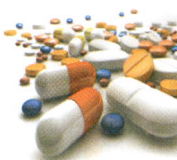

- This drug is recently approved in Europe, Canada, and UK for the treatment of chronic constipation in females.
- It is given in a dose of 2–4 mg orally OD.
- It has low affinity for cardiac potassium channels and does not prolong Q-T interval unlike cisapride and tegaserod.
- The common side effects are abdominal pain, headache, dizziness, and fatigue.

Castor Oil

- It is also a natural product, obtained from the seeds of *Ricinus communis*.
- It is the powerful and one of the oldest purgatives.
- It is hydrolyzed in the small intestine to its active form ricinoleic acid, which stimulates intestinal contractions by irritating the GI mucosa and decreasing the intestinal absorption of water and electrolytes.
- It also acts like detergent and softens the stools by lowering surface tension.
- Dose: Adult: 15–25 mL
  Children: 5–15 mL
- It should be taken in the morning, as it takes 2–3 hours to perform purgation.

Osmotic Purgatives

- Osmotic purgatives are soluble but non-absorbable compounds that result in increased stool liquidity by osmotic activity (Table).
- These drugs draw water from the lumen, distend the bowel and stimulate peristalsis causing evacuation of watery stools within 1–3 hours.
- These are most powerful and rapidly acting agents.
- The commonly used osmotic purgatives are magnesium sulphate, magnesium hydroxide, magnesium citrate, sodium phosphate and lactulose.

Doses of Various Osmotic Purgatives/Day

- Mag. sulfate (Epsom salt): 5–15 g.
- Sod. sulfate (Glauber's salt): 10–15 g.
- Sod. phosphate: 6–12 g.
- Sod. phosphate: 6–12 g
- Sod. pot. tartrate (Rochelle salt): 8–15 g

Magnesium Hydroxide (Milk of Magnesia)

- It is a commonly used osmotic purgative.
- In patients with renal impairment, it should not be used for prolonged periods as it causes hypomagnesemia.
- It is also used as an antacid.
- It is given as 8% W/W flavored suspension in a dose of 30 mL/day.

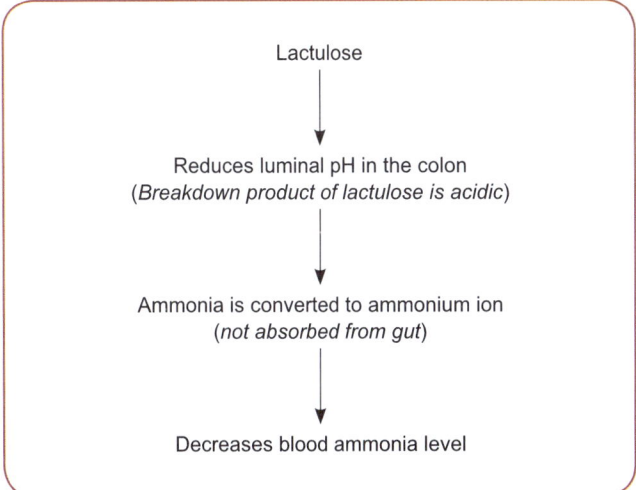

FIG. 4.2: Mechanism of blood ammonia level reduction by lactulose

Lactulose

- Lactulose is non-absorbable sugar used to prevent or treat chronic constipation.
- It is metabolized by colonic bacteria.
- It is also used to treat and prevent constipation in pregnant and lactating mothers.
- In addition to its purgative effects, it also reduces blood ammonia level in patients with *hepatic encephalopathy* (Fig. 4.2).
- The common side effects are flatus and abdominal cramps.
- For purgative action, it is given in a dose of 10 g BD with plenty of water.
- In hepatic encephalopathy, 20 g TDS is given but causes loose motions.

Polyethylene Glycol

- Lavage solutions containing **polyethylene glycol (PEG)** are used for complete colonic cleansing prior to surgical, radiological and endoscopic procedures of GI tract.
- It is non-absorbable, osmotically active sugar with sodium sulfate, sodium chloride, sodium bicarbonate, and potassium chloride.
- It is safe for all patients, as it does not cause electrolyte imbalance.
- 2–4 L of PEG is given over 2–4 hours with plenty of water or juice.
- It is also used for treatment or prevention of chronic constipation in smaller doses of 17 g mixed with lot of water or juice and ingested daily.
- PEG does not produce significant cramps or flatus as compared to lactulose.

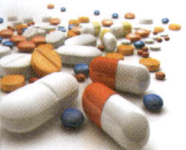

 ## Nursing Implications

⟲ **Purgatives and laxatives**

☞ Assess for fecal impaction or intestinal obstruction, which could be exacerbated if purgatives are given.

☞ Do not administer laxatives more than the prescribed dose.

☞ Arrange for appropriate fiber diet for these patients.

☞ Encourage fluid intake throughout the day as appropriate to maintain fluid balance and improve GI movement.

☞ Administer bulk laxatives with plenty of water. If only a little water is used, it may absorb enough fluid in the esophagus to swell into a gelatin-like mass that can obstruct the esophagus and cause severe problems.

☞ Insert rectal suppositories high into the rectum; encourage patients to retain enemas or rectal solution as long as possible to improve effectiveness.

☞ Monitor patient response to the drug (relief of GI symptoms, absence of straining, evacuation of GI tract) and keep a written record.

☞ Monitor fluid intake, output and electrolyte levels.

☞ Evaluate effectiveness of the teaching plan (patient can name drug, dosage, possible adverse effects to watch for, and specific measures to help avoid adverse effects).

ANTACIDS

Antacids are weak basic salts, which neutralize gastric acid and raise gastric pH.

They do not affect the acid production, however only temporarily increases the gastric pH. They act only when the gastric pH is more acidic, i.e., less than 4. When the gastric pH increases more than 4, gastrin is released reflexly which causes 'rebound acidity'.

Antacids, when taken in empty stomach act for 30–60 minutes only, whereas they act for at the most 2–3 hours when taken with meals.

The antacids are classified as systemic and non-systemic antacids.

SYSTEMIC ANTACIDS

- They are highly water-soluble and are rapidly absorbed from the gut.
- They rapidly neutralize acid in the stomach and locally act only for shorter duration.
- Systemically, these drugs act for longer duration; therefore may cause metabolic alkalosis.
- They produce CO_2, which may cause abdominal discomfort, distension, belching and bloating and may cause rebound acidity.

Sodium Bicarbonate

- It is a powerful and rapid acid neutralizer.
- It is also used for alkalinize urine and to treat acidosis.
- It increases sodium load, which may lead to edema; therefore, it is contraindicated in pulmonary edema, severe hypertension and chronic heart failure.
- 1 g of sodium bicarbonate neutralizes 12 mEq HCl.

Sodium Citrate

- It is having similar properties to sod. bicarbonate.
- It does not produce carbon dioxide.
- 1 g neutralizes 10 mEq HCl.

NON-SYSTEMIC ANTACIDS

- They are insoluble basic compounds and neutralize acid in the stomach.
- They are poorly absorbed from the gut and do not cause any systemic acid-base disturbance.
- Magnesium and aluminum salts are commonly used as antacids, and their combination have following advantages:
  - Magnesium salt causes diarrhea, while aluminum salt causes constipation; so they antagonize the adverse effects of each other.
  - Aluminum hydroxide acts slowly, while magnesium hydroxide acts rapidly; so the combination produces rapid and sustained effects.
  - In combination, they produce synergistic effects at low doses; therefore produce minimum systemic toxicity. Whereas, individually they have to be administered in higher doses for proper action.

Magnesium Hydroxide

- 1 g neutralizes 30 mEq HCl.
- Mild rebound acidity may occur.
- Its aqueous suspension is called milk of magnesia, which is available as 0.4 g/5 mL suspension.

Magnesium Trisilicate

- 1 g neutralizes 10 mEq HCl, but its clinical efficacy is very less [1 g neutralizes 1 mEq only].

Aluminum Hydroxide Gel

- 0.3 g/5 mL of its suspension may neutralize just 1 mEq HCl.
- It is also used therapeutically in hyperphosphatemia as it binds with phosphates in the intestine and inhibits the absorption of phosphates.
- It is contraindicated in osteoporosis as it inhibits calcium absorption from intestine.
- It may cause osteomalacia *de novo*.

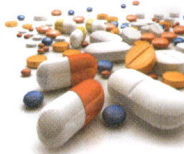

Magaldrate

- It is a hydrated complex of aluminum and magnesium salts; that is why it is a good antacid with rapid and sustained neutralizing action with minimal side effects.
- Dose: 400 mg tab, 400 mg/5 mL suspension.

Calcium Carbonate

- It is a potent and rapidly acting acid neutralizer.
- 1 g neutralizes 20 mEq HCl. but clinical efficacy is very less.

Milk Alkali Syndrome

When a large quantity of milk is taken with calcium carbonate [CaCO$_3$] (or NaHCO$_3$) for peptic ulcer, the combination often produces a syndrome which is characterized by abdominal distension, belching and bloating, headache, anorexia, weakness and renal stones. It occurs due to alkalosis and hypercalcaemia. This is known as Milk alkali syndrome. It is rarely seen these days.

ANTIFOAMING AGENTS

Methylpolysiloxane [Simethicone, Dimethicone]

- They are inert, insoluble, and non-toxic in nature.
- They are antifoaming agents and relieve flatulence.
- They form a thin layer on surface of bubbles and collapse them.
- They reduce the side effects of antacids.
- They are commonly available in combination with megaldrate.
- **Dose:** 25–40 mg four times daily.
- **Preparation for lithotripsy:** Dimethicone in a dose of 300 mg TDS for 5 days has been advocated for the patients undergoing lithotripsy as it helps to lessen the gas in the intestinal loops and makes the vision clear in the C-arm.

 Nursing Implications

☞ **Antacids**

- ☞ Administer antacids at least 1 hour before or 2 hours after any other medication to ensure adequate absorption of the other medications.
- ☞ Advise the patient to chew tablets thoroughly.
- ☞ Monitor patient response to the drug (relief of GI symptoms caused by hyperacidity).
- ☞ Shake well the syrup or gel bottle before use.
- ☞ Evaluate effectiveness of the teaching plan (patient can name drug, dosage, possible adverse effects to watch for, and specific measures to help avoid adverse effects).

HISTAMINES

- Most of the *Histamine* is present within storage granules of *mast cells*.
- Histamine-rich tissues are skin, gastric and intestinal mucosa, lungs, liver and placenta.
- Non-mast cell histamine is found in brain, epidermis, gastric mucosa and growing regions.
- *Histamine* is also present in blood, most body secretions, venoms and pathological fluids.
- *Histamine* acts through various receptors known as histaminic receptors.

Histamine Receptors

Four types of histaminergic receptors are there; H1, H2, H3 and H4 receptors.

All have different physiological and pathophysiological roles.

Pharmacological Actions of Histamine

- Histamine causes marked dilatation of smaller blood vessels, including arterioles, capillaries and venules. It constricts the larger blood vessels.
- When injected intradermally, it elicits the *triple response which* consists of Red spot, Wheal and Flare.
  - *Red spot* occurs due to intense capillary dilatation.
  - Wheal occurs due to exudation of fluid from capillaries and venules.
  - *Flare* (redness) in the surrounding area occurs due to arteriolar dilatation mediated by axon reflex.
- It causes constriction in the bronchial smooth muscles.
- It causes increase in gastric, bronchial, salivary and lacrimal secretions.

Pathophysiological Roles

- **Gastric secretion:** Histamine has important physiological role in mediating secretion of HCl in the stomach.
- **Allergic phenomena:** It is involved in mediation of many hypersensitivity reactions.
- **As transmitter:** Histamine is the afferent transmitter in initiation of the sensation of itch and pain at sensory nerve endings.
- **Inflammation:** Histamine is a mediator of vasodilatation and other changes that take place during inflammatory process.
- **Tissue growth and repair:** It has been suggested that it plays an essential role in the process of growth and repair because growing and regenerating tissues contain high concentrations of histamine.

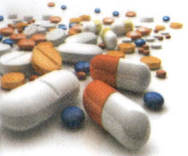

Uses of Histamine

Histamine has no therapeutic use.

In the past it was used to test acid-secreting capacity of stomach, bronchial hyperreactivity in asthmatics, and for diagnosis of pheochromocytoma, but obsolete now.

BETAHISTINE

It is an orally active, somewhat H1 selective histamine analogue, which is used to control vertigo in patients of Meniéré's disease: Possibly acts by causing vasodilatation in the internal ear.

It is contraindicated in asthmatics and ulcer patients.

 Nursing Implications

☞ **Histamines**

  ☞ Administer the drug apart from any other oral medications approximately 1 hour before or 2 hours after to ensure adequate absorption of the other medications.

  ☞ Administer drug before meals to ensure the therapeutic effectiveness of the drug.

  ☞ Monitor the patient continually if giving IV doses to allow early detection of potentially serious adverse effects, including cardiac arrhythmias.

  ☞ Assess the patient carefully for any potential drug–drug interactions if given in combination with other drugs because of the drug effects on liver enzyme systems.

  ☞ Monitor the patient's nutritional status; use of small frequent meals may be helpful if GI upset is a problem.

  ☞ Advise the patient to avoid alcohol, NSAIDs and food that may cause GI irritation.

  ☞ Nurse should arrange bland diet for these patients.

  ☞ Evaluate effectiveness of the teaching plan (patient can name drug, dosage, possible adverse effects to watch for, and specific measures to help avoid adverse effects).

ANTIHISTAMINES

H_1 ANTIHISTAMINICS

(Refer to Chapter 5)

H_2 ANTAGONISTS OR H_2 ANTIHISTAMINICS

- H_2 receptors are present in the parietal cells of gastric mucosa. The histamine binds to the H_2 receptors and stimulates acid secretion.
- H_2 antagonists competitively block H_2 receptors and suppress the acid secretion.
- They inhibit meal-stimulated acid secretion and basal nocturnal acid secretion in a linear and dose-dependent manner; therefore best efficacy is achieved when taken at bedtime.
- They also decrease the volume and concentration of gastric acid secretion.
- They do not affect the absorption of vitamin B-12.
- H_2 antagonists are cimetidine, ranitidine, famotidine roxatidine and nizatidine.
- Cimetidine was the first H_2 antagonist developed in 1970, but obsolete nowadays due to its side effects (antiandrogenic effects mainly gynecomastia).
- All H_2 antagonists undergoes first pass hepatic metabolism, while nizatidine have little first pass metabolism.
- The plasma t½ of H_2 antagonists ranges between 1–4 hours.
- Dose reduction is required in patients with hepatic or renal impairment.
- They are well-tolerated and the common side effects are bowel upset, dry mouth, headache and dizziness.

Some clinically important H_2 Antagonists are Cimetidine, Ranitidine, Famotidine, Roxatidine and Nizatadine. The details of commonly used H_2 antihistaminics are given in Table 4.4.

TABLE 4.4: Important H_2 antagonists

Drug	Usual dose for hyperacidity	Dose for acute duodenal or gastric ulcer	Dose for gastroesophageal reflux disease	Dose for prevention of stress induced bleeding
Cimetidine*	400–800 mg	800 mg HS or 400 mg BD	800 mg BD	50 mg/h continuous infusion
Ranitidine	150 mg	300 mg HS or 150 mg BD	150 mg BD	6.25 mg/h continuous infusion or 50 mg IV every 6–8 hours
Famotidine	20 mg	40 mg HS or 20 mg BD	20 mg BD	20 mg IV BD
Roxatidine	75 mg	150 mg HS or 75 mg BD	75 mg BD	–
Nizatidine	150 mg	300 mg HS or 150 mg BD	150 mg BD	–

* Obsolete nowadays (having only historic importance).

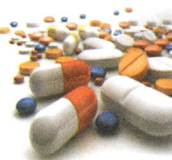
The main indications of H_2 antagonists are:

- Duodenal ulcer
- Gastric ulcer
- Stress ulcers and gastritis
- Zollinger-Ellison syndrome
- Gastroesophageal reflux disease (GERD)
- Prophylaxis of aspiration pneumonia
- Other uses: H_2 blockers have adjuvant beneficial action in certain cases of urticaria who do not adequately respond to an H_1 antagonist

PROTON PUMP INHIBITORS (PPIs)

- The parietal cells of the stomach secrete H^+ (Proton) with the help of an enzyme H^+/K^+ ATPase (proton pump). This membrane-bound enzyme plays an important role in the final step of gastric acid (HCl)secretion due to many stimuli.
- PPIs are the most powerful inhibitor of gastric acid secretion by inhibiting proton pump.
- These drugs should be administered approximately 1 hour before breakfast because they inhibit only those acid secretory proton pumps which are in active stage.
- As such, inhibition of HCl secretion occurs within 1 hour, reaches maximum at 2 hours, is still half maximal at 24 hours and lasts for 2–3 days. Since only actively acid secreting proton pumps are inhibited, and only few pumps may be active during the brief interval that the PPI is present (all have 1–2 hours plasma t½), antisecretory

action increases on daily dosing to reach a plateau after 4 days. At steady state all PPIs produce 80–98% suppression of 24 hour acid output with conventional doses. Secretion resumes gradually over 3–5 days of stopping the drug.

- These drugs are relatively safe in renal and mild to moderate hepatic impairment, while in severe hepatic impairment dose should be monitored.
- They are microsomal enzyme inhibitors; therefore cause many drug interactions. They increase the plasma levels of warfarin, benzodiazepine and phenytoin, which may lead to toxicity.
- These are well tolerated; the common side effects are loose stools, abdominal pain, joint pains, headache and dizziness.
- Prolonged use of PPI may cause atrophic gastritis, Achlorhydria, hypogastrinemia and vitamin-B12 deficiency.

Some clinically important PPIs are omeprazole, esomeprazole, lansoprazole, dexlansoprazole pantoprazole, rabeprazole, dexrabeprazole, ilaprazole, etc. The details of commonly used PPIs are given in Table 4.5.

> The main indications of proton pump inhibitors are:
> - Peptic ulcer
> - Bleeding peptic ulcer
> - Stress ulcers
> - GERD
> - Zollinger-Ellison syndrome
> - Aspiration pneumonia

TABLE 4.5: Clinically important proton pump inhibitors

Drug	t½	Dosage and route	Special features
Omeprazole	0.5–1.0	20–40 mg OD, oral and IV	• More effective than H2 blockers • Relief of pain and healing is rapid and excellent
Esomeprazole	1.5	20–40 mg OD, oral and IV	• It is S-enantiomer of omeprazole • It has higher oral bioavailability, slow elimination and longer t1/2 than omeprazole
Lansoprazole	1.0–2.0	30 mg OD, oral	• More potent than omeprazole • It has higher oral bioavailability, faster onset of action, slow elimination and longer t½ than omeprazole
Dexlansoprazole	1.0–2.0	30–60 mg OD, oral	• It is a dextro-isomer of Lansoprazole
Pantoprazole	1.0–1.9	40 mg OD, oral and IV	• More acid stable and has higher oral bioavailability • It is also available for IV administration • Specially used in bleeding peptic ulcer and for prophylaxis of acute stress ulcers
Rabeprazole	1.0–2.0	20 mg OD, oral and IV	• Causes fastest acid suppression otherwise potency and efficacy are similar to omeprazole
Dexrabeprazole	24	20–30 mg OD, oral	• It is the active dextro-isomer of rabeprazole, producing similar acid suppression at half the dose
Ilaprazole	8.1	5–10 mg OD, oral	• Latest PPI

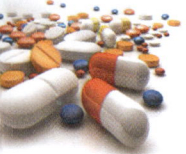

ULCER PROTECTIVES

SUCRALFATE

- It is a basic aluminum salt of sulfated sucrose.
- It forms sticky gel in stomach after being mixed with gastric secretions. This gel forms a layer over the ulcerative region of the stomach, forms a pseudo-barrier and protects it at least for 6 hours.
- It does not neutralize acid in the stomach but delays the gastric emptying, which prolongs its stay over the ulcer area; thereby increasing the duration of action.
- It also promotes the secretion of mucosal prostaglandin and bicarbonate for better healing.
- The GIT absorption is poor; the maximum amount of sucralfate is excreted through feces.
- The major indications are:
  - Upper GI bleeding.
  - Prevention of stress induced GI bleeding.
  - Gastritis
  - Gastropathy due to bile reflux.
  - Gastric and duodenal ulcer.
- It is given in a dose of 1 g QID in empty stomach (at least 1 hour before meals) followed by maintenance dose at 1 g BD.
- Topical application of sucralfate is used in burns, bedsores, diabetic/radiation ulcers, excoriated skin, etc. where it forms a protective layer.
- The common side effects are constipation and dry mouth.

COLLOIDAL BISMUTH SUBCITRATE (CBS; TRIPOTASSIUM DICITRATOBISMUTHATE)

- The CBS is water-soluble and works at pH < 5.
- Probably it acts like sucralfate; protects GI erosion and promotes local synthesis of prostaglandins.
- It is given in a dose of 120 mg QID preferably in empty stomach.
- The common side effects are diarrhea, headache and dizziness.

DRUG THERAPY FOR HELICOBACTER PYLORI (*H. pylori*) INFECTION

- *H. pylori* is a Gram-negative bacillus and found as commensal in 20–70% of normal population.
- Besides, it is also involved in the pathogenesis of peptic ulcer, gastritis, gastric lymphoma and cancer. Approximately all patients with gastric and duodenal ulcer are positive to *H. pylori* infection.

- It affects the surface of gastric epithelium beneath the mucous membrane and produces ammonia by urease activity; that protects the bacteria from HCl.
- The management of *H. pylori* infection involves concurrent therapy of PPI/H₂ antagonist with antimicrobial antibiotics (AMAs).
- Among antibiotics, the commonly used AMAs are amoxicillin, clarithromycin, tetracycline, and metronidazole/tinidazole.
- Ulcer protective agents are also used in combination with AMAs.
- PPI or H₂ antagonist decrease the gastric acidity and help AMAs to act better on *H. pylori*.

The various regimes used to treat *H. pylori* infection are shown below Table 4.6.

Commonly used 1 week and 2 weeks triple drug regimens
- **The US-FDA approved regimen**:
  Lansoprazole 30 mg + Amoxicillin 1000 mg + Clarithromycin 500 mg, all given twice daily for 2 weeks.
- **National Formulary of India (NFI, 2010)**:
  Omeprazole 40 mg OD + Metronidazole 400 mg TDS + Amoxicillin 500 mg TDS 1 week regimen.
- **Quadruple drug regimen** is advocated when triple drug regimen fails. Commonly employed quadruple drug regimen is CBS 120 mg QID + Tetracycline 500 mg QID + Metronidazole 400 mg TDS + Omeprazole 20 mg BD.

These drugs are used as triple drug regimen or quadruple drug regimen for 1–2 weeks depending upon the severity of illness followed by 1 PPI for a minimum period of 2–6 weeks.

TABLE 4.6: British National Formulary regimen

Anti-H. pylori Regimens			
Proton pump inhibitor	Amoxicillin	Clarithromycin	Metronidazole/Tinidazole
One week-twice daily			
Omeprazole (20 mg) or Esomeprazole (20 mg) or Lansoprazole (30 mg) or Pantoprazole (40 mg) or Rabeprazole (20 mg)	1.0 g	500 mg	—
	—	250 mg	400 mg/500 mg
	1.0 g	—	400 mg/500 mg
	—	—	—
	—	—	—
Two weeks-twice daily			
Omeprazole (20 mg) or Lansoprazole (30 mg) or Pantoprazole (40 mg)	750 mg	—	400 mg/500 mg
	—	250 mg	400 mg/500 mg
	750 mg	—	—

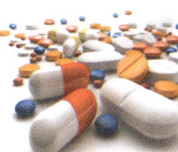

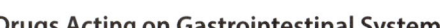

GASTROESOPHAGEAL REFLUX DISEASE (GERD)

- Reflux is a very common problem presenting as 'heart-burn', acid eructations, sensation of stomach contents coming back in the foodpipe. These symptoms are more especially after a large meal and aggravated by stooping or lying flat.
- The management of GERD depends upon the severity of disease.
- The severity of GERD and respective management is given in Table 4.7.

TREATMENT OF GERD

- Treatment of GERD is individualized according to the causative factors involved in an individual, severity and stage of the disorder.
- Dietary modifications, like avoidance of tea, coffee, alcohol, smoking, spicy foods, and taking light early dinner are advocated.
- Lifestyle measures, like daily light exercises, weight reduction, avoidance of precipitating factors and raising head end of bed must be taken.
- Different classes of drugs used in GERD are:
  - Proton pump inhibitors (PPIs)
  - H_2 receptor antagonists
  - Antacids
  - Prokinetic drugs

TABLE 4.7: Management of GERD according to severity

Severity of GERD	Medical management
Stage I • Sporadic uncomplicated heartburn, often in setting of known precipitating factor • Less than 2–3 episodes per week. • Often not the chief complaint and no additional symptoms are there	• Lifestyle modifications, including diet, positional changes, weight loss, etc. • Antacids and/or histamine H_2 receptor antagonists as needed
Stage II • Frequent symptoms, with or without esophagitis • Greater than 2–3 episodes per week	• Proton pump inhibitors more effective than histamine H_2 receptor antagonists
Stage III • Chronic, unrelenting symptoms; immediate relapse when off therapy • Esophageal complications (e.g., stricture, Barrett's metaplasia)	• Proton pump inhibitor either once or twice daily • Treatment of complications

ANTIDIARRHEALS

As per WHO, diarrhea is defined as 3 or more times passage of loose or watery stools within 24-hour period. It may occur due to bacterial/viral/protozoal infections, certain pathological conditions such as IBD, toxins, drugs, anxiety, electrolyte imbalance, worm infestations, etc.

- *In developing countries, childhood (<5 years of age) diarrhea is the major cause of morbidity and mortality, which is accounting approximately 1.5–2.5 million deaths per year.*
- In India, around 1000 children die every day due to diarrhea.
- Most of the deaths in diarrhea occur due to dehydration which is preventable if timely action is taken. Diarrhea may be acute or chronic.
- **Acute diarrhea**
  Diarrhea of less than 2 weeks' duration is known as acute diarrhea and it is most commonly caused by invasive or non-invasive pathogens and their enterotoxins.
  - **Acute non-inflammatory diarrhea is** watery, non-bloody, usually mild, self-limited and is caused by a virus or non-invasive bacteria. Diagnostic evaluation is limited to patients with diarrhea that is severe or persists beyond 7 days.
  - **Acute inflammatory diarrhea is accompanied with** blood or pus and fever. It is usually caused by an invasive or toxin-producing bacteria.
- **Chronic diarrhea**
  Diarrhea which is present for more than 4 weeks duration is known as chronic diarrhea. Common causes including medications, chronic infections, and irritable bowel syndrome, etc.

MANAGEMENT OF DIARRHEA

- Mostly, the diarrhea is self-limiting in nature. If not controlled itself, the proper management of diarrhea depends upon establishing the underlying cause and instituting specific therapy.
- Therapeutic measures may be grouped into:
  - Rehydration by replacement of fluids and electrolytes, treatment of shock, acidosis and maintenance of nutrition.
  - Treatment of the underlying cause
  - Drug therapy.

Rehydration

In majority of cases, this is the only measure required. Rehydration can be done orally (*in mild to moderate dehydration*) or by intravenous route (*in severe dehydration*).

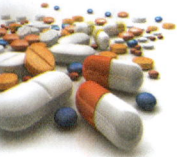

Oral Rehydration

- This is carried out with the help of Oral Rehydration Solution (ORS) which is prepared by adding 1 L of potable water in one packet of oral rehydration salts.
- It is the best choice to rehydrate the patient suffering from mild to moderate dehydration.
- In 2002, WHO has replaced standard (310 mOsm/L) ORS formula by a new formula known as *New formula WHO-ORS* (245 mOsm/L) which contains low Na^+ and low glucose.

New formula WHO-ORS			
Content		**Concentrations**	
NaCl	: 2.6 g	Na^+	— 75 mM
KCl	: 1.5 g	K^+	— 20 mM
Trisod. citrate	: 2.9 g	Cl^-	— 65 mM
Glucose	: 13.5 g	Citrate	— 10 mM
Water	: 1 L	Glucose	— 75 mM
		Total osmolarity 245 mOsm/L	

Rationale of ORS composition

- Oral rehydration solution contains glucose, Na^+, K^+, Cl and bicarbonate or citrate Na^+.
- A rational combination has been made to maintain normal body electrolyte levels.
- Glucose with sodium enhances glucose coupled Na^+ absorption.
- Potassium is an important constituent of ORS since in most acute diarrheas, K^+ loss is substantial.
- The base (bicarbonate, citrate, lactate) is added to correct acidosis due to alkali loss in stools. In addition, it may independently promote Na^+ and water absorption.

Administration of Oral Rehydration Therapy (ORT)

- ORT is not designed to stop diarrhea, but to restore and maintain hydration, electrolyte and pH balance until diarrhea ceases.
- Patients are encouraged to drink ORS at ½–1 hourly intervals.
- Initially, volume of ORS equal to 5–7.5% of body weight is given in 2–4 hours (5 mL/kg/hr in children). Subsequently it may be left to demand, but should at least cover the rate of fluid loss in stools.
- In a weak child who refuses to drink ORS at the desired rate, it can be given by intra-gastric drip through Ryle's tube with the aim of restoring hydration within 6 hours.

Non-diarrheal uses of ORT

- *Post-surgical, post-burn and post-trauma maintenance of hydration.*
- *Heat stroke.*
- *During change over from intravenous to enteral alimentation.*

Intravenous Rehydration

- Intravenous rehydration is instituted when the fluid loss is severe, i.e., >10% body weight or if patient is losing >10 mL/kg/hr, or is unable to take enough oral fluids due to weakness, stupor or vomiting.
- If the severe dehydration is not promptly corrected, it leads to hypovolemic shock and death.
- Volume equivalent to 10% body weight should be infused over 2–4 hours; the subsequent rate of infusion is matched with the rate of fluid loss avoiding fluid overload.
- In most of the cases, oral rehydration can be instituted after the initial volume replacement.
- There are three types of IV fluids depending on osmolality. These are isotonic, hypotonic and hypertonic solutions.
- Isotonic solution has osmolality of 310 mEq/L e.g., 0.9% NS and Ringer's lactate. These have osmolality nearly equal to extracellular fluid. When given intravenously, it increases the plasma volume by 25% only and remaining fluid diffuses in the extracellular fluid. Ringer's lactate solution contains sodium chloride, potassium, calcium and lactate. The lactate provides bicarbonate and helps to correct acidosis.
- Hypotonic solution has osmolality of <250 mEq/L e.g., 0.45%NS
- Hypertonic solution has osmolality of >375 mEq/L e.g., 10% dextrose, DNS

> ✔ **Nutrition During Diarrheal Episodes**
>
> Patients of diarrhea should never be starved. Fasting decreases brush border disaccharidase enzymes and reduces absorption of salt, water and nutrients. It leads to malnutrition if diarrhea is prolonged or recurrent. Feeding during diarrhea increases intestinal digestive enzymes and cell proliferation in mucosa.
>
> **Patients are advised:**
> - To take adequate oral fluids containing glucose and electrolytes.
> - Simple foods like boiled potato, rice, curd, khichadi, sago, banana, etc.
> - Frequent feedings of tea, beverages, easily digested foods (e.g., soups, toast, etc.) are encouraged.
> - To avoid fats, milk products, caffeine, and alcohol.

Treatment of the Underlying Cause

If the cause of diarrhea is identifiable, it should be taken care of along with correction of dehydration.

Drug Therapy (Antidiarrheal Agents)

Antimicrobial therapy should be considered when the suspected cause of diarrhea/dysentery is bacterial, protozoal or mixed.

The oral drugs of choice for empiric treatment are:

- Fluoroquinolones (Ciprofloxacin 500 mg, Ofloxacin 200 mg, or norfloxacin 400 mg, twice daily) for 5–7 days.
- Rifaximin, 200 mg three times daily for 3 days, is approved for empiric treatment of non-inflammatory traveller's diarrhea.
- Nitroimidazoles (metronidazole 400 TDS, tinidazole 500 mg BD, Ornidazole 500 mg BD) for 5–7 days and secnidazole 2 g stat.
- Nitazoxanide 500 mg BD for 5–7 days.(covers both protozoal and helminths)
- Quiniodochlor 250 mg TDS for 7 days.
- Furazolidone 100 mg TDS for 5–7 days
- Loperamide 4 mg orally initially, followed by 2 mg after each loose stool (maximum: 16 mg/24 hours).
- **Combination of prebiotics and probiotics in diarrhea:** Probiotics are microbial cell preparations. These are either live cultures or lyophillized powders and are intended to restore and maintain healthy gut flora. Most commonly used organisms are *Lactobacillus sp.*, *Bifidobacterium*, *Streptococcus faecalis*, *Enterococcus sp.* and the yeast *Saccharomyces boulardii*, etc. Curd is an abundant source of lactic acid producing organisms. Probiotics are safe and useful adjuncts to conventional therapy of acute infectious diarrhea. **Prebiotics** are a source of food for probiotics to grow, multiply, and survive in the gut. Prebiotics are the fibers, which cannot be absorbed or broken down by the body and therefore, serve as a great food source for probiotics to colonies better. The natural sources of prebiotics are onion, garlic, leek, asparagus, artichoke, etc. In formulations, fructo-oligosaccharide is commonly used as prebiotic.
- **Use of zinc in pediatric diarrhea:**
  - Zinc along with low osmolarity ORS reduces the duration and frequency of acute diarrhea episodes in children below 5 years of age. Zinc should be supplemented for 10–14 days following the episode of diarrhea.
  - It reduces the recurrence of diarrhea for the next 2–3 months.
  - The GoI has initiated providing zinc in addition to ORS through its National Rural Health Mission.
  - Zinc probably reduces fluid secretion in the intestine by indirectly inhibiting cAMP dependent Cl^- transport across the mucosa through an action on the basolateral membrane K^+ channels.
  - It also helps in regeneration of intestinal epithelium and strengthens the immune response.
  - Zinc is available as syrup, dispersible tablets and capsule form.
  - Dose for 0–6 month-age is 10 mg/day and for 6 month to 5 years of age is 20 mg/day for 10–14 days.

Nursing Implications

☞ **Anti-diarrheal**
- ☞ Administer the ORS after each loose stool to ensure therapeutic effectiveness.
- ☞ Maintain intake, output chart properly as it is a significant tool in the management of diarrhea patient.
- ☞ Keep track of the exact amount given to ensure that the dose does not exceed the recommended daily maximum dose.
- ☞ Monitor the response carefully; note the frequency and characteristics of the stool. If no response is seen within 48 hours, the diarrhea could be related to an underlying medical condition. Arrange to discontinue the drug and arrange for medical evaluation to allow for the diagnosis of underlying medical conditions.
- ☞ Monitor the patient response to the drug (relief of diarrhea).
- ☞ Evaluate effectiveness of the teaching plan (patient can name drug, dosage, possible adverse effects to watch for, and specific measures to help avoid adverse effects).

ANTISECRETORY DRUGS

RACECADOTRIL

It is a prodrug, given orally and is rapidly converted to its active form *thiorphan*.

- It prevents degradation of endogenous enkephalins (ENKs) by inhibiting enkephalinase.
- Endogenous enkephalines have antisecretory action.
- It increases water absorption at colon level without decreasing the intestinal motility; therefore does not cause constipation.
- It is indicated in acute secretary diarrheas for short duration only.
- The plasma t½ is 3 hours.
- The common side effects are nausea, vomiting, flatulence and drowsiness.
- Dose: Children: 1.5 mg/kg TDS for 7 days.
  Adults: 100 mg TDS for 7 days.

OCTREOTIDE

It is an analogue of somatostatin having longer plasma half life (90 minutes).

- It has potent antisecretory and antimotility action.
- It is indicated in diarrhea associated with carcinoids, AIDS, cancer chemotherapy, and diabetes.
- Control of diarrhea is due to suppression of hormones which enhance intestinal mucosal secretion.
- It is given subcutaneously in a dose of 50–100 mcg BD/TDS depending upon severity.

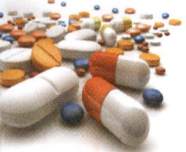

Drug Interactions

- Metoclopramide facilitates the gastric emptying and increases the absorption of many drugs such as aspirin, diazepam, etc.
- Prokinetic agents reduce the absorption of digoxin as stomach gets less time for the absorption of this drug.
- By blocking DA receptors in basal ganglia, metoclopramide abolishes the therapeutic effect of levodopa.
- Docusate sodium should not be co-prescribed with liquid paraffin as they may cause profound diarrhea.
- Antacids interfere with the absorption of digoxin, tetracycline, iron salt, INH, phenytoin, TCA and indomethacin.
- Antacids reduce the absorption of H_2 antihistaminics by raising the gastric pH.
- Antacids reduce the absorption of H_2 antihistaminics and PPIs by raising the gastric pH.
- PPIs may decrease the absorption of ketoconazole, iron salt and digoxin.
- PPIs may enhance the effect of warfarin, phenytoin carbamazepines, etc. by inhibiting the oxidation of these drugs.
- Clarithromycin increases the plasma level of rabeprazole or omeprazole by inhibiting their metabolism.
- Metronidazole causes disulfiram-like reaction when used with alcohol.
- The effect of oral anticoagulants may increase in dehydrated patients; hence, dose may have to be decreased.

Assess Yourself

Long and Short Answer Questions

1. What is the medical importance of emetic agents?
2. What are antiemetics? Classify them.
3. Describe the drugs used for chemotherapy induced vomiting.
4. What is lactulose? Describe its uses and mode of action.
5. What are anticholinergic drugs? Describe atropine.
6. Name any four common side effects of antihistaminic drugs.
7. Write short notes on:
   a. Prokinetics
   b. 5-HT$_3$ antagonist
   c. Bisacodyl
   d. Bulk forming laxative
   e. Proton pump inhibitors
   f. H$_2$ antihistaminics
8. Explain the role of zinc in pediatric diarrheas.
9. Write the composition of ORS and its use.

Multiple Choice Questions

1. **Which of the following drugs is not an antiemetic?**
   a. Ondansetron
   b. Domperidone
   c. Metoclopramide
   d. Cinnarizine

2. **The antiemetic drug which has been banned is:**
   a. Cisapride
   b. Mosapride
   c. Itopride
   d. Ondasetron

3. **Metoclopramide:**
   a. Increase lower esophageal sphincter tone
   b. Prokinetic action is blocked by atropine
   c. Increase gastric peristalsis
   d. Increase large intestinal peristalsis

4. **Stimulant purgatives are contraindicated in:**
   a. Bed ridden patients
   b. Before abdominal radiography
   c. Subacute intestinal obstruction d. All of these

5. **Laxative acting by opening of chloride channels:**
   a. Docusate
   b. Anthraquinone
   c. Lubiprostone
   d. Bisacodyl

6. **Mosapride is a:**
   a. 5HT$_4$ Agonist
   b. 5HT$_3$ Agonists
   c. 5HT$_3$ Antagonists
   d. 5HT$_4$ Antagonists

Answer Key

1.	d.	2.	a.	3.	a.	4.	c.	5.	c.	6.	a.

Drugs used on Respiratory System

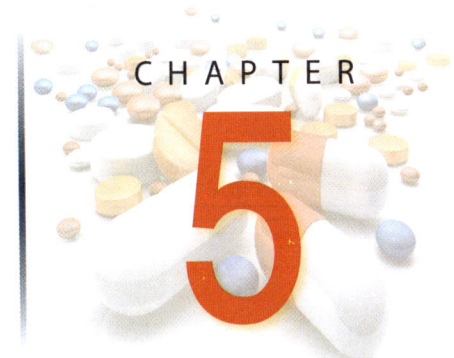

ANTI-ASTHMATICS

The drugs used to treat the bronchial asthma are called **anti-asthmatics**.

Asthma is a chronic inflammatory disease of the airways. It occurs due to hyper responsiveness of tracheobronchial tree to various allergic stimuli. It is characterized by:
- Dyspnea
- Wheeze
- Dry cough

These symptoms occur due to bronchospasm, increased bronchial secretions and edema of the bronchial mucosa.

Simplified View of Allergic Inflammation in the Airways

Asthma is an episodic narrowing of the bronchi thought to be caused by an underlying chronic inflammatory disorder. In allergic asthma, inhaled allergen initiates the inflammatory response by interacting with IgE bound to basophils and mast cells. This leads to a cascade of events involving other immune cells and release of various inflammatory mediators into the interstitial space, where they influence the growth and function of cell types within the airway wall. The drugs available for the treatment of asthma are targeted at inhibiting the inflammatory responses and/or relaxing the bronchial smooth muscle (Fig. 5.1). The various classes of drugs used in treating asthma are β_2 adrenergic agonists; corticosteroids; leukotriene modifiers; muscarinic receptor antagonists; cromolyn; theophylline; anti-IgE therapy.

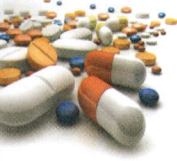

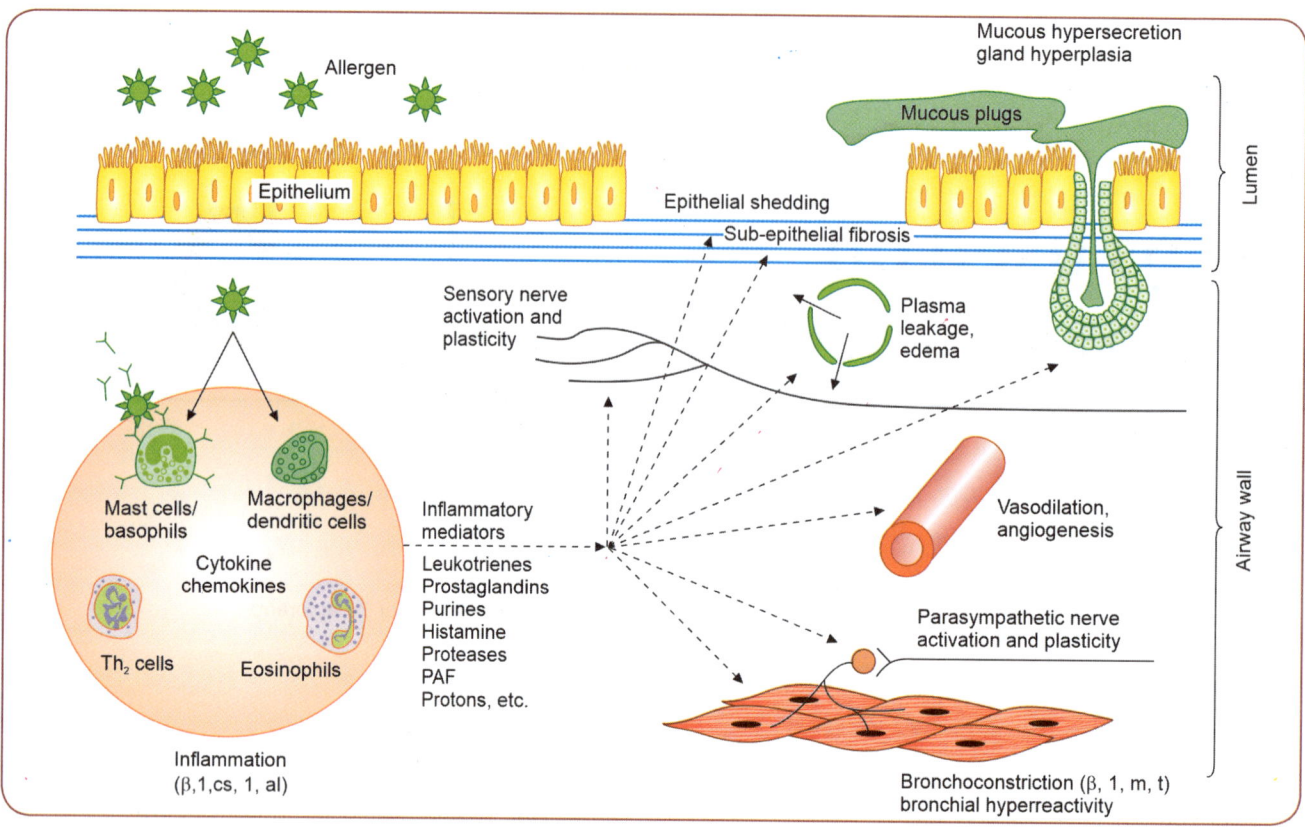

FIG. 5.1: Sites of action of various classes of drugs used in the treatment of asthma.

TABLE 5.1: Differences between extrinsic and intrinsic asthma

	Extrinsic Asthma	Intrinsic Asthma
Time of onset	Childhood	Late/adulthood
Allergy	Personal history or strong family history	No H/O allergy
Level of IgE and eosinophils	Increased	Normal
External stimulus	Required	May or may not be required
Status asthmatics	Less frequent	More frequent

Asthma is divided into two categories: Extrinsic and Intrinsic asthma (Table 5.1)

TRIGGER FACTORS

- Upper respiratory tract infection (Intrinsic asthma).
- Allergens. **Examples:** pollen grains, house dust or smoke, etc.
- Drugs such as Aspirin, nonselective beta-blocker (propranolol), opioids
- Cold or dry air
- Exercise induced (sign/symptoms develop when person takes rest after exercise).

DRUGS USED IN THE TREATMENT OF BRONCHIAL ASTHMA

- **Bronchodilators**
  - **Sympathomimetics:** Salbutamol, terbutaline, salmeterol, formoterol, bambuterol and ephedrine.
  - **Methylxanthines:** Theophylline, aminophylline, doxophylline, acebrophylline
  - **Anticholinergics:** Tiotropium bromide and ipratropium bromide
- **Leukotriene antagonists:** Zafirlukast and montelukast.
- **Mast cell stabilizers:** Ketotifen and sodium cromoglycate.
- **Corticosteroids**
  - **Systemic:** Prednisolone, hydrocortisone and deflazacort, etc.
  - **Inhalational:** Budesonide, fluticasone, beclomethasone and ciclesonide.
- **Anti-IgE antibody:** Omalizumab

BRONCHODILATORS

It is a very important class of drugs used in the management of bronchial asthma.

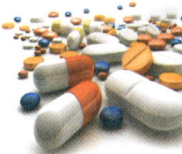

LEUKOTRIENE (LTs) ANTAGONISTS (MONTELUKAST AND ZAFIRLUKAST)

- The pharmacological actions and uses of both these drugs are same.
- Both these agents exhibit competitive antagonism. They antagonize LTs receptor mediated bronchoconstriction, airway mucous secretion, increased vascular permeability and recruitment of eosinophils.

Pharmacokinetics

- These drugs have good oral absorption with high plasma protein binding.
- The metabolism occurs in liver.
- The plasma t½ of montelukast is 3–6 hours and zafirlukast is 8–12 hours.

Indications

- Mild-to-moderate asthma as alternatives to inhaled glucocorticoids.
- Severe asthma (additive effect with inhaled steroids).
- Effective in aspirin-induced asthma and exercise-induced asthma.
- No value in chronic obstructive pulmonary disease.

Side Effects

Headache, rashes and eosinophilia.

Dose

The dose of leukotriene antagonists is given in Table 5.2

TABLE 5.2: Dose of leukotriene antagonists

Drugs	Dose
Montelukast	Adults: 10 mg once daily Children: (age group 2–5 year): 4 mg once daily, (age group 6–14 year): 5 mg once daily *To be given in the evening.*
Zafirlukast	Adults: 20 mg twice daily Children (age group 5–11 year): 10 mg twice daily

MAST CELL STABILIZERS

Cromoglycate Sodium

- It inhibits degranulation of mast cells and reduces the bronchial hyperreactivity.
- Bronchospasm induced by allergens, irritants, cold air and exercise is decreased.
- It does not have a therapeutic effect during an asthmatic attack.
- It is not a bronchodilator-like salbutamol.

Pharmacokinetics

It is not absorbed orally. Hence, given by metered dose inhaler for direct effect on bronchi.

Uses

- **Bronchial asthma:** It is used for the prophylaxis of exercise-induced asthma and mild-to-moderate asthma.
- **Allergic rhinitis:** Some symptomatic improvement seen after 4–6 weeks.
- Cromoglycate Sodium eye drops are given for the prophylaxis of **chronic allergic conjunctivitis**.

Dose

- Metered dose inhaler 1 mg and 5 mg/puff, 2 puffs 4 times daily.
- 2% nasal spray, two spray in both nostrils QID.
- 2% and 4% eye drops: 1 drop in each eye QID.

Adverse Effects

- Systemic toxicity is minimal.
- Other side effects are dizziness, headache, nasal congestion, rashes, arthralgia, etc.

Ketotifen

- It is an antihistaminic (H_1) and not a bronchodilator.
- It is given orally.
- It has some mast cell stabilizing effect also.

Indications

Bronchial asthma, urticaria, food allergy, conjunctivitis, perennial rhinitis and atopic dermatitis.

Adverse Effects

- Generally well tolerated.
- The other side effects are dry mouth, nausea, sedation, dizziness, increase in weight.

Dose

In adults 1–2 mg twice daily and in children 0.5 mg twice daily.

CORTICOSTEROIDS

- **Systemic:** Prednisolone, deflazacort, hydrocortisone, etc.
- **Inhalational:** Budesonide, fluticasone, beclomethasone, etc.
- **Mechanism of action**
  - Glucocorticoids do not have bronchodilatory effects.
  - These agents decrease the bronchial tree hyper-reactivity and mucosal edema by their potent anti-inflammatory actions.

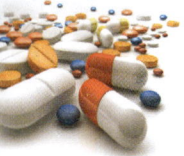

Systemic Steroids

- The various indications of systemic steroidal therapy in asthma are as follows:
  - **Severe chronic asthma:** Prednisolone is started in a dose of 20–60 mg (or equivalent) daily. (*If, the severe/recurrent episodic attacks of asthma are not controlled by steroidal inhaler and bronchodilator*).
  - **Status asthmaticus/acute asthma exacerbation.**
  - **Chronic obstructive pulmonary disease (COPD):** Short-term (1–3 weeks) therapy of oral glucocorticoids can be beneficial during exacerbation of COPD.

Inhalational Steroids

The following inhalational steroids are used frequently in the patients of asthma:

- Fluticasone
- Budesonide
- Ciclesonide
- Beclomethasone

These inhalational steroidal agents are used in aerosol form as they have good topical activity on tracheobronchial tree. Their systemic action is poor because of high first pass metabolism.

The airway inflammation in COPD is not very responsive to corticosteroids.

Adverse Effects

The common side effects are dysphonia, hoarseness of voice, oropharyngeal candidiasis, sore throat and oral thrush.

(These above-mentioned side effects can be controlled by the use of a spacer device and normal saline gargling after every dose)

ANTI-IgE ANTIBODY

Omalizumab

- Omalizumab acts against IgE by binding and neutralizing the free IgE in blood circulation.
- It is a humanized monoclonal antibody and given by subcutaneous route.
- It does not activate mast cells and other inflammatory mediating cells.
- Omalizumab reduces the exacerbations and the requirement of steroidal therapy in severe allergic asthma.
- It is very costly. Therefore, reserved for resistant cases only.
- It should be given only after sensitivity test.

Drugs Used by Inhalational Route for Asthma Treatment

- The following types of antiasthmatic drugs are available in inhalational forms.
  - *Glucocorticoids* (Beclomethasone, Fluticasone, Budesonide, Ciclesonide)
  - *β₂ agonists* (Salbutamol, Terbutaline, Salmetrol, etc.)
  - *Anticholinergics* (Ipratropium bromide, Tiotropium bromide)
  - *Cromoglycate sodium*
- Currently, inhalational agents are the preferred drugs for both short and long-term management of asthma.
- Drugs given by inhalational route have the following advantages over that given by oral route:
  - The drug is delivered directly at the site of action.
  - Prompt action is achieved.
  - Minimal systemic side effects than oral anti-asthamatics.
  - Inhalational doses are lower than oral doses of the same drug.

MANAGEMENT OF ASTHMA

The immediate treatment of asthma is guided by the severity of the signs and symptoms of patient. The main aim of the treatment is to relieve the bronchospasm and prevent the further damage to the respiratory tract. After the asthma is under control for 3–6 months, the medications are reduced in a stepwise manner (Table 5.3).

Aerosols

These are the drug preparations which can be converted into vapor form for their maximum effect in the tracheobronchial tree.

Aerosols are of two types:

1. **Drug in solution:** Pressurized metered dose inhaler (pMDI), nebulizers.
   - **Metered dose inhalers:** They are the small handy devices, which can be carried in pockets and used on '*as and when required basis*'.
   - **Nebulizers:** It is an electrical drug delivery device, which converts the nebulizing solution into aerosol forms for inhalation with the help of mask. It provides immediate local action on the tracheobronchial tree. It is used at bedside in patients of all age groups.
2. **Drug as dry powder:** Spinhaler, rotahalers.
   - **Dry powder inhalers:** They are also a portable handy drug delivery devices in which the drug-containing capsule is fitted in a pit. The rotation of the device breaks the capsule, which releases the aerosolized drug. The patient has to take deep inspiration through this device, which carries the aerosolized drug directly to the site of action.

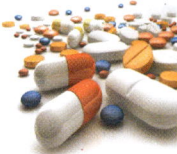

Refer to Table 5.3 for management of various types of asthma.

TABLE 5.3: Management of various types of asthma

Type of asthma	Management
Seasonal asthma (Symptoms seen in particular seasons only due to allergens/cold climatic conditions)	• Inhaled short-acting β_2 receptor agonist • Inhaled steroid in low-dose • Cromoglycate sodium (should be given 3–4 weeks before the onset of seasonal attacks and continued till 3–4 weeks after the season is over)
Mild episodic asthma (Symptoms < 1 per day, asymptomatic in between attacks)	• Inhaled short-acting β_2 receptor agonist at the onset of each episode
Mild chronic (persistent) (Acute exacerbation)	• Regular low-dose inhaled steroid • Inhaled cromoglycate sodium • Oral theophylline • Episode treatment with inhaled short acting β_2 receptor agonist
Moderate asthma (attacks occur >1 per day or mild baseline symptoms)	• Slightly higher dose of inhaled steroid + inhaled long-acting β_2 receptor agonist • Sustained release theophylline may be used in addition • Leukotriene receptor antagonist may be used in addition
Severe asthma (continuous symptoms; activity limitation; frequent exacerbations/ hospitalization)	• High dose of inhaled steroid administered regularly by a large volume spacer device + inhaled long-acting β_2 receptor agonist (salmeterol) twice daily • Leukotriene antagonist/sustained release oral theophylline/oral β_2 receptor agonist/inhaled ipratropium bromide • Rescue treatment with short-acting inhaled β_2 receptor agonist • Humidified oxygen inhalation

STATUS ASTHMATICUS/REFRACTORY ASTHMA

It is also known as acute severe asthma. It is a life-threatening condition and mostly occurs due to precipitation of chronic asthma by acute respiratory infection.

Patient presents with following signs/symptoms:

- Unable to speak a sentence due to severe dyspnea.
- Severe cyanosis.
- Pulsus paradoxus (inspiratory fall in systolic blood pressure ≥10 mm Hg).
- Silent chest (No pathological sign during auscultation).
- Encephalopathy, seizure, coma and death if not treated appropriately within the golden period.

Management of Status Asthmaticus

- Hydrocortisone 100 mg intravenously given stat, then 100–200 mg 4–8 hourly infusion (or equivalent dose of another glucocorticoid). The onset of action of hydrocortisone takes about 6 hours.
- 2.5–5 mg of nebulized salbutamol + 0.5 mg of ipratropium bromide.
- Administration of humidified oxygen in high flow.
- Salbutamol/terbutaline 0.4 mg intramuscularly or subcutaneously can be given for its better therapeutic effect.
- In severe respiratory distress, intubation and mechanical ventilation is advocated.
- Broad spectrum antibiotic therapy is required to control the chest infection.
- Correction of electrolyte imbalance.
- Correction of acidosis with sodium bicarbonate/lactate infusion.
- If hypokalemia is detected, correct with potassium chloride infusion.
- Recording and maintenance of vitals.

MUCOLYTICS

(*muco*— mucous; *lytic*— to break)

These are the drugs, which liquefy the sputum by breaking down the disulfide bonds in mucopolysaccharide strands. The thick tenacious sputum/secretions are very difficult to expel out in cough. These drugs help in easy expulsion of thick, tenacious secretions by decreasing the viscosity of sputum.

The following drugs act as Mucolytics:

Bromhexine, ambroxol, acetylcysteine, carbocysteine, dornase alfa.

BROMHEXINE

- It is a potent mucolytic and mucokinetic, capable of inducing thin copious bronchial secretion.
- It is given orally.
- It breaks down the network of fibers in tenacious sputum by depolymerizing mucopolysaccharides and also by liberating lysosomal enzymes.

Dose

- Adults: 8 mg thrice daily.
- Children (1–5 years): 4 mg twice daily and for 5–10 years 4 mg thrice daily.

Side Effects

- Rhinorrhea
- Lacrimation

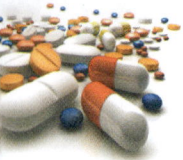

- Nausea and gastric irritation
- Hypersensitivity

AMBROXOL

- It is a metabolite of bromhexine.
- It is given orally.
- Its mucolytic action, uses and side effects are similar to bromhexine.

Dose

15–30 mg thrice daily.

ACETYLCYSTEINE

- A good mucolytic available in solution and tablet form.
- It is administered directly into the respiratory tract by injectable solution, which is given by nebulization or by instilling through tracheostomy tube.
- It opens disulfide bonds in mucoproteins present in sputum and makes it less viscid.
- It is also used as antidote in paracetamol poisoning.

Dose

- By nebulization, 2–20 mL of 10% solution 2–6 hourly.
- By direct instillation in lungs, 1–2 mL of 10–20% solution 1–4 hourly.
- Tablet: 600 mg thrice daily.

CARBOCYSTEINE

- It liquefies viscid sputum in the same way as acetylcysteine.
- It is administered orally.
- Specially given in patients of chronic bronchitis.
- Most effective in *smoker's cough*.

Dose

250–750 mg thrice daily.

Side Effects

- Rashes.
- Gastric discomfort hence, contraindicated in peptic ulcer.

Other Uses

Bronchitis, bronchiectasis, sinusitis, etc.

DORNASE ALFA

- It is a mucolytic prepared by recombinant DNA technique.

- It selectively breaks down respiratory tract mucus by separating extracellular DNA from proteins.
- Dornase alfa has a long duration of action.
- It is used in:
  - Cystic fibrosis, which is characterized by thick, tenacious mucous production.
  - Post-operative patients such as patients with tracheostomy to facilitate airway clearance and suction.
  - Clearing of secretions for diagnostic tests (e.g., diagnostic bronchoscopy).

Dose

2.5 mg once daily inhaled through nebulizer, may increase to 2.5 mg twice daily if needed.

Contraindications and Cautions

- In patients of acute bronchospasm, the increased secretions can aggravate the problem. Hence, contraindicated.
- Cautious use in patients suffering from peptic ulcer and esophageal varices, because these drugs can break the gastric mucosal barrier.

DECONGESTANTS

- These are the drugs, which decrease the overproduction of secretions by causing local vasoconstriction in the nasal mucosa.
- These drugs provide relief from the discomfort of blocked nose by promoting drainage of secretions and thereby improving airflow.
- Topical decongestants are sympathomimetics, meaning that they imitate the effects of the sympathetic nervous system to cause vasoconstriction.
- They are available as nasal drops and nasal sprays.
- These are used to relieve the discomfort of nasal congestion that accompanies the common cold, sinusitis, and allergic rhinitis.

The commonly used nasal decongestants are:

- **Topical Nasal Decongestants:** Ephedrine, Xylometazoline, Phenylephrine, Oxymetazoline, etc. (Table 5.4).
- **Oral Decongestants:** Pseudoephedrine (Table 5.5).
- **Topical Steroid Nasal Decongestants:** Beclomethasone, Flunisolide Dexamethasone, Budesonide, Triamcinolone, etc. (Table 5.6).

Indications

- Nasal congestion related to the common cold, sinusitis, and allergic rhinitis.
- To relieve the pain and congestion of otitis media.

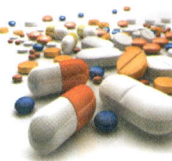

TABLE 5.4: Topical nasal decongestants

Drugs	Dosage
Ephedrine	• Instill solution in each nostril 4 hourly • Do not use for children <6 years unless advised by physician
Xylometazoline	• Adult: Two to three sprays or two to three drops in each nostril 8 hourly (0.17% solution) • Pediatric (2–12 years): Two to three drops of 0.05% solution 8–12 hourly
Phenylephrine	• Adult and pediatric (>6 years): One to two sprays in each nostril 3–4 hourly • Pediatric (2–6 years): Two to three drops of 0.125% solution in each nostril 4 hourly
Oxymetazoline	• Adult and pediatric (>6 years): Two to three sprays or drops in each nostril 12 hourly • Pediatric (2–5 years): Two to three drops of 0.05% solution in each nostril 12 hourly

TABLE 5.5: Oral decongestants

Drug	Dosage
Pseudoephedrine	• Adult: 60 mg 4–6 hourly • Pediatric: 6–12 years 30 mg 4–6 hourly • 2–5 years 15 mg 4–6 hourly • 1–2 years 0.02 mL/kg 4–6 hourly • 3–12 months: three drops/kg 4–6 hourly

TABLE 5.6: Topical steroid nasal decongestants

Drug	Dosage
Beclomethasone	• Adult: One to two inhalations in each nostril 12 hourly • Pediatric (6–11 years): One inhalation in each nostril 12 hourly
Flunisolide	• Adult: Two sprays in each nostril 12 hourly • Pediatric (6–14 years): one spray in each nostril 8 hourly to two sprays in each nostril 12 hourly
Dexamethasone	• Adult: Two sprays in each nostril BD to TDS • Pediatric: one to two sprays in each nostril 12 hourly
Budesonide	• Adult and pediatric (>6 years): two sprays in each nostril morning and evening or four sprays in each nostril in the morning
Triamcinolone	• Adult: Two sprays in each nostril every day

Pharmacokinetics

• **Topical Nasal Decongestants:** The onset of action is almost immediate. These are not generally absorbed systemically. The metabolism occurs in the liver and excretion through kidneys, if the drug is absorbed.

TABLE 5.7: Contraindications and cautions of decongestants

Drugs class	Contraindications and cautions
Topical nasal decongestants	• Erosion in the mucous membranes. • Glaucoma, diabetes, coronary disease, hypertension thyroid disease, or prostate hypertrophy
Oral decongestants	• Glaucoma, diabetes, coronary disease, hypertension thyroid disease, or prostate hypertrophy
Topical steroid nasal decongestants	• Active infection such as tuberculosis • Chicken pox or Measles

TABLE 5.8: Adverse effects of decongestants

Drugs class	Adverse effects
Topical nasal decongestants	• Local stinging and burning • Rebound congestion • Sympathomimetic effects (e.g., increased pulse rate and BP; urinary retention) seen in some patients only
Oral decongestants	• Rebound congestion • Sympathomimetic effects such as anxiety, restlessness, tremors, hypertension, arrhythmias, sweating, and pallor
Topical steroid nasal decongestants	• Local irritation, headache and dryness of the mucosa • Delayed healing in nasal surgery or trauma

• **Oral decongestants:** Pseudoephedrine is well absorbed and attains peak levels quickly in 20–45 minutes. The metabolism occurs in the liver and excretion through kidneys.

• **Topical steroid nasal decongestants:** The onset of action is not immediate. These drugs may require up to 1 week to produce their effect. The drug should be discontinued, if no effects are seen after 3 weeks. These drugs are not generally absorbed systemically. The absorbed drug (if any) is metabolized in the same way as other steroids.

The contraindications, and adverse effects of various decongestants are given in Tables 5.7 and 5.8, respectively

EXPECTORANTS

(Mucokinetics, muco—mucous, kinetics—movement)

• Expectorants are also called *Mucokinetics*.
• Expectorants are the drugs which increase the bronchial secretions.
• These drugs also reduce the viscosity of these secretions thereby helping in easy expulsion of the sputum.
• These are included in expectorant formulations in combination with antitussives and antihistaminics.

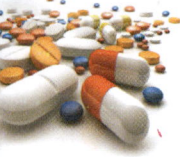

Examples are:
- **Bronchial secretion enhancers:** Guaiphenesin, Sodium or Potassium citrate, potassium iodide, ammonium chloride, vasaka.
- **Mucolytics:** Acetyl cysteine, ambroxol, bromhexine, carbocisteine.

MECHANISM OF ACTION OF EXPECTORANTS

The mechanism of action of expectorants is given in Table 5.9.

INDICATIONS

In the treatment of productive cough accompanied with excessive, thick and difficult to remove secretion/sputum.

ADVERSE EFFECTS

- GI symptoms such as nausea, vomiting, and anorexia (most common).
- Headache, dizziness or both.

PRECAUTIONS

- The most important consideration in the use of these drugs is identifying the exact cause of the underlying cough.
- Prolonged use of the OTC (cough syrup) preparations could result in the masking of important symptoms of a serious underlying disorder.
- These drugs should not be used for more than 1 week; if the cough persists, encourage the patient to seek health care.

TABLE 5.9: Mechanism of action of expectorants

Drug	Dosage	Mechanism of action
Sodium and potassium citrate	1–2 g	Increase bronchial secretion by salt action
Ammonium chloride	300 mg	Reflexly increase respiratory secretions
Potassium iodide	200–300 mg	Irritate the airway mucosa as it is secreted by bronchial glands
Guaiphenesin (most commonly used)	**Adult and pediatric** (>12 years): 200–400 mg PO 4 hourly **Pediatric:** 6–12 years 100–200 mg 4 hourly 2–6 years 50–100 mg 4 hourly	Enhance mucociliary excretory function as these are secreted by tracheobronchial glands

The various drugs classes and their sites of action on respiratory tract are shown in Figure 5.2.

ANTITUSSIVES

The drugs used to control the dry cough are known as antitussives.
- These drugs act directly on the cough center in the medulla of the brain to depress the cough reflex and raise the threshold of cough center.
- Act peripherally in the respiratory tract to reduce cough impulses, or both these actions.

The aim of giving antitussives is to control rather than eliminate cough.

CLASSIFICATION OF ANTITUSSIVES

Antitussives can be classified into:
- **Opioids:** Codeine, Pholcodeine, Ethyl morphine
- **Non-opioids:** Noscapine, dextromethorphan, chlophedianol

Opioids

Codeine (Methyl Morphine)

- An opium alkaloid, similar to but less potent than morphine.
- More selective for cough center.
- Codeine is regarded as the standard antitussive.
- Suppresses cough for about 6 hours.
- Abuse liability is low, but present.

Side Effects and Precautions

- Constipation.
- Respiratory depression (at higher dosage).
- It causes drowsiness. Hence, cautionary advised for drivers.
- It is contraindicated in asthmatics.
- It should be avoided in children.
- Not to be used in head injury patients.

Dose

- Adult: 10–20 mg orally 4–6 hourly.
- Pediatric (6–12 years): 5–10 mg orally 4–6 hourly.
- Pediatric (2–6 years): 2.5–5 mg orally 4–6 hourly.

Pholcodeine

- It is similar to codeine in efficacy as antitussive.
- It is longer acting and acts for 12 hours.
- It has no analgesic or addicting property.

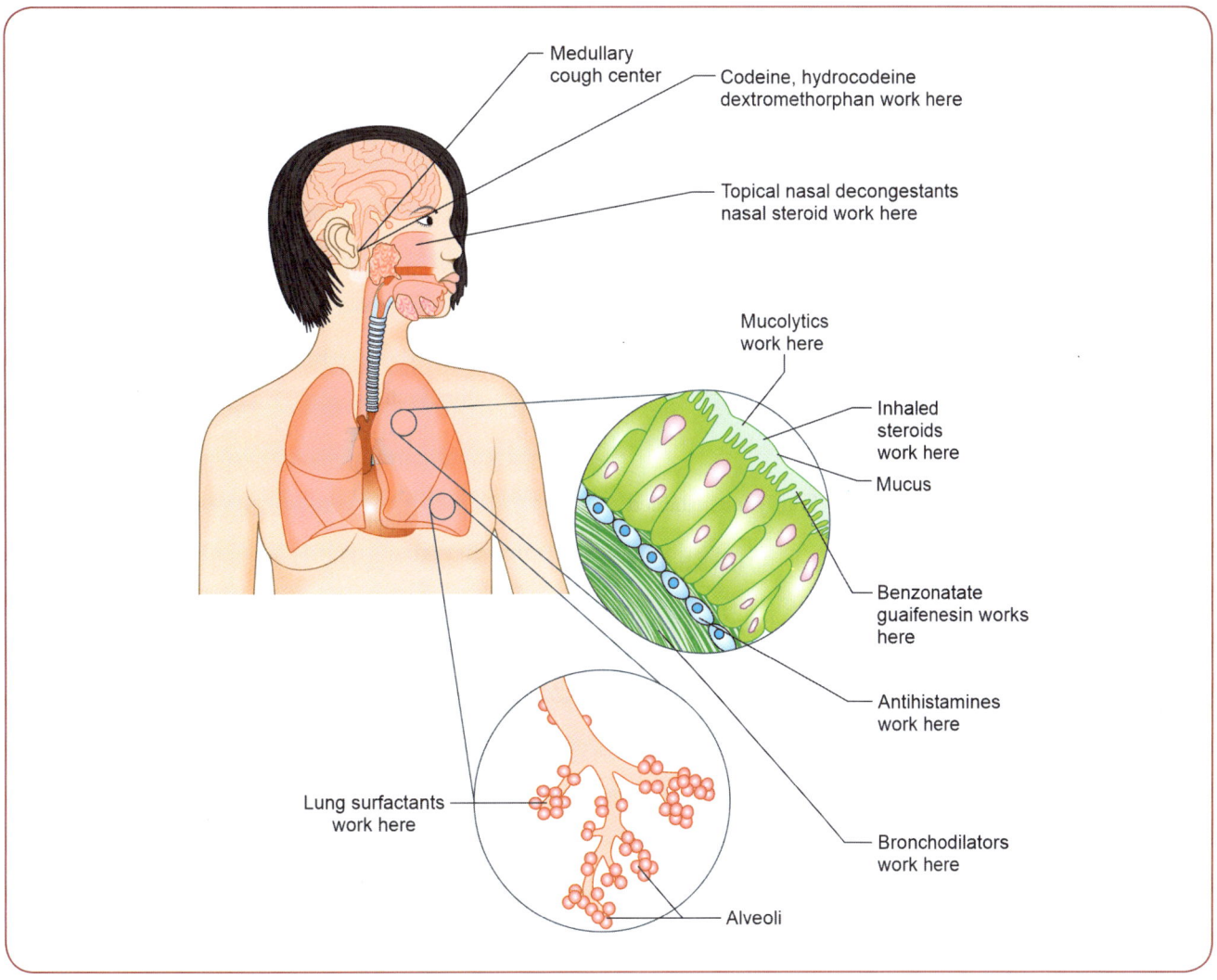

FIG. 5.2: Site of action of various drugs on respiratory tract

Dose

10–15 mg 12 hourly.

Ethyl Morphine

It is similar to codeine in all actions except constipation, which is less with it.

Dose

10–30 mg 8 hourly.

Nonopioids

Noscapine (Narcotine)

- It is nearly equipotent antitussive as codeine.

- It depresses the cough center.
- It has no narcotic, analgesic or dependence inducing properties.
- Useful in spasmodic cough.

Side Effects

- Headache and nausea
- Bronchoconstriction in asthmatics.

Dose

- Adults: Given in a dose of 15–30 mg 3–4 times daily.
- Children (2–6 years): Given in a dose of 7.5 mg 3–4 times daily.
- Children (6–12 years): Given in a dose of 15 mg 3–4 times daily.

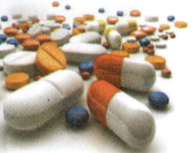

Dextromethorphan

- The antitussive action of dextromethorphan is similar to codeine.
- It is a synthetic and centrally acting NMDA (N-methyl D-aspartate) receptor antagonist.
- Constipation not seen.
- Non-addicting.

Side Effects

- Dizziness
- Nausea
- Drowsiness
- Ataxia and hallucinations (at high doses)

Dose

- **Adult:** 10–30 mg 4–8 hourly; 60 mg 8 hourly for sustained action
- **Pediatric (6–12 years):** 5–10 mg 4 hourly; 30 mg 8 hourly for sustained action
- **Pediatric (2–6 years):** 2.5–7.5 mg 4–8 hourly; 15 mg 8 hourly for sustained action

Chlophedianol

- It is an antitussive having central action.
- It has slow onset of action with longer duration.

Side Effects

The common side effects are vertigo, irritability, sedation and dryness of mouth.

Dose

20–40 mg 2–3 times daily.

Pharmacokinetics

- All antitussives are rapidly absorbed orally.
- The metabolism occurs in liver, and excretion through kidneys.
- It crosses the placenta barrier and secretes in breast milk.

Contraindications and Cautions

- Patients with asthma and emphysema because cough suppression in these patients could lead to an accumulation of secretions.
- Patients who are hypersensitive to or have a history of addiction to narcotics.
- During driving, as these drugs can cause sedation and drowsiness.

- **Pregnancy and lactation:** These drugs are having potential for adverse effects on the fetus or baby, including sedation and CNS depression.

BRONCHODILATORS

These are the drugs having ability to dilate the bronchi, which are in a state of bronchospasm. The bronchospasm is due to the contraction/constriction of bronchial smooth muscles which lead to decreased air entry into the tracheobronchial tree resulting in dyspnea and difficult respiration.

There are various classes of drugs which act as bronchodilators such as:

- **Sympathomimetics:** Salbutamol, salmeterol, terbutaline, formoterol, bambuterol, ephedrine.
- **Methylxanthines:** Theophylline, aminophylline, doxophylline, acebrophylline
- **Anticholinergics:** Ipratropium bromide, tiotropium bromide.

SYMPATHOMIMETICS (MIMICKING SYMPATHETIC SYSTEM)

- These are the drugs which are having actions similar to sympathetic stimulation.
- These drugs are potent bronchodilators.

Mechanism of Bronchodilatation

- β_2 **receptor are present in the bronchi.**
- The stimulation of these β_2 receptors leads to bronchodilatory effect.
- The bronchodilatory effect is good in constricted bronchi.
- The main mechanism operating at cellular level is as follows:

Adrenergic drugs and β2 receptor agonists → stimulation of β2 receptor → increased cAMP formation in bronchial muscle cell → bronchodilatatory effect.

- In addition, the inflammatory mediator release is also decreased.
- These drugs are the drug of choice due to their effectiveness and rapid bronchodilatory effect in reversible airway obstruction. Preferably, these drugs are given in inhalational form for prompt relief. Details of the sympathomimetic drugs are given in Table 5.10.

Adrenaline, Ephedrine and isoprenaline: Although these drugs are bronchodilators, these are not preferred due to low efficacy, risk of adverse effects and availability of better drugs.

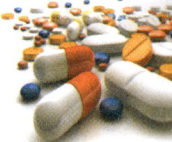

TABLE 5.10: Sympathomimetics

Comparison	Salbutamol	Terbutaline	Salmeterol	Formoterol
Dosage and route of administration	• **Adult and >12 years** 2–4 mg TDS or BD orally. 100–200-mcg by inhalation • **Pediatric:** 2–6 years 0.1 mg/kg TDS orally 6–12 years 2 mg TDS or QID orally. (inhaled 15 min before exercise)	• **Adult and pediatric** (>15 years): 5 mg QID orally. 250-mcg by inhalation • **Pediatric** (12–15 years): 2.5 mg TDS orally	• **Adult and pediatric** (≥12 years): 25-mcg pMDI two puff 12 hourly • **Pediatric** (4–12 years) one inhalation BD	• **Adult and pediatric** (>5 years): 12-mcg capsule 12 hourly, *(capsule inhaled using the Aerolizer inhaler, at least 15 minutes before exercising)*
Indications	• Long-acting treatment • Prophylaxis of bronchospasm	• Treatment and prophylaxis of bronchospasm in patients >12 years of age	• Prevention of asthma due to exercise • As a maintenance therapy and nocturnal asthma • COPD	• Prevention of asthma due to exercise • As a maintenance therapy and nocturnal asthma • COPD
Special points	• Inhaled salbutamol delivered mostly from pressurized metered dose inhaler (pMDI) produces broncho-dilatation within 5 minute and the action lasts for 2–4 hours • Levo-Salbutamol has equal action at half dose	• Use of inhalers should be restricted to symptomatic relief of wheezing	• Long acting selective beta 2 agonist • Onset of action is slow • Mostly used in combination inhaled steroids	• Long acting selective beta 2 agonist • It has faster onset of action than Salmeterol • Specially used for round the clock bronchodilatation

COPD, Chronic obstructive pulmonary disease

Side Effects

The side effects are commonly seen with the short acting β_2 receptor agonists such as salbutamol and terbutaline and less commonly with the long acting β_2 receptor agonists such as salmeterol and formoterol. Some commonly seen side effects are muscle tremors, palpitation, restlessness, nervousness, throat irritation, ankle edema and hypoklemia.

METHYLXANTHINES

• The xanthines have been in use for the treatment of bronchospasm and asthma since ancient times.
• Theophylline and caffeine are methylxanthines obtained from natural sources. However, because they have a relatively narrow margin of safety and interact with many other drugs, they are no longer considered the first choice bronchodilators.
• Xanthines, used to treat respiratory diseases include theophylline, aminophylline, and doxophylline.

Mechanism of Action

• **Inhibition of phosphodiesterase (PDE):** PDE enzyme degrades cyclic AMP and methylxanthines inhibits this enzyme, thereby increasing cAMP levels. This increase in cAMP causes bronchodilation.
• **Blockade of adenosine receptors:** Adenosine contracts smooth muscles by acting as a local mediator. Methylxanthines produce opposite effects.
• The calcium (in skeletal and cardiac muscle) from sarcoplasmic reticulum is released. This action is seen in higher dose only.

At normal therapeutic doses, bronchodilation occurs due to mechanism 1 and 2. Action number 3 is observed only at toxic doses.

Theophylline

Pharmacokinetics

• Theophylline is well absorbed orally
• It is widely distributed in all compartments of body.

135

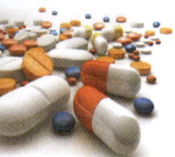

TABLE 5.11: Side effects of theophylline according to serum levels of theophylline

Serum level (mcg/mL)	Side effects
≤20	Uncommon
>20–25	Nausea, vomiting, diarrhea, insomnia, headache, irritability
>30–35	Tachycardia, arrhythmias, hypotension, hyperglycemia, seizures, brain damage, death

- It also crosses the placental barrier and is secreted in milk.
- The metabolism occurs in liver and excretion occurs through kidneys.
- In higher doses, the kinetics of theophylline change from first order kinetics to zero order kinetics due to saturation of metabolizing enzyme of liver. Hence, accumulation of drugs occurs which can lead to severe toxicity.

Dose

100–300 mg orally, thrice daily.

Side Effects

Theophylline has a narrow margin of safety. Side effect profile is different at different serum levels (Table 5.11).

Aminophylline

- It is a water-soluble drug.
- It is given by slow intravenous route in acute attack of asthma not responding to beta 2 agonist.
- It should be given slow intravenously in a dose of 250 mg over 15–20 minutes.
- Rapid IV injection may cause hypotension, arrhythmias which may lead to convulsions, collapse and death.
- It is not given by IM/SC route due to its highly irritating nature.
- In children, the recommended dose is 7.5 mg/kg intravenously.

Hydroxyethyl Theophylline (Etophylline, 80% Theophylline)

- It is administered by intravenous, intramuscular and oral route in a dose of 250 mg.
- It has low irritating nature.

Doxophylline

- It is a methylxanthine with long duration of action and given by oral route.
- It neither interferes with sleep nor stimulates gastric secretion.

Dose

- **Adult:** 400 mg once or twice daily.
- **Children:** 12 mg/kg daily.

ANTICHOLINERGICS

- These are the drugs which block the action of acetylcholine on muscarinic receptors.
- M_3 cholinergic receptors are present in larger airways and their stimulation causes bronchoconstriction.
- Anticholinergic drugs block M_3 receptors and cause bronchodilation.
- These drugs relax bronchial smooth muscles but response is slower than sympathomimetics.
- These drugs are given by inhalational route.
- These are the bronchodilators of choice in COPD.
- The anticholinergics show a good effect in patients of COPD, asthmatic bronchitis and psychogenic asthma.
- The synergistic effect is obtained by combining the ipratropium bromide with a β_2 agonist in the form of prolonged and potentiated bronchodilatation.
- *Ipratropium bromide* is a short acting (duration 4–6 hours), while *Tiotropium bromide* is long acting (duration 24 hours).
- Available in inhalers, rotacaps and solution forms.

BRONCHOCONSTRICTORS

- The drugs which cause constriction of bronchi (bronchospasm) are called bronchoconstrictors.
- Bronchoconstriction is never induced as apart of any treatment, except in experimental animals to check the effectiveness of bronchodilators.
- In experimental animals *histamine* is commonly used as bronchoconstriction inducing agent.
- Some other bronchoconstrictors are 5HT, LTC_4, LTD_4, $PGF_2\alpha$, PGD_2, PAF and TXA_2.
- Bronchoconstriction due to histamine causes symptoms of dyspnea, which are antagonized with antihistaminics and adrenaline, which act as physiological antagonist.

ANTIHISTAMINICS

The drugs which competitively antagonize the actions of histamine on histaminic receptors are called antihistaminic drugs.

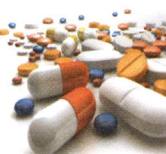

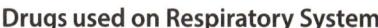

HISTAMINE

- A major amount of histamine is present in the mast cells.
- The tissues containing maximum histamine are skin, gastric mucosa, intestinal mucosa, liver, placenta and lungs.
- Brain, gastric mucosa, epidermis and growing regions contain non-mast cell histamine.
- Some other sites where histamine is found are body secretions, blood, pathological fluids and venoms of snake and scorpions.
- *Histamine* acts through various receptors known as histaminic receptors.

Histamine Receptors

The histamine receptors are of four types: H_1, H_2, H_3 and H_4 (Table 5.12).
- The antihistaminic term is conventionally used for H_1 antagonists only.
- The drugs which antagonize H_2 receptors are called H_2 receptor blockers. H_2 receptor blockers are specifically used for acid suppression in gastric mucosa and are *studied in detail with GIT system.*
- H_3 and H_4 antagonists have not been ascribed any specific clinical utility yet.

ANTIHISTAMINICS (H$_1$ ANTAGONISTS)

- The H_1 antagonistic drugs act at H_1 receptors and antagonize the actions of histamine competitively.
- The H_1 antihistaminics have many common properties except they differ in their sedative actions mainly.

TABLE 5.12: Histamine receptors

Receptor	Distribution in body	Actions
H$_1$ receptor	Airway, intestinal and uterine smooth muscle	Contractions
	Blood vessels	Vasodilatation due to release of nitrous oxide
	Larger blood vessels (smooth muscles)	Vasoconstriction
H$_2$ receptor	Gastric glands	Increase acid secretion
	Blood vessels	Vasodilatory effect
	Brain	Increase synapse transmission
H$_3$ receptor	Brain	Sedation
	Lung, spleen, skin and gastric mucosa	Reduction of histamine release
H$_4$ receptor	Eosinophil, mast cells and basophils	Chemotaxis effect

Classification of Antihistaminics

- First Generation: mild, moderate and highly sedative
- Second Generation or non-sedative

First Generation Antihistaminics

The first compound of this group was introduced in the late 1930s. These were very frequently used before introduction of less sedating/non-sedating 2nd generation antihistaminics. Some of these drugs are still used for a variety of purposes (Table 5.13).

Pharmacological Actions

- **Histaminic antagonizing effects:** The bronchoconstriction and the triple response due to histamine are antagonized. The triple response consists of wheal, flare and itch.
- **Antiallergic effects:** The manifestations of immediate hypersensitivity (type I reactions) are suppressed. They are having a good role in the treatment of urticaria, itching and angioedema.
- **Anticholinergic effects:** The acetylcholine produces muscaranic effects through H_1 receptor, which are antagonized by these drugs.
- **CNS effects:** The older antihistaminics show sedative effects, whereas these effects are rarely or not at all seen with the newer second generation antihistaminics drugs.
- **CVS effects:** No CVS effects are seen on oral administration. Fast IV administration of these drugs can produce sudden hypotension.

Pharmacokinetics

- By both oral and parenteral routes, the absorption of these drugs is optimal.
- The metabolism occurs in liver and excretion occurs through urine.

TABLE 5.13: First generation of antihistaminics

Drugs	Dose and route of administration
Mild sedatives	
Chlorpheniramine	2–4 mg orally and intramuscularly
Dexchlorpheniramine	2 mg, by oral route
Triprolidine	2.5–5 mg, by oral route
Clemastine	1–2 mg, by oral route
Moderate sedative	
Pheniramine	20–50 mg orally and intramuscularly
Cinnarizine	
Cyproheptadine	25–50 mg, by oral route 4 mg, by oral route
Highly sedative	
Diphenhydramine	25–50 mg, by oral route
Promethazine	25–50 mg orally and intramuscularly
Hydroxyzine	25–50 mg, by oral route

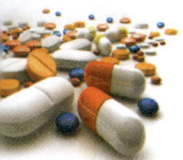

TABLE 5.14: Second generation antihistaminics

Drug	Dosage	Specific points
Fexofenadine	120–180 mg orally, once daily	• Safe in cardiac patients, doesn't cross blood brain barrier
Loratadine	10 mg orally, once daily	• Fast acting, with longer t½ of 17 hours
Desloratadine	5 mg orally, once daily	• Effective at half the dose of loratadine
Cetirizine	10 mg orally, once daily	• Metabolite of hydroxyzine • Mild sedation in some recipients • Attains high concentration in skin
Levocetirizine	5–10 mg orally, once daily	• It is the active enantiomer of cetirizine • Effective at half the dose of cetirizine • Less sedative
Azelastine	4 mg orally, once daily; 0.28 mg intranasally	• Good topical activity antagonizes LT and PAF • Provide quick symptomatic relief when given by intranasal route
Rupatadine	10 mg orally, once daily	• Additional PAF antagonistic property

- These agents show wide distribution in the body tissues and also penetrates the blood brain barrier.
- The 2nd generation agents have poor or absent penetration of blood brain barrier. Hence, have minimal or no sedative effect.

Side Effects

Side effects of first generation H_1 antihistaminics are frequent, but generally mild.

- Some tolerance to side effects develops on repeated use.
- The common side effects are sedation, reduced alertness and ability to concentrate, tendency to fall asleep, headache, listlessness.
- Regular use of conventional antihistamines may interfere with learning due to CNS depressant property hence, not advisable in children.
- Some other side effects due to anticholinergic activity are xerostomia, visual disturbance, GI disturbances and urinary hesitation.

Second Generation Antihistaminics

The H_1 receptor blockers which were marketed after 1980 are called second generation antihistaminics (SGAs). The dosage and their specific points are given in Table 5.14.

These have one or more of the following properties:
- No sleepiness due to absence of CNS depression.
- No anticholinergic side effects due to highly H_1 selectivity.
- Additional anti-allergic mechanisms such as antagonizing leukotrienes and PAF.
- Poor anti-pruritic, antiemetic and antitussive actions.

Major Indications

- **Nose:** Allergic rhinitis, pollinosis, (to control sneezing, runny but not blocked nose).
- **Eye:** Conjunctivitis, red, watering and itchy eyes.
- **Skin:** Atopic eczema, urticaria, dermographism, hay fever.
- **General:** Drug and food allergy.

Uses of Antihistaminics

- **Allergic disorders** of eye (*allergic conjunctivitis, angioedema of eyelids, etc*), nose (*rhinitis, sneezing, etc*) and skin (*angioedema of lips, itching urticaria, hay fever, etc*) and other general allergic disorders.
- **Pruritis:** Antihistaminics, like cholpheniramine, diphenhydramine and cyproheptadine are very commonly used in idiopathic pruritic cases.
- **Common cold:** Second generation antihistamines are less effective in this respect. First generation antihistaminics provide only symptomatic relief by anticholinergic (reduce rhinorrhea) effect, but do not alter the course of the illness.
- **Motion sickness:** Promethazine, diphenhydramine and dimenhydrinate. These drugs should be taken at least one hour before starting journey to get the best effects.
- **Vertigo:** Cinnarizine is commonly used in Meniere's disease and other types of vertigo.

Drug Interactions

- The metabolism of theophylline is enhanced by smoking, phenytoin and rifampicin by microsomal enzyme induction; hence, either dose of theophylline should be increased or the combination should be avoided.
- The metabolism of theophylline is decreased by allopurinol, ciprofloxacin erythromycin and oral contraceptives; hence, either dose of theophylline should be decreased or the combination should be avoided.
- The effects of oral anticoagulants, digitalis, furosemide and oral hypoglycemic are enhanced by theophylline.
- Injection of aminophylline interacts with phenytoin, insulin, erythromycin, tetracyclines, etc. Hence, mixing in the same infusion bottle should be avoided.
- Sodium cromoglycate potentiates the effect of sedatives, hypnotics, antihistaminics and alcohol.

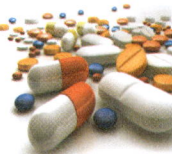

 Nursing Implications

- ☞ Teach the use of inhalers to patients. Advise the patient to brush the teeth after using inhalers to prevent infections in mouth (steroid inhaler cause fungal infection in mouth).
- ☞ During aminophylline infusion, keep a check on heart rate as HR >120/min is a sign of toxicity.
- ☞ Advise patient not to crush the tablet in mouth except chewable tablets.
- ☞ Do not use decongestants in hypertensive patients.
- ☞ After administering liquid preparation for cough, advise patient not to take any liquids for 20–30 minutes.
- ☞ As some antihistaminics cause sedation, advise patient to take these drugs at bedtime only.
- ☞ Provide steam inhalations with care whenever advised.
- ☞ Keep a close look on vitals of the patient when administering intravenous medications.
- ☞ Be well conversant with proper use of inhalers, rotahalers and nebulizers.
- ☞ Monitor patient response to the drug (improvement of respiratory symptoms and loosening of secretions).
- ☞ Monitor for adverse effects (CNS effects, skin rash, bronchospasm, and GI upset).
- ☞ Do perform postural drainage (with tapping) wherever recommended by the physician.
- ☞ Avoid combining the mucolytic agents with other drugs in the nebulizer to avoid the formation of precipitates and potential loss of effectiveness of either drug.
- ☞ Provide other measures to help relieve cough (e.g., humidity, cool temperatures, fluids, use of topical lozenges) as appropriate.

Assess Yourself

Long and Short Answer Questions

1. What are bronchodilators?
2. Classify the drugs used for the treatment for bronchial asthma.
3. Explain pharmacological management of status asthmaticus.
4. Write short notes on:
   a. Methylxanthines
   b. Montelukast
   c. Sodium cromoglycate
   d. Salbutamol
   e. Codeine
5. What are the differences between inhaler and nebulizers?
6. What are the nasal decongestants? Describe their uses and side effects.
7. Describe the drugs used in dry cough.

Multiple Choice Questions

1. **Which of the following is not a mucolytic?**
   a. Ambroxol
   b. Codeine
   c. Carbocisteine
   d. Bromhexine

2. **Which drug is not used for acute bronchial asthma?**
   a. Salmeterol
   b. Formeterol
   c. Salbutamol
   d. Corticosteroids

3. **Mechanism of action of theophylline in bronchial asthma is:**
   a. Inhibition of phosphodiesterase-IV
   b. Beta 2 antagonism
   c. Anticholinergic action
   d. Inhibition of mucocillary clearance

Contd...

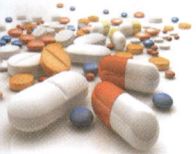
4. Complications of aerosol steroids used include:
   - a. Oral candidiasis
   - b. Cushing's syndrome
   - c. Decreased ACTH
   - d. Systemic complications

5. Which of the following is not a bronchodilator?
   - a. Ipratropium bromide
   - b. Methylxanthines
   - c. Steroids
   - d. Anticholinergic

6. Drug inhibits histamine release:
   - a. d-penicillamine
   - b. Tubocurarine
   - c. Atracurium
   - d. Nedocromil sodium

7. Leukotriene receptor antagonist used in the management of bronchial asthma:
   - a. Sodium cormoglycate
   - b. Zafirlukast
   - c. Zileuton
   - d. Ketotifen

8. Leukotriene receptor antagonist:
   - a. Zafirlukast
   - b. Nedocromil
   - c. Latanoprost
   - d. Zileuton

Answer Key

1.	b.	2.	a.	3.	a.	4.	a.	5.	c.	6.	b.	7.	b.
8.	a.												

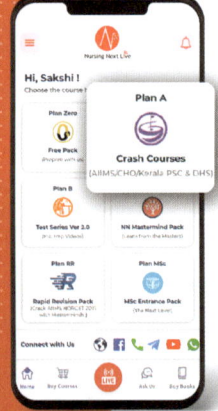
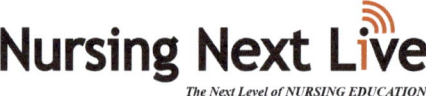
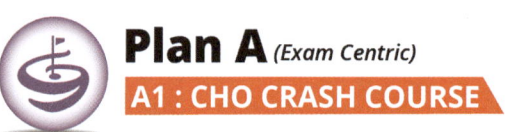
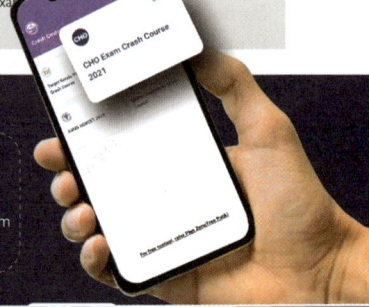

Drugs used on Urinary System

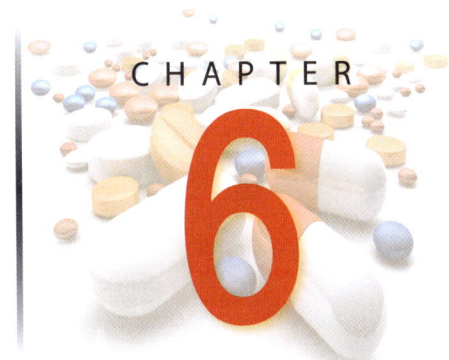

DIURETICS AND ANTIDIURETIC DRUGS

RENAL PHYSIOLOGY

Kidney is the main excretory organ of our body. Normally, we have a pair of kidneys. *Nephron* is the smallest functional unit of kidney. Approximately 1–1.5 million nephrons constitute one kidney.

The main functions of kidneys are:

- **Excretory function:** Excretion of nitrogenous wastes such as urea, uric acid, creatinine, etc.
- **Regulatory function:** It regulates and maintains the balance of fluid and electrolyte mainly. It also maintains the blood pressure and acid-base balance.
- **Hormonal function:** Production of erythropoietin and renin, activation of Vitamin-D.
- The kidneys receive approximately 20–25% of cardiac output, out of which 10% is filtered in the glomeruli and is known as *glomerular filtrate*.
- Normally both kidneys filter nearly 125 mL fluid per minute. This is called *glomerular filtration rate*.
- The kidneys filter approximately 180 L of fluid/day, out of which 99% is reabsorbed and 1% (i.e., 1.8 L) is excreted out in the form of urine.

Urine formation involves mainly three processes:

- **Glomerular filtration:** It is a process of filtration of plasma through the glomerulus into tubules of nephron.
- **Selective tubular reabsorption:** It is a process of selective water and solutes reabsorption from the tubular fluid.
- **Tubular secretion:** It is a process where solutes are secreted into the tubular fluid. Mostly, those solutes are secreted which cannot be filtered through glomerulus.

The net volume of urine formation is affected by above the three processes mentioned above.

The diuretic and antidiuretic drugs affect the urine formation by acting at the different parts of nephron. The drugs mainly affect selective reabsorption process.

The different sites of drug action are as follows:

- **Site I:** Proximal convoluted tubule
- **Site II:** Thick ascending limb of loop of Henle
- **Site III:** Cortical diluting segment of loop of Henle
- **Site IV:** Distal convoluted tubule and collecting duct.

DIURETICS

The drugs, which increase the excretion of urine by their action on the kidneys (specifically nephrons), are called diuretics. This is achieved mainly by increasing the loss of sodium and water.

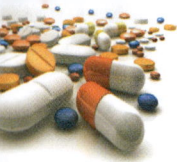

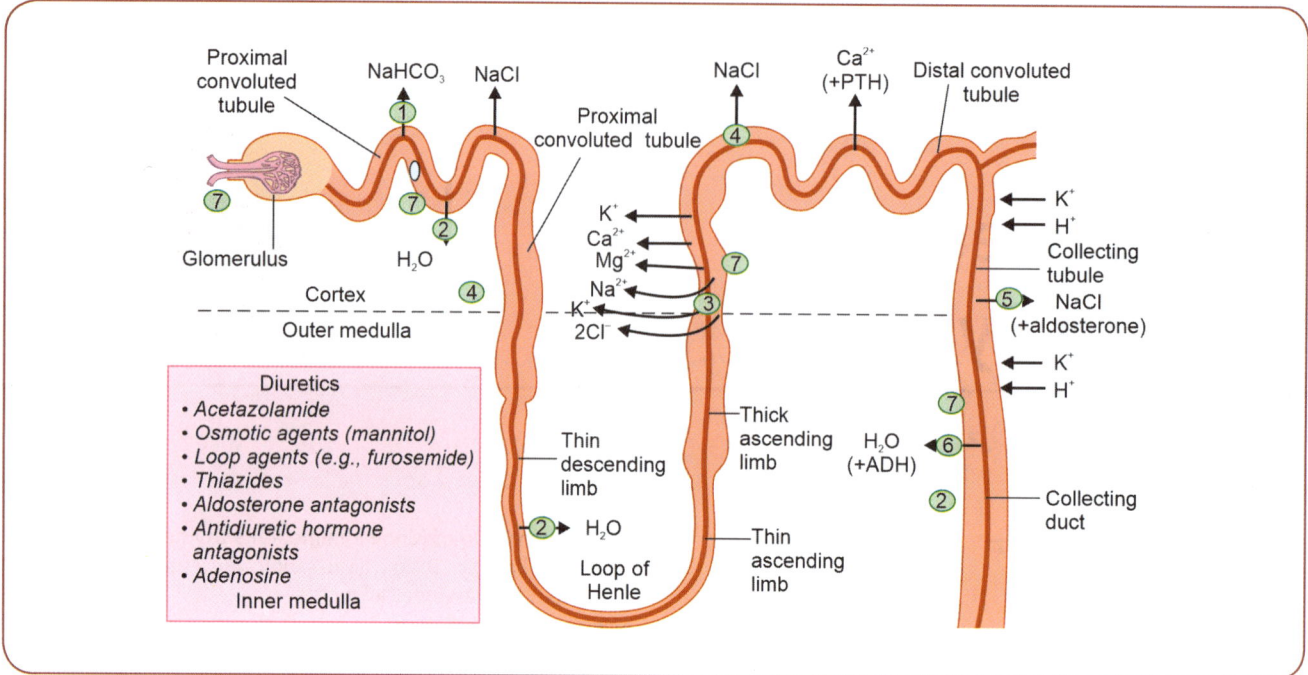

FIG. 6.1: Action of diuretics on tubular transport system

Classification of Diuretics

The classification of diuretics is based upon the site of nephron on which they act (Fig. 6.1). The different diuretics are as follows:

- **Drugs acting on Site I or proximal convoluted tubule or** *Carbonic anhydrase inhibitors:* Acetazolamide
- **Drugs acting on Site II or thick ascending limb of loop of Henle or Loop diuretics:** Furosemide, Bumetanide, Torasemide, Ethacrynic acid, Indacrinone.
- **Drugs acting on Site III: Cortical diluting segment of loop of Henle or early DCT or thiazides and thiazide like diuretics:**
  - **Thiazide diuretics:** Hydrochlorothiazide, chlorthiazide, clopamide, bendroflumethiazide, benzthiazide.

- **Thiazide like diuretics:** Chlorthalidone, indapamide, xipamide, metolazone, quinethazone.
- **Drugs acting on Site IV: Late DCT and collecting duct (CD) or Potassium sparing diuretics:**
  - **Aldosterone receptor antagonists:** Spironolactone and Eplerenone.
  - **Na⁺ channel inhibitors (at collecting duct):** Triamterene and Amiloride.
- **Drugs acting on entire nephron or osmotic diuretics:** Mannitol, isosorbide, glycerol, etc.

Classification of diuretics according to their efficacy is given in Table 6.1.

Drugs Acting on Site I or Proximal Convoluted Tubule

[Weak or adjunctive diuretics or (carbonic anhydrase inhibitors)]

TABLE 6.1: Classification according to efficacy of diuretics

High efficacy diuretics	Medium efficacy diuretics	Weak or adjunctive diuretics
Na⁺–K⁺–2Cl⁻ cotransport inhibitors	Na⁺Cl⁻ symport Inhibitors	• Inhibitors of carbonic anhydrase enzyme: Acetazolamide
• Furosemide	**Thiazides diuretics:**	• **Potassium sparing diuretics:**
• Torasemide	• Hydrochlorothiazide	▪ Aldosterone receptor antagonist
• Bumetanide	• Chlorthiazide	▪ Spironolactone
• Indacrinone	• Benzthiazide,	▪ Eplerenone
• Ethacrynic acid	• Hydroflumethiazide, bendroflumethiazide	

Contd...

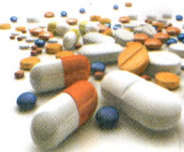

High efficacy diuretics	Medium efficacy diuretics	Weak or adjunctive diuretics
	Thiazide-like diuretics: • Chlorthalidone • Indapamide • Xipamide • Metolazone • Quinethazone	• **Na⁺ channel inhibitors (at collecting duct):** ▪ Triamterene ▪ Amiloride • **Osmotic diuretics:** ▪ Mannitol ▪ Glycerol ▪ Isosorbide

Carbonic Anhydrase (CAse) Inhibitors (Acetazolamide)

- Carbonic anhydrase inhibitors are weak diuretics and have some other pharmacological actions also.
- The various sites where carbonic anhydrase enzyme is present are:
  - Kidney: Renal tubular cells of proximal tubules
  - GIT: Gastric mucosa exocrine pancreas
  - Eye: Ciliary body of eye
  - Brain
  - Blood: RBCs
- In these tissues, a gross excess of CAse is present and more than 99% inhibition is required to produce clinical effects. Methazolamide and dichlorphenamide are some other systemic CAse inhibitors, whereas, dorzolamide and brinzolamide are topical case inhibitors used in glaucoma.

Mechanism of action

- Acetazolamide is a non-competitive reversible inhibitor of both membrane-bound and cytoplasmic forms of carbonic anhydrase in PCT.
- Inhibition of carbonic anhydrase enzyme causes increased excretion of bicarbonates with Na⁺, K⁺ and water.
- The net result is excretion of alkaline urine due to retention of HCO_3^- in the tubular lumen.

Extra-renal Effects of Acetazolamide

- It decreases intraocular pressure by reducing the formation of aqueous humor.
- It decreases the pH and raises CO_2 in brain; that may lead to sedation and seizures.
- It may cause CO_2 transport alteration in lungs.

Pharmacokinetics

It is well absorbed orally and excreted via tubular secretion. The efficacy decreases on prolonged use. It has effects on choroid plexus and ciliary body also. It is given in a dose of 250 mg OD/BD.

Indications

Because of self-limiting action (refractoriness), production of acidosis and hypokalemia, acetazolamide is not used as diuretic.

Its current clinical uses are:

- **Glaucoma:** As adjuvant to other ocular hypotensives. (Dorzolamide and Brinzolamide are used topically).
- **To increase urinary pH:** Increasing urinary pH helps to treat urate calculi, cystinuria and urinary tract infections
- **Mild metabolic alkalosis:** It can be treated as they cause hyperchloremic acidosis.
- **Epilepsy:** As adjuvant in absence seizures when primary drugs are not fully effective.
- **Acute mountain sickness syndrome:** It has both prophylactic and therapeutic value.

Adverse Effects

- The common side effects are hyperchloraemic acidosis, drowsiness, paraesthesias, fatigue, hypokalemia and abdominal discomfort.
- Refractoriness is also a major disadvantage.
- Acetazolamide is contraindicated in hepatic cirrhosis patients.

Drugs Acting on Site II or Thick Ascending Limb of Loop of Henle

OR

Loop Diuretics/High Efficacy Diuretics/High Ceiling Diuretics

(Inhibitors of Na⁺- K⁺-2Cl⁻ cotransport)

- All the drugs of this class primarily act on the site II or the thick ascending limb of Henle's loop. Therefore, these are called *loop diuretics.*
- The diuretic response increases as we go on increasing the dose, hence called *high ceiling diuretics.*
- The efficacy of these drugs has been rated as highest amongst all diuretic agents, hence also called *high efficacy diuretics.*
- These drugs are capable of producing up to 10 L of urine in a day.
- These agents have very fast and short duration of action.

Mechanism of Action

- When given by oral/IM or IV route, these drugs on reaching the circulation get bound to plasma proteins and cannot pass through glomerulus.
- These drugs reach their site of action (thick ascending limb of loop of Henle) by the process of proximal tubular secretion and act from the luminal side.
- These drugs inhibit Na^+–K^+–$2Cl^-$ cotransport at site II and inhibit the reabsorption of NaCl out of the tubule into the interstitial space. Thus, the increased Na^+ and Cl^- reach the distal tubule and promote the loss of H^+ and K^+ along with increased loss of water causing profuse diuresis.
- The excretion of calcium and magnesium also increases.
- Intravenous furosemide transiently decreases preload by increasing systemic venous capacitance or peripheral pooling. This action is prostaglandin mediated and is responsible for the quick relief in left ventricular failure and pulmonary edema.

Indications

- **Edematous conditions:** Associated with hepatic, renal or cardiac origin. These drugs are very effective in relieving the symptoms of congestive cardiac failure, cirrhosis of liver and nephrotic syndrome immediately. Thiazides may be given later on for maintenance purpose.
- **Acute pulmonary edema:** Intravenous administration of furosemide or its congeners produces prompt relief.
- **Hypertension:** High ceiling diuretics are indicated in hypertension only in the presence of renal insufficiency, Congestive heart failure, or in resistant cases and in hypertensive emergencies; otherwise thiazides are preferred.
- **In massive blood transfusions:** Diuretics are given during massive blood transfusions to prevent renal overload.
- **Acute renal failure:** In renal failure cases, these drugs can convert oliguric phase of renal failure to non-oliguric phase.
- **Cerebral edema:** Intracranial pressure can be lowered by these drugs but osmotic diuretics are preferred.
- **Acute hypercalcemia:** The calcium excretion and urine flow is increased.

Adverse effects

- Electrolyte disturbances such as hypoklemia, hyponatremia, hypocalcemia, hypomagnesemia.
- Metabolic disturbances such as hyperglycemia, hyperuricemia, hyperlipidemia.
- General disturbances such as nausea, vomiting, diarrhea, headache, giddiness, myalgia, etc.
- Reversible ototoxicity.
- Hypersensitivity reactions.

Furosemide or Frusemide

- It is the most efficacious of all diuretics.

- It is well absorbed orally with 60% of bioavailability.
- It is highly plasma protein bound and eliminated partly through glomerular filtration and partly through tubular secretion. Some part is directly excreted in intestines through bile also.
- It has very rapid onset of action, i.e., within 2–5 minutes after IV administration, 10–20 minutes after IM route and 20–40 minutes after oral administration.
- The t½ is 1–2 hours with maximum duration of action 3–6 hours.
- It is given in a dose of 20–80 mg by oral route once daily in the morning.
- In pulmonary edema, it is given in a dose of 40–80 mg IV.

Bumetanide

- It is 40 times more potent than furosemide with other pharmacological properties similar to furosemide.
- It is also well absorbed orally with 80–100% of bioavailability.
- The plasma t½ is 60 minutes and may prolong in patients with kidney or liver impairment.
- It is preferred in furosemide non-responders or furosemide allergic patients.
- Bumetanide is given in a dose of 1–5 mg oral route once daily in the morning and 1–4 mg by IM or IV route.

Torasemide (Torsemide)

- It is three times more potent and longer acting than furosemide.
- It is rapidly and completely absorbed by oral route with a t½ of 3.5 hours.
- The duration of action is 4–8 hours.
- It is given in a dose of 2.5–5 mg OD for hypertension and 5–20 mg/day in edema.

Ethacrynic Acid

Due to its ototoxic and hepatotoxic side effects, it has gone *out of use.*

Indacrinone

- Indacrinone is an ethacrynic acid analogue and is a uricosuric diuretic.
- It inhibits the absorption of uric acid at proximel convolnted tuble besides inhibiting Na^+–K^+–$2Cl^-$ convoluted at site II.
- It is usually preferred in the gout patients requiring diuretic therapy.

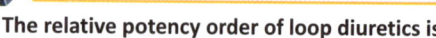

The relative potency order of loop diuretics is:
Bumetinide > torasemide > furosemide > ethacrynic acid = indacrinone

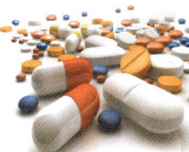

Drugs Acting on Site III: Cortical Diluting Segment of Loop of Henle or Early DCT

OR

Medium Efficacy Diuretics/Thiazides and Thiazide like Diuretics

(Na$^+$ Cl$^-$ symport inhibitors)

- **Thiazide diuretics:** Hydrochlorothiazide, chlorthiazide, clopamide, bendroflumethiazide, benzthiazide.
- **Thiazide-like diuretics:** Chlorthalidone, indapamide, xipamide, metolazone, quinethazone.
- All the drugs of this class primarily act on the site III or cortical diluting segment of loop of Henle or early distal convoluted tubule.
- These are the less powerful than loop diuretics but, more powerful than other diuretic groups, hence also called as *medium efficacy diuretics.*
- They have a longer duration of action as compared to loop diuretics.

Mechanism of Action

- When given by oral route, these drugs on reaching the circulation get bound to plasma proteins and cannot pass through glomerulus.
- These drugs also reach their site of action (early distal convoluted tubule) by the process of proximal tubular secretion and act from the luminal side.
- These drugs inhibit Na$^+$Cl$^-$ symporter at site III and also inhibit the reabsorption of NaCl out of the tubule into the interstitial space. This increases the loss of NaCl with water in the form of urine.
- Some of the thiazides and related drugs have additionally weak carbonic anhydrase inhibitory action in proximal convoluted tubule.
- They inhibit urinary excretion of calcium and uric acid.
- There are no injectable preparations of these drugs.

Hydrochlorothiazide

- The t½ of hydrochlorothiazide is 3–6 hours.
- In hypertension, it is given in a dose of 12.5–50 mg/day.
- In edema patients, it is given in a dose of 25-100 mg/day

Chlorthalidone

- It is a non-thiazide, but thiazide-like diuretic and behaves pharmacologically like hydrochlorothiazide.
- The plasma t½ is 40–50 hours.
- In hypertension, it is given orally in a dose of 12.5–50 mg once daily, preferably in the morning.

Metolazone

- Metolazone has a special property that it works even in severe renal failure patients with a GFR of ≤15 mL/minute.

- It has a synergistic effect when given with furosemide.
- In edema, it is given orally in a dose of 5–10 mg/day.
- In hypertension, it is given orally in a dose of 2.5–5 mg/day.

Xipamide

- Its pharmacological action is similar to low doses of furosemide.
- Its duration of action is approximately 12 hours and is given in a dose of 20–40 mg/day.
- The dose given in hypertension is 10–20 mg/day and in edema is 40–80 mg/day.
- It may cause severe hypokalemia sometimes.

Indapamide

- It is a lipid soluble thiazide and has very little diuretic action, but retains some antihypertensive action for which it is still used in some cases.
- It is given in a dose of 2.5–5 mg OD and has duration of action 12–34 hours.

> The relative potency of Thiazides and thiazide-like diuretics is:
> *Indapamide > Bendroflumethiazide > Metolazone > Hydrochlorthiazide = Chlorthalidone > chlorthiazide*
>
> **The duration of action rank order of Thiazides and thiazide-like diuretics is:**
> *Chlorthalidone > Indapamide = Metolazone > Bendroflumethiazide > Hydrochlorthiazide > Chlorthiazide*

Indications

- **Hypertension:** Thiazides and related diuretics, especially chlorthalidone and hydrochlorthiazide are one of the first line drugs in hypertension in elderly. The fall in BP develops gradually over 2–4 weeks. The maximum antihypertensive efficacy is reached at a dose of 25 mg/day.
- **Edema:** Thiazides may be used for mild to moderate cases. To start with, more efficacious diuretics are preferred to mobilize the edema fluid and thiazides are used for maintenance therapy. They act best in cardiac edema and are less effective in hepatic or renal edema.
- **Diabetes insipidus:** Thiazides reduce the urine volume in patients of diabetes insipidus. This is a paradoxical effect. These are the only drugs effective in nephrogenic diabetes insipidus. However, these drugs reduce the volume of urine in patients of central diabetes also.
- **Hypercalciuria:** Thiazides inhibit urinary Ca$^+$ excretion and are useful in idiopathic hypercalciuria. Therefore, these drugs are beneficial for patients suffering from recurrent calcium oxalate stones.

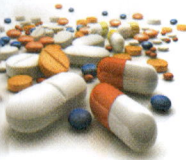

Adverse Effects

- Electrolyte disturbances such as hypokalemia, hyponatremia, hypomagnesemia. In contrast to loop diuretics, these cause hypercalcemia. So, electrolyte monitoring should be done regularly.
- Metabolic disturbances such as hyperglycemia, hyperuricemia, hyperlipidemia are similar to loop diuretics.
- Hypersensitivity reactions such as rashes and photosensitivity reactions occur in sulphonamide sensitive patients.
- General disturbances such as nausea, vomiting, diarrhea, headache, giddiness, myalgia, etc.
- Reversible erectile dysfunction is seen as a idiosyncratic reaction in some patients.

Differences between high and moderate efficacy diuretics are given in Table 6.2.

- Loop diuretics are the drugs, which cause maximum sodium loss.
- Ethacrynic acid causes maximum loss of chloride ions in urine.
- Acetazolamide causes maximum loss of potassium and uric acid in urine and this is only drug that causes chloride reabsorption.

TABLE 6.2: Differences between high and moderate efficacy diuretics

Properties	High efficacy diuretics	Moderate efficacy diuretics
Mode of action	$Na^+- K–2Cl^-$ cotransport inhibitors	$Na^+–Cl^-$ symport inhibitors
Site of action	Thick ascending loop of henle	Distal convoluted tubule
Role in calcium metabolism	Increase Ca^+excretion	Increase Ca^+reabsorption
Ototoxicity	+++	+
Role in CHF	Commonly used	Not used; but Indapamide may be useful
Role in renal failure	Most preferred diuretics	Not used; but Metolazone may be used.
Role in hypertension	Not preferred	Most preferred diuretics; it decreases the total peripheral resistance resulting decrease in BP.
Hyperuricaemia	Most preferred	Not preferred

Both groups of drugs may cause hypomagnesemia, hyponatremia, hypokalemia, hyperuricemia, hyperlipidemia and hyperglycemia.

Drugs Acting on Site IV: Late DCT and Collecting Duct (CD)

OR

Potassium Sparing Diuretics

These drugs retains K^+ ions while maintain the diuretic effects. These are preferably given along with loop diuretics to prevent the potassium loss.

- **Aldosterone receptor antagonists:** Spironolactone and Eplerenone.
  Spironolactone and Eplerenone produce diuretic effects by antagonizing mineralocorticoid receptors.
- **Na⁺ channel inhibitors (at collecting duct):** Triamterene and Amiloride.
  Amiloride and Triamterene produce diuretic effects by antagonizing luminal sodium channel at distal part and collecting tubules.

Aldosterone Receptor Antagonists (Spironolactone and Eplerenone)

Spironolactone

- It is a competitive inhibitor of mineralocorticoid receptors.
- Spironolactone competitively antagonizes the aldosterone. Hence, prevent the sodium and water reabsorption and causes diuresis.
- As sodium reabsorption is inhibited, the concomitant potassium secretion into the tubules does not take place. Hence, the potassium sparing effect is obtained.

Pharmacokinetics

- It is partially absorbed with only 65% of bioavailability (*the microfine form of tablet has 75% bioavailability*).
- It is metabolized in liver converted to active metabolite '*Canrenone*'.
- It also undergoes enterohepatic circulation.
- The t½ of spironolactone is 1–2 hours, while that of canrenone is ~18 hours.
- The t½ may increase in case of cirrhosis.
- It is given in a dose of 25–50 mg BD–QID and the maximum dose ≤200 mg/day.

Indications

- It is used in combination with high efficacy diuretics to compensate the K^+ loss in urine.
- Edema due to cirrhosis of liver and nephrotic syndrome: *Aldosterone levels are high in these conditions.*
- Congestive heart failure and hypertension: As an adjuvant to other diuretics to prevent hypokalemia.
- Conn's syndrome.
- Ectopic aldosterone production (secondary aldosteronism).

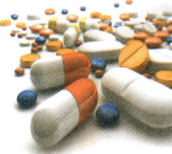

Adverse effects

- The common side effects are hyperkalemia, epigastric distress, loose motions, and mental confusion.
- It may also cause gynecomastia and erectile dysfunction in males, while menstrual irregularities in females.

Eplerenone

- It is a newer agent having more specific antagonistic property towards the mineralocorticoid receptors. Therefore, the incidence of hormonal adverse effects is lesser than spironolactone.
- The oral absorption is good, metabolism occurs in liver and excretion through urine and feces.
- The plasma t½ is 4–6 hours.
- It is given orally in a dose of 25–50 mg BD.

Indications

- Acute myocardial infarction with left ventricular systolic dysfunction.
- Congestive heart failure
- Hypertension

Na⁺ Channel Inhibitors (Act at Collecting Duct) (Triamterene and Amiloride)

Mechanism of Action

- These drugs act by inhibiting the renal epithelial Na⁺ channel and increase Na⁺ excretion with retention of K⁺ ions.
- They also reduce the excretion of Ca^{2+} and Mg^{2+} ions without changing renal hemodynamics.

Indications

These drugs are indicated in:
- In combination with thiazide these drugs are used to treat refractory edema.
- In hypertension, to prevent hypokalemia induced by loop diuretics.
- Lithium induce diabetes insipidus (it blocks entry of lithium by sodium channels in the collecting duct).
- Some case of cystic fibrosis.

Triamterene

- Its oral absorption is partial.
- It is metabolized in liver and excretion occurs through urine with t½ of 4 hours.
- It is given orally in a dose of 50–100 mg OD.
- The common side effects are nausea, muscle cramps and dizziness.

Amiloride

- It is 10 times more potent than triamterene.
- The oral absorption is very poor.
- The metabolism occurs in liver and excretion occur through urine.
- The plasma t½ is 20 hours. It is given orally in a dose of 5–10 mg OD/BD.
- The common side effects are hyperuricemia, headache, nausea and diarrhea.

Drugs Acting on Entire Nephron or Osmotic Diuretics

(Mannitol, Isosorbide, Glycerol)

- These drugs mainly act in the PCT and the descending limb of loop of Henle.
- The effect of anti-diuretic hormone in the collecting duct is also decreased by these agents.
- These agents also inhibit the normal water reabsorption by their osmotic effects and lead to increased urine excretion.
- The Na⁺ and water reabsorption is inhibited because these drugs decrease the contact time between tubular epithelium, causing natriuresis and excessive water loss.

Mannitol

It is pharmacologically inert substance (neither absorbed nor metabolized) and administered in high dose to produce osmotic effects on tubules and/or plasma fluids. The route of administration is intravenous only (10–20% strength). The plasma t½ is 0.5–1.5 hours.

Mechanism of action is shown here as follows:

Renal	Extra-renal
Increased osmotic pressure of glomerular filtration	When osmolarity increase in blood
↓	↓
Increases osmolality of tubular fluid	Increase intravascular volume
↓	↓
Decrease reabsorption of water and Na⁺	Increase renal blood flow
↓	↓
Diuresis	Decrease renin production
	↓
	Decrease aldosterone production
	↓
	Diuresis

Indications

For decreasing intracranial tension (ICT) and intraocular tension (IOT):

1–2 g/kg; it takes 60–90 minutes to reduce ICT/IOT. It decreases the cerebral and ocular edema.

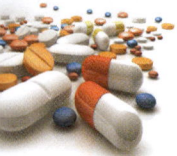

Adverse Effects

- The most common side effect is headache; while other side effects are nausea, vomiting, dehydration, hyperkalemia, hyponatremia and pulmonary edema.
- It is contraindicated in pulmonary edema, established renal failure, acute left ventricular failure, cerebral hemorrhage and congestive heart failure.

Isosorbide and Glycerol

- These osmotic diuretics can be administered by oral route.
- These are indicated in the case of cerebral edema or acute congestive glaucoma to reduce ICT or IOT, respectively.
- These are given in a dose of 0.5–1.5 g/kg as oral solution.

ANTIDIURETICS

Antidiuretics are the drugs that reduce urine volume. Their primary indication is *diabetes insipidus*.

Antidiuretic drugs are divided in three groups:

- **Antidiuretic hormone** [Antidiuretic hormone, argenine vasopressin (AVP)], lypressin, terlipressin, desmopressin.
- **Thiazides and Amiloride.**
- **Other drugs:** Indomethacin, chlorpropamide, carbamazepine.

Antidiuretic Hormone (ADH/AVP)

- Antidiuretic hormone is synthesized in the supraoptic and paraventricular nucleus of hypothalamus and secreted by the posterior pituitary along with oxytocin.
- It is secreted under some physiological stimuli such as rise in plasma osmolarity and contraction of extra-cellular fluid or falling blood pressure.
- Osmoreceptors regulate the rate of their release.
  Table 6.3 enlists the factors affecting antidiuretic release.
- The human ADH is 8-arginine-vasopressin, hence also called *AVP*.
- It has a role in long-term blood pressure control by increasing the water reabsorption from the collecting duct.
- It can raise blood pressure by constricting the blood vessels, hence also called *vasopressin*.

TABLE 6.3: Factors affecting antidiuretic hormone release

Increase ADH secretion	Decrease ADH secretion
Histamine	Ethanol
NeuropeptideY	Gamma-aminobutyric acid
Angiotensin II	Atrial natriuretic peptide
Prostaglandins	Phenytoin
High dose morphine	Low dose morphine
Acetylcholine	Haloperidol

> **Osmoreceptors**
>
> These are sensory receptors, which are present in the hypothalamus, hepatic portal system, pulmonary veins, left atrium and ventricles. The change in osmotic pressure in our body is detected by these receptors and the fluid balance is maintained by regulating the rate of ADH release.
>
> When the blood plasma is more diluted or concentrated, the osmoreceptors expand or contract, respectively. This leads to hyperactivation of afferent neurons and send signals to the hypothalamus, which increases or decreases the secretion of antidiuretic hormone from posterior pituitary to maintain normal blood concentration.

ADH exerts its effects by acting through V_1 **and** V_2 receptors.

V_1 **receptors** are located in vascular smooth muscle (including that of vasa recta in renal medulla), uterine and other visceral smooth muscles, interstitial cells in renal medulla, cortical collecting duct cells, adipose tissue, brain, platelets, liver, anterior pituitary, certain areas in brain and in pancreas, etc.

Their clinical importance lies in the constriction of blood vessels mainly.

V_2 **receptors** are located in the collecting duct cells, ascending limb of loop of Henle cells and the endothelium of blood vessels.

Their clinical importance lies in the antidiuretic effect by increasing the water permeability of collecting duct.

Other actions of AVP are:

- Increased GI peristalsis (large intestine).
- Uterine contractions are increased like oxytocin.
- Regulation of temperature, systemic circulation and adrenocorticotropic hormone release.
- Learning of tasks.

Pharmacokinetics

- AVP is inactive orally because it is degraded by trypsin; therefore, it is given parenterally by IV, SC or intranasal route in a dose of 10 U/day.
- The plasma t½ is 25 minutes.

Vasopressin Analogues (Lypressin, Terlipressin, Desmopressin)

Lypressin (8-lysine Vasopressin)

- The potency of lypressin is lesser than AVP.
- The pharmacological actions are exerted on both V_1 and V_2 receptors.
- The duration of action is about 4–6 hours.

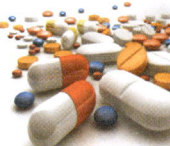

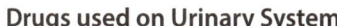

- It is given IM/SC in a dose of 10 IU
- The IV infusion of 20 IU diluted in 200 mL of dextrose is given over 10–20 minutes.

Desmopressin

- Desmopressin is 10–12 times more potent than vasopressin and is a selective V_2 receptor agonist.
- It is longest acting ADH (8–12 hours) with a plasma t½ of 1–2 hours.
- It is available in intranasal, oral, subcutaneous and parenteral forms.
- It is given in different doses which are as follows:
  - **Orally:** 0.1–0.2 mg thrice daily.
  - **Parenterally:** 2–4 µg/day by SC/IV route in divided doses.
  - **Intranasally:** Adults: 10–40 µg/day in divided doses. Pediatric: 5–10 µg at night (HS).

Terlipressin

- It is a synthetic prodrug of vasopressin.
- The most common indication of terlipressin is bleeding esophageal varices.
- It is given in a dose of 2 mg IV may be repeated in a dose of 1–2 mg every 4–6 hours, if required.

Indications of ADH and Vasopressin Analogues

- **Diabetes insipidus:** Highly effective in central or neurogenic diabetes insipidus, whereas ineffective in renal or nephrogenic diabetes insipidus.
- **Nocturnal enuresis:** Intranasal or oral desmopressin at bedtime controls primary nocturia by reducing urine volume.
- **Hemophilia and von Willebrand's disease:** AVP releases von Willebrand's factor and factor VIII, which are helpful in controlling bleeding.
- All the above actions are based on V_2 receptor activation and Desmopressin is the drug of choice.
- **Bleeding esophageal varices:** Vasopressin analogues stop bleeding by constricting mesenteric blood vessels and reducing blood flow through the liver to the varices, allowing clot formation.
- This action is based upon V_1 receptor activation and Terlipressin is the drug of choice.

Adverse Effects

- **Local side effects:** Nasal congestion, rhinitis and epistaxis.
- **Systemic side effects:** Headache, flushing, nausea, urticaria, abdominal cramps, backache in females (due to uterine contraction) and hyponatremia.

Vasopressin Receptor Antagonists (Conivaptan, Tolvaptan)

Conivaptan

- **Mechanism of action is** antagonism of vasopressin V_{1a} and V_2 receptors.
- **Its main effects are** to antagonize the action of vasopressin (ADH).
- **Clinically useful in managing** hyponatremia in hospitalized patients.
- **Indicated in** syndrome of inappropriate ADH secretion (SIADH) and congestive heart failure due to ADH excess.
- **Route of administration** is intravenous only.
- **Common complication** is infusion site reaction.

Tolvaptan

Tolvaptan is similar to conivaptan, but more selective for vasopressin V_2 receptors; can be given orally.

THIAZIDE DIURETICS, AMILORIDE

- Thiazides reduce the urine volume in patients of diabetes insipidus. This is a paradoxical effect.
- Hydrochlorothiazide 25–50 mg TDS or equivalent dose of a longer acting agent is commonly used.
- These are the only drugs effective in nephrogenic diabetes insipidus. However, these drugs reduced the volume of urine in patients of center diabetes also.
- They are valuable in renal diabetic insipidus as AVP is ineffective.
- Mechanism of action: Thiazides induce a state of sustained electrolyte depletion so that glomerular filtrate is more completely reabsorbed iso-osmotically in PT. Furthermore, because of reduced salt reabsorption in the cortical diluting segment, a smaller volume of less dilute urine is presented to the collecting ducts and the same is passed out.
- Secondly, thiazides reduce glomerular filtration rate (GFR) and thus, the fluid load on tubules.
- High ceiling diuretics are also effective but are less desirable because of their short and brisk action.

In lithium induced nephrogenic diabetes insipidus, *Amiloride* is the most preferred drug.

Other drugs: Indomethacin, Chlorpropamide, Carbamazepine.

- **Indomethacin** reduces renal prostaglandin synthesis. It is used in combination with thiazide/amiloride in nephrogenic diabetes insipidus. Other non-steroidal anti-inflammatory dimetics (NSAIDs) are less active.
- **Chlorpropamide** sensitizes the kidneys to ADH actions. It acts by reducing urine formation at pituitary level.

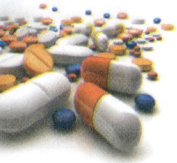

- **Carbamazepine** is an anticonvulsant agent. It decreases the volume of urine in central or neurogenic diabetes insipidus. The probable mechanism of action is reduction of urine formation at pituitary level. Higher doses are needed for this effect.

Nursing Implications

☞ **Diuretics and anti-diuretics**
- ☞ Assess for contraindication or cautions of diuretic use.
- ☞ Continuously monitor urinary output, cardiac response, and heart rhythm of patients receiving intravenous diuretics to monitor for electrolyte disturbances leading to cardiac arrhythmia.
- ☞ If patient is not catheterized, administer oral/injectable diuretics early in the day so that increased urination will not interfere with sleep.
- ☞ Monitor for adverse effects of diuretic therapy and take timely action accordingly.
- ☞ Patient should be educated that, thiazide diuretics may cause photosensitivity.
- ☞ The pulse of the patient on diuretic therapy should be palpated carefully to assess the ectopic beats and if noted should be brought into the notice of physician.
- ☞ Evaluate the effectiveness of the teaching plan (patient can name drug, dosage, adverse effects to watch for, and specific measures to avoid them).

URINARY ANTISEPTICS

Conditions affecting the urinary tract and bladder are quite common in clinical practice. These conditions include urinary tract infections, bladder spasms, bladder pain, and benign prostatic hyperplasia (BPH).

Drugs acting on urinary bladder, urethra and prostate are mentioned in Figure 6.2.

The following group of people are vulnerable to UTIs:
- Females, due to shorter perineal area and short urethra.
- Patients with indwelling catheters or intermittent catheterizations often develop bladder infections or cystitis, which can result from bacteria introduced into the bladder by these devices.
- Blockage anywhere in the urinary tract can lead to backflow problems and the spread of bladder infections into the kidney (pyelonephritis).
- Patients with anatomical abnormalities of urinary tract.

The signs and symptoms of urinary tract infection include: Increased frequency of micturition, urgency, burning micturition (associated with cystitis), chills, fever, flank pain, and tenderness (associated with acute pyelonephritis).

To treat these infections, clinicians use specific urinary tract anti-infectives, which include antibiotics, as well as some specific agents that alter the urinary pH.

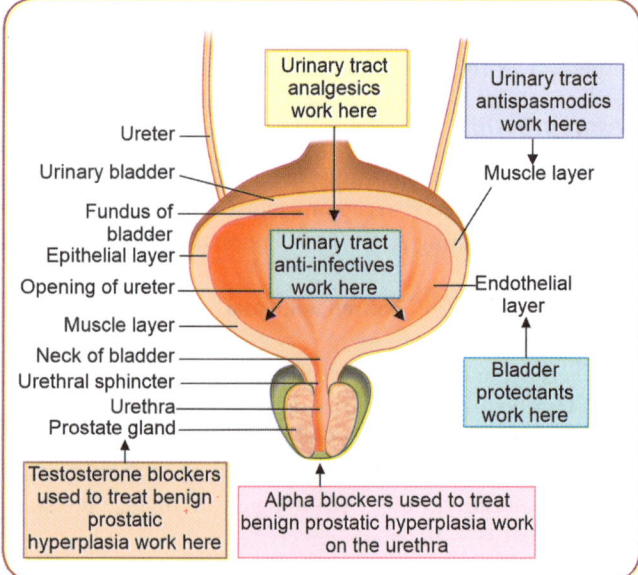

FIG. 6.2: Drugs acting on urinary bladder, urethra and prostate

The orally administered anti-microbial agents (AMAs), which attain good antibacterial concentration only in urine, with little or no systemic antibacterial effects are called *urinary antiseptics*. This is equivalent to a form of local therapy. These drugs are excreted unchanged via renal route and are useful mainly in lower urinary tract infections. Examples: Nitrofurantoin, nalidixic acid and methenamine, etc.

Some other drugs, which are also useful in treating urinary tract infections, are known as urinary anti-infective drugs.

Urinary tract anti-infectives are:

The antibiotics used specifically to treat urinary tract infections are as follows:
- Nitrofurantoin (urinary antiseptics)
- Fluroquinolones: Norfloxacin, ofloxacin, ciprofloxacin, prulifloxacin, etc.
- Cephalosporins: Cefixime, cefuroxime, ceftriaxone, ceftazidine, etc.
- Aminoglycosides: Amikacin, gentamicin, etc.
- Sulphonamides: Cotrimoxazole, etc.
  - These drugs are preferred in the treatment of urinary tract infections but used for treating other infections also.
  - In complicated urinary tract infections and pyelonephritis, drugs are used mainly in injectable form to achieve good bioavailability and early minimum inhibitory concentration for attaining maximum efficacy and early response.
  - *The above list of drugs is for empirical use only and the specific urinary tract infections treatment should be based upon urine culture sensitivity report only.*

The details of these drugs have been described in Antimicrobial agents.

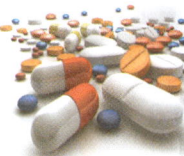

Nursing Implications

☞ **Urinary antiseptics, acidifiers and alkalinizers**

☞ Ensure that culture and sensitivity tests are performed before therapy begins and are repeated if the response is not as expected to ensure appropriate treatment of the infection.

☞ Patient should be educated about the importance and proper technique of urine sample collection. Midstream urine should be collected in the sterile container.

☞ Catheter care should be properly done and nurse should keep a record of the exact date of catheterization, as catheter needs to be changed within 2–3 weeks.

☞ Encourage the patient to drink lots of fluids (unless contraindicated by other conditions) to promote flushing of the bladder and prevent urinary stasis and to avoid citrus juices and antacids, which promote alkaline urine and provide opportunity for bacteria growth.

☞ Provide or assist with perineal hygiene as indicated to reduce the risk of reinfection or prevent transmission of infection.

☞ Monitor patient response to the drug (resolution of UTI and relief of signs and symptoms); repeat culture and sensitivity tests as recommended for evaluation of the effectiveness of all these drugs.

☞ Evaluate the effectiveness of the teaching plan (patient can name drug, dosage, adverse effects to watch for, specific measures to avoid them, and measures to take to increase the effectiveness of the drug).

CHOLINERGIC AND ANTICHOLINERGIC DRUGS

CHOLINERGIC DRUGS (CHOLINOMIMETIC, PARASYMPATHOMIMETIC)

The drugs which produce acetylcholine like actions on different organ systems are known as cholinergic drugs. These drugs act either by directly interacting with cholinergic receptors or by increasing availability of acetylcholine (ACh) at these sites. Drugs acting directly on cholinergic receptors are known as cholinergic agonists (e.g., bathenechol) and the drugs which increase availability of ACh by inhibiting cholinesterase enzyme are known as anticholinesterases (e.g., neostigmine).

Cholinergic Receptors

There are two types of cholinergic receptors: *muscarinic and nicotinic.*

- **Muscarinic receptors:** have been divided into five subtypes M_1, M_2, M_3, M_4 and M_5. These are located on heart, blood vessels, eye, smooth muscles and glands of gastrointestinal, respiratory and urinary tracts, sweat glands, etc.

- In the urinary system, the cholinergic drugs act through M_3 receptors. These have a role in visceral smooth muscle contraction and glandular secretions. Some of the actions are also mediated through M_2 receptors.
  Smooth muscles in ureter and detrusor muscle in urinary bladder are contracted through M_3 receptors. Peristalsis in ureter is increased. The detrusor muscle contracts while the bladder trigone and sphincter relax which leads to micturition.

- **Nicotinic receptors** are present at skeletal muscle end plate and autonomic ganglia.

Cholinergic drugs useful in urinary system: *Bethanechol and Neostigmine*
Acetylcholine is not used clinically due to non-selective and extremely short duration of action.

- **Bethanechol:** It initiates micturition by increasing the tone of detrusor muscle. It is indicated in postoperative/postpartum non-obstructive urinary retention and neurogenic bladder.
  It is given in a dose of 10–50 mg orally and 2.5–5 mg subcutaneously. Commonly seen side effects are abdominal cramps, involuntary urination and defecation, vasodilation, sweating, hypotension and may precipitate asthma, etc.

- **Neostigmine:** Neostigmine is an anticholinesterase and given in a dose of 0.5–1 mg subcutaneously in cases of postoperative urinary retention. It should not be given in the cases of organic obstruction in the urinary tract.

ANTICHOLINERGIC DRUGS (MUSCARINIC RECEPTOR ANTAGONISTS, ATROPINIC, PARASYMPATHOLYTIC)

The drugs which block actions of ACh on autonomic effectors are known as *'anticholinergic drugs'.* The effects are exerted through antagonism at the level of muscarinic receptors.

The anticholinergic drugs useful for urinary system disorders are:

- **General antispasmodics:** Dicyclomine, Valethamate.
- **Drugs acting specifically on urinary system [Vasicoselective drugs]:** Oxybutynin, Flavoxate, Tolterodine, Darifenacin and Solifenacin.

Mechanism of Action

- The anticholinergic drugs have a relaxant effect on all the visceral smooth muscles that receive parasympathetic motor innervations.
- Anticholinergic drugs have relaxant action on ureter and urinary bladder. Clinically, this effect is beneficial

151

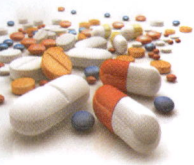

in increasing bladder capacity by decreasing the tone of detrusor muscles.

- This also controls detrusor hyper-reflexia in patients suffering from neurogenic bladder or enuresis.

General Antispasmodics (*Dicyclomine, Valethamate*)

- **Dicyclomine:** In addition to weak anticholinergic effects, it also has direct smooth muscle relaxant action. It is used in renal colic in a dose of 10–20 mg oral/IM for adults and 5–10 mg for children.
- **Valethamate:** It is useful as antispasmodic in a variety of colics such as urinary, biliary and intestinal colic. Primarily, it is used, as a smooth muscle relaxant to hasten dilatation of cervix during delivery. It is given in a dose of 8 mg IM and 10 mg orally BD.

Drotaverine

- It is an effective *non-anticholinergic spasmolytic drug*. It causes smooth muscle relaxation by inhibiting phosphodiesterase-4 (PDE-4) enzyme.
- It is used both orally and parenterally for intestinal, biliary and renal colics, irritable bowel syndrome, uterine spasms, etc.
- It is given in a dose of 40–80 mg BD/TDS orally and 20–40 mg IM BD/TDS.

Drugs Acting Specifically on Urinary System [Vesicoselective Drugs] (Oxybutynin, Flavoxate, Tolterodine, Darifenacin and Solifenacin)

- **Oxybutynin:** It has selective action on bladder and is useful in patients suffering from vesical spasm, urinary frequency, neurogenic bladder and nocturnal enuresis. It is given in a dose of 5 mg BD/TDS orally in adults and 2.5 mg BD in children above 5 years.
- **Flavoxate** is prescribed in urinary frequency, urgency and dysuria associated with lower urinary tract infection. It is given in a dose of 200 mg TDS.
- **Tolterodine:** It is M_3 selective muscarinic antagonist with specific action on urinary bladder. The anticholinergic side effects are less. It is prescribed in overactive bladder with urinary frequency and urgency. It is given in a dose of 1–2 mg BD or 2–4 mg OD orally.
- **Darifenacin** and **Solifenacin** are other relatively M_3 subtype selective antimuscarinics useful in bladder disorders.

ACIDIFIERS AND ALKALINIZERS

Acidifiers and alkalinizers are the agents, which are used or can be used to acidify or alkalinize the urine, respectively as per requirement. As these agents are given systemically, they

temporarily alter the pH of blood also, may it be for a short duration only, as the compensatory mechanisms of the body immediately respond and maintain the normal pH of blood and other body fluids.

Certain AMAs act better in acidic urine, while others work better in alkaline urine. However, specific intervention to produce urine of desired pH is rarely required because most of the drugs used in UTI attain high concentration in urine and minor changes in urinary pH do not affect clinical outcome. In case of inadequate response or in complicated cases, measurement of urinary pH and appropriate corrective measure may help.

The AMAs which work better in acidic pH are: Nitrofurantoin, tetracyclines, cloxacillin, etc.

The AMAs which work better in alkaline pH are: Cephalosporins, fluoroquinolones, aminoglycosides, cotrimoxazole, etc.

ACIDIFIERS

- These are the drugs, which are used or can be used to acidify urine whenever required for therapeutic purpose.
- Renal excretion of basic drugs (e.g., amphetamine) can be enhanced by acidification of urine.
- Ammonium chloride, potassium chloride and ascorbic acid can be used for this purpose. Rarely required practically.

ALKALINIZERS

- These are the drugs, which are used or can be used to alkalinize urine whenever required for therapeutic purpose.
- Renal excretion of acidic drugs (e.g., salicylates) can be enhanced by acidification of urine.
- Potassium citrate, magnesium citrate, sodium citrate and tricitrate solutions of these compounds can be used for this purpose.

Mechanism of Action of Alkalinizers

After oral administration, these agents are absorbed systemically and increase the plasma bicarbonate levels; *blood pH is raised*. In case of patients suffering from acidosis, the excess hydrogen ions are buffered and the clinical manifestations of acidosis are reversed.

These agents are metabolized to bicarbonates, which are excreted as free bicarbonate ions in the urine and increase the urinary pH. Theses make the urine alkaline and helps in dissolution of uric acid and cystine stone.

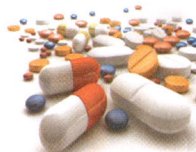

Pharmacokinetics

- These agents are given orally in tablet form or solution form. After oral administration, these are absorbed systemically and converted to sodium and potassium bicarbonates.
- These are excreted via renal route in the form of bicarbonates. Less than 5% is excreted in unchanged form.
- These agents have quick onset of action within 1 hour of administration and remains up to 12 hours.
- Alkalinizers when given in a dose of 10–15 mL QID: maintain a urine pH of 6.5–7.4 and when given in a dose of 15–20 mL QID maintain a urine pH of 7.0–7.6

The alkalinizing effect remains up to 24 hours after the last dose.

Indications

- To treat UTIs along with AMAs, which work better in alkaline urine.
- To treat the symptoms of systemic acidosis for shorter durations. Higher doses are needed for this purpose.
- For prevention and treatment of uric acid and calcium oxalate stones.

- For symptomatic improvement in burning micturition in case of cystitis and urethritis.
- To enhance the excretion of acidic drugs (phenobarbitone, salicylates) in case of poisonings. Intravenous soda bicarbonate is used. It can be tried but only when renal functions are not compromised. It is rarely practised now.

Drug Interactions

- Loop diuretics and spironolactone enhance the digitalis toxicity by causing hypokalemia.
- The levels of lithium are raised by loop diuretics. Hence, the combinations should be avoided.
- Thiazides or high ceiling diuretics are intentionally given in combination with anti-hypertensive to obtain synergistic effects.
- The combinations of high ceiling diuretics and aminoglycoside antibiotics should be avoided as both are ototoxic and nephrotoxic in nature.
- NSAIDs decrease the effect of high ceiling diuretics by inhibiting prostaglandin synthesis in the kidney. Hence, the combinations should be avoided.
- Spironolactone should not be given with angiotensin converting enzyme inhibitors/angiotensin II receptor blockers as fatal hyperkalemia may occur.

Assess Yourself

Long and Short Answer Questions

1. What are diuretic agents? Classify them, describe loop diuretics.
2. Describe the complications of diuretic therapy.
3. What is the rational of combination of potassium sparing diuretic with loop diuretics?
4. Describe the diuretics, which are used as therapy for hypertension.
5. Why the loop diuretics are called high ceiling diuretics?
6. Why mannitol is used in head injury?
7. Write short note on:
   - a. Urinary antiseptics
   - b. Bethanechol
   - c. Alkalinizers
   - d. Furosemide
   - e. Spironolactone

Multiple Choice Questions

1. **The site of action of the loop diuretic furosemide is:**
   - a. Thick ascending limb of loop of Henle
   - b. Descending limb of loop of Henle
   - c. Proximal tubule
   - d. Distal tubule

2. **Thiazides can cause:**
   - a. Hyperkalemic paralysis
   - b. Hypouricemia
   - c. Hypolipidemia
   - d. Impotence

3. **Thiazides diuretics causes all except:**
   - a. Hyperglycemia
   - b. Increased calcium excretion
   - c. Useful in congestive heart failure
   - d. Decreased uric acid excretion

4. **Mannitol is not useful for:**
   - a. Glaucoma
   - b. Raised ICT
   - c. Impending renal failure
   - d. Pulmonary edema

Contd...

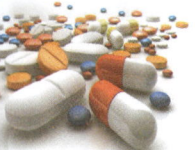

5. Potassium sparing diuretics acts on:
    a. $Na^+ K^+$ pump
    b. Aldosterone receptor
    c. Carbonic anhydrase
    d. $Na^+–Cl^-$ symporter

6. Loop diuretics act by
    a. Inhibition of $Na^+–Cl^-$ Symport
    b. Inhibition of $Na^+–K^+–2\ Cl^-$ cotransport
    c. Inhibition of $Na^+–K^+$ ATPase
    d. Inhibition of $H^+–K^+$ ATPase
    e. Inhibition of renal epithelial Na^+ channel

7. Which of the following is a aldosterone antagonist?
    a. Eplerenone
    b. Amiloride
    c. Triamterene
    d. All of the above

8. Loop diuretics act on:
    a. PCT
    b. DCT
    c. Thick ascending loop of Henle
    d. Collecting duct

Answer Key

1. a.	2. d.	3. b.	4. d.	5. b.	6. b.	7. a.
8. c.						

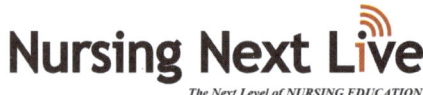

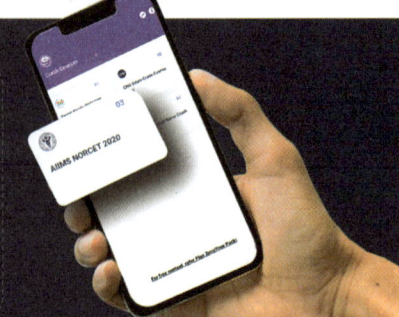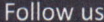

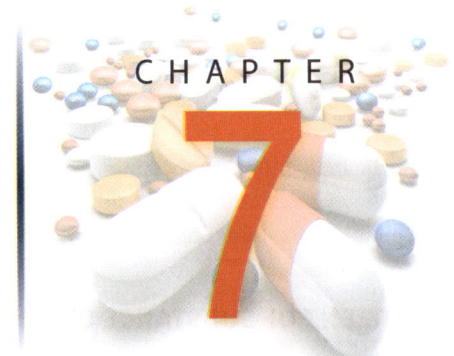

Miscellaneous Drugs

 CHAPTER OUTLINE

Drugs for De-addiction
- Treatment of Substance use Disorders
- Drugs used in De-addiction
- Cardiopulmonary Resuscitation
- Drugs Required for the Management of Various Emergencies

Vitamins and Minerals
- Minerals

Immunosuppressants

Antidotes
- Types of Antidotes

Anti Venom
- Production of Antivenom
- Storage of Antivenom

- Principle of Antivenom
- Route of Administration
- Mechanism of Action
- Antisnake Venom (ASV) Serum Polyvalent

Vaccine and Sera
- Vaccines
- Sera
- Immunity
- Vaccines
- Antisera and Immunoglobulins

DRUGS FOR DE-ADDICTION

Addiction means excessive, recurrent and compulsive use of drug/drugs to obtain pleasurable effects. The addicted individuals become so obsessed to these drugs that it becomes their primary aim to procure and use these drugs. This behavioral change disrupts their ability to adjust in the family, workplace and society.

Addiction involves the following features:
- There is always intense craving for the drugs. *Craving means intense desire to take the drug by any means.*
- There is a need to increase the dose of drugs to get the same level of pleasure due to development of tolerance.
- Appearance of life-threatening withdrawal symptoms if the dose of addictive drug is missed or ceased, which forces the individual to take the drug again and again.
- The detrimental effects of the drug harm the individual, family and society as well.

There are various terms, which are used in relation to the excessive and compulsive use of the drugs such as habituation, drug dependence and drug addiction.

- *Habituation* means that a person is in the habit of taking the substance without any detrimental effects on his body or society and there is no craving, tolerance and withdrawal symptoms. Examples: tea, coffee, etc.
- **Drug dependence** means the state of a person arising after repeated and continuous use of a substance in which all-detrimental effects and craving appears. There is a psychological and physical need to continue the drug for the fear of getting the withdrawal symptoms.
- **Psychological dependence** means the behavior involved in procurement of the drug.
- **Physical dependence** means body demands the presence of substance in the blood to continue the various physiological processes, hence also called **Physiological dependence.** Withdrawal symptoms appear on discontinuance of the drug.

The *diagnostic and statistical manual of mental disorders* (DSM-V) has included all the above terms in a single term **"substance use disorder,"** ranging from mild to severe. This was done to remove the confusion of using above-mentioned different and various terms.

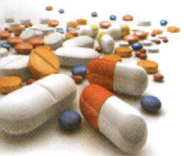

The different substances which can produce addiction or substance-used disorders are as follows:

- Tea, coffee, tobacco in various forms such as bidi, cigarette, gutka, khaini, etc. These cause mild form of substance use disorders.
- Marijuana (sulfa), amphetamine, cocaine, nicotine due to excessive use of >20 cigarettes/day.
- Opioids, benzodiazepines, alcohol, etc.

TREATMENT OF SUBSTANCE USE DISORDERS

Goal of Treatment

- The ultimate goal of treatment program is to achieve a drug free status as early as possible and to prevent relapse.
- The drug free status is achieved with the help of pharmacotherapy.
- The prevention of relapse is achieved by a combination of behavioral treatment, rehabilitation program, psychosocial interventions and pharmacotherapy.

DRUGS USED IN DE-ADDICTION

Opioid De-addiction Drugs

Methadone

- Methadone is a long-acting synthetic opioid agonist medication that can prevent and reduce the craving and withdrawal symptoms in opioid-addicted individuals. It is a type of substitution therapy.
- It also blocks the effects of illicit opioids.
- It is used in the treatment of opioid dependence in adults.
- Methadone maintenance is more effective when it is combined with behavioral treatment.
- It is given orally in a dose of 10 mg OD.

Buprenorphine

- It is also a synthetic opioid medication that acts as a partial agonist at opioid receptors.
- It does not produce the euphoria and sedation caused by heroin or other opioids but is able to reduce or eliminate withdrawal symptoms associated with opioid dependence and carries a low risk of overdose.
  Buprenorphine maintenance Therapy is currently used in India as a part of opioids de-addiction regimen.
- Buprenorphine is available in two formulations that are taken sublingually:
  - Buprenorphine tablet alone (8 mg).

- Combination of buprenorphine (8 mg) with naloxone (2 mg), an antagonist (or blocker) at opioid receptors.

LAAM

- It is levo-alfa-acetyl-methadol.
- It is a long acting analogue of methadone.
- It is given thrice weekly in a dose of 20–40 mg in those patients who had not been initiated with methadone and up to 120 mg to methadone receiving patients.
- It has minimum abuse potential.
- It may cause arrhythmia and QT prolongation, which needs regular monitoring.
- *It has been banned in few countries.*

Naloxone

- It is a synthetic pure opioid antagonist.
- It is competitive antagonist to all opioids receptors.
- It also blocks the action of endogenous opioids such as endorphins and encephalins.
- It immediately antagonizes all the action of opioids.
- It is given in a dose of 0.1–0.4 mg IV until the desirable effects are achieved.

Naltrexone

- Naltrexone is a synthetic opioid antagonist.
- It blocks opioids from binding to their receptors and thereby prevents their euphoric and other effects.
- The de-addiction treatment with naltrexone should ideally begin in a residential setting in order to prevent withdrawal symptoms. But, it can be prescribed in outpatient medical settings also.
- Before initiation of therapy, the patient should be opioid free for at least 7–10 days. The therapy is started orally with 25 mg initially under supervision, then 50 mg daily till the patient stabilizes and then, 100 mg three times a week.
- Recently, a long-acting injectable version of naltrexone has been approved to treat opioid addiction. It only needs to be delivered once a month to improve compliance.

Tramadol

- Tramadol is a synthetic opioid agonist.
- It prevents and reduces the craving and withdrawal symptoms in opioid-addicted individuals.
- It is a type of substitution therapy.
- Initially, it is given in a dose of 50 mg BD, then 50 mg TDS, then tapering to 50 mg BD and 50 mg OD for a few days. Then, it is withdrawn in a tapering fashion.

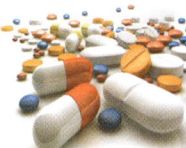

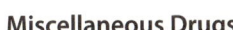

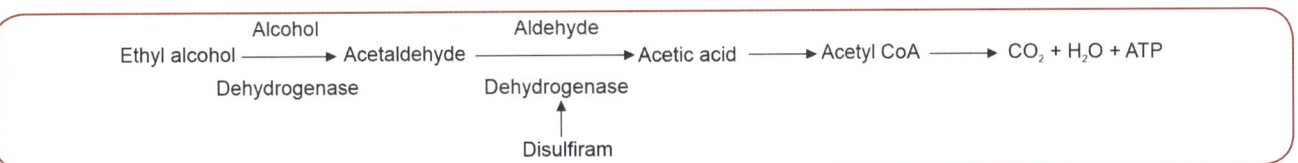

FIG. 7.1: Mechanism of action of Disulfiram.

Ethyl alcohol → Acetaldehyde (Alcohol Dehydrogenase) → Acetic acid (Aldehyde Dehydrogenase) → Acetyl CoA → $CO_2 + H_2O + ATP$. Disulfiram acts on Aldehyde Dehydrogenase.

Tobacco De-addiction Drugs

Nicotine Replacement Therapy (NRT)

A variety of formulations of nicotine replacement therapies (NRTs) now exist, including the transdermal nicotine patch, nicotine spray, nicotine gum, and nicotine lozenges. Because nicotine is the main addictive ingredient in tobacco, the rationale for NRT lies in providing the stable low levels of nicotine to prevent withdrawal symptoms. It helps to keep people motivated to quit. *Research shows that combining the patch with another replacement therapy is more effective than the single therapy alone.*

Bupropion

- It is an antidepressant drug.
- It produces mild stimulant effects by blocking the reuptake of certain neurotransmitters, especially norepinephrine and dopamine.
- It is quite effective in suppressing tobacco craving, helping them quit smoking without weight gain.
- It is given orally in a dose of 150 mg OD for three days, then 150 mg BD for at least 7 weeks.

Varenicline

- It is the most recently FDA-approved medication for smoking cessation.
- It acts on a subset of nicotinic receptors in the brain thought to be involved in the rewarding effects of nicotine.
- It also blocks the ability of nicotine to activate dopamine, interfering with the reinforcing effects of smoking, thereby reducing cravings and supporting abstinence from smoking.
- This is given initially 0.5 mg once daily for one week, then 1 mg BD for 6 months.

Each of the above pharmacotherapy is recommended for use in combination with behavioral interventions, including group and individual therapies, as well as telephone quitlines.

Alcohol De-addiction Drugs

Naltrexone

- It blocks opioid receptors that are involved in the rewarding effects of drinking and the craving for alcohol.
- It has been shown to reduce relapses.

- It is given three times a week in a dose of 100–150 mg or 50 mg OD or in the form of depot injection on monthly basis.

Acamprosate

- It acts on the gamma-aminobutyric acid (GABA) and glutamate neurotransmitter systems and is thought to reduce symptoms of protracted withdrawal, such as insomnia, anxiety, restlessness, and dysphoria.
- It is given for maintenance therapy of alcohol abstinence.
- It is given in a dose of 666 mg two to three times in a day.
- It can be given for several weeks to months, and it may be more effective in patients with severe dependence.

Disulfiram (Aversion Therapy)

- It interferes with degradation of alcohol by inhibiting aldehyde dehydrogenase enzyme which is required for metabolism of alcohol as given in Figure 7.1.
- This results in accumulation of acetaldehyde which, in turn, produces a very unpleasant reaction, known as *aldehyde syndrome*. This reaction may be seen in mild to severe form depending upon the amount of alcohol consumed during disulfiram therapy. Patients with this reaction may need to be hospitalized in case of severe reactions. Therefore, this drug is always given under supervision to well-motivated patients after counseling.
- It is given in a dose of 500 mg/day for a week, followed by 250 mg daily.
- Another regimen is 1000 mg on 1st day, 750 mg on 2nd day, 500 mg on 3rd day and 250 mg subsequently.
- Sensitization to alcohol develops after 2–3 hours of 1st dose and lasts for several days after stopping the drug.

Topiramate

- It can be used for the treatment of alcohol dependence on OPD basis.
- It modulates the gamma aminobutyric acid (GABA) adrenergic transmission in the central amygdala, a brain center implicated in the regulation of emotions and alcohol intake.
- It is given in a dose of 150–300 mg/day.

CARDIOPULMONARY RESUSCITATION

Cardiopulmonary resuscitation (CPR) is a technique of basic life support (BLS) for the purpose to restore the normal cardiopulmonary function.

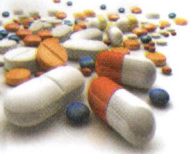

CPR is an emergency procedure that combines chest compression often with artificial ventilation in a manual effort to preserve oxygenation to the heart, lungs and brain until further measures are taken to restore spontaneous blood circulation and breathing in a person who is in cardiac arrest.

Resuscitation is a continuous process from basic life support (BLS) to advance cardiac life support (ACLS). Cerebral resuscitation is the most important goal of advanced cardiac life support. BLS initiates the process of resuscitation and ACLS restores and maintains the spontaneous respiration and circulation.

History of CPR
- 5000 BC: First artificial mouth-to-mouth respiration.
- 3000 BCL: Ventilation.
- 1780: First attempt of newborn resuscitation by blowing.
- 874: First experimental cardiac massages.
- 1901: First successful direct cardiac massage in man.
- 1946: First experimental indirect cardiac massage and defibrillation.
- 1960: Indirect cardiac massage.
- 1980: Development of cardiopulmonary resuscitation due to works of Peter Safar.

Stages of Resuscitation (ABCDE)

- **Airway:** Ensure open airway by preventing the falling back of tongue and tracheal intubation, if possible.
- **Breathing:** Start artificial ventilation of lung by either mouth to mouth or mouth to nose technique.
- **Circulation:** By external cardiac massage or manual heart compression.
- **Drugs and defibrillation:** By use of different medications or electric defibrillation in case of ventricular fibrillation.
- **Establish the components of advanced life support**
- **Establish oxygen administration to correct hypoxia**
- **Establish an IV line to administer drugs**
- **Electrocardiogram (ECG) monitoring**
- **Endotracheal intubation**, if required.

According to the latest CPR guidelines, 2015 by American Heart Association, the sequence employed for CPR is C-A-B, i.e., first perform chest compression to maintain circulation, followed by airway patency checking followed by breathing by either mouth to mouth or mouth to nose technique.

Drugs Used in CPR

It is based upon the underlying cause of cardiac arrest and other associated conditions.

The main drugs used in CPR and post resuscitation are as follows:

Adrenaline

Route and Dose	Indications	Actions
1 mg IV* OR 2–5 mg IV* via ETT (Intracardiac injection is strictly contraindicated now)	Any pulseless rhythm	Increases perfusion to myocardium and to brain by increasing peripheral vascular resistance

*Every 3–5 minutes.

Nor Adrenaline

Route and Dose	Indications	Actions
2–4 µg/min IV infusion*	Hypotension	Vasopressor (predominately an α-agonist)

*To be titrated to effect

Atropine

Route and Dose	Indications	Actions
1.0 mg IV push q 5 minutes, to maximum of 3 mg*	Bradycardia, asystole	Parasympatholytic, eliminates vagal tone

*May be repeated if required.

Dopamine and Dobutamine

Route and Dose	Indications	Actions
2–20 µg/kg/min*	Hypotension	Inotropic agent (β-agonist)

*Low doses are predominantly β; high doses become predominantly α action.

Soda Bicarbonate

Route and Dose	Indications	Actions
50 mEq in the IV fluid*	Metabolic acidosis	Corrects metabolic acidosis

*To be titrated with the pH.

Esmolol

Route and Dose	Indications	Actions
0.5 mg/kg bolus over 1 minute followed by 0.05–0.02 mg/kg/min*	Supraventricular tachycardia, atrial fibrillation or flutter	Reduce heart rate, blood pressure and arrhythmia β-blocker (short acting)

*May be given as another bolus if desired effect not achieved; start drip 50 µg/kg/minutes.

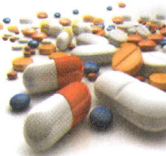

Metoprolol

Route and Dose	Indications	Actions
5 mg IV* push	Supraventricular tachycardia, myocardial infarction	β-Blocker (β1 selective)

*Repeat twice at 5 minutes intervals, then give 50-mg oral load.

Lignocaine

Route and Dose	Indications	Actions
1.0–1.5 mg/kg IV* push	Ventricular fibrillation, pulseless ventricular tachycardia, ventricular tachycardia with a pulse	Class IB antiarrhythmic; suppresses ventricular activity and electrical conduction

*Second and subsequent doses of 0.75 mg/kg every 5 minutes to a total dose of 3 mg/kg.

Procainamide

Route and Dose	Indications	Actions
17 mg/kg IV slow bolus at maximum rate of 50 mg/min*	Ventricular tachycardia with a pulse	Decreases myocardial excitability and conduction velocity

*Continue infusion (4 mg/min) until QRS widening >50%, dysrhythmia terminated, onset of hypotension; or 17 mg/kg infused.

Vasopressin

Route and Dose	Indications	Actions
40 units IV*	Ventricular fibrillation, pulseless ventricular tachycardia	Increases peripheral vascular resistance

*Single dose, may be followed at 10 minutes by epinephrine.

Adenosine

Route and Dose	Indications	Actions
6 mg rapid IV* push through proximal peripheral line; central line dose is one-half	Supraventricular tachycardia	Endogenous nucleoside causing brief asystole allowing dominant pacemaker to resume function

*If needed, second dose of 12 mg (pediatric, double initial dose up to 12 mg); third dose of 12–18 mg.

Amiodarone

Route and Dose	Indications	Actions
For ventricular fibrillation or pulseless ventricular tachycardia: 300 mg IV* push	Ventricular fibrillation, pulseless ventricular tachycardia, ventricular tachycardia with a pulse, Supraventricular tachycardia	Predominately class III antiarrhythmic, but has sodium, potassium channel, and α and β receptor blockade

*May use second dose of 150 mg for recurrent ventricular fibrillation/ventricular tachycardia. In children may be repeated in 5 mg/kg.

Magnesium

Route and Dose	Indications	Actions
1–2 g IV* slow push	Torsade de pointes, known hypomagnesemia	Can cause cutaneous flush, apnea, and hyperreflexia, if given too quickly

*Single dose.

DRUGS REQUIRED FOR THE MANAGEMENT OF VARIOUS EMERGENCIES

- The requirement of drugs differs for various emergencies. As the treatment and handling of the emergency depends upon the cause and extent of the problem, the organ systems involved and the facilities available at the place of treatment.
- Most of the above mentioned drugs are helpful in managing emergencies.
- In addition to above mentioned drugs, here is a list of some important drugs which prove to be helpful in managing emergencies.
- Inj. hydrocortisone, Inj. dexamethasone, Inj. methylprednisolone sodium succinate, Inj. CPM, Inj. Frusemide, Inj. deriphylline, Inj. KCl, Inj. calcium gluconate, 25% dextrose, IV fluids (normal saline, dextrose and sodium chloride solution, ringa's lactate dextrose 5%,), Inj. diazepam, Inj. phenytoin sodium, Inj. ranitidine or pantoprazole.

The dosages of these drugs have been given in respective chapters.

VITAMINS AND MINERALS

Vitamins are organic substances that are essential for carrying out the normal biochemical processes and physiological functions of body. These are non-energy compounds and required in very small quantities. The vitamins generally serve as cofactors for the enzymes required in intermediary metabolism.

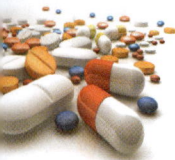
The main source of vitamins is diet. A balanced diet supplies adequate amounts of vitamins to fulfill the daily requirements. Humans cannot synthesize vitamins in the body except some vitamins such as Vitamin D in skin, and nicotinamide from tryptophan.

Lack of particular vitamin leads to specific deficiency syndromes. Vitamin deficiencies occur due to inadequate intake, malabsorption, increased tissue needs, increased excretion, certain genetic abnormalities and drug-vitamin interactions.

There are numerous single and multivitamin preparations, which one may have to take when the daily requirement is not fulfilled from the diet alone. The vitamins may have to be supplemented for prophylactic as well as for therapeutic purpose.

The vitamins have been broadly divided into two groups:
- **Fat-soluble vitamins:** Vitamins A, D, E and K. These vitamins are stored by the body, mainly in the liver. Excessive intake of these can lead to toxicity due to accumulation, known as hypervitaminosis.
- **Water-soluble vitamins:** Vitamin B complex group and vit. C. These vitamins are least stored and toxicity does not occur. The excess of vitamins is rapidly metabolized and readily excreted in the urine.

Vitamers

The different chemical forms and precursors of a vitamin are known as *Vitamers* of that particular vitamin. These vitamers have generally similar molecular structure and show vitamin-activity in a vitamin deficient biological system. All vitamers may not possess equal vitamin potency.

Examples of vitamers include **cyanocobalamin, hydroxy-cobalamin, methylcobalamin and 5-deoxyadenosylcobalamin which are all vitamers of Vitamin B_{12} and all possess B_{12} activity. Similarly, both niacinamide and nicotinic acid are vitamers of Vitamin B_3 (Niacin).**

These vitamins need to be activated to their active forms in the body for their actions. The active forms of some of the vitamins are given in Table 7.1.

TABLE 7.1: Active forms of various vitamins

Vitamins	Active forms
Vitamin A	Retinal (stored as retinol)
Vitamin D	1,25 dihydrocholecalciferol
Vitamin E	α-tocopherol
Vitamin K	Napthaquinone
Vitamin C	L-ascorbic acid
Vitamin B1 (Thiamine)	Thiamine pyrophosphate

Contd...

Vitamins	Active forms
Vitamin B2 (riboflavin)	Flavin-mononucleotide (FMN)
Vitamin B3 (niacin)	Nicotinamide adenine dinucleotide (NAD)
Vitamin B5 (pantothenic acid)	Coenzyme-A
Vitamin B6 (pyridoxine)	Pyridoxal phosphate
Vitamin B9 (folic acid)	Tetrahydrofolate
Vitamin B12 (cynocobalamin)	5-methyl cobalamin

Fat Soluble Vitamins

Vitamin-A

There are various natural forms of Vitamin A (vitamers) such as Retinol (Vitamin A_1), Dehydroretinol (Vitamin A_2) and carotenoids.

Dietary Sources

Carrot (richest plant source), red cabbage, turnip, spinach, mango, etc., are some of the plant sources. Marine fish liver oil such as cod, halibut (richest animal source), fresh water fish, egg yolk, milk, cheese, butter are some of the animal sources.

Physiological Functions

- Essential for proper functioning of *Rod cells* in the visual cycle; hence the night vision (Fig. 7.2). Vision in the dim light depends upon proper functioning of *rods*. Prevents night blindness and Xerophthalmia.
- Maintenance of normal epithelium all over body.
- As antioxidants (*Vitamins A, C, E are more potent antioxidants in nature*) and anti-cancer properties.
- Enhances immune functions and prevents recurrent infections like measles, malaria and diarrhea, etc.
- In reproduction, for normal spermatogenesis and fetal development.
- Bone growth in children.

Deficiency Symptoms

These are seen when there is a long term deprivation and the stores are depleted. A disturbance in the physiological roles manifests as the deficiency symptoms.

Some of the symptoms are:
- **Eye:** Xerosis (dryness) of eye, 'Bitot's spots', keratomalacia (softening of cornea), corneal opacities, night blindness (nyctalopia) progressing to total blindness.
- **Epithelium:** Dry and rough skin with papules (phrynoderma), hyperkeratinization, atrophy of sweat glands, keratinization of bronchopulmonary epithelium. Increased tendency to urinary stone formation due to shedding of ureteric epithelial lining which acts as a nidus.

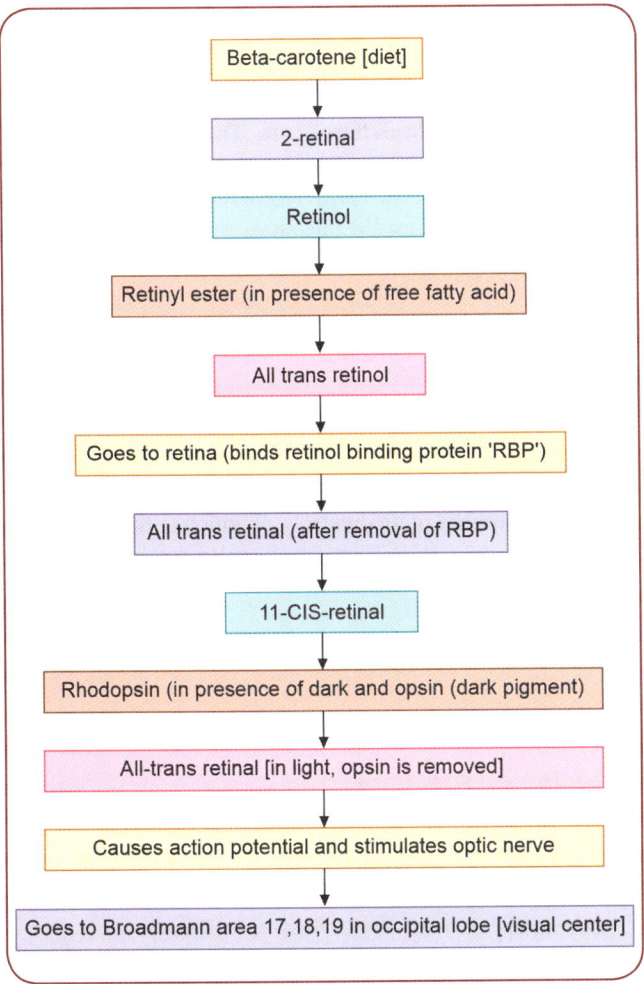

FIG. 7.2: Action of retinal in night vision

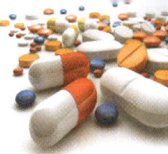

commonly seen are nausea, vomiting, headache (due to increased intracranial tension and also known as Pseudotumor-cerebri), itching, erythema, dermatitis, exfoliation, hair loss, bone and joint pains, loss of appetite, irritability, etc. Daily intake should not exceed 20,000 IU.

Vitamin-A has been included in National Immunization Program of India.
- A total 17-lac unit of vitamin-A is supplemented to child.
- A total of 9 mega doses are to be given from 9 months of age to 5 years.
- 100,000 IU at 9 months with measles immunization,
- 200,000 IU at 16-18 months with DPT booster,
- 200,000 IU every 6 months upto the age of 5 years.

Vitamin D

Vitamin D is the collective name given to antirachitic substances found in foods and synthesized in the body and activated by UV radiation.

- **D1:** Mixture of antirachitic substances found in food—only of historic interest.
- **D2:** Ergocalciferol or calciferol is made by ultraviolet irradiation, e.g., ergosterol in plants and also present in irradiated foods such as yeasts, fungi, bread, milk, etc.
- **D3:** Cholecalciferol synthesized in the skin under the influence of UV rays.

Vitamin D2 and D3 undergo two successive hydroxylations—first in the liver to form 25-hydroxy cholecalciferol and second in the proximal tubules of the kidney to form 1,25-dihydroxy cholecalciferol which is the most physiologically active form of the Vitamin D, i.e., *calcitriol* (Fig. 7.3).

- **Immunity:** Increased susceptibility to infection such as diarrhea, measles, etc.
- **Reproduction:** Sterility due to faulty spermatogenesis, abortions, fetal malformations and growth retardation, etc.

Recommended Dietary Allowance (RDA)

- **Daily requirement and for prophylaxis of Vitamin A deficiency** (during infancy, pregnancy, lactation, hepatobiliary diseases, steatorrhea): 3000–5000 IU/day.
- **Treatment of established Vitamin A deficiency:** 50,000–100,000 IU IM or orally for 1–3 days followed by intermittent supplemental doses.
- **Skin diseases like acne, psoriasis, ichthyosis:** Retinoic acid and 2nd or 3rd generation retinoids are used.

Hypervitaminosis-A

It can occur due to regular intake of excessive vit-A >100,000 IU/day for more than three weeks. The toxicity symptoms

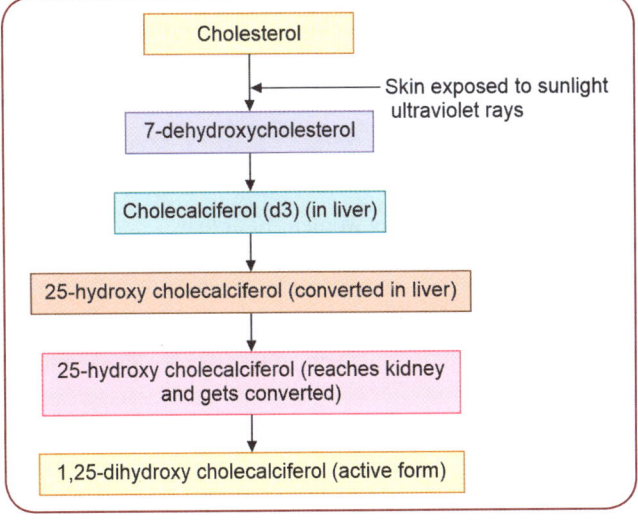

FIG. 7.3: Formation of active form of Vitamin D in liver

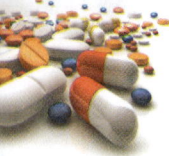

Dietary Sources

Halibut liver oil (richest source), codfish liver oil, other animal's liver oil and synthesis in body as explained above.

Physiological Functions

- Vitamin D increases absorption of calcium and phosphates from GIT and tubular reabsorption from renal tubules.
- It increases both serum, calcium and calcitonin levels.
- It increases the bone mineralization and thus, bone-mineral-density (BMD) (deficiency leads to rickets in children and osteomalacia in adults).
- Some other important actions such as actions of calcitriol on immunological cells, lymphokine production, proliferation and differentiation of epidermal and certain malignant cells, neuronal and skeletal muscle function have also been demonstrated recently.

Deficiency Symptoms

Deficiency may occur in cases of malnutrition, poor sun exposure, intestinal malabsorption, chronic liver disease and chronic renal failure cases. Manifestations may be in the form of:

- Rickets in children which may present in the form of various bony deformities such as bow legs, bossing of skull, chest deformities, etc.
- Osteomalacia in adults which may present in the form of bone tenderness and decreased BMD and predisposition to fractures.

Recommended Dietary Allowance (RDA)

- Prophylactic dose is 400 IU/day and
- Therapeutic dose of nutritional Vitamin D deficiency is 3000–4000 IU/day. This is given to prevent and treat rickets in children and osteomalacia in adults.
- 300,000–600,000 IU can be given orally or IM once in 2–6 months.
- Recommended Daily Allowance if Sun exposure is adequate:
  - Children: 5 µg/day,
  - Adult: 2.5 µg/day,
  - Pregnant/Lactating women: 10 µg/day
  1 µg of cholecalciferol = 40 IU of Vitamin D.

Hypervitaminosis-D

It can occur due to chronic take of large doses approximately 50,000 IU/day.

Manifestations are hypercalcemia, weakness, fatigue, vomiting, diarrhea, sluggishness, polyuria, albuminuria, ectopic Ca^{2+} deposition in soft tissues, blood vessels, parenchymal organs (calcinosis), renal stones or nephrocalcinosis, hypertension, growth retardation in children.

Vitamin D Preparations

Supplementation is required in many cases. A few preparation of Vitamin D are as follows:

- **Calciferol (Ergocalciferol, vit. D2):** Filled in gelatin capsules 25,000 and 50,000 IU caps.
- **Cholecalciferol (vit. D3):** As granules for oral ingestion and oily solution for IM injection.
- **Calcitriol:** 0.25–1 µg orally daily or on alternate days
- **Alfacalcidol:** It is 1 α-OH D3—a prodrug that is rapidly hydroxylated in the liver to the active form of Vitamin D, i.e., 1,25 (OH)$_2$ D3 or calcitriol. Available in capsule form.
- **Calcipotriol** is a preparation for local use and useful in the treatment of psoriasis.

Vitamin E

There are a number of tocopherols, of which α-tocopherol has the most potent Vitamin E activity. It is also the most abundant form of Vitamin E.

Dietary Sources

Wheat germ oil is the richest source, others are cereals, nuts, spinach and egg yolk.

Physiological Functions

- It is the most powerful antioxidant.
- It protects the unsaturated lipids in cell membranes from free radical oxidation damage. Also protects oxidation of coenzyme Q.
- It plays an important role in preventing the risk of myocardial infarction, Alzheimer's disease, etc.
- It is a lipotropic and has some role in reducing the low density lipoproteins (LDL)-cholesterol levels.
- It stabilizes RBC membrane and also enhances the use of Vitamin A.

Deficiency Symptoms

Deficiency of this vitamin may lead to hemolytic anemia, retinopathy, skeleton myopathy and peripheral neuropathy with spinocerebellar degeneration.

Recommended Dietary Allowance (RDA)

The estimated daily requirement of Vitamin E is 10 mg.
1 mg of α-tocopherol = 1.49 IU of Vitamin E.
Some conditions where Vitamin E is useful are:
- **G-6-PD deficiency:** 100 mg/day
- **In Retrolental fibroplasia,** in premature infants exposed to high oxygen concentrations can be reduced by 100 mg/kg/day oral vitamin E.
- **Acanthocytosis:** 100 mg /week IM.
- **Fibrocystic breast disease, nocturnal muscle cramps and intermittent claudications:** 400–600 mg/day.

Hypervitaminosis-E

No toxicity has been reported even with large doses of vit-E for long periods.

Some side effects are abdominal cramps, loose motions and lethargy.

Vitamin K

- Vitamin K (koagulation vitamin) is essential for the coagulation process. It is not directly involved in the clotting process but required for the synthesis of four clotting factors in the liver cell: Factor II, VII, IX and X. It occurs naturally in two forms: Phylloquinone (K_1) from plant source and menaquinone (K_2) which is synthesized by colonic bacteria (*E. coli*) in the colon.
- K_3 is the synthetic form and is available as Fat-soluble forms (Menadione, Acetomenaphthone) and water-soluble forms (Menadione sod. Bisulfate and Menadione sod. Diphosphate).

Dietary Sources

Green leafy vegetables such as cabbage, spinach and liver, cheese, cereals, nuts, and egg yolk, etc. Wheat germ oil is the richest source.

Physiological Functions

Vitamin K is essential for formation of clotting factor-II, VII, IX, X, protein-C and S.

Deficiency Symptoms

- Vitamin K is only temporarily concentrated in liver and this store can be exhausted within one week.
- The deficiency of Vitamin K occurs due to liver disease, obstructive jaundice, malabsorption, long-term antimicrobial therapy which alters intestinal flora.
- The most important manifestation is bleeding tendency due to lowering of the levels of prothrombin and other clotting factors in blood. Hematuria is usually first to occur; other common sites of bleeding are gastrointestinal tract, nose and under the skin where it presents in the form of hemorrhagic spots.

Recommended Dietary Allowance (RDA)

- Normal adult requirement is 50–100 µg/day.
- As it can be synthesized in the colon, even 3–10 µg/day may be sufficient.

Some conditions where Vit-K is useful are:

- **For prevention of hemorrhagic disease of the newborn:** All newborns especially premature infants have low levels of prothrombin and other clotting factors. Vitamin K 1 mg IM soon after birth has been recommended routinely.
- Alternatively, 5–10 mg IM to the mother 4–12 hours before delivery can be given. Hemorrhagic disease of the newborn can be effectively prevented/treated by such medication.
- Menadione (K3) should not be used for this purpose as patients with G-6-PD deficiency and neonates are especially susceptible. In the newborn menadione or its salts can precipitate kernicterus.
- As an antidote in overdose of oral anticoagulants.
- In patients suffering from liver disease (cirrhosis, viral hepatitis).
- Patients on prolonged antimicrobial therapy.
- Patients with obstructive jaundice or malabsorption syndromes (sprue, regional ileitis, steatorrhoea, etc). The therapy given is Vit-K 10 mg i.m./day, or orally along with bile salts for better absorption.

Hypervitaminosis-K

- It has not been reported.
- Only severe allergic or anaphylactoid reactions can occur with IV injection of Vitamin K formulations.

Water-Soluble Vitamins

B Complex Group of Vitamins

- The vitamins of this group all generally found together in the food; hence are collectively termed as vitamin B-complex. Most of these are found in both vegetarian and non-vegetarian sources except Vitamin B_{12}, which is not found in vegetable sources, but is found only in various non-vegetarian sources.
- The B-complex vitamins have been divided conventionally into three subgroups according to the major functions in which they are involved.
- These are:
  - Energy forming B-complex vitamins: Vitamin B1, B2, B3, B5, B6, B7 (Biotin)
  - Hematopoietic B-complex vitamins: Folic acid (vitamin B9), B12
  - Non B complex group: Vitamin C or ascorbic acid.

Thiamin or Vitamin B₁ or Aneurine

Dietary sources: Cereals, pulses, nuts, green vegetables, yeasts, egg and meat. It is found in the outer layers of the cereals and is heat labile.

Physiological functions

- Its active form thiamin pyrophosphate acts as a coenzyme in the carbohydrate metabolism.
- It also plays some role in nerve conduction.

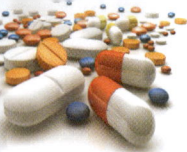

TABLE 7.2: Differences between dry and wet beriberi

Dry Beriberi	Wet Beriberi
• Mostly involves peripheral nervous system. • The common signs and symptoms are: peripheral neuropathy, muscles atrophy, muscles weakness, wrist and foot drop (due to involvement of radial and deep peroneal nerve respectively)	• Mostly involves cardiovascular system. • The common signs and symptoms are: tachycardia, edema, cardiomegaly, high output cardiac failure.

Deficiency symptoms

Deficiency is mainly dietary in nature. In addition, raw fish, shellfish, coffee and tea inhibit the absorption of vitamin B_1. Some common manifestations are:

- **Beriberi** (acute manifestation of B_1 deficiency) (Table 7.2) The treatment involves IV/IM injection of vitamin-B_1 given in a dose of 2–10 mg OD, till the symptomatic improvement occurs. Then treatment is given orally.
- **Infantile beriberi:** In this condition, newborn of vitamin B1 deficient mother presents with signs and symptoms of BeriBeri.
  To manage this condition, prophylactically 2–10 mg/day vitamin B_1 is supplemented to pregnant mother or infants.
- **Wernick's encephalopathy:** It is most commonly seen in severe alcoholic individuals. Patient presents with global confusion, opthalmoplegia and cerebral ataxia and these features combined with psychosis are called Koraskoff's psychosis.
  To prevent this condition thiamine is given in a dose of 100 mg/day intravenously.

Transketolase (product of HMP shunt) test is done to detect vitamin-B1 deficiency.

Recommended dietary allowance (RDA): 1–2 mg/day.

Therapeutic uses

- **Prophylactically:** 2–10 mg daily is given in infants, pregnant women, chronic diarrhea and patients on parenteral alimentation.
- **Beriberi:** 100 mg/day IM or IV till symptoms regress. After it, maintenance doses are given orally.
- **Acute alcoholic intoxication:** Thiamine 100 mg is added to each vac of glucose solution infused. In Korsakoff's psychosis, 100 mg/day is given parenterally.
- **In neurological disorders.**

Adverse effects

Thiamine is non-toxic. Sometimes, hypersensitivity reactions can occur on parenteral injection.

Riboflavin or Vitamin-B$_2$

- **Dietary sources:** Dairy milk products, liver, meats, egg, cereals, pulses, yeast, green vegetables and sprouts, etc.
- **Physiological functions:** Its active form acts as coenzyme in the oxidation-reduction reactions and carbohydrate metabolism.

Deficiency symptoms

Ariboflavinosis: The deficiency of vitamin-B_2 usually presents with angular stomatitis, cheilosis, seborrheic dermatitis and geographical ulcer on tongue.

- **Recommended dietary allowance (RDA):** 1–2 mg/day.
- **For therapeutic purpose in ariboflavinosis:** Riboflavin is given in a dose of 2–20 mg/day oral or parenteral till the symptoms subside.

Niacin or Vitamin-B$_3$

Dietary sources

Liver, meats, egg, fish, cereals, wholegrains, nuts, etc.

Physiological functions

Nicotinic acid is readily converted to its amide which is a component of the coenzyme Nicotinamide-adenine-dinucleotide (NAD) and its phosphate form (NADP) involved in oxidation-reduction reactions involved in cellular respiration, glycolysis and fatty acid oxidation.

Nicotinic acid is also a lipid-lowering agent.

Deficiency symptoms

- **Pellagra:** A deficiency of Niacin may present with **4 Ds: diarrhea, dermatitis, dementia and death**. Along with these features, anemia and hypoproteinemia are also seen. These features are commonly seen in malnourished and alcoholic individuals.
  To treat this condition, niacin is given twice daily in a dose of 200–500 mg orally.
- **Hartnup's disease:** Another deficiency of Niacin, particularly by tryptophan, which is a precursor of niacin formation. Supplementation of niacin is curative.

Recommended dietary allowance (RDA)

15–20 mg/day.

Therapeutic uses

- **Pellagra treatment:** Niacin is given twice daily in a dose of 200–500 mg orally.

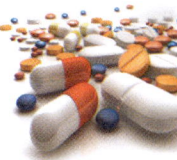

- **Dyslipidemia:** Nicotinic acid also used for managing dyslipidemia in a dose of 250 mg BD to 2.0 g/day in sustained release form or three divided doses.
- **Hartnup's disease:** In which tryptophan transport is impaired, need niacin supplementation.

Pantothenic Acid or Vitamin B$_5$

- **Dietary sources:** Liver, meats, egg yolk, fish, cereals, wholegrain, nuts, vegetables, etc.
- **Physiological functions:** It is a component of coenzyme-A which functions in carbohydrate, fat, steroid and porphyrin metabolism.

Deficiency symptoms

- It has been thought to be one of the causing factor of leg cramps, paraesthesia and flatulence.
- **Burning Foot Syndrome (Nutritional megalalia)** may occur due to deficiency of pantothenic acid and seen in individuals expose to heavy antibiotic therapy or colonic resection or severe malnutrition.

Recommended dietary allowance (RDA)

2–7 mg/day.

Therapeutic uses

- For the treatment of burning foot syndrome, 50–100 mg/day is given.
- Sometimes it is used to treat post-operative paralytic ileus.

Pyridoxine or Vitamin B$_6$

Pyridoxine, pyriodoxal and *pyridoxamine* are related naturally occurring pyridine compounds that have vitamin B$_6$ activity and are vitamers of vitamin B$_6$.

Dietary sources

Widely distributed in the food products of plant and animal origin such as vegetables, soybean, wholegrain, eggs, liver, meat, etc.

Physiological functions

Pyridoxine is converted to its coenzyme form, i.e., pyridoxal phosphate. Pyridoxal phosphate dependent enzymes (*transaminases, hydroxylases and decarboxylases*) are involved in synthesis of non-essential amino acids, GABA and aminolevulinic acid (first step in the synthesis of heme).

Deficiency symptoms

- **Peripheral neuropathy:** Presents with tingling sensations of lower limbs. Isoniazid and oral contraceptive pills produce a pyridoxine deficiency state.

- **Sideroblastic anemia:** Can be treated by administration of 50–200 mg/day pyridoxine phosphate.
- Seborrheic dermatitis, glossitis, growth retardation, premenstrual tension, mental confusion, lowered seizure threshold and convulsions.

Recommended dietary allowance (RDA)

0.8 mg/1000 kcal (2 mg/day).

Therapeutic uses

- **Prophylactically in alcoholics, infants and patients with deficiency of other B complex vitamins:** 2–5 mg daily.
- **To prevent and treat isoniazid, hydralazine and cycloserine induced neurological disturbances:** 10–100 mg/day.
- **To treat mental symptoms in women on oral contraceptives:** 50 mg daily.
- **Pyridoxine responsive anemia may be benefited by large doses of pyridoxine:** 50–200 mg/day.

Biotin or Vitamin B$_7$ or Vitamin H

Biotin is a sulfur containing organic acid found in many food items. Some intestinal bacteria synthesize biotin which is also absorbed. Its deficiency can be caused by eating raw egg white for months to years. Egg white contains a protein named "Avidin" which binds biotin strongly and prevents its absorption.

Dietary sources

Liver, egg yolk, meat, nuts are the other source.

Physiological functions

Biotin is a coenzyme for five carboxylases in the body and is essential for amino acid catabolism, gluconeogenesis and fatty acid metabolism. It is also essential for gene stability because it is covalently attached to histones.

Deficiency symptoms

Deficiency can occur due to regular raw egg white intake, colonic resection or severe malnutrition or heavy exposure to antibiotics. Symptoms are: Anorexia, glossitis, seborrheic dermatitis, alopecia, fatigue and muscular pain.

Recommended dietary allowance (RDA)

0.2 mg/day. Therapeutic dose in case of deficiency symptoms is 10–20 mg/day.

Folic acid or Vitamin B$_9$

In 1941, Mitchell isolated an antianemia principle from spinach and called it 'folic acid' (from leaf). Folic acid is present in the

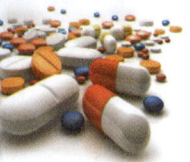

food as polyglutamates. Each folic acid molecule may have 2–8 molecules of glutamic acid. The additional glutamate residues are split off primarily in the upper intestine before absorption.

Dietary sources

Green leafy vegetables (spinach), liver, egg, meat, milk. It is also synthesized by gut flora, but this is largely unavailable for absorption.

Physiological functions

Folic acid is inactive as such and is reduced to the coenzyme form in two steps:

FRase DHFRase
FA ⟹ DHFA ⟹ THFA
FA: folic acid, DHFA: dihydrofolic acid, THFA: tetrahydrofolic acid
Frase; folic acid reductase, DHFRase: dihydrofolic acid reductase.

- FA is converted to DHFA by folate reductase (FRase) and then to THFA by dihydrofolate reductase (DHFRase).
- THFA mediates a number of one carbon transfer reactions which are essential in the synthesis of purines and pyrimidines. These purines and pyrimidines are essential in DNA synthesis.

Deficiency symptoms

These can occur due to dietary deficiency, malabsorption syndrome, excessive demand, liver diseases or drug induced.
The manifestations are:
- Megaloblastic anemia
- **Neural tube defects:** Neural tube defects, including spina bifida in the offspring, due to maternal folate deficiency. This can be prevented by administration of folic acid started 3 months before conception till first trimester followed by iron with calcium.
- **Epithelial damage:** Glossitis, enteritis, diarrhea, steatorrhea, etc.
- General debility, weight loss, sterility.

Recommended dietary allowance (RDA)

2–5 mg/day, prophylactic 0.5 mg/day.

Therapeutic uses

- Megaloblastic anemias, Nutritional folate deficiency,
- **Increased demand:** Pregnancy, lactation, infancy, during treatment of severe iron deficiency anemia, hemolytic anemias.
- Pernicious anemia.
- **Malabsorption syndromes:** Tropical sprue, coeliac disease, idiopathic steatorrhea, etc.

- **Antiepileptic therapy:** Patients on prolonged phenytoin/phenobarbitone therapy
- **Prophylactic of folate deficiency:** During pregnancy to prevent neural tube defects in fetus.

Vitamin B$_{12}$

Cyanocobalamin and hydroxocobalamin are complex cobalt containing compounds present in the diet and referred to as vitamin B$_{12}$.

Dietary sources

Richest source is liver, which contains large deposit of vitamin-B$_{12}$ and that is sufficient for 2–5 years. Other sources are kidney, sea fish, egg yolk, meat, cheese. The only vegetable source is legumes (pulses) which get it from microorganisms harbored in their root nodules. Vitamin B$_{12}$ is synthesized by the colonic microflora, but this is not available for absorption in man. The commercial source is *Streptomyces griseus*.
Animal food product contain higher amount of Cyanocobalamin than plant products.

Physiological functions

- Vitamin B$_{12}$ is intricately linked with folate metabolism.
- The active coenzyme forms of B$_{12}$ generated in the body are *deoxy-adenosyl-cobalamin* (DAB$_{12}$) and *methyl-cobalamin* (methyl B$_{12}$).
- It links the carbohydrate and lipid metabolisms.
- It is needed in the synthesis of phospholipids and myelin sheath.
- Vit-B$_{12}$ is essential for cell growth and multiplication.

Deficiency symptoms

Vitamin B$_{12}$ deficiency may occur due to strict vegetarian diet, pernicious anemia, severe malabsorption, surgical resection of terminal ileum or stomach.
Deficiencies of vitamin B$_{12}$ manifest as:
- Megaloblastic anemia.
- Subacute combined degeneration of spinal cord (SACD).
- Peripheral neuritis which usually presents with loss of fine touch, vibration and proprioception, paresthesias and depressed stretch reflexes. If these features are present with psychosis, it is called *megaloblastic madness*. To prevent this condition administer 1000 µgm vitamin B$_{12}$ weekly for 8 weeks.
- Glossitis, gastrointestinal (GI) disturbances and damage to epithelial structures.

Recommended dietary allowance (RDA)

Adult: 1–3 µg/day, pregnancy and lactation 3–5 µg/day.

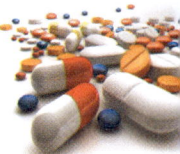

Oral vitamin B12 is not dependable for treatment of confirmed vit B12 deficiency because its absorption from the intestine is unreliable.

Injected vitamin B12 is a must when deficiency is due to lack of intrinsic factor (pernicious anemia, other gastric causes), since the absorptive mechanism is totally non-functional.

Various regimens are in use:

- In Britain—*hydroxocobalamin* 1 mg IM/SC daily for 2 weeks or till neurological symptoms subside, followed by 1 mg injected every 2 months for maintenance.
- In USA—*cyanocobalamin* 100 μg IM/SC daily for 1 week, then weekly for 1 month, and then monthly for maintenance indefinitely.
- *Methylcobalamin* (methyl B12) is the active coenzyme form of vitamin B12 for synthesis of methionine and S-adenosyl methionine that is needed for integrity of myelin. This preparation of vitamin B12 in a dose of 1.5 mg/day has been especially promoted for correcting the neurological defects in diabetic, alcoholic and other forms of peripheral neuropathy.

Therapeutic uses

- **Treatment of vitamin B_{12} deficiency:** Vitamin B_{12} is used along with 1–5 mg of oral folic acid and an iron preparation to get best results.
- **Prophylaxis:** When there are definite predisposing factors for development of deficiency.
- **Tobacco amblyopia:** Hydroxocobalamin provides some benefit by trapping cyanide derived from tobacco to form cyanocobalamin.
- **Mega doses of vitamin B_{12}** have been used in neuropathies, psychiatric disorders, cutaneous sarcoid and as a general tonic to allay fatigue, improve growth. The value of these uses is questionable.

Adverse effects

Even large doses of vitamin B_{12} are quite safe. Allergic reactions have occurred on injection, probably due to contaminants. *It should never be used by IV route.*

Vitamin-C

Ascorbic acid is an organic acid with structural similarity to glucose. It is a potent reducing agent and *l*-form is biologically active. Vitamin C is sensitive to heat.

Dietary Sources

Citrus fruits (lemons, oranges), black currants, crane- berry, ley berry, guava, tomato, leafy vegetables, sprouts, mango and green chilies. Breast milk contain more vit-C than cow's milk. *Indian gooseberry (Amla) is the richest source of vitamin C.*

Physiological Functions

- Vitamin C plays an important role in many oxidative and other metabolic reactions.
- It is essential for the formation and stabilization of collagen. Therefore, it plays essential role in tissue repair and formation of cartilage, bone and teeth.
- It acts as an antioxidant, improves immunity and prevents cataract formation also.
- It plays an important role in absorption of iron and conversion of folic acid to folinic acid; therefore helps in RBC production (erythropoeisis).
- It plays an important role in biosynthesis of adrenal steroids, catecholamines, oxytocin, vasopressin and bile acid.

Deficiency Symptoms

Scurvy (swollen and bleeding gums), delayed wound healing, anemia, growth retardation, brittle bones, etc.

Recommended Dietary Allowance (RDA)

40–60 mg/day.

Therapeutic uses

- **Prophylactic dose** (in deficiency susceptible individuals) is 50–100 mg daily.
- **Therapeutic dose** in scurvy treatment is 500–1500 mg/day.
- **To acidify urine in UTI treatment:** 1 g TDS.
- **Anemia:** To enhance the iron absorption [500 mg BD; along with iron tablets].
- To improve immunity and wound and fracture healing after surgery, injury, etc., given in a dose of 500 mg daily along with zinc.

Adverse Effects

Renal oxalate stone formation can occur when higher doses are taken for longer durations.

MINERALS

Minerals are the naturally occurring inorganic substances found in the forms of ores. They are purified by metallurgic process for the human consumption. These constitute 5% of human body. These are essential for normal physiological functions. The study of minerals is called mineralogy.

Minerals are present in the body in an optimum range. Any deviation from the normal (high or low) levels is pathological.

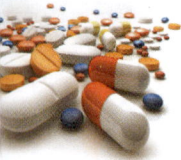

Classification

- **Principle minerals:** The RDA is usually ≥100 mg/day. Contains 60–80% of total minerals. Examples: calcium, magnesium, phosphate, sodium, potassium, chloride, etc.
- **Trace elements:** RDA is usually ≤100 mg/day
  - **Essential trace elements:** Molybdenum (Mo), manganese (Mn), copper (Cu), chromium (Cr), iron (I), zinc (Zn), fluoride (F), etc.
  - **Possible trace element:** Nickel (Ni) cadmium, (Cd), selenium (Si).
  - **Toxic elements:** Lead, aluminum, Mercury.

Sodium

- Sodium is mainly present in the extracellular fluid.
- It is mainly involved in maintaining the ECF volume, fluid and electrolyte balance and excitability of muscle and tissues.
- Common sources of sodium are common salt (sodium chloride), vegetables, sea-foods, junk foods [kurkure, chips], aachar, papad, chuttni, etc. These contain sodium in large quantities; hence should be avoided by hypertensive patients.
- Daily requirement of sodium is 5–15 g/day.
- In tropical or coastal areas, more sodium is required as it is excreted in sweat.
- The normal serum sodium level is 135–145 mEq/L.
- Hyponatremia/hypernatremia both are pathological conditions and demand timely correction and close monitoring.

Potassium

- Potassium is mainly present in the intracellular fluid.
- It is mainly involved in maintaining the fluid and electrolyte balance, acid base balance and excitability of muscle and tissues.
- **RDA:** 3–5 g/day.
- **Sources:** Banana, guava, pomegranate, tender coconut water, fresh fruits, cereals, pulses, vegetables, nuts and oilseeds.
- Normal plasma level: **3.3–5.5 mEq/L**
- Hypokalemia/hyperkalemia both are pathological conditions and fatal if not timely corrected as it directly affects the functioning of heart. Close monitoring of the levels is required.

- **Hypokalemia:** Electrocardiogram (ECG) changes like **U**-wave pattern and T-wave inversion are seen. The management is done by administering oral potassium chloride solution or slow IV KCl infusion.
- **Hyperkalemia:** ECG changes like Tall T-wave are seen. The management is done by administering loop diuretics, which promote potassium excretion.

Calcium

- Calcium is an important mineral and constitutes about 2% of body weight.
- An average human adult has 1–2 kg of calcium in the body 99% of this is stored in bones and remaining 1% is distributed in plasma and all tissues and cells.
- It is essential for tissue excitability, excitation-contraction-coupling (nerve conduction, muscular contraction).
- In addition, it acts as intracellular messenger for hormones, autacoids and transmitters as well as controls impulse generation and A-V conduction in heart.
- It is required for the smooth functioning of clotting mechanism.
- It is an integral part of bone and teeth.
- **RDA:** 400–500 mg/day
- **Source:** Milk and milk products sitaphal, green vegetables, cereals, millets, singhada, etc.
- The normal plasma level of calcium is 9–11 mg/dL. The normal levels of calcium are regulated by vitamin D, parathyroid hormone and calcitonin.
- Hypocalcemia may lead to Tetany, which is presented as muscles spasms.
- Deficiency in children causes rickets and in adults osteoporosis.
- Chronic hypercalcemia may cause nephrolithiasis.

Phosphorus

- Phosphorus is present in many food items such as milk, fish, meat, cereals, pulses and nuts.
- Human body contains approximately 500–600 g of phosphorus.
- The daily requirement of phosphorus is about 900–1000 mg/day.
- It is an important constituent of bone and teeth and also required for various phosphorylation reactions.

Magnesium

- Magnesium maintains normal nerve and muscle function, normal heart conduction, blood glucose levels, improve immune system and maintain bones healthy.
- The normal plasma level is 1.8–2.4 mg/dL.
- The various sources are vegetables, cereals, nuts, fish, meat, etc.
- **RDA:** 300–340 mg/day.
- Its main uses are:
  - Oral: As antacid, purgative.
  - Topically: To reduce the local edema.
  - Parenterally: In eclampsia, anticonvulsion, cardiac arrhythmia and as tocolytic agents.

Iron

(Described in Detail in Chapter 10)

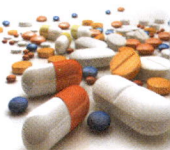

Iodine

- Iodine is an element which is essential for thyroid hormone (T_3, T_4) formation. Nearly 150 µg/day is required for normal functioning of thyroid. Iodine in food is present in several chemical forms including sodium and potassium salts, inorganic iodine, iodate and iodine.
- Main sources are sea food, iodized salt, dairy products and plants grown in iodine rich soil.
- Excessive cauliflower intake inhibits iodine absorption. Many months of iodine deficiency leads to goiter or hypothyroidism. Deficiency happens more commonly in pregnant women and children. The fetus of iodine deficient pregnant women suffer from congenital hypothyroidism and the children suffer from a form of physical and intellectual disability known as cretinism.
- The daily requirement for infants is 110–130 µg/day, children require 90–120 µg/day, Adults require 150 µg/day, pregnant females require 220 µg/day and lactating females require 290 µg/day.
- It is found in the form of iodides in nature.
- It has a variety of uses such as;
  - Prophylaxis of endemic goiter (as "iodized salt").
  - As antiseptic (tincture iodine, povidone iodine).
  - In thyroid storm (Lugol's iodine).
  - In pre-operative preparation for thyroidectomy in Graves' disease (Iodine is generally given for 10 days just preceding surgery. It makes the gland firm, less vascular and easier to operate on.
  - Its radioactive isotopes (^{131}I, ^{125}I, ^{123}I) also have quite a lot of medicinal importance.

Zinc

- Zinc is an important trace mineral to stay healthy. It is found in the cells throughout the body and is needed for the immune system to work efficiently.
- It has a role in cell division, cell growth, wound healing and the breakdown of carbohydrates, insulin synthesis and action.
- It is also needed for the sense of smell and taste.
- It reduces the duration of diarrhea and common cold.
- Food sources are animal proteins, beef, pork, lamb, dark meat of chicken, nuts, whole grains, legumes and yeast. Vegetables are not a good source.
- Deficiency symptoms are; frequent infections, loss of hair, poor appetite, anosmia, skin sores and wounds taking long time to heal.
- Its daily requirement is 10–12 mg/day. It has to be taken either in diet or in capsules/tab/syrup formulations in deficient state.

Copper

- Copper is an important mineral and found in many foods such as meat, seafood's, nuts, seeds, grain products, soya flour, almonds, avocados, mushrooms and cocoa products.
- The body stores copper mainly in liver, brain, heart, kidneys, bones and muscles. Copper is required for following functions in the body such as efficient utilization of iron, catecholamine synthesis, as cofactor in various enzymes, collagen synthesis, and superoxide dismutase activity.
- It is transported in the blood along with a plasma protein, ceruloplasmin.
- The daily requirement in adults is 900 µg/day
- Deficiency of copper is rare. It may occur in patients of intestinal bypass surgery, malnourished infants, persons consuming high doses of zinc and vitamin C.
- The deficiency symptoms present as anemia, neutropenia, hypothermia, brittle bones, osteoporosis, low resistance to infections and thyroid disorders.
- Copper is also used for improving wound healing and osteoporosis.
- Wilson's disease occurs due to deficiency of ceruloplasmin due to which copper levels in the blood rise and copper gets deposited in liver, basal ganglia and other parts of brain. (Penicillamine is used to treat this condition).

Chromium

- Chromium is required for carbohydrate, lipids and protein metabolism.
- It is required for action of insulin.
- It plays very important role in gene regulation.
- Low level of chromium may result in infertility as it decreases the sperm count.

Molybdenum

- This trace element is required in very small quantities.
- In the human body, it is found in bones, liver and kidneys.
- The major food sources are legumes [beans, peas], brown rice, whole grains, liver, nuts and dark green leafy vegetables.
- The RDA is 40–50 µg/day.
- It plays an important role as a co-factor for the essential enzymes involved in carbohydrate metabolism, utilization of iron and sulfide detoxification.
- The deficiency may result in tachypnea, tachycardia, mouth and gum disorders and sexual impotence in older males.

Cobalt

- It is an essential component of the structure of vitamin-B_{12}, also called as cobalamin.

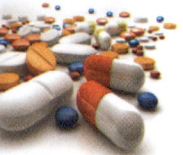

- Food sources of cobalt are clams [rich source of cobalt], organ [liver] meat, oysters, poultry, and milk.
- As it is a factor of B_{12}, the daily-recommended intake of cobalt is expressed in units of B_{12}.
- The average adult needs 2.4 μg/day.
- The deficiency is mostly seen in strict vegetarians, malabsorptive condition and in post gastrectomy patients and presents as macrocytic anemia.

Fluoride

(Described in Chapter 3)

In addition,

- The main source of fluoride is drinking water. It is added in toothpastes and mouth washes to prevent tooth decay/ dental caries.
- The higher doses can weaken bones, cause muscular weakness and neuropathies, known as fluorosis.
- Concentration of ≃1PPM has no side effects.
- Higher concentration show dose dependent adverse effects, such as
  - ≥2 PPM may lead to GIT adverse effects.
  - ≥10 PPM may lead to dental adverse effects.
  - ≥20 PPM may lead to skeleton fluorosis.

Selenium

- Selenium acts as a cofactor for various enzymes involved in lipid metabolism, especially *Glutathione peroxidase*.
- It is a very good antioxidant and has a role in prevention of various cancers.
- Selenium is found in two forms, selenium cysteine and selenium methionine.
- Its daily requirement is 200–300 μg/day.
- *Keshan disease* occurs due to deficiency of selenium, most commonly seen in Korean and Chinese individuals who are deficient of selenium.

IMMUNOSUPPRESSANTS

Refer to Chapter 2.

ANTIDOTES

- **Antidotes** are agents/substances used to neutralize or counteract the ill effects of poison/drug. Nearly all the drugs used for therapeutic purpose; if taken at their toxic doses have the potential to act as poisons.
- A proper history of the poisoned patients should be taken to know the exact nature and the amount of poison/drug

taken. This is must to chalk out the best treatment plan for a particular patient, as the antidotes are different for different poisons/drugs. As antidotes are not available for all poisons/drugs; stress is given on general supportive measures, which include maintenance of vitals and symptomatic management.

- The antidotes are life saving, if administered timely.
- If antidotes are available, they should be invariably used.
- Antidotes work best when administered in the *golden period* of management.
- The list of poisonings along with their antidotes with exact dosage schedule should be available in emergency department at all times.

TYPES OF ANTIDOTES

Antidotes have been divided into the following types:

- **Physical antidotes:** These agents prevent the further absorption of poison by adsorption mechanism. Examples egg albumin and activated charcoal are physical antidotes for alkaloid poisonings.
- **Chemical antidotes:** These agents react chemically and form a complex with poison and inactivate it or oxidize the poison to non-toxic and easily excretable form. Examples: chelating agents bind heavy metals; antacids neutralize the acid in stomach.
- **Physiological antidotes:** These agents act at a different receptor than poison and counteract the effects of poison by having an opposite physiological action. Example: hypoglycemia induced by excessive dose of insulin is counteracted by glucagon, adrenaline counteracts histaminic effects in respiratory tract.
- **Pharmacological antidotes:** These agents compete with poison for binding to the same receptor site where the poison binds and antagonizes the effects of poison/drug. These are divided into two types:
  1. Competitive type
  2. Non-competitive type
- **Universal antidotes:** These agents are given when the details of ingested poison are unknown. Universal antidotes usually act by decreasing the further absorption of ingested poison and do not have any effect on the already absorbed part.

Composition of universal antidote is: Powdered activated charcoal (2 parts) + Magnesium oxide (1 part) + Tannic acid (1 part).

(Its use is not advocated much these days as advantage is unproven.)

A few toxicity-causing agents with their specific antidotes are given in Table 7.3.

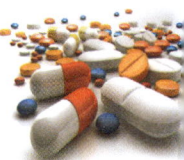

TABLE 7.3: Common toxicity-causing agents with their specific antidotes

Toxicity causing agents	Antidotes	Dose and Route	Mechanism of action
Iron	Desferrioxamine	10–15 mg/kg/hr IV (max 75 mg/day) Or 50 mg/kg IM	Chelates ferrous ions and enhances its elimination in the urine.
Streptokinase overdose	Epsilon-amino-caproic acid (EACA)	5 g oral/IV, followed by 1 g hourly till bleeding stops (max 30 g in 24 hours)	Inhibits plasminogen activation.
Methotrexate overdose	Leucovorin or folinic acid	3.0 mg IV to be repeated as required.	Being active coenzyme form protects the healthy cells from the effects of methotrexate.
Methanol poisoning	Fomepizole	Loading dose: 15 mg/kg IV Maintenance dose: 10 mg/kg every 12 hours till serum methanol falls below 20 mg/dL,	A competitive inhibitor of the enzyme alcohol dehydrogenase and prevents toxic metabolites formation.
Cyanide poisoning	Sodium nitrite or amyl nitrite and sodium thiosulfate	Sod. nitrite: 10 mL of 3% sol. IV then, Sod. thiosulfate: 50 mL 25% sol. IV	Sod. nitrite forms methemoglobin, which binds to cyanide and forms cyano-methemoglobin, which is converted to easily excretable form Sod. thiocyanate by Sod. thiosulfate
Lead poisoning	Calcium disodium edetate.	1 g is diluted to 200–300 mL in saline or glucose solution and infused IV over 1 hour twice daily for 3–5 days	Chelation of lead ions
Heparin overdose	Protamine sulfate	1 mg IV for every 100 units of heparin	Protamine forms a stable complex with heparin and neutralizes it
Copper	d-Penicillamine	100 mg/kg/day orally in 4 divided doses for 3–7 days	Chelation of copper ions
Organophosphate poisoning	Atropine Oximes	**Atropine:** 2 mg IV repeat every 10 minutes. **Pralidoxime:** 30 mg/kg IV loading dose, followed by 8–10 mg/kg/hour continuous infusion till recovery	**Atropine:** Anti-muscarinic **Oxime::** Reactivation of ChE enzyme. (No role in carbamate poisoning)
Morphine overdose	Naloxone	0.4–0.8 mg IV every 2–3 minutes: max 10 mg	Competitive antagonist on all types of opioid receptors
Warfarin overdose	Vitamin-K or fresh frozen plasma	10 mg IM followed by 5 mg 4 hourly for one day then 5 mg OD to be titrated with response	Induces synthesis of clotting factors
As, Hg, Au, Bi, Ni, Sb poisoning	Dimercaprol (British antilewisite; BAL)	5 mg/kg *stat* followed by 2–3 mg/kg every 4–8 hours for 2 days, then once or twice a day for 10 days	Chelation of ions
Belladona poisoning (Atropine)	Physostigmine	0.5–2 mg IV repeated as required	Reversible anti-cholinesterase effect
Paracetamol poisoning	Acetylcysteine	Orally 140 mg/kg, followed by 70 mg/kg every 4 hours for 17 doses. Or IV 150 mg/kg infusion over 15 minutes may be repeated; if required	Restores depleted glutathione stores
Benzodiazepines	Flumazenil	1 mg over 1–3 minutes; maximum dose 1–5 mg given over 2–10 minutes	Competitive benzodiazepine inhibitor
Curare (arrow poison)	Neostigmine	0.5–2.0 mg (30–50 mg/kg) IV, preceded by atropine or glycopyrrolate 10 mg/kg	Anti-cholinesterase at neuromuscular junction
Digitalis	Digoxin immune fab	Parenteral: 38 or 40 mg per vial with 75 mg sorbitol lyophilized powder to reconstitute for IV injection Each vial will bind approximately 0.5 mg digoxin or digitoxin	Binds free glycosides in plasma, complex excreted in urine easily
Carbon monoxide	Oxygen	100% oxygen by high flow non breathing mask	Competitive displacement of carbon monoxide

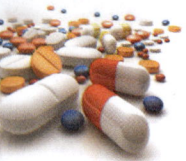

ANTI VENOM

- Venom is a form of toxin secreted by an animal for the purpose of self-protection and causing harm to another animal. Venom is injected into the victims by means of a bite, sting or other sharp body feature, which differentiate it from poison (that is absorbed, consumed or inhaled). *'Every venom is a poison, but every poison is not a venom'.*
- The potency of different venom varies amongst each other. The potency of a venom is characterized by median lethal dose (LD_{50}) which is expressed as milligram of toxin per kilogram of body mass.
- **Venomous invertebrates include**
  - **Spiders** (*use fangs to inject venom and black widow spider is most venomous*).
  - **Centipedes** (*use forcipules to inject venom*),
  - **Scorpions and stinging insects** (*use stings to inject venom*),
  - Bees and wasp (*use ovipositor to inject venom*),
  - Box jellyfish (*use harpoon to inject venom* and it is *most venomous jellyfish*)
  - Snakes (vertebrate) (*use fangs to inject venom.*)
- In India, snakebites are the most commonly encountered fatal venomous accidents. Snake venom is produced by mandibular glands situated below the eyes. Snake venom contains a variety of peptide toxins including proteases, nucleases, and neurotoxins.
- Depending upon the species of snake, the bites can be haemotoxic, neurotoxic and vasculotoxic.
- Venomous snake bites may cause a variety of symptoms depending upon the type of snake and the quantity of venom injected. The symptoms include severe pain, swelling, tissue necrosis, hypotension, seizures, hemorrhage, respiratory paralysis, kidney failure, coma and death.
- The composition and potency of snake venom differs from species to species. The habitat of poisonous and non-poisonous snakes is different, which defines the lethality of venom.
- *The venom has therapeutic uses also. Such as the venom of Russel's viper is a source of an enzyme complex known as hemocoagulase, it is useful in promoting coagulation by shortening the bleeding and clotting time. It converts fibrinogen to fibrin. It is available for topical, IV, IM and SC administration.*

PRODUCTION OF ANTIVENOM

- Antivenom is a biological product used in the treatment of venomous bites or stings.
- Antivenom is produced by administering a small amount of targeted venom into the animals such as sheep, horse, goat or rabbit. The immune system of the animal responds to the venom's active molecules and produces antibodies.
- These antibodies from animal's blood are extracted out, refined, packed and stored as antivenom.
- The anti venom (antibodies) is injected into bite victim to antagonize the ill effects of venom.

STORAGE OF ANTIVENOM

Antivenom for therapeutic use is often preserved as freeze-dried ampules and some as liquid forms, which have to be kept refrigerated.

PRINCIPLE OF ANTIVENOM

- The principle of antivenom is based upon both active and passive immunity.
- The active immunity against the venom is induced in the animal (sheep, horse, goat or rabbit) by injecting smaller doses of venom. It simulates vaccination process and the antibodies against venom are produced.
- The passive immunity is provided to the bite victim in the form of hyperimmunized serum or antibodies, which had been obtained from the animal's blood.

ROUTE OF ADMINISTRATION

The majority of antivenom is administered intravenously after proper dilutions as advised by the manufacturer.

MECHANISM OF ACTION

- Antivenom should be administered intravenously as per the administration guidelines/instructions as early as possible after the *venomous bite*.
- The antivenom binds to the venom molecules present in the blood as well as the local site of bite. It neutralizes the venom and halts the further damage. It does not reverse the damage, which has been already done by the venom. **Antivenoms can be classified into monovalent and polyvalent antivenom.**
- **Monovalent antivenom** is effective against the venom of a single species. It is used only when the species of biting snake has been identified.
- **Polyvalent antivenom** is effective against the venom of a variety of species. These days, polyvalent antivenom is most commonly used because, catching the snake after bite and identifying the species is not that easy and practicable.

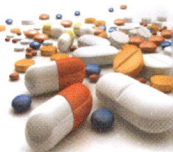

ANTISNAKE VENOM (ASV) SERUM POLYVALENT

It is available as lyophilized form in the vials, with 10 mL ampoule of distilled water.

After reconstitution, each mL neutralizes:

- 0.6 mg of standard Cobra (*Naja naja*) venom.
- 0.6 mg of standard Russel's viper (*Vipera russelli*) venom.
- 0.45 mg of standard Sawscaled viper (*Echis carinatus*) venom.
- 0.45 mg of standard Krait (*Bungarus caeruleus*) venom.

Indication and Method of ASV Administration

ASV is indicated in the presence of signs and symptoms of systemic envenomation. Because majority of snakes are non-poisonous and chances of pseudobites are more.

- The ASV is reconstituted as per the instructions given by the manufacturer. 20 mL IV infusion at a rate of 1 mL/min is given every 1–6 hourly intervals till symptoms of envenomation disappear.
- It is important to continue ASV treatment till evidence of envenomation persists.
- In case of viper bite, some serum should also be infiltrated around the site of bite to prevent venom-induced gangrene.

Adverse Effects of Antivenoms and their Management

- The antivenom should be used with caution as administering antivenom has also some inherent dangers. Although, antivenom is purified by several processes but it still contains some serum proteins, which can act as antigens.
- Some individuals may react to the antivenom with an immediate hypersensitivity reaction (anaphylaxis) or sensitization can develop to antivenom due to repeated exposures and causes serum sickness.
- Preferably, sensitivity test should be done before administering antivenom. An antihistaminic and a glucocorticoid may also be given prophylactically to avoid hypersensitivity reaction. Adrenaline may be injected SC/IM, if required.
- Supportive measures such as maintenance of vitals and empathetic counseling of patient should also be done simultaneously as most of the deaths occur due to neurogenic shock.

VACCINE AND SERA

Vaccines and immune sera, including antivenom and antitoxins, are usually referred to as biologicals. These have a common use to reinforce the immunological defense of the body against foreign agents such as microorganisms (bacteria or virus) or their toxins.

VACCINES

- Vaccines are used to stimulate the production of antibodies and provide active immunity to the individual.
- These antibodies provide the immunity specific to that antigen only.
- Administering vaccines is frequently called **artificial active immunization** because they stimulate immunity.
- Vaccines are routinely administered to children (and adults in some special cases) to provide prophylactic medical care for prevention of some vaccine preventable diseases.
- Artificial active immunization provides memorized long-term immunity.

SERA

- Sera are used to provide preformed antibodies and provide passive immunity to the individual.
- Administering immune sera is called artificial passive immunization because they provide readymade antibodies.
- Sera are used after exposure to antigens or toxins or after bites from poisonous snakes or spiders to make diseases less invasive and aggressive or to prevent clinical problems from developing at all.
- Sera provides non-memorized short-term immunity.

When both vaccine and sera are administered simultaneously in the same patient, it is called combined immunization.

IMMUNITY

Immunity is defined as the state of relative resistance to a disease that develops after exposure to the specific antigen.

Active immunity is defined as the production of antibodies by the immune system of host against antigen or specific protein of pathogen. These antibodies are specific to the antigen. If the specific foreign protein is reintroduced into the body, the memory cells react immediately to release antibodies.

Passive immunity is defined as the administration of preformed/readymade antibodies into the body.

- The colostrum contains antibodies and the infant received the passive immunity in the form of breast feed.
- Passive immunity is also transferred transplacently.
- The circulating antibodies act in the same manner as those produced from plasma cells, recognizing the foreign protein and attaching to it, rendering it harmless.
- The passive immunity lasts only as long as the circulating antibodies last because the body does not produce its own antibodies.
- Sometimes, the host human responds to the circulating injected antibodies by producing its own antibodies to the injected antibodies (*as sera are also foreign proteins to the host's body*). This results in **serum sickness**, a massive

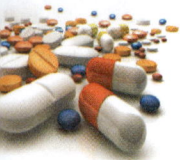

immune reaction manifested by fever, arthritis, flank pain, myalgia, and arthralgia.

- **Immunization** is defined as the process in which disease specific vaccines/protein are administered to produce active immunity.
- The proteins used in manufacturing/synthesizing the vaccine could be a weakened bacterial cell membrane, the protein coat of a virus, or a virus that has been chemically weakened so that it cannot cause disease.

VACCINES

The word vaccine is derived from the Latin word for smallpox, *vaccinia*.

- Vaccines contain weakened or altered protein antigens that stimulate the formation of antibodies against a specific disease.
- They are used to promote active immunity.
- Vaccines can be made from chemically inactivated (attenuated) microorganisms or from live, weakened viruses or bacteria.
- Toxoids are vaccines that are made from the toxins produced by the microorganisms.
- Some vaccines require booster doses—doses that are given a few months after the initial dose to further stimulate the formation of antibodies.

Patients should be advised to keep a written record of all immunizations or immune sera used. Booster doses for various vaccines may be needed to further stimulate antibody production.

Vaccines are divided in three groups

1. **Live attenuated vaccines**
   - **Bacterial:** Bacillus Calmette-Guérin (BCG), Typhoid.
   - **Viral:** OPV (Sabin), Measles, Mumps, Rubella, (MMR), Varicella, Yellow fever.
2. **Killed vaccines**
   - **Bacterial:** Typhoid-paratyphoid (TAB), Vi Typhoid polysaccharide Cholera, Pertussis (whooping cough), Meningococcal, *Hemophilus* influenzae type b [Hib],
   - **Viral:** Poliomyelitis, Rabies, Influenza, Hepatitis A, Hepatitis B, etc.
   - **Toxoids:** Diphtheria, Tetanus.

3. **Combined vaccines**
   - **Bivalent vaccine: D**iphtheria toxoid + **T**etanus toxoid (DT)
   - **Trivalent vaccine:**
     - **D**iphtheria + **P**ertussis + **T**etanus (DPT)
     - **M**easles+ **M**umps+ **R**ubella (MMR)
   - **Pentavalent vaccine** (DPT + Hepatitis B + *H. influenzae* type b)

Vaccines under Universal Immunization Program (UIP)

- BCG
- DPT
- OPV
- Measles
- Hepatitis B
- TT
- Hib (DPT + Hep B + Hib) pentavalent vaccine.
- Vaccine JE (in selected high disease burden districts only)

Refer to Table 7.4 for universal immunization program (UIP)

Rotavirus Vaccine

Rotavirus infection is one of the leading cause of diarrhea, dehydration and deaths in children below 1 year. According to Indian academy of Pediatrics (IAP), Rotavirus vaccination should also be ensured to children below one year.

Other important vaccines are given in Table 7.5

Viral Vaccines

Poliomyelitis

- *Oral poliovirus vaccine (OPV; Sabin vaccine [described above])*
- *Inactivated poliomyelitis vaccine (IPV, Salk vaccine):* It is inactivated suspension of the virus. Three doses of 1 mL each are injected subcutaneously in the deltoid region at 4–6 week intervals and fourth dose is given 6–12 months later. In every 5 years booster doses are given.

TABLE 7.4: Universal immunization program (UIP)

Vaccine	Protection	Dose and route	No. of doses	Vaccination schedule
BCG	Tuberculosis	0.1 mL, intradermal, left deltoid muscles	1	At birth (less than 1 year)
OPV	Polio	Oral route Only two drops	5	At birth Primary doses at the age of 6, 10, 14 week, one booster dose at the age of 16 months-2 year

Contd...

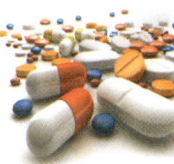

Vaccine	Protection	Dose and route	No. of doses	Vaccination schedule
Hep B	Hepatitis B	Intramuscularly 0.5 mL in the anterolateral aspect of thigh	4	Birth dose within 24 hours of birth Primary doses at 6, 10, 14 weeks
DPT	Diphtheria, Pertusis Tetanus	Intramuscularly 0.5 mL in the anterolateral aspect of thigh	5	Primary doses at the age of 6, 10, 14 weeks, First booster dose at the age of 16 months-2 years, second booster dose at the age of 5–6 years
Measles	Measles	0.5 mL, subcutaneously thigh/ deltoid	2	First dose at the age of 9 months–1 year Second dose at the age of 16 months–2 years
TT	Tetanus	Intramuscularly 0.5 mL deltoid	2	At the age of 10 years and 16 years, In pregnant female, 2 doses (If immunized within last 3 years only single dose is preferred)
Hib	Hib pneumonia and Hib meningitis	Intramuscularly 0.5 mL in the anterolateral aspect of thigh	3	At the age of 6, 10 and 14 weeks
JE*	Japanese encephalitis (brain fever)	1–3 years: 0.5 mL ≥3 years: 1.0 mL Subcutaneously, deltoid	2	At the age of 9 months–1 year, 2nd dose at the age of 16 months–2 years

Japanese encephalitis vaccine is contraindicated when Hypersensitivity to the first dose appears.

TABLE 7.5: Other vaccines

Vaccine	Protection against disease	Dose and route	No. of doses	Vaccination schedule
Varicella*	Herpes	Subcutaneously 0.5 mL, deltoid	2	Single dose between 1 and 12 years, More than 13 years—two dose at 1 month interval
Hepatitis A	Hepatitis A	Intramuscularly 0.5 mL in the anterolateral aspect of thigh	2	After 1 year of age, 2 doses at 6–12 month interval
Typhoid Vi antigen vaccine	Typhoid	Intramuscularly 0.5 mL, deltoid	–	First dose after 2 year, booster every 3 year
Typhoid oral vaccine	Typhoid	Oral	3	One capsule on alternate days in between meals (days 1, 3 and 5) Not indicated for age <5 years and in pregnant women
Meningococcal vaccine	Meningitis	Intramuscular/subcutaneos 0.5 mL, thigh/deltoid	3	2 years and above during epidemics
Pneumococcal 23 valent vaccine	Pneumonia	Intramuscularly/subcutaneously 0.5 mL in the anterolateral aspect of thigh	1	Single dose in high risk children ≥2 year
Rabies**	Rabies	1.0 mL IM	Based upon schedule followed	Any age Post-exposure: 0, 3, 7, 14, 28 days. Pre-exposure: 0, 7 and 28
Cholera vaccine	Cholera	Intramuscularly/ subcutaneously 0.5 mL	2	Primary dose: 0.5 mL Second dose: 1 mL 1–4 weeks later

All the above vaccines are stored at the temperature of +2°C to +8°C.

*Vericella vaccine is contraindicated when hypersensitivity to neomycin is there.

** Other schedule described below.

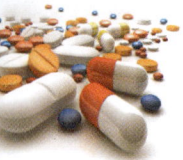

Rabies

There are three type of rabies vaccine, they are:

- Purified chick embryo cell vaccine (PCEV).
- Human diploid cell vaccine (HDCV)
- Purified vero cell rabies vaccine (PVRV)

Post-exposure Prophylaxis in Unvaccinated Person

- Intramuscular regimen: 1mL PCEV/HDCV or 0.5 mL PVRV. Any one of these to be given on deltoid region on days 0,3,7,14,30,90.
- Intradermal regimen: 0.1 mL PCEV/PVRV or 0.2 mL HDCV. Any one of these to be given on both deltoid region on days 0, 3, 7 and on one deltoid region on days 30, 90.

Post-exposure Prophylaxis in Already Vaccinated Person

This is given when an immunized person is bitten by a suspected animal. It is administered as 0.1 mL intradermal injections on days 0, 3 and 7. Any one of above mentioned rabies vaccines can be used.

Local Treatment of Bite Wound

- Early local treatment of bite wound is essential in addition to the vaccine ± rabies immunoglobulin (RIG).
- The wound should be thoroughly washed with soap under running water for at least 5 minutes, followed by application of an antiseptic (alcohol/povidone iodine/cetrimide). Cauterization with carbolic acid is contraindicated.
- In category III bites, RIG should be infiltrated locally in the depth and around the wound to inactivate the locally present virus.
- Suturing of the wound should be avoided.
- RIG is given in a dose of 20 IU/kg body weight and the maximum dose is 1500 IU.

ANTISERA AND IMMUNOGLOBULINS

Antisera are the drugs that are obtained from the *serum of the horses*, which have been already immunized against the specific antigen.

- The serum extracted from horse is purified and the required antibodies are extracted out. These antibodies are marketed in a concentrated form.
- Sensitivity test should be performed before injecting these agents, as they can be antigenic and can cause hypersensitivity reactions.

Immunoglobulins (IGs) are separated *human gamma globulins*, which carry the antibodies.

- These are *more efficacious* than the corresponding antisera.
- These may be non-specific (normal) or specific (hyperimmune) against a particular antigen.

- Sensitivity test need not to be done, as hypersensitivity reactions are very rare with these agents.

> **Covishield Vaccine**
>
> Serum Institute of India's COVID-19 vaccine, called Covishield, is a version of the Oxford-AstraZeneca vaccine that is manufactured in India. According to AstraZeneca's primary analysis of phase 3 trial data, the vaccine has a 76% efficacy rate after both doses.

Antisera (Horse)

- **Tetanus antitoxin (ATS):**
  - **Prophylactic dose:** 1500–3000 IU, intramuscularly/subcutaneosly
  - **Therapeutic dose:** 50,000–100,000 IU partly intravenously and rest by intramuscularly.
- **Diphtheria antitoxin (ADS):** It is always given for therapeutic purpose. 20,000–40,000 IU intravenously/intramuscularly. Higher dose may be required in severe cases.
- **Antirabies serum (ARS):** It is also called as 'Equine Rabies Immune-Globulin' (ERIG). It is given along with rabies vaccine in non-immunized persons. A total of 40 IU/kg dose is given. Some amount is injected around the bite wound and the rest is injected intramuscularly. Only single dose at the start of therapy is given. It is inferior to human rabies immune globulin.
- **Gas gangrene antitoxin (AGS):**
  - Prophylactic dose: 10,000 IU subcutaneously/intravenously/intramuscularly
  - Therapeutic dose: 30,000–75,000 IU subcutaneously/intravenously/intramuscularly
- **Antisnake venom polyvalent:** It is available as lyophilized powder form in a vial. This is reconstituted with 10 mL distilled water. 20 mL of the reconstituted solution is given intravenously at a rate of 1 mL/min and repeated at 1–6 hours interval. This therapy is given till disappearance of envenomation symptoms. Maximum up to 300 mL of ASV can be given.

Immunoglobulins (Human)

- **Tetanus immunoglobulin:** It is indicated in patients who are not immunized and having highly contaminated wound with a risk of developing tetanus.
  - **Prophylactic dose:** 250–500 IU, intramuscularly
  - **Therapeutic dose:** 3000–6000 IU intramuscularly and/or 250–500 IU intrathecally
- **Normal human gamma globulin:**
  - **Prophylactic uses:** Viral hepatitis A and B, measles, mumps, poliomyelitis and chickenpox and burns patients.
  - **Therapeutic use:** Agammaglobulinemia, premature infants and patients undergoing immunosuppression therapy. It improves the response to antibiotics in debilitated patients with bacterial infections.

Refer to Table 7.6 for various antisera immunoglobulins.

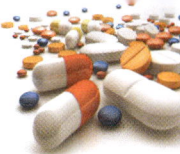

TABLE 7.6: Various antisera and immunoglobulins

Antisera (from horse)	Immunoglobulins (from human)
• Tetanus antitoxin (ATS)	• Tetanus immunoglobulin
• Diphtheria antitoxin (ADS)	• Normal human gamma globulin
• Antirabies serum (ARS)	• Hepatitis-B immunoglobulin
• Gas gangrene antitoxin (AGS)	• Rho(D) immunoglobulin
• Antisnake venom polyvalent	• Rabies immunoglobulin

The total dose is 2 g/kg body weight, which is to be given by IV route in divided doses in five days.

- **Rabies immune globulin (HRIG):** It is superior to ERIG. The dose is 20 IU/kg body weight and the maximum dose is 1500 IU. The required dose according to number and size of bite is infiltrated round the bite wound and the rest is injected by IM route. The injection site for the vaccine and HRIG should be different.
- Rho(D) immuneglobulin: (Refer to Chapter 2)
- **Hepatitis B immuneglobulin:** It is indicated in individuals acutely exposed to HBsAg positive blood or blood products. It should be administered intramuscularly as early as possible or within 7 days of exposure in a dose of 1000–2000 IU for adults and 32–48 IU/kg for children. Simultaneously, immunization of the individual with Hepatitis B vaccine is mandatory. The site of immunoglobulin and vaccine administration should be different.

 Nursing Implications

- Assess for contraindications or any known allergies to any vaccines or to the components.
- Nurse should keep a check during vaccination that the child is not suffering from active viral/bacterial infection. Do not administer if the patient exhibits signs of acute infection or immune deficiency because the vaccine can cause a mild infection and can exacerbate acute infections.
- Arrange for proper preparation and administration of the vaccine; check on the timing and dose of each injection because dose, preparation, and timing vary with individual vaccines.
- Provide a written record of the immunization, including the need to return for booster immunizations and timing of the boosters, if necessary, to increase patient compliance with medical regimens.
- Immunoglobulins should be administered slowly.
- Do not administer vaccine if the patient has received blood, blood products, or immunoglobulin within the last 3 months because a severe immune reaction could occur.
- In combined immunization, vaccine and immunoglobulin should not be administered at same site.
- Maintain emergency equipment on standby, including adrenaline, in case of severe hypersensitivity reaction.
- Evaluate the effectiveness of the teaching plan (patient can name drug, dosage, adverse effects to watch for; has written record of immunizations; can state when to return for the next immunization or booster if needed).
- During the administration of antidotes and antivenom, proper dilution, dose and administering regimen should be strictly followed. The vitals should be recorded regularly for early diagnosis of any adverse or anaphylactic reactions.

Assess Yourself

Long and Short Answer Questions

1. What are the goals of treatment in substance used disorders?
2. Enumerate the drugs used in de-addiction.
3. Why is buprenorphine used in opioids addiction?
4. Enumerate drugs, which are required in the emergency tray for CPR?
5. What are the stages of resuscitation?
6. What are the adverse effects of antivenom and describe their management?
7. What are the roles of nurses in the management of poisoning?
8. What is antidote? Describe their types and name at least 10 antidotes.
9. What are vitamins? Classify them and describe folic acid and B12.
10. Write short notes on:
    a. Disulfiram
    b. Naltrexone
    c. Calcium
    d. Vitamin K
    e. Vitamin A
    f. Vitamin D
    g. Storage of vaccine, immunoglobulin, and antivenoms
    h. Vaccines
    i. Immunoglobulins

Contd...

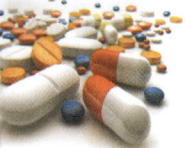

Multiple Choice Questions

1. **Which of the following is not an opioid de-addiction drug?**
   a. Methadone
   b. Buprenorphine
   c. Bupropion
   d. Naloxone

2. **Which of the following is fat soluble vitamin?**
   a. Folic acid
   b. Ascorbic acid
   c. Biotin
   d. Tocopherol

3. **Which of the following is the most powerful antioxidant?**
   a. Vit. A
   b. Vit. E
   c. Vit. C
   d. Vit B_{12}

4. **Beriberi occurs due to deficiency of:**
   a. Vitamin B complex.
   b. Thiamine
   c. Pyridoxine.
   d. Riboflavin

5. **Antidote for lead poisoning is:**
   a. Calcium disodium edetate
   b. Fomepizole
   c. Neostigmine
   d. Naloxone

Answer Key

1. c.   2. d.   3. b.   4. b.   5. a.

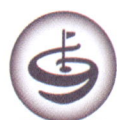

Drugs used on Skin and Mucous Membranes

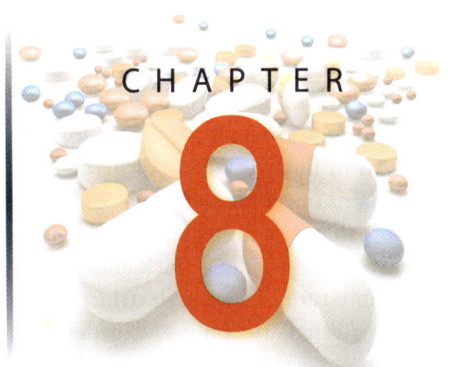

TOPICAL USES OF DRUGS

- Skin is the largest organ in the body. It is a highly efficient self-repairing organ, which plays an important role in regulating heat and water loss.
- It prevents the entry of microorganisms and chemicals by acting as barrier. The principle barrier to penetration resides in the multilayered lipid rich stratum corneum layer of skin.
- **Several drugs** are used topically for their local action on the skin and mucous membranes to treat/cure the dermatological conditions as well as for intentional systemic absorption [transdermal patches].
- The systemic absorption of topically applied drug varies with the site of application and molecular size of drug. Example: Least absorption occurs from the palm and sole, whereas the absorption increases progressively on the forearm, trunk, head and neck. Scrotum and vulva have highest level of absorption.
- **The absorption of the drug increases:**
  - Ten times when the occlusive dressing (impermeable plastic membrane cover) has been applied.
  - When the skin is damaged by inflammation, burns or exfoliation.
  - When hot fomentation has been done prior to applying the topical agents.
- The absorption of drug also depends upon the physiochemical nature and molecular size of the drug. Lipophilic drugs utilize the intracellular route because they readily cross cell membrane, whereas the hydrophilic drugs principally take the intercellular route, diffusing in the fluid filled spaces between cells.
- *Smaller the molecular size of drug, better will be the absorption.*

> The drugs for topical application are presented in vehicles or bases. Along with drug, the vehicle is the chief ingredient of a topical formulation. The vehicles are designed to vary in the extent to which they increase hydration of the stratum corneum.

A few commonly used vehicles for topically applied drugs are as follows:

- **Emulsion:** It is the mixture of two immiscible liquids in which droplets of one liquid are dispersed throughout the body of second liquid, e.g., castor oil emulsion.
- **Lotion:** This is usually aqueous solution or suspension intended for local administration, e.g., calamine lotion.

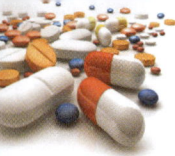

- **Ointment:** This is a semi-solid water in oil preparation for external application. It forms a protective oil film on skin. It is greasy to very greasy and can stain clothes, e.g., Povidone iodine ointment.
- **Dusting powder:** It is a dosage form, when a solid drug is given in finely divided powdered state. A simple powder contains one ingredient and a compound powder contains more than one ingredient, e.g., Clotrimazole powder.
- **Paste:** It is usually a thick and stiff non-greasy ointment like mixture of starch, dextrin, zinc oxide, etc. These are for external use only and penetrate the skin less than ointment, e.g., Toothpaste.
- **Liniments:** These are mixture of medicinal substance in oily, alcoholic solutions of soap or emulsions. These are applied with friction and rubbing, e.g., turpentine liniment.
- **Cream:** Cream is a semi-solid oil in water type emulsion containing suspension or solution of medicament for external application. It spreads and can be removed easily without leaving a greasy feel. It leaves concentrated drug at skin surface, e.g., Silver-sulfadiazine cream.
- **Paint:** They are simple solutions of drug in glycerine or liquid paraffin, e.g., Mandl's paint.
- **Gel:** These are greaseless non-staining water soluble emulsions.

There are variety of drugs which are applied topically on the skin and mucous membranes to produce therapeutic effects locally on the skin and mucous membranes. Sometimes, these topical agents can also be applied to get some special systemic effects. The drugs for topical use are manufactured/synthesized in such a way that they are able to produce the desired effects. This is done by adding vehicle/base and some other adjuvant in such a way that the drug can penetrate the stratum corneum easily and produce the desired effects.

Mechanism of percutaneous absorption has been described in Figure 8.1.

The various preparations for topical use on skin and mucous membranes are as follows:

- **Topical anti-infective preparations**
  - Topical antibacterial preparations
  - Topical antiviral preparations
  - Topical antifungal preparations
  - Topical antiparasitic/antiscabies preparations
- Topical steroids
- Emolients, keratolytics and cleansers
- Drugs acting on skin vasculature
- Drugs for acne-vulgaris
- Sunscreens
- Demelanizing agents

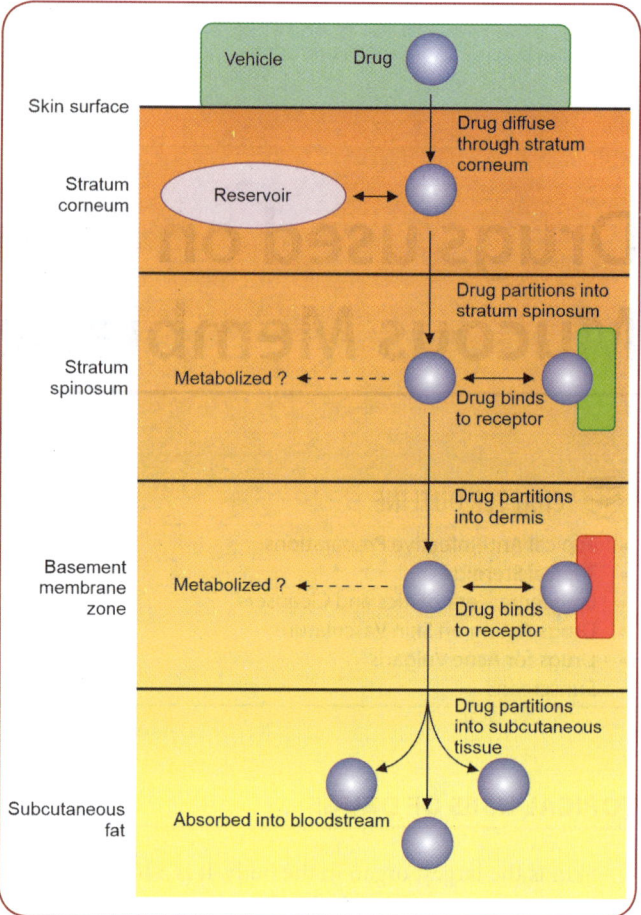

FIG. 8.1: Schematic diagram of percutaneous absorption

- Melanizing agents
- Anti-seborrheics.

The preparations for topical use on eye are as follows:
- Anti-infective eye preparations
- Anti-inflammatory and anti-allergic preparations
- Mydriatics and cycloplegics
- Anti-glaucoma
- Vitreous substitutes
- Tear substitute
- Miscellaneous eye drops

The preparations for topical use in ear and nose are as follows:
- Aural preparations: Antibiotics and antifungals
- Nasal decongestants.

The preparations for topical use in buccal cavity are as follows:
- Mouthwashes
- Gumpaints
- Medicated toothpastes.

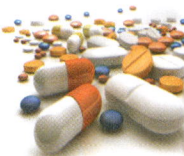

ANTIPRURITICS

These group of drugs are used as antipruritics. Here a separate discussion is not done as these drugs are already discussed in this and other chapters. The antipruritic drugs fall under the following group of drugs:

- Antihistamines
- Topical steroids or oral steroids
- Topical non-steroid creams, such as cooling gels, anti-itching medicines, or capsaicin
- Antidepressant medications
- Immunosuppressant medications, such as cyclosporine A

TOPICAL ANTI-INFECTIVE PREPARATIONS

These drugs are used topically to treat various bacterial, viral, fungal and parasitic infections. For minor infections, topical therapy alone is sufficient, but when these infections occupy a large skin area or show systemic symptoms also, additional oral or systemic treatment is also required.

Various topical anti-infective preparations are given in Tables 8.1 to 8.4.

TABLE 8.1: Topical antibacterial preparations

Drugs	Preparation and Dose	Indications	Special features
Mupirocin	2% w/w ointment and cream TDS for 10–14 days	Minor skin infections, impetigo, foliculitis furuncolosis, cuts and wounds	No cross resistance with other antibiotics is seen
Fusidic acid	2% w/w ointment and cream TDS for 7–10 days	Skin infections by *Staphylococcus* and *Streptococcus* both	Use with caution in pregnancy, pediatric patient and patient with hepatic disease
Nadifloxacin	1% w/w cream BD for 7–10 days	Acne vulgaris, folliculitis, suspected bacterial infections	Caution required in pregnant and pediatric patients
Sisomicin	1% w/w cream BD for 7–10 days	Susceptible bacterial infections	Cover the area with a gauge piece
Neomycin	0.5% w/w cream 1–4 times/day for 7–10 days	Minor skin infections	Commonly indicated in history of hypersensitivity to any aminoglycosides
Gentamicin	0.5% w/w cream 3–4 times/day for 7–10 days	Susceptible bacterial and superficial skin infections	Nephrotoxic potential on excessive use
Silver sulfadiazine	1% w/w cream BD for 7–10 days	Prevention and treatment of 2nd and 3rd degree burns	Caution required in pregnant, pediatric patients and patients allergic to sulfa drugs
Providone iodine	1% gargles, 5% and 10% w/w cream and oint., 5% sol. and powder, 7.5% scrub	Burns, ulcers, boils, furnculosis surgical scrub and for dressing the wounds, etc.	Sensitivity reaction and thyroid dysfunction on prolonged use may occur
Chlorhexidine	1% w/w cream, 1.5% sol., 2–4 times a day	As germicidal skin cleanser	Main use as surgical scrub and wound cleaning
Cetrimide	5% lotion, 15–20% v/v soln. 2–4 times/day	Disinfecing and cleansing wounds, pre-operative skin preparation	Low conc.-bacteriostatic, High conc.- bactericidal
Nitrofurazone	0.2%w/w, once daily	2nd and 3rd degree burns and skin grafting	With caution use in patients with renal disease and G-6-PD deficiency
Retapamulin	1% ointment BD for 5 days	Impetigo	It is not effective against MRSA

TABLE 8.2: Topical antiviral preparations

Drugs	Preparation and Dose	Indications	Special features
Acyclovir	3% and 5% w/w cream. Apply every 3–4 hours for 5–7 days	Initial and recurrent mucosal and cutaneous herpes simplex	Should be used in addition to oral antiviral treatment

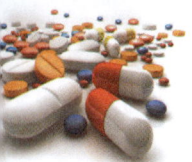

TABLE 8.3: Topical antifungal preparations

Drugs	Preparation and dose	Indications	Special features
Clotrimazole	1% w/w cream and powder,1%w/v lotion, 2% cream. BD for 3–4 weeks	Susceptible fungal infections of skin, hair and vagina. Powder for athlete's foot and ringworms	It should be used along with oral antifungal agents
Miconazole	2% w/w cream, 2% lotion and 2% gel 2% powder BD up to 1 month	Vulvovaginal candidiasis, tinea infection including skin and mucous membrane	Full course of therapy should be done. Avoid direct contact with eyes
Ketoconazole	2% w/w cream, 2% w/w ointment and 2% w/v solution: 1–2 times/day 2 % w/v shampoo: twice weekly for 4 week	Susceptible fungal infection as above	Cautious use while giving terfenadine, astemazole and cisapride may cause cardiac arrhythmias
Oxiconazole nitrate	1% w/w cream and 1% w/v lotion. Twice daily for 2–4 weeks	*Tinea pedis, T. cruris, T. corporis*	Hypersensitivity may occur
Ciclopirox olamine	Cream 1% w/w Solution 8% w/v (only for nails) Twice daily for 4 weeks	*Tinea pedis, T. cruris, T. corporis* Onychomycosis of finger and toe nails	Not to be used below 10 years of age
Econazole	Cream 1% w/w Twice daily for 2–4 weeks	*Tinea pedis, T. cruris, T. corporis.*	
Butenafine	Cream 1% w/w Twice daily for 2–4 weeks	*Tinea pedis:* BD for 1 week. *T. cruris* and *T. corporis:* OD for 2 weeks	Avoid direct contact with eyes
Terbinafine	Cream 1% w/w Lotion 1% w/v Twice daily for 2–4 weeks	*Tinea pedis, T. cruris, T. corporis, Candida albicans,* pitryasis vesicolor	Avoid direct contact with eyes. Alopecia pruritus and contact dermatitis can occur
Tolnaftate	Cream 5 mg/g Solution 10 mg/mL Twice daily for 2–4 weeks	*Tinea pedis, T. cruris, T. corporis.*	Cream not recommended for nail and scalp infection
Quiniodochlor	Cream: 3%, 4% and 8%. BD-TDS for 2–4 weeks	Dermatophytosis, seborrheic dermatitis, pitryasis vesicolor	Has weak antibacterial activity also
Bifonazole	Cream 1% w/w OD for 21 days	*Tinea pedis, T. cruris, T. corporis.* pitryasis vesicolor	Avoid direct contact with eyes

TABLE 8.4: Topical antiparasitic/anti scabies preparations

Drugs	Preparation and dose	Indications	Special features
Gamma benzene hexa chloride [GBHC]	Lotion 1 % w/v Cream 1% w/w	Scabies and pediculosis	Application schedule should be strictly followed Avoid direct contact with eyes and face
Benzyl benzoate	Lotion 125% w/v	Scabies and pediculosis	Application schedule should be strictly followed Avoid direct contact with eyes and face
Crotamiton	Lotion and cream 10% w/w and w/v	Scabies, pruritus and lice infestation	Application schedule should be strictly followed Avoid direct contact with eyes, face and broken skin
Permethrin	Cream 5% w/w Lotion 1% w/v	Scabies, pediculosis	Application schedule should be strictly followed Avoid direct contact with eyes and face

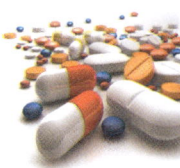

TOPICAL STEROIDS

GENERAL PRINCIPLES OF TOPICAL STEROID THERAPY

- Topical glucocorticoids are used for various dermatological conditions by virtue of their anti-inflammatory, immuno-suppressive and anti-proliferative properties. The topical steroids have been classified according to their potency and efficacy as high efficacy, intermediate efficacy and low efficacy steroids. The potency and efficacy of these steroids depends upon the chemical composition as well as percentage of a given formulation. For example, 0.05% betamethasone dipropionate is more potent than 0.1% betamethasone valerate due to its chemical composition.
- Topical steroids are available as different formulations such as lotion, cream, spray, and ointment. The type of formulation also plays an important role in efficacy.
- Penetration and absorption of steroids varies at different sites.
- The penetration is maximum at axilla, groin, face, scalp and scrotum due to high vascularity and thin skin at these areas. Therefore, we should avoid applying highly potent preparations at these areas to avoid the adverse effects of steroid applications. Mild corticosteroid should be opted for these sites. For infants and young children also, mild corticosteroid should be opted because at this age, the skin is very thin and absorption is maximum.
- The penetration is intermediate at limbs and trunk and low in sole, elbow, palm, knee, etc. Intermediate and high efficacy steroids respectively should be opted for these sites.
- Hyperkeratinized areas have lowest penetration and absorption. These areas require high efficacy steroids either alone or in combination with some keratolytic agent.
- Therapy should not be started with high efficacy steroids; if initiated it should be short term in continuation with mild efficacious steroids.
- The sudden discontinuation of steroids should be avoided. Common topical glucocorticoids are given in Table 8.5.

- **Common indications of topical steroids:** Eczema, psoriasis, otitis externa, lichen simplex and planus, contact dermatitis, seborrhoeic dermatitis and steroid responsive dermatoses.
- **Common contraindications of topical steroids:** Scabies, acne, furunculosis, chicken pox, herpes, untreated fungal and bacterial infections, etc.
- **Common side effects of topical steroids:** Skin atrophy, thinning of epidermis, easy bruising, delayed wound healing, superimposed fungal and bacterial infections and sometimes if used for prolonged periods, systemic side effects can also appear.

EMOLIENTS, KERATOLYTICS AND CLEANSERS

EMOLIENTS

These are bland oily substances which soothen and soften the skin.

TABLE 8.5: Topical glucocorticoids

High efficacy steroids		Intermediate efficacy steroids		Low efficacy steroids	
Drug	Conc.	Drug	Conc.	Drug	Conc.
Betamethasone dipropionate	0.05%	Betamethasone valerate	0.1%	Betamethasone valerate	0.01%
Halobetasol propionate	0.05%	Mometasone	0.1%	Methylprednisolone acetate	1.0%
Clobetasol propionate	0.05%	Hydrocortisone valerate	0.2%	Hydrocortisone	0.25–2.5%
Fluocinonide	0.05%	Fluticasone	0.05	Prednisolone	0.5%
Desoximetasone	0.25%	Prednicarbate	0.1–0.25%	Dexamethasone	0.1%
Triamcinolone acetonide	0.5%	Triamcinolone	0.05–0.1%	Triamcinolone acetonide	0.025%
Fluocinolone acetonide	0.2%	Fluocinolone acetonide	0.025%	Fluocinolone acetonide	0.01%
Beclomethasine dipropionate	0.025%				

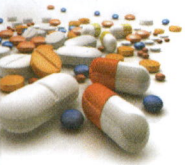

Indications

They form an occlusive film over the skin, prevent evaporation of moisture and restore elasticity of cracked and dry skin. They are used as vehicle for topically applied medicaments.

Examples: Coconut oil, olive oil, vegetable oil, coco-butter, soft-paraffin, hard-paraffin and liquid paraffin.

KERATOLYTICS

Keratolytics are the agents, which dissolve the intracellular substance in the horny layer of skin. The epidermal cells swell, soften and then desquamate.

Indications

These drugs are commonly indicated in hyperkeratotic lesions like corns, warts, psoriasis, chronic dermatitis, ringworm, athlete's foot, etc.

Examples

Salicylic acid, Resorcinol, Urea.

CLEANSERS

These are soap free and lipid free emolient lotions. After application, they form an emulsifying complex on the skin. The cleaning effect on the skin is obtained by the emulsifying complex.

Indications

Oily skin, skin damaged by adverse weather conditions, patients suffering from ichthyosis.

Preparation and Dose

Cetyl alcohol 2.6% w/w and stearyl alcohol 0.26% w/w. It should be applied in the morning and in the evening with gentle swirling with fingers. Remove it gently with cotton or damp cloth or rinse with water after 5–10 minutes.

DRUGS ACTING ON SKIN VASCULATURE

MINOXIDIL

It is a vasodilator. It increases cutaneous blood flow and stimulates the resting hair follicles.

Indications

Androgenic alopecia and Alopecia areata.

Preparation and Dose

Available as 2% and 5% w/v solution and spray form. It should be applied twice daily on bald area of the scalp for minimum 4 months. Continuous application is required to maintain the hair growth.

Side Effects

Headache, edema, chest pain, hypotension, etc.

HEPARIN TOPICAL

It is an anticoagulant and useful in thromboembolic conditions.

Indications

Hematomas, superficial thrombophlebitis, tenosynovitis, sprain and bruises.

Preparation and Dose

It is available in cream, gel, and lotion forms. It is applied twice/thrice daily with gentle massage.

Side Effects

Hypersensitivity may occur.

DRUGS FOR ACNE VULGARIS

- Acne vulgaris is a skin disease of sebaceous follicles of face and neck.
- There is increased production of sebum by the sebaceous follicles due to hyperandrogenic stimulation, which is infected by bacteria and yeast (*Propionibacterium acnes, Staphylococcus. epidermidis, Pityrosporum ovale*).
- It is most commonly seen in adolescent girls and boys.

The management of acne vulgaris includes:

Application of topical anti-acne agents, oral drugs or a combination of both. A few commonly used drugs are as follows:

- **Retinoic acid and derivatives, isotretinoin, adapalene, tazarotene**
- **Benzoyl peroxide**
- **Azelaic acid**
- **Topical antibiotics (clindamycin, erythromycin, metronidazole, sodium sulfacetamide).**
- **Topical steroids**

Drugs for acne should be applied strictly locally on acne only avoiding normal skin.

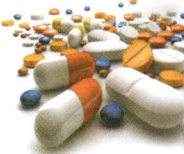

RETINOIC ACID AND DERIVATIVES

- Retinoic acid is also called *all-trans*-retinoic acid and is an effective topical treatment for acne vulgaris.
- On topical application, <10% of retinoic acid is absorbed in systemic circulation. It is metabolized by liver and excreted through kidney and bile.
- **Mechanism of action:** It is comedolytic in action. It decreases cohesion between epidermal cells and increases the epidermal cell turnover. It leads to expulsion of open comedones and the transformation of closed comedones into open ones.
- **Preparation and dose:** To startwith, the low concentration cream (0.025%) is applied once daily and if tolerated well, followed by high concentration cream (0.05%) for a period of 6–10 weeks.
- The most common side effects of topical retinoic acid therapy are erythema and dryness of skin, which occurs during first few weeks of use and resolve with continued therapy.

ISOTRETINOIN

- Isotretinoin is an analog and synthetic derivative of vitamin A. It is given orally for various dermatologic diseases. It is well absorbed orally with plasma t ½ is 10–20 hours.
- It reduces sebum production by inhibiting the sebaceous gland size and function.
- It is indicated in severe cystic acne in a dose of 0.5–1 mg/kg BD for 4–5 months.
- Some other possible uses are in the treatment and prevention of skin cancer, to treat actinic keratosis, oral leucoplakia and other premalignant skin lesions.
- The common side effects are itching and dryness of skin, while pseudotumor cerebri, anorexia, alopecia, muscle and joint pains are rare.
- Being highly teratogenic drug, it is contraindicated in pregnancy.

ADAPALENE

- It is similar to retinoic acid for treating acne.
- It is available as a 0.1% gel, cream, or lotion and a 0.3% gel form.
- It should be applied once daily at bedtime after washing the affected area.
- It is stable with benzoyl peroxide and can be combined with it.
- It is most effective in patients with mild to moderate acne vulgaris and is less irritant than tretinoin.

Tazarotene

It is available as a 0.1% gel and cream form. It should be applied once daily in the evening. It is used to treat mild to moderately severe facial acne and psoriasis.

BENZOYL PEROXIDE

- Benzoyl peroxide possesses comedolytic, keratolytic and antimicrobial activity against *P. acnes*. It is most effective topical agent for the treatment of acne vulgaris.
- It penetrates the stratum corneum or follicular openings and liberates nascent oxygen, which kills the anaerobic bacteria.
- It is available in 2.5% and 5% concentration in cream and gel form.
- **The method of application:** Apply and leave on skin for 15 minutes the first evening. Increase the length of exposure by 15 minutes until application is tolerated for 2 hours without burning sensation. Then, it may be left overnight for further applications.
- It is well tolerated with mild local irritation, dryness of skin and erythema.

AZELAIC ACID

It is obtained from *Pityrosporum ovale*. It is available as 20% cream or 15% gel and is applied twice daily for 4–6 weeks. It is effective in inflammatory acne and melasma. The common side effects are mild irritation, redness, and dryness of skin.

TOPICAL ANTIBIOTICS ESPECIALLY USEFUL IN ACNE VULGARIS

- Many systemic as well as topical antibiotics are used for the management of acne vulgaris.
- Currently, clindamycin, erythromycin, metronidazole, nadifloxacin, fusidic acid and sulfacetamide are used to treat acne.

Refer to Table 8.6 for topical antibiotics for acne vulgaris

TABLE 8.6: Topical antibiotics for acne vulgaris

Drugs	Dose	Special feature
Clindamycin	1% gel	The common side effects are local irritation, burning sensation
Erythromycin	2% lotion and ointment	The common side effects are local irritation, dryness and burning sensation of skin
Metronidazole	1% gel	The common side effects are local irritation, dryness and burning sensation of skin.
Sulfacetamide	4% lotion and 10% face wash	Used in acne vulgaris and acne rosacea Contraindicated in patient with history of hypersensitivity to sulfonamides
Nadifloxacin	1% cream	It is a newer agent for inflamed acne and folliculitis
Fusidic acid	2% ointment and cream	It is also used in boil, foliculitis, psychosis barbae and other cutaneous infections

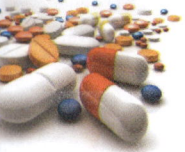

TOPICAL STEROIDS IN ACNE VULGARIS

Commonly, mild efficacy topical steroids in combination with topical antibacterial agent are used to reduce the inflammation and to treat acne.

SUNSCREENS

- Sunscreens are the topical medications that protect the skin from harmful effects of sunlight by absorbing ultraviolet light.
- The sunscreens are of two types: Chemical and physical sunscreens.
- The most commonly used **chemical sunscreen** agents are:
  - Para-aminobenzoic acid (PABA)
  - Benzophenones (Oxybenzone, Dioxybenzone, and Sulisobenzone)
  - Dibenzoylmethanes
- PABA is most effective against erythema and sunburn associated with sun exposure and tanning (Table 8.7).
- **Benzophenones** (oxybenzone, dioxybenzone, and sulisobenzone): They are used to treat erythema but are less effective than PABA.
- **Dibenzoylmethanes:** They are used to treat polymorphous light eruption, cutaneous lupus erythematosus and drug-induced photosensitivity.

PHYSICAL SUNSCREENS

- Titanium dioxide, zinc oxide petroleum jelly and calamine are opaque substances used to protect the skin from harmful UV rays. They are also called 'sun shades' and have to be applied as a thick lotion/cream, which may be cosmetically disagreeable.

Sun Protection Factor (SPF) (Table 8.8)
- The efficacy of sunscreen is quantified by its SPF.
- It measures sunscreen protection from UV-B rays, which is responsible for sunburn and skin cancer.
- It does not measure how well a sunscreen will protect from UVA rays, which are also damaging and dangerous.
- SPF-15 or SPF-30 is recommended as sunscreen. Higher SPFs do not give much more protection.
- Once applied, the sunscreen protects skin for 80-90 minutes. If the sun-exposure is going to remain for a longer duration, repeated application is required.

TABLE 8.7: Drugs efficacy according to UV rays wavelength

Ultraviolet rays	Wavelength	Drugs effective
Ultraviolet-A (UVA)	320–400 nm	• Dibenzoylmethanes • Benzophenones
Ultraviolet-B (UVB)	280–320 nm	• P-aminobenzoic acid (PABA) • Benzophenones
Ultraviolet-C (UVC)	100–280 nm	• Benzophenones

TABLE 8.8: The SPF (Sun protection factor) scale

Sunscreen with SPF	Protection against UVB
SPF 15	93%
SPF 30	97%
SPF 50	98%

Indications

Chemical sunscreens are used as adjuncts in vitiligo therapy, drug induced phototoxicity and to facilitate tanning while preventing sunburn. There is some evidence that they can prevent skin cancer and premature ageing of skin.

DEMELANIZING AGENTS

HYDROQUINONE, MONOBENZONE, AND MEQUINOL

- These drugs are used for the reduction hyperpigmentation of the skin.
- These are indicated in melasma and chloasma of pregnancy.
- Hydroquinone inhibits the tyrosinase enzyme; hence the biosynthesis of melanin is inhibited.
- Monobenzone has anti-melanocytic action as it causes permanent destruction of melanocytes.
- Topical application of hydroquinone and mequinol cause temporary lightening of skin color, while monobenzone lead to irreversible depigmentation.
- **Hydroquinone:** Available as 2%, 4% cream, solution and ointment to be applied two times daily.
- **Monobenzone:** Available as 5% lotion and 20% ointment to be applied 3 times daily.
- **Azelaic acid:** Available as 10% and 20% cream to be applied 2 times daily.
- **Glycolic acid:** Available as 10-20% lotion to be applied two times daily.

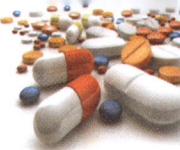

MELANIZING AGENTS

(Psoralen, Trioxsalen and Methoxsalen)
These are the drugs that increase sensitivity of skin to solar radiations (UV) and promote repigmentation of hypopigmented, depigmented and vitiligenous area. These drugs stimulate melanocytes on photo activation and induce their proliferation also.

PSORALEN

- **Topical therapy:** The solution/ointment is carefully applied on the small well defined vitiliginous lesion—which is then exposed to sunlight for 1 minute and then occluded by bandage or sun screen ointment. Weekly treatment with longer exposures is given. Pigmentation usually begins to appear after a few weeks; months are needed for satisfactory results. Then periodic maintenance treatment may be needed. This therapy should be undertaken only under direct supervision of physician because longer exposure causes burning and blistering.
- **Oral therapy:** The drug is given orally in the morning in a dose of 0.3–0.6 mg/kg (usually 20 mg). After 2 hours of an oral dose of a psoralen, skin is exposed to sunlight (or artificial UV light), initially for 15 minutes—gradually increasing to 30 minutes over days. The therapy is given on alternate days.
- Eyes, lips and other normally pigmented areas should be protected during exposure to sunlight.
- It is available as 5 and 10 mg tablet, 0.25% solution and ointment and 1% ointment.

TRIOXSALEN AND METHOXSALEN

Trioxsalen and methoxsalen are synthetic psoralens, which are used in combination with photochemotherapy for repigmentation of depigmented macules of vitiligo. They are combined with ultraviolet rays–A (UVA) ranging from 320–400 nm.

DECAPEPTIDE (BASIC FIBROBLAST GROWTH FACTOR)

It is applied locally and stimulates the multiplication of melanocytes. It is available as lotion. Method of applying: Apply 1–2 hours before going to bed, expose to sunlight next morning for 15 minutes. It has good results in vitiligo treatment.

ANTI-SEBORRHEIC AGENTS

- These agents are effective in seborrheic dermatitis.
- Seborrheic dermatitis affects areas rich in sebaceous glands (scalp, face, trunk) and is characterized by erythematous, scaling lesions.
- Dandruff is the commonest complaint.
- Drugs used are enlisted in Table 8.9.

PREPARATIONS FOR TOPICAL USE ON EYE

Drugs used for topical use on eye are given in Tables 8.10 to 8.16.

TABLE 8.9: Anti-seborrheic agents

Drug	Dose and preparation	Special features
Selenium sulfide	2.5% lotion or shampoo Apply on scalp twice weekly and then as required	• It is an anti-keratolytic and fungicidal to *P. ovale* • Relapse is seen in ≥50% individuals after discontinuation of therapy
Zinc pyrithione	1% shampoo Apply on scalp twice weekly and then as required	• Reduces epidermal turnover and inhibits *P. ovale* • Usually combined with ketoconazole
Ketaconazole	2% cream/shampoo/scalp gel Apply on scalp twice weekly and then as required	• Ketoconazole (KTZ) is most effective against *P. ovale* • It has better efficacy with negligible side effects
Corticosteroids	2% cream/shampoo Apply on scalp twice weekly and then as required	• It is highly effective against seborrheic dermatitis including dandruff • Relapse is high after discontinuation of therapy • Prolonged use may lead to purpura and poor healing

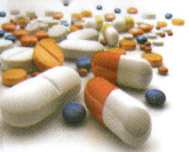

TABLE 8.10: Anti-infective eye preparations

Drug	Preparation and dose	Indications
Sulfacetamide	Eye drops: 10,20, 30% 1–2 drops to be apply QID	Trachoma blepharitis, conjunctivitis, ophthalmia neonatorum, for prophylaxis of ocular infection after burn and injury, before and after ocular surgery
Chloramphenicol	Ointment and eye drops: 1%, 0.5% w/v 1–2 drops to be apply TDS- QID	Corneal ulcer, bacterial conjunctivitis, trachoma, ocular infections
Gentamicin	Eye drops: 0.3% w/v 1–2 drops to be apply TDS- QID	External bacterial infection of eye and lid, pre- or post-operative ocular surgery
Tobramycin	Eye drops and ointment: 0.3% w/v 1–2 drops to be apply QID	Ocular bacterial infection
Neomycin	Eye drops: 0.1% w/v 1–2 drops to be apply QID	Ocular bacterial infection
Ciprofloxacin	Eye drops and ointment: 0.3% w/v 1–2 drops to be apply TDS-QID	Bacterial conjunctivitis, keratitis, corneal ulcer and pre- or post-operative ocular surgery
Ofloxacin	Eye drops: 0.3% w/v 1–2 drops to be apply TDS-QID	Bacterial conjunctivitis, blepharitis, bacterial corneal ulcer and pre or post-operative ocular surgery
Moxifloxacin	Eye drops and ointment: 0.5% w/v 1 drop to be apply TDS-QID	Bacterial conjunctivitis, keratitis, corneal ulcer and pre or post-operative ocular surgery
Polymyxin-B	Ointment: 5000 IU Eye drops: 5000/10000 IU 1–2 drops to be apply TDS-QID	Superficial ocular infection
Acyclovir	Eye drops and ointment: 0.3% w/v 1–2 drops to be apply 5 times a day	Herpes simplex keratits
Fluconazole	Eye drops: 0.3% w/v 1–2 drops 4 times daily	Fungal infection of eye

TABLE 8.11: Anti-inflammatory preparations

Drug	Preparation and dose	Indications
Steroidal anti-inflammatory agents		
Dexamethasone	Eye drops: 0.1% w/v 1–2 drops 4-6 times daily	Non-infected steroid responsive inflammatory eye conditions such as uveitis, marginal keratitis, allergic conjunctivitis and scleritis
Betamethasone	Eye drops: 0.5% w/v 1–2 drops 4–6 times daily	Same as above
Hydrocortisone	Eye drops: 0.25% w/v 1–2 drops 4–6 times daily	Same as above
Prednisolone	Eye drops: 0.1% w/v 1–2 drops 4–6 times daily	Same as above
Fluorometholone	Eye drops: 0.1% and 0.25% w/v Instill one drop in to the conjunctival sac QID. During the initial 12–40 hours, the dosage may be increased to one application every 4 hours	Steroid responsive inflammation of the palpebral and bulber conjunctiva, cornea and anterior segment of eye
Triamcinolone	Eye drops: 0.1% w/v 1 drop 2–3 times daily	Ocular inflammation
Loteprednol	Eye drops: 0.05% w/v 1 drop 4 times daily	Seasonal allergic conjunctivitis

Contd...

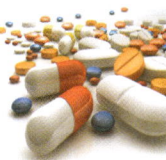

Non-steroidal anti-inflammatory agents		
Flurbiprofen	Eye drops: 0.03%, 0.3% w/v 1–2 drops every ½ hourly, 2–3 hours before ocular surgery to prevent intraoperative miosis	Postlaser and post-operative anterior segment inflammation of eye
Ketorolac	Eye drops: 0.5% w/v 1 drop to the affected eye	Seasonal allergic conjunctivitis
Diclofenac	Eye drops: 0.1%, 0.2% w/v 1 drop every ½ hourly, 2–3 hours before and 3 hour after ocular surgery	Post-operative inflammation after cataract surgery. Also used to prevent miosis and other inflammatory condition of eye
Nepafenac	Eye drops: 0.1% w/v 1 drop 3 times a day for 3 weeks	Post-operative pain and inflammation after cataract surgery

TABLE 8.12: Anti-allergic preparations

Drug	Preparation and dose	Indications
Sodium cromoglycate	Eye drops: 2% w/v 1–2 drops 4 times a day	Keratoconjunctivitis, allergic vernal heratoconjunctivits and hay fever
Azelastine	Eye drops: 0.05% w/v 1–2 drops 4 times a day	Ocular allergy
Olopatadine	Eye drops: 0.1% w/v 1–2 drops twice daily	Seasonal allergic conjunctivitis
Ketotifen	Eye drops: 0.025% w/v 1–2 drops 2–3 times a day	Ocular allergy

TABLE 8.13: Mydriatics and cycloplegics

Drug	Preparation and dose	Indications
Atropine	Eye drops: 1% w/v	Allergic conjunctivitis, corneal burn, uveitis, refraction in children, keratitis, suppression amblyopia, pre- and post-operative use after surgery
Homatropine	Eye drops: 2% w/v	Corneal burn, uveitis, refraction, post-operative use after surgery
Tropicamide	Eye drops: 0.8, 1% w/v 1 Drop 6–8 times a day	Pre- and post-operatively, for mydriasis in diagnostic procedure
Cyclopentolate	Eye drops: 0.5, 1% w/v	Refraction, retinal examination and used in post-operatively
Phenylephrine	Eye drops: 5%, 10% w/v	Ocular examination, vasoconstriction in uveitis, pupil dilation, surgery, ptosis-Horner's or Raeder's syndrome

TABLE 8.14: Anti-glaucoma preparation

Drug	Preparation and dose	Indications
Pilocarpine	Eye drops: 0.5, 1%,2%, 4% w/v 1–2 drops instill in to conjuctivial sac	Glaucoma
Carbachol	Eye drops: 1.5% w/v 1–2 drops instill in to conjuctivial sac	Glaucoma
Dipivefrine	Eye drops: 0.1% w/v 1–2 drops instill in to conjuctivial sac	Chronic open angle glaucoma
Timolol	Eye drops: 0.25%, 0.55% w/v 1 drop twice daily	Chronic open angle glaucoma, aphakic glaucoma, secondary glaucoma
Betaxolol	Eye drops: 0.25%, 0.55% w/v 1 drop twice daily	Chronic open angle glaucoma
Levobunolol	Eye drops: 0.5% w/v 1–2 drops once daily	Chronic open angle glaucoma, ocular hypertension

189

Contd...

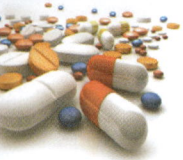

Drug	Preparation and dose	Indications
Acetazolamide	Tablet/capsule: 250 mg 1–4 tablets daily in divided dosage	Chronic open angle glaucoma
Dorzolamide	Eye drops: 2% w/v 1 drop thrice daily or twice daily with other adjunctive therapy	Ocular hypertension, open angle glaucoma
Brimonidine	Eye drops: 0.15%, 0.2% w/v 1 drop twice daily	Ocular hypertension, open angle glaucoma
Apraclonidine	Eye drops: 0.5%, 1% w/v One drop of solution should be starting instilled in the schedule operative eye one hour before anterior segment laser surgery and second drop to the same eye instilled immediately after surgery	For control of intraocular tension following anterior segment laser surgery
Latanoprost	Eye drops: 0.005% w/v 1 drop once daily in the evening	Ocular hypertension, open angle glaucoma
Travoprost	Eye drops: 0.004% w/v 1 drop once daily in the evening	Ocular hypertension, chronic open angle glaucoma

TABLE 8.15: Vitreous substitutes

Drug	Preparation and dose	Indications
Polydimethyl siloxane	Injection: 10 mL	Complex retinal detachment, severe diabetic tractional retinal detachment, giant tear and traumatic retinal detachment

TABLE 8.16: Tear substitutes

Drug	Preparation and dose	Indications
Hydroxyl propyl methyl cellulose	Eye drops: 0.7% w/v 1–2 drops thrice daily	Anterior segment surgical procedure (cataract and IOL implantation) Also use in gonioscopy for glaucoma and artificial tear
Carboxy methyl cellulose	Eye drops: 1% w/v. 1-2 drops thrice daily.	Anterior segment surgical procedure (cataract and IOL implantation) Also use in gonioscopy for glaucoma and artificial tear

PREPARATIONS FOR TOPICAL USE IN EAR AND NOSE

Refer to Tables 8.17 and 8.18 for preparations for topical use in ear and nose

TABLE 8.17: Aural preparations

Drug	Preparation and dose	Indications
Chloramphenicol	Ear drops and solution: 5% w/v Adult: 2–3 drops 3–4 times a day Children: 1–2 drops 3 times a day	Otitis externa, chronic otits media, pre and post aural or mastoid surgery
Gentamicin	Ear drops and Solution: 0.3% w/v 2–3 drops 3–4 times a day	Otitis externa and ear infections
Ciprofloxacin	Ear drops: 0.3% w/v 2–3 drops 2–3 hourly as required	Otitis media and externa
Ofloxacin	Ear drops: 1% w/v 2–3 drops 3–4 times a day	Fungal infection of external ear

Contd...

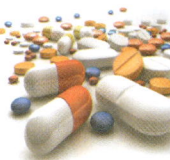

Drug	Preparation and dose	Indications
Neomycin	Ear drops: 3400 U 2–3 drops 3–4 times a day	Otitis externa and ear infections
Polymyxin-B	Ointment: 5000 IU Eye drops: 5000/10000 IU 1–2 drops to be apply TDS-QID	Superficial ocular infection
Cotrimazole	Ear drops: 1% w/v 2–3 drops 3–4 times a day	Fungal infection of external ear
Sodium fluoride	Tablet: 20 mg 1 tablet after meals, twice daily for 6 month- 2 years	Otosclerosis, conductive deafness

Topical steroids like Betamethasone, dexamethasone, prednisolone, etc. are available in combination with above AMAs and lignocaine also. These are to be used as per the diagnosis and prescription by the ENT specialist only.

CERUMENOLYTICS (Ear wax dissolving agents)

Paradiachlorobenzine 2% w/v + benzocaine 2.5% w/v + chlorbutol 5% w/v + terpentoin oil 15% w/v: *This combination is used to soften the impacted wax and facilitate its removal from the ear. Instillate 5-10 drops.*

TABLE 8.18: Nasal drops

Drug	Preparation and dose	Indications
Xylometazoline	Nasal drops: 0.05,1% w/v Adult and children >6 years: Instill 2–3 drops into each nostril BD or TDS Children <6 years: Instill 2–3 drops into each nostril BD or TDS, duration not to exceed >7 days	Nasal congestion
Oximetazoline	Nasal drops: 0.01, 0.025, 0.05, 0.1% w/v Adult and children >6 years: Instill 2–3 drops into each nostril BD or TDS Children <6 years: Instill 2–3 drops into each nostril BD or TDS, duration not to exceed >7 days	Nasal congestion
Sodium chloride	Nasal drops: 0.65% w/v Instill 2–3 drops into each nostril BD or TDS	Nasal congestion
Phenylephrine	Nasal drops: 0.25% w/v. Instill 4–5 drops into each nostril every 4-6 hours	Nasal congestion
Naphazoline	Nasal drops: 0.01% w/v Instill 2–3 drops into each nostril every 4–6 hours	Nasal congestion
Sodium chromoglycate	Nasal drops: 2% w/v. Instill 2–3 drops into each nostril every 8/12 hours Inhaler: 2 mg/MDI, BD/TDS Spray: 2.8 mg/dose, BD/TDS.	Allergic rhinitis
Ephedrine	Nasal drops: 0.075, 0.5% w/v Instill 2–3 drops into each nostril every twice/thrice a day	Nasal congestion
Fluticasone nasal spray	Nasal spray: 0.05% w/v Use 1–2 spray in each nostril	Allergic/inflammatory nasal congestion
Budesonide nasal spray	Nasal spray: 100 µg Use 1–2 spray in each nostril	Allergic/inflammatory nasal congestion
Mometasone nasal spray	Nasal spray: 50 µg Use 1–2 spray in each nostril	Allergic/inflammatory nasal congestion
Azelastine nasal spray	Nasal spray and solution: 0.1% Use 1–2 spray in each nostril	Allergic nasal congestion

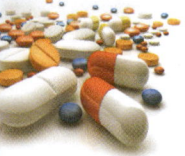

PREPARATIONS FOR TOPICAL USE IN BUCCAL CAVITY

Refer to Table 8.19 for preparations for topical use in buccal cavity.

TABLE 8.19: Oro pharyngeal preparations

Drug	Preparation and dose	Indications
Chlorhexidine	Mouthwash: 0.12, 0.2, 0.25% v/v	Stomatitis, tonsillitis, gingivitis and oral bacterial infection of mouth
Povidine iodine	Mouthwash: 1% w/v	Stomatitis, tonsillitis, gingivitis and oral candidal or bacterial infection of mouth
Triamcinolone	Mouthwash: 0.1% w/v	Stomatitis, tonsillitis, gingivitis and oral candidal or bacterial infection of mouth
Benzocaine	Mouthwash: 2.7% w/v	Stomatitis, tonsillitis, gingivitis and oral candidal or bacterial infection of mouth
Benzydamine	Mouthwash: 0.15% w/v	Stomatitis, tonsillitis, gingivitis and oral candidal or bacterial infection of mouth
Sodium fluoride	Mouthwash: 0.2% w/v	Stomatitis, tonsillitis, gingivitis and oral candidal or bacterial infection of mouth
Mandl's paint	Iodine + potassium iodide + glycerin	Stomatitis, tonsillitis, gingivitis and oral candidal or bacterial infection of mouth
Tannic acid	A component of gum paint available as 2–20% w/v	Stomatitis, tonsillitis, gingivitis and oral candidal or bacterial infection of mouth
Potassium nitrate	Toothpaste: 5% w/w Oral solution/rinse: 3% w/v	Stomatitis, tonsillitis, gingivitis and oral candidal or bacterial infection of mouth

 ## Nursing Implications

- Universal precautions should be strictly followed during topical application of different drugs.
- Every nurse should be well aware of the proper technique of topical applications of drugs on skin, eye, ear, nose, etc. Nurse should not hesitate to learn the procedures from their seniors.
- Nurse should educate the patients that if any irritation occurs on application of topical cream or ointment; they should immediately discontinue the drugs and report to the physician.
- Nurse should educate the patients with history of photosensitivity, to wear protective clothes or apply sunscreen before going outdoors.
- Nurse should wear gloves and mask during dressings of burn patients.
- Nurse should check the expiry date of all the medicines.

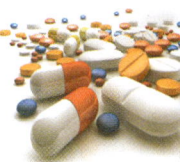

Assess Yourself

Long and Short Answer Questions

1. Write down the methods to facilitate the absorption of topical applications on skin.
2. Classify topical antifungal agents. Describe ketoconazole.
3. What are the anti-seborrheic agents? Describe their method of application.
4. Classify topical steroidal agents and their contraindications.
5. Write short notes on:
   a. Keratolytic agents   b. Benzoyl peroxide   c. Isotretinoin   d. Sunscreen
   e. Psoralen   f. Ivermectin

Multiple Choice Questions

1. Which of the following is not a contraindication of topical steroids?
   a. Scabies   b. Psoriasis   c. Herpes   d. Chicken pox

2. Which of the following is not a keratolytic agent?
   a. Salicylic acid   b. Lactic acid   c. Ethacrynic acid   d. Glycolic acid

3. Which of the following drugs is contraindicated in pregnancy?
   a. Azelaic acid   b. Isotretinoin   c. Adapalena   d. Benzoyl peroxide

4. Which of the following is indicated in otitis media?
   a. Ciprofloxacin   b. Prednisolone   c. Cotrimazole   d. Sodium fluoride

5. Which of the following is not indicated in seasonal allergic conjunctivitis?
   a. Triamcinolone   b. Loteprednol   c. Ketorolac   d. Olopatadine

Answer Key

1. b.   **2.** c.   **3.** b.   **4.** a.   **5.** a.

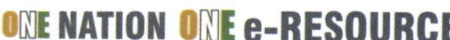

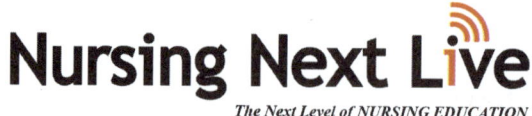
Nursing Next Live
The Next Level of NURSING EDUCATION

PREPARE ANYTIME, ANYWHERE FOR
Nursing Officer/Staff Nurse/CHO/ Nursing Undergraduate & Postgraduate Exams

Undergraduate Packs
By **THE MASTERMINDS**

Undergraduate Pack - 1st Year

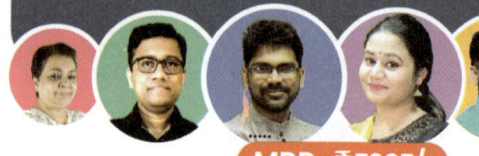

MRP ₹ 7997/-
Validity: 18 months

What all you will get

Main Subjects	Video Duration	No. of Questions
Anatomy	60+ Hours	600+ Qs
Physiology	60+ Hours	600+ Qs
Biochemistry & Nutrition	50+ Hours	500+ Qs
Microbiology	50+ Hours	500+ Qs
Fundamentals of Nursing	200+ Hours	400+ Qs

Bonus Subjects:- Computers & Psychology

Undergraduate Pack - 2nd Year

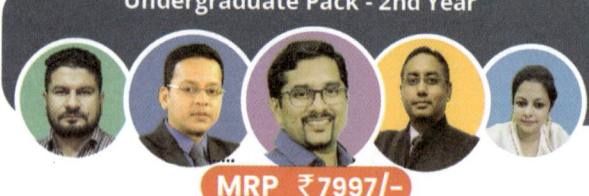

MRP ₹ 7997/-
Validity: 18 months

What all you will get

Main Subjects	Video Duration	No. of Questions
Pharmacology	50+ Hours	800+ Qs
MSN - Medicine	90+ Hours	900+ Qs
MSN - Surgery	50+ Hours	600+ Qs
Community Health Nursing	90+ Hours	900+ Qs
Sociology	40+ Hours	250+ Qs

What all you will get

Main Subjects	Video Duration	No. of Questions
Pediatric Nursing	80+ Hours	900+ Qs
Midwifery & Obstetrical Nursing	100+ Hours	1000+ Qs
MSN - Medicine	90+ Hours	900+ Qs
MSN - Surgery	50+ Hours	600+ Qs
Mental Health Nursing	90+ Hours	900+ Qs
Community Health Nursing	90+ Hours	900+ Qs
Nursing Research & Statistics	35+ Hours	400+ Qs

Bonus Subjects:- Nursing Managment & Nursing Education

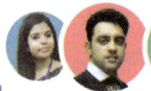 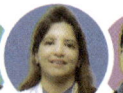 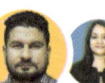

MRP ₹ 12992/-
Validity: 24 months

Special Features

- Handwritten Notes of Videos in PDF Format
- Monthly Mega Assessment Tests
- Best Guidance & Support
- IBQs/VBQs Discussion Videos of above mentioned Subjects
- Monthly Live Doubt Session/Live Classes/Live Webinar by MM Faculty
- Get your query directly resolved by MM faculty

Scan the QR Code to download the app

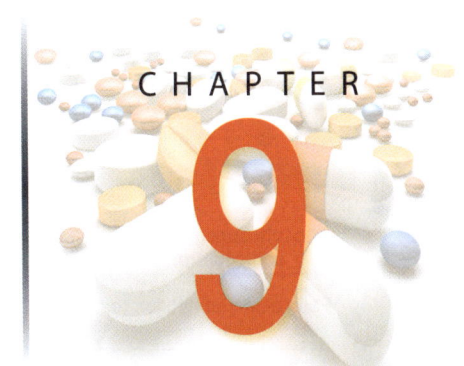

Drugs Acting on Nervous System

CHAPTER 9

 CHAPTER OUTLINE

- Analgesics or Non-steroidal Anti-inflammatory Drugs (NSAIDs)
- Tranquilizers or Anxiolytic Drugs and Hypnotics
- General and Local Anesthetics
- Gases (Oxygen, Nitrous Oxide, Carbon Dioxide)
- Cholinergic and Anticholinergic Drugs
- Adrenergic System and Drugs

- Skeletal Muscle Relaxants
- Antipsychotics or Major Tranquilizers or Neuroleptic Drugs
- Anticonvulsants
- Antidepressants
- Central Nervous System Stimulants

ANALGESICS OR NON-STEROIDAL ANTI-INFLAMMATORY DRUGS (NSAIDs)

The word analgesic is derived from Greek word *an–without + algesic–pain*. Meaning *without pain*.

- By definition, analgesics are the drugs having the property to provide relief from pain.
- These drugs provide symptomatic relief from pain, with or without any therapeutic effect on the basic pathology of the pain.
- Management of pain is one of the clinical medicine's greatest challenges.

> Pain is defined as an unpleasant sensation that can be either acute or chronic and is a consequence of complex neurochemical processes in the peripheral and central nervous systems (CNS). It is subjective, and the clinician must rely on the patient's perception and description of pain.

Depending upon their site of action, analgesic drugs have been divided broadly into two types:

1. **Non-narcotic or Non-opioid analgesics or Non-steroidal Anti-Inflammatory Drugs (NSAIDS):** These drugs act at peripheral level pain mechanisms to provide the pain relief.

2. **Narcotics or opioids analgesics:** All opioid analgesics act by binding to the specific opioid receptors in the CNS to produce analgesic effects. Although, the opioids have a broad range of effects, their primary usefulness is in providing relief from intense pain, whether that pain results from surgery, injury, or chronic disease.

NON-STEROIDAL ANTI-INFLAMMATORY DRUGS (NSAIDS)

Common Properties of NSAIDs

- Non-steroidal anti-inflammatory drugs (NSAIDs) are having analgesic, antipyretic and anti-inflammatory actions mostly at peripheral level and to a lesser extent in the CNS also. In CNS, they have a role in raising the pain threshold.
- Unlike opioid analgesics, these drugs neither have a CNS depressant effect nor physical/psychological dependence or addiction of any type, hence known as **non-narcotic or non-opioid analgesics**.
- None of these drugs is steroid in nature, hence known as **non-steroidal anti-inflammatory drugs**.
- Most of these agents act by inhibiting prostaglandin (PG) synthesis except a few drugs, which have additional mechanisms too.

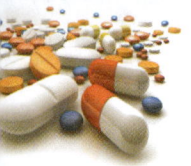

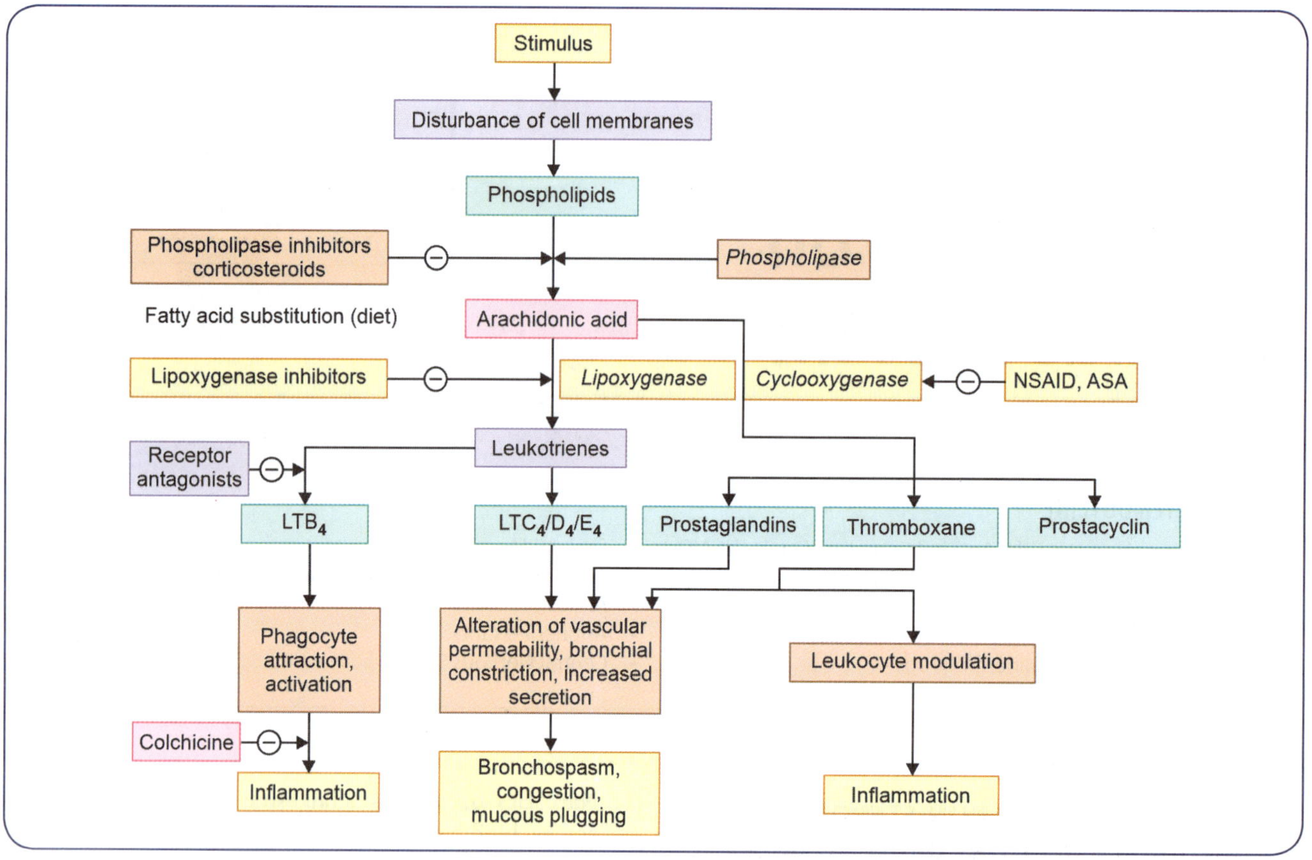

FIG. 9.1: Prostaglandins and leukotrienes synthesis pathway with the site of action of some related drugs

Abbreviations: ASA, acetyl salicylic acid; NSAID, non-steroidal anti-inflammatory drugs

Whenever a tissue injury occurs by any mechanical, chemical or biological stimuli, the phospholipase-A enzyme gets activated and converts the membrane phospholipids into arachidonic acid. This arachidonic acid is converted into PGs, prostacyclins and thromboxane by cyclooxygenase (COX) enzyme through cyclooxygenase pathway and into leukotrienes by lipooxygenase enzyme through lipooxygenase pathway (Fig. 9.1).

- PGs have two major actions:
  1. They are mediators of inflammation, stimulate sensory nerve endings and cause pain.
  2. They also allow the movement of other inflammatory mediators like histamine and bradykinins at the site of inflammation and aggravate the pain.
- The main mechanism involved in providing pain relief requires inhibition of formation of PGs and other inflammatory mediators, which can be achieved by inhibiting the different enzymes involved in their synthesis.
- Therefore, it can be achieved by inhibition of Phospholipase A, COX enzyme and LOX enzyme, which arrests the further pathway of events.

- Phospholipase-A is inhibited by steroids.
- COX enzymes (COX-1 and COX-2) are inhibited by different NSAIDs.
- LOX enzyme is inhibited by Zileuton.
- COX and LOX both are inhibited by Licofelone.

In relation to NSAIDs, COX enzymes need a detailed study.

- There are two types of cyclooxygenase enzymes, namely COX-1 and COX-2.
  1. COX-1: It is constitutively present in most of the cells and is known as housekeeping enzyme.
  2. COX-2: It is inducible in the cells which are affected by inflammatory processes.
     Recently a spliced variant of COX-1 has been identified and named as COX-3 enzyme. It has COX like enzymatic activity and is known to be involved in pain perception and fever but not inflammation. Paracetamol is a selective COX-3 inhibitor.
- Comparison of COX-1 and COX-2 enzymes is given in Table 9.1.

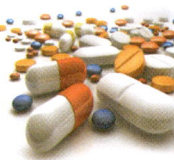

TABLE 9.1: Differences between COX-1 and COX-2 enzymes

Properties	COX-1	COX-2
Site of action	Found in many tissues, important for homeostasis	Induced by inflammatory stimuli at the site of inflammation
Effects of activation	• Converts arachidonic acid to inflammatory prostaglandins • Maintains renal function • Provides integrity to gastric mucosa (cytoprotective) • Promotes vascular homeostasis • Autocrine effects cause fever	• Increases pain, inflammation • Vasodilatory effects • Blocks platelet clumping
Effects of blocking	• Decreases swelling, pain and • Inflammation	• Decreases pain and inflammation
Effects of blocking for a prolonged period leads to adverse effects like	• Damage to renal system (acute tubular necrosis may occur). • Sodium retention, edema, increased blood pressure • Gastrointestinal erosions (ulcer) and bleeding, etc. • Decreases fever	• Prevents protective vasodilation • Allows platelet clumping, which can lead to myocardial infarction, cerebrovascular accidents. (on prolonged use)

Classification of Nsaids

Depending upon the specificity of COX inhibition, the NSAIDs have been broadly classified as given in Table 9.2.

Most of the above NSAIDs have some actions in common.

Common Pharmacological Characteristics of NSAIDs

- **Antipyretic effects:** Any infection or tissue injury produces pyrogens including interleukins (ILs), tissue necrosis factor (TNF-α), interferons, etc. which interfere with thermoregulatory center in the hypothalamus and cause hyperthermia. The NSAIDs inhibit the action of these pyrogens. The antipyretic action is exhibited only when pyrogens are present. They do not cause hypothermia in normothermic individuals.
- **Analgesic effects:** NSAIDs inhibit the generation of mediators of pain, e.g., PGs, bradykinin, TNF-α and ILs; thereby produce analgesic effects and increase pain threshold without causing sedation, tolerance, and drug dependence.
- **Anti-inflammatory effects:** NSAIDs inhibit the generation of PGs at the site of injury. (*PGs are mainly responsible for the inflammation process after any tissue injury*). They do not inhibit the generation of other mediators of inflammation like leukotrienes (LTs), platelets activating factor (PAF), cytokines, etc.
- **Platelet anti-aggregatory effects:** NSAIDs predominantly inhibit the synthesis of thromboxane A_2 (TXA_2), and cause increase in bleeding time. TXA_2 *is responsible for platelets aggregation*. Only selective NSAIDs produce this effect.
- **Effects on GI mucosa:** Traditional non-steroidal anti-inflammatory drugs [tNSAIDs] inhibit the generation of gastroprotective PGs, (COX-1 inhibitory effect) resulting in erosion of gastrointestinal (GI) mucosa and ulcer formation. COX-2 selective drugs are safe for GI mucosa as they do not inhibit gastroprotective PGs.

TABLE 9.2: Classification of NSAIDs

Types of NSAIDs	Drugs
Nonselective COX inhibitors (traditional NSAIDs)	Aspirin, ibuprofen, ketoprofen, naproxen, flurbiprofen, mephenamic acid, piroxicam, tenoxicam, ketorolac, indomethacin, nabumetone, phenylbutazone, oxyphenbutazone.
Preferential COX-2 inhibitors:	Nimesulide, diclofenac, aceclofenac, etodolac, meloxicam, etc.
Selective COX-2 inhibitors:	Celecoxib, etoricoxib, parecoxib.
Analgesic-antipyretics with poor anti-inflammatory action:	Paracetamol (acetaminophen), metamizol, nefopam, propiphenazone, etc.
Both COX and LOX inhibitors:	Licofelone

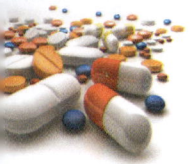

- **Effects on kidneys:** Prolonged use of tNSAIDs may lead to impairment of renal functions. Renal blood flow is decreased due to inhibition of cytoprotective and vasodilatory effects of PGs. This occurs due to COX-1 inhibition. COX-2 inhibition results in sodium and water retention. Prolonged use of NSAIDs also contributes to renal papillary necrosis. These effects are markedly seen in patients with chronic renal disease, congestive heart failure, cirrhosis, and hypovolemia, but rarely in normal individuals.
- **Analgesic nephropathy:** Analgesic nephropathy is a condition which involves renal papillary necrosis

and renal tubular atrophy followed by renal fibrosis. This condition occurs due to heavy and prolonged consumption of NSAIDs. Recovery of renal functions occurs if the condition is recognized early and the NSAIDs are discontinued.

Like all other drugs, NSAIDs also have both beneficial and toxic effects. To summarize, some of these effects are given in Table 9.3.

The chemical group to which they belong, $t_{1/2}$, dose schedule and route of administration of some commonly used NSAIDs are given in Table 9.4.

TABLE 9.3: Effects of NSAIDs

Beneficial effects	Toxic effects
<ul><li>Anti-inflammatory</li><li>Antipyretic</li><li>Analgesic effects</li><li>Antithrombotic</li><li>Closure of ductus arteriosus in newborn</li></ul>	<ul><li>GI ulcer</li><li>Asthma precipitation</li><li>Anaphylactic reaction in susceptible individuals</li><li>Rash and pruritus</li><li>Sodium and water retention, hyperkalemia, and proteinuria.</li><li>Delay/prolongation of labor</li><li>Bleeding [Prolong bleeding time]</li><li>Abnormal liver function tests</li></ul>

TABLE 9.4: t½ dose and route of administration of commonly used NSAIDs

Nonselective COX inhibitors (Traditional NSAIDs)			
Groups	**Drug name**	**t½ [hours]**	**Dose**
Salicylates	Aspirin	0.25-5 [dose dependent]	<ul><li>As antiplatelet: 40–80 mg/day</li><li>In pain/fever: 325–650 mg QID</li><li>In rheumatic fever: 1 g every QID</li><li>In rheumatoid arthritis: 3–5 g, OD</li><li>As anti-inflammatory: 1.2–1.5 g, TDS</li><li>Children: 10 mg/kg every QID</li><li>All above doses are oral</li></ul>
Propionic acid derivatives	Ibuprofen	2–4	400–600 mg TDS, oral
	Naproxen	14	250 mg BD/TDS, oral
	Ketoprofen	1.8	50–100 mg BD/TDS, oral
	Flurbiprofen	6	50 mg BD/QID, oral
Fenamate	Mephenamic acid	2–3	250–500 mg TDS, oral
Enolic acid derivatives	Piroxicam	57	20 mg OD/BD, oral, 20 mg/1 mL, IM
Acetic acid derivatives	Ketorolac	4–6	10–20 mg QID, oral 30 mg/1 mL IV/IM
	Indomethacin	2.5	25–50 mg BD/QID, oral
	Nabumetone	24	500 mg OD, oral
	Sulindac	7	150–200 mg BD, Oral
Pyrazolone derivatives	Phenylbutazone, propiphenazone, oxyphenbutazone, metamezol, etc.		

Contd...

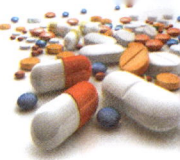

Preferential COX-2 inhibitors		
Drug name	**t½ [hours]**	**Dose**
Nimesulide	2–5	100 mg BD, oral
Diclofenac	1–2	50 BD/TDS, oral 75 mg IV/IM, 1% topical gel
Aceclofenac	—	100 mg BD, oral
Meloxicam	15–20	7.5–15 mg OD, oral
Piroxicam	45–50	20 mg/day OD, oral
Etodolac	7	200–400 mg BD/TDS, oral
Selective COX-2 inhibitors		
Celecoxib	6–12	100–200 mg BD, oral
Etoricoxib	24	60–120 mg OD, oral
Parecoxib	—	40 mg BD-QID, IV, IM, oral
Analgesic-antipyretics with poor anti-inflammatory action		
Paraaminophenol derivative	Paracetamol (Acetaminophen) 2	500 mg QID, oral. 300 mg/2 mL IM
Pyrazolone derivatives	Metamizol —	0.5–1.5 g oral/IM/IV
	Propiphenazone —	300–600 mg TDS
Benzoxazocine derivative	Nefopam	20–60 mg TDS 20 mg IM QID

NONSELECTIVE COX INHIBITORS (TRADITIONAL NSAIDS)

These drugs inhibit both COX-1 and COX-2 enzymes non-selectively.

Salicylates (Aspirin)

Important Historical Points

- *Salicylates were prepared from the glycoside obtained from Willow bark (Salix alba). Willow bark was in use as analgesic for centuries without knowing the exact active principle.*
- *Vane and coworkers (in 1971) were the first scientists to make an observation that Aspirin and some NSAIDs act by blocking PGs generation.*

Aspirin

Aspirin is one of the oldest analgesic-anti-inflammatory drugs. The chemical name of aspirin is acetylsalicylic acid. It is converted in the body to salicylic acid to produce its effects.

Pharmacological Actions

- Aspirin has a good *anti-inflammatory* and *antipyretic effect*, but weak *analgesic* activity. Anti-inflammatory and

analgesic activities are mediated by inhibition of peripheral PGs synthesis, whereas antipyretic effect is mediated by resetting the hypothalamic thermostat mechanism.

- **Effects on Blood and CVS:** Aspirin is used at low doses for the prevention of *thrombo-embolic phenomena* in the patients of hypertension, dyslipidemia and coronary artery disease. It inhibits the *platelet aggregation* by irreversibly blocking the synthesis of TXA_2. This mechanism operates in the portal circulation. The acetyl salicylate molecules passing through portal circulation bind to the COX enzyme present on the platelets and inhibit it irreversibly. This effect remains for the life period of platelets, i.e., one week.
- At higher doses, aspirin stimulates respiratory center (central response) leading to *hyperventilation*.
- Aspirin causes *nausea, vomiting and epigastric distress* by irritating the gastric mucosa. The *gastrointestinal (GI) bleed* may occur at higher dose of aspirin.
- Urate excretion: Aspirin has *anti-uricosuric effect*, i.e., it inhibits the excretion of urate in urine. Therefore, it is contraindicated in the patient suffering from gout.
- This effect is dose dependent and is described in Table 9.5.

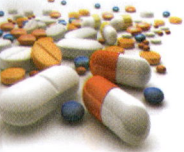

TABLE 9.5: Dose effects of aspirin on urate excretion

Dose effects	
<2 g/day	Urate retention and antagonism of all other uricosuric drugs.
2–5 g/day	Variable effects, often no change.
5 g/day	Increased urate excretion.

Pharmacokinetics

- It is rapidly absorbed from the stomach and upper small intestines.
- It is deacetylated to its active form salicylic acid in liver, plasma and other tissues and excreted through glomerular filtration and tubular secretion.

Indications

- Prophylactically used in post myocardial infarction and stroke patients (most common indication)
- Acute rheumatic fever
- Rheumatoid arthritis (not a first choice drug)
- As analgesic for various aches (not for visceral pain)
- Osteoarthritis (not a first choice drug)

Adverse Effects

- **At low doses, i.e., 0.3–1.5 g/day:** It may lead to nausea, vomiting, epigastric pain and occult blood loss in stools. This occurs due to gastric mucosal damage.
- **Hypersensitivity reactions:** Present as rashes, urticaria, angioedema, asthma and anaphylactic reaction.
- **Salicylism:** It is a milder form of salicylate toxicity, which occurs at doses of 3–5 g/day for a prolonged period. It presents as headache, confusion, vertigo, temporary visual and hearing impairment, electrolyte imbalance, hyperventilation, etc. Stopping or tapering the therapy causes decreasing the signs and symptoms of salicylism.
- **Reye's syndrome:** It is a rare condition, seen in children. It occurs when salicylate is given in children suffering from viral infection (varicella, influenza, etc.). It results in liver damage and hepatic encephalopathy; hence, salicylate is contraindicated in children with viral infections.

Acute Salicylate Poisoning

Cause: Overdosing of salicylates. In adults, the fatal dose is 15–30 g and less in children (but the poisoning is common in children). Seen only when the plasma level of salicylate exceeds ≥50 mg/dL.

Contd...

Clinical features: Vomiting, hyperpyrexia, electrolyte imbalance, dehydration, hyper/hypoglycemia, delirium, convulsions, coma, cardiovascular collapse and death due to respiratory failure.

Management: There is no specific antidote available to manage acute salicylate poisoning.

The management is as follows:

- Hospitalization
- IV fluid administration for correction of dehydration and electrolyte imbalance.
- External cooling in the form of cold sponging.
- Gastric lavage to remove the unabsorbed drug.
- Intravenous infusion of sodium bicarbonate for metabolic acidosis.
- Hemodialysis in severe cases and administration of vitamin-K in case of bleeding.

Contraindications and Precautions

- Patient with history of GI bleeding, peptic ulcer.
- Children with viral infections.
- It should be stopped one week before elective surgical procedures.
- It should be avoided in pregnancy.

Propionic Acid Derivatives

Ibuprofen, Naproxen, Ketoprofen, Flurbiprofen

- These drugs are better tolerated than aspirin and have analgesic, anti-inflammatory and antipyretic effects.
- Naproxen is the most potent of all propionic acid derivatives.

Pharmacokinetics

- All these drugs are well absorbed orally.
- These drugs enter the blood-brain barrier, synovial fluids and crosses placenta.
- They are metabolized in liver and excreted in urine and by bile.

These drugs interfere with the action of oral anticoagulants and oral hypoglycemic agents; hence, concomitant use should be avoided.

The commonly used propionic acid derivatives with their indications are given in Table 9.6.

Fenamate (Mephenamic Acid)

- It is a weak anti-inflammatory and good analgesic and antipyretic agent.
- It inhibits both central and peripheral pain receptors.
- The oral absorption is slow but complete.
- It is metabolized in liver and excreted through urine and bile.

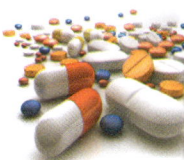

TABLE 9.6: Commonly used propionic acid derivatives

Drugs	Indications	Special feature
Ibuprofen	Fever, pain, dysmenorrhea, rheumatoid arthritis, osteoarthritis, musculoskeletal disorders, fractures and tooth extraction related pain.	It is available as OTC drug.
Naproxen	Rheumatoid arthritis, ankylosing spondylitis and migraine	It has longer t½ than other propionic acid derivatives. It has less renal side effects. Anti-inflammatory effects appear after 2–4 weeks.
Ketoprofen	Rheumatoid arthritis, ankylosing spondylitis and migraine	Additional action to stabilize lysosomes and LOX inhibition.
Flurbiprofen	Rheumatoid arthritis, ankylosing spondylitis and migraine and inflammatory eye conditions	It is also available in 0.03% in ophthalmic solution.

- It is indicated in dysmenorrhea and to provide relief in pain originating from muscles, joint and soft tissues.
- It is also used in rheumatoid arthritis and osteoarthritis but less preferred.
- The common side effects are diarrhea, epigastric pain, rash and dizziness.

Enolic Acid Derivatives

(Piroxicam, Tenoxicam, Meloxicam)

Piroxicam

- It is a long-acting potent NSAID that has good anti-inflammatory, analgesic and antipyretic action.
- It is a nonselective, reversible COX inhibitor.
- It attains good concentration in synovial fluid and decreases the production of IgM rheumatoid factor and leukocyte chemotaxis. This prevents the inflammatory damage to synovial membrane.
- It is completely absorbed with a plasma t½ of 2 days; Hence, OD dose is sufficient.
- It is metabolized in liver and excreted through urine and bile.
- It is indicated in rheumatoid arthritis, osteoarthritis, ankylosing spondylitis, gout and musculoskeletal disorders.

- It is well tolerated with few side effects like rashes and pruritus.
- The GI erosion is less common.

Tenoxicam and Meloxicam

- They have similar pharmacological properties as piroxicam.
- Tenoxicam is given in a dose of 20 mg OD.
- Meloxicam inhibits COX-2 preferentially and is given in a dose of 7.5–15 mg OD.

Acetic Acid Derivatives

(Ketorolac, Indomethacin, Nabumetone, Sulindac)

Ketorolac

- It is a potent analgesic.
- It is well absorbed orally, metabolized in liver and excreted through urine.
- It is indicated in:
  - Post-operative pain (as its efficacy equals morphine): 15–30 mg IM/IV QID (max. 90 mg/day).
  - Renal colic, migraine, pain due to bony metastasis, dental pain and musculoskeletal pain.
  - Non-infective ocular inflammatory conditions: 0.5% eye drops; 1–2 drops BD-QID.
- It should not be used for more than five days as side effects start appearing.
- The common side effects are nausea, dyspepsia, gastric ulceration, abdominal pain, headache, nervousness, pruritus and pain at injection site.

Indomethacin

- It has potent anti-inflammatory and antipyretic action.
- It is highly effective in pain induced by inflammation or tissue injury.
- It is well absorbed orally, metabolized in liver and excreted through kidney.
- It is most commonly used drug for medical closure of patent ductus arteriosus given in a dose of 0.1–0.2 mg/kg IV BD.
- Other indications are inflammations associated with psoriatic arthritis, ankylosing spondylitis, acute gout or rheumatoid arthritis, which are non-responsive to other NSAIDs.
- The common side effects are gastric irritation and bleeding, nausea, anorexia and diarrhea.
- It may also cause headache, confusion, hallucinations and depression, hence, contraindicated in pregnant women, children, machinery operators and patient with epilepsy and psychiatric illness.

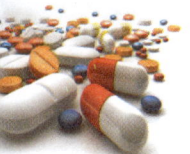

Pyrazolones

(Phenylbutazone, Oxyphenbutazone, Metamizol, Propiphenazone)

- These drugs were earlier indicated to treat pain and fever but due to their excessive side effects (agranulocytosis and bone-marrow depression), they have been banned nowadays.
- Only two pyrazolones are available in India, they are metamizol and propiphenazone. Rarely used now.

PREFERENTIAL COX-2 INHIBITORS

These drugs inhibit COX-2 enzymes preferentially.
The commonly used preferential COX-2 inhibitors with their indications are given in the Table 9.7.

Common adverse effects of preferential COX-2 inhibitors: Nausea, loose motions, pruritus, rash, etc.

SELECTIVE COX-2 INHIBITORS

- These drugs selectively inhibit COX-2 enzymes.
- These are devoid of the side effects seen with non-specific COX inhibitors.
- They have analgesic, antipyretic and anti-inflammatory actions similar to non- selective NSAIDs.

- These drugs can be given in the patients suffering from gastric ulcer, gastritis, peptic ulcer and ulcer bleeds, as they do not inhibit the COX-1 protective actions in GIT.
- These drugs reduce PGI_2 production and do not inhibit platelet aggregation. This effect produces prothrombotic conditions and cardiovascular risk, which are important limiting side effects of these drugs. Rofecoxib and Valdecoxib were withdrawn due to this limitation only.
- Nowadays, only three COX-2 inhibitors (Celecoxib, Etoricoxib and Parecoxib) are available in the market for clinical use (Table 9.8).

Common Adverse Effects of Selective COX-2 Inhibitors

The common side effects are mild hypertension, pedal edema, rash, dyspepsia, mild diarrhea, dry mouth, dysgeusia and aphthous ulcers.

Celecoxib and parecoxib are sulfonamide derivatives and may cause skin rash whereas etoricoxib is structurally related to diclofenac; hence, hepatic functions should be monitored.

***Licofelone** is a dual inhibitor of the COX and 5-LOX pathways.*

Differences between selective COX-2 and nonselective COX inhibitors are enlisted in Table 9.9.

TABLE 9.7: Preferential COX-2 inhibitors

Drugs	MOA	Indications	Special features
Nimesulide	Inhibits COX-2 selectively, PAF and TNF-α	Short lasting painful inflammatory conditions such as dental pain, dysmenorrhea, ENT disorders, bursitis	• Pediatric use is banned in India and many countries due to fulminant liver disease • No cross reactivity with other NSAIDs; so, can be given to asthma patients also
Diclofenac	COX-2 selective inhibition. Reduction of inflammatory mediators locally	Rheumatoid, osteoarthritis, bursitis, ankylosing spondylitis, toothache, dysmenorrhea, renal colic, post-traumatic and post-operative inflammatory conditions	• It has good tissue penetrability • It remains in synovial fluid in 3 times higher concentration than plasma; hence effective in joint inflammation
Aceclofenac	Moderately COX-2 inhibitor	Same as above	• Chondroprotective in nature
Etodolac	Moderately COX-2 inhibitor	Used as post-operative analgesic Rheumatoid arthritis, osteoarthritis and musculoskeletal pain	• It is better tolerated at low doses than other NSAIDs • Relatively safer in renal patients

Abbreviations: COX-1, cyclooxygenase-1; COX-2, cyclooxygenase-2; PAF, platelets activating factor; PGs, prostaglandin; TNF-α, Tumor necrotic factor-α; TXA2, thromboxane A2

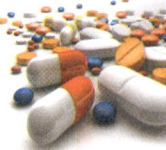

TABLE 9.8: Selective COX-2 inhibitors

Drug name	MOA	Indications	Special features
Celecoxib	Modest COX-2 selective inhibition	Rheumatoid arthritis, osteoarthritis and inflammatory conditions in GI ulcer patients	It does not interfere in platelets aggregation
Etoricoxib	Highest COX-2 selective inhibition	Rheumatoid arthritis, gout, ankylosing spondylitis, dysmenorrhea and osteoarthritis	It does not affect the gastric mucosa and platelets function
Parecoxib	Modest COX-2 selective inhibition. (Prodrug of valdecoxib)	Short-term use for post-operative pain	It is available in injectable form

TABLE 9.9: Differences between nonselective COX and selective COX-2 inhibitors

Pharmacological features	Non-selective COX	Selective COX-2
Antipyretic effects	Yes	Yes
Analgesic effects	Yes	Yes
Anti-inflammatory effects	Yes	Yes
Effect on gastric mucosa	Yes	No
For closure of ductus arteriosus	Yes	No
Precipitation of asthma	Yes	No
Risk of bleeding	Yes	No
Cardiovascular toxicity	Less	More
Hepatotoxicity	Less	More
Renal toxicity	More	Less

MANAGEMENT OF RHEUMATOID ARTHRITIS

- *Rheumatoid arthritis* (RA) is a chronic autoimmune disease, which involves joint inflammation, synovial proliferation and destruction of synovial cartilage with bony erosions.
- It is most commonly seen in middle age females.
- There is IgM mediated overproduction of inflammatory cytokines such as TNF-α, IL-1 and PGs. These inflammatory mediators lead to erosion and damage of cartilage and pain in joints (by PGs synthesis).
- NSAIDs are first line drug therapy for the management of pain, joint swelling, and morning stiffness but do not reduce the progression of disease.
- In addition to NSAIDs, the drugs are given to modify the disease process. These drugs which can suppress the rheumatoid process and bring about a remission in the disease process are called **D**isease **M**odifying **A**nti-**R**heumatic **D**rugs (DMARDs).

The aims of anti rheumatoid treatment are:
- To reduce pain, swelling and joint stiffness.
- To prevent articular cartilage damage and bony erosions.
- To prevent deformity and preserve joint function.

Disease Modifying Anti-Rheumatic Drugs (DMARDs)

- The early or mild symptoms are treated by NSAIDs only.
- DMARDs are indicated only when the patient is diagnosed to have RA.
- Nowadays, DMARDs are used in combination of ≥2 drugs for early and better-prognosis.
- Does, route and special features of DMARDs are given in Table 9.10.

Biological Agents as DMARDs

- *Gold and d-penicillamine are obsolete DMARDs.*
- Does, route and special features of biological agents as DMARDs are given in Table 9.11.

MANAGEMENT OF GOUT

- Gout is a metabolic disorder characterized by increased uric acid levels. The normal plasma uric acid level is 2–6 mg/dL.
- Hyperuricemia does not always present as gouty arthritis.
- Uric acid is a product of purine metabolism.

203

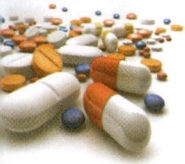

TABLE 9.10: Disease modifying anti-rheumatic drugs (DMARDs)

Drugs	Dose and Route	Special features
Hydroxy-chloroquine	Initial: 400 mg OD for 4–6 weeks, orally (≤6.5 mg/kg) Maintenance: 200 mg OD	• It may cause irreversible retinal damage
Sulfasalazine	Initial: 500 mg BD, orally Maintenance: 1–1.5 g BD daily	• It may lead to hemolytic anemia with granulocytopenia
Methotrexate	7.5–15 mg/week, orally. *Folic acid 1 mg OD to reduce toxicity*	• It may cause hepatotoxicity, bone marrow suppression and infection
Azathioprine	1–2.5 mg/kg/day orally	• Additionally, used in prevention of rejection in renal transplants • Never combined with Methotrexate • Has steroid sparing effect
Cyclosporine	3–5 mg/kg OB/BD, orally *Not used nowadays*	• It may cause anemia, leukopenia and thrombocytopenia • At high dose, may cause cardiotoxicity and sterility especially in women
Leflunomide	100 mg for 3 days, then 20 mg daily, orally	• Inhibits T-cell proliferation; thereby inhibits IgM production by B-cells • It can be given along with methotrexate and sulfasalazine

TABLE 9.11: Biological agents as DMARDs

Drugs	Dose and Route	Special features
Etanercept	25 mg subcutaneous twice weekly or 50 mg subcutaneous once a week.	• Effective in patients unresponsive to other therapy • Also indicated in ankylosing spondylosis, psoriatic arthritis • Clinical benefits increase when given with methotrexate
Infliximab	3–5 mg/kg IV at 0,2,6 weeks then every 8 weeks May increase the dose up to 10 mg/kg every 4 weeks	• It may increase the risk of bacterial and fungal infection • It may also reactivate latent TB
Adalimumab	40 mg SC every other week.	• It may increase the risk of bacterial and fungal infection • It may also reactivate latent TB
Anakinra (IL-1 antagonist)	100 mg SC daily	• Reduction of signs and symptoms of rheumatoid arthritis in patients >18 years if one or more arthritis agents have failed
Adjuvant drugs		
Prednisolone	7.5 mg OD preferably in morning before 8 am	• Should be used for short period only just to control the acute inflammation. • Long-term use may lead to osteoporosis.

- Increase levels of uric acid deposit in joints, subcutaneous tissue (as tophi) and kidneys.

Gout is classified as acute and chronic gout

- **Acute gout:** It is sudden in onset with inflammation of joints (especially in first metatarso-phalangeal joint of great toe) due to precipitation of urate crystals in the joint space. It usually present as swelling and severe pain around the joints involved. It requires immediate attention.
- **Chronic gout:** The gout is called chronic when pain and stiffness persist in a joint in between the attacks. It presents as high plasma uric acid levels with tophi (chalk-like stones

under the skin in pinna, eyelids, around joints) and urate stones in the kidney.

Commonly used drugs in management of gout are given in Table 9.12.

TABLE 9.12: Drugs used in management of gout

Acute gout	Chronic gout	
	Uricosurics	**Synthesis inhibitors**
• NSAIDs • Colchicine • Corticosteroids	• Probenecid • Sulfinpyrazone	• Allopurinol • Febuxostat

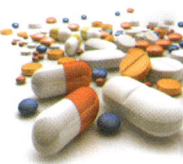

Acute Gout Management

NSAIDs

- Being good anti-inflammatory agents, these drugs provide quick relief in pain. Most commonly used NSAIDs are indomethacin, etoricoxib, piroxicam, diclofenac and naproxen.
- These drugs are given for terminating the acute attack and used at their maximum tolerable doses for shorter period only.
- The response comes after 12–24 hours; they may be continued at lower doses for 3–4 weeks after the attack is subsided.

Colchicine

- It is an alkaloid, obtained from Colchicum autumnale.
- It has anti-inflammatory action against gout specifically.
- It does not interfere with uric acid production or excretion. Hence, no effect on plasma uric acid levels is seen.

Mechanism of action

- It blocks the release of chemotactic factors and glycoprotein, which are responsible for inflammation.
- It also inhibits the migration of granulocytes to inflamed joints and interferes with progression of disease.

Pharmacokinetics

- It is rapidly absorbed orally.
- It is partially metabolized in liver and excreted through bile; undergoes enterohepatic circulation.

Indications and doses

- **For management of acute gout:**
  - *Starting dose:* 0.5 mg 1–3 hourly with a total of 3 doses in a day; maximum 6.0 mg for 3–4 days, and the second course should not be started before 3–7 days.
  - *Maintenance doses:* 0.5–1 mg/day for 4–8 weeks.
- **Prophylaxis:** *Colchicine* 0.5–1 mg OD, for prevention of further attacks.

Adverse effects

- The side effects are usually dose dependent; they are nausea, vomiting, abdominal pain and diarrhea.
- Overdose of colchicine may lead to CNS depression, intestinal bleed, renal damage. If not timely managed, muscle paralysis and respiratory failure lead to death.

Corticosteroids

- Corticosteroid is a reserve drug, used in patients not tolerating NSAIDs/colchicines.

- Most commonly used corticosteroid is prednisolone in a dose of 40–60 mg/day and should be tapered over few weeks. These are rarely required.
- Intra-articular injection of triamcinolone acetate is used to treat symptoms of acute mono-articular gout.

Chronic Gout Management

Uricosuric Drugs

Probenecid

- It is a competitive inhibitor of active transport of organic acids by Organic anion-transporting polypeptide (OATP).
- It has high lipid solubility, developed in 1951 to prolong the duration of action of penicillin by inhibiting its excretion from renal tubules.
- It enhances the excretion of uric acid from kidneys; therefore, used as uricosuric drug for chronic gout management.
- It has neither analgesic nor anti-inflammatory effects.

Pharmacokinetics

- It is well absorbed orally with high plasma protein binding (≥90%).
- It is metabolized in liver and excreted through kidneys.
- The plasma t½ is 6–8 hours.

Indications and doses

Chronic gout and hyperuricemia: It is a second line drug therapy for chronic gout [first line: allopurinol] given in a dose of 0.25 g BD and increased to 0.5 g BD with concomitant therapy of colchicine or NSAIDs for prevention of acute gout attack.

Adverse effects

- The most common side effect is dyspepsia; hence should be avoided in patients with peptic ulcer disease.
- Other side effects like hypersensitivity and skin rash are uncommon.

Sulfinpyrazone

- It is another uricosuric agent, related to Phenylbutazone.
- It inhibits the tubular reabsorption of uric acid and at low dose, it reduces the urate excretion.
- It has similar uricosuric action as Probenecid.
- It is not used nowadays due to serious GI side effects.

Uric Acid Synthesis Inhibitors

Allopurinol

- It is a competitive inhibitor of xanthine oxidase; an enzyme responsible for uric acid synthesis while in higher concentration, it behaves as noncompetitive inhibitor.

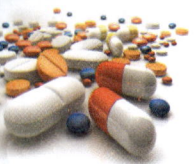

- It is well absorbed orally with no plasma protein binding.
- The plasma t½ is 2 hours while its major metabolite alloxanthine has t½ of 24 hours.
- It is metabolized by xanthine oxidase and has longer duration of action; hence given in OD basis.

Dose regimen

The treatment is started with an initial dosage of 100 mg OD and is increased to 300 mg daily until the satisfactory results are achieved (≤6 mg/dL).

Indications

- Chronic gout (as a first line therapy)
- Secondary hyperuricemia due to cancer chemotherapy/ radiations.

Adverse effects

- It is well tolerated with very uncommon side effects; they are nausea, vomiting, diarrhea, bone marrow suppression and rarely aplastic anemia.
- Hypersensitivity like pruritic maculopapular rash may occur in some individuals.

Febuxostat

- It is newer non-purine xanthine oxidase inhibitor.
- It is more potent than allopurinol in reducing plasma uric acid levels.
- It is well absorbed orally, metabolized in liver and excreted through kidneys.
- The plasma t½ is 6 hours.
- It is indicated in chronic gout as an alternative to allopurinol.
- It is not given in malignancy associated hyperuricemia.
- It is given in a dose of 40–80 mg OD with concomitant use of NSAIDs or colchicine at least for initial 1–2 months.
- The common side effects are nausea, diarrhea, headache and hepatotoxicity. Regular monitoring of liver enzymes is advised.

Rasburicase

- It is a newer recombinant xanthine oxidase enzyme that oxidizes uric acid to soluble and easily excretable form, allantoin.
- The only indication of its use is in prevention of chemotherapy associated hyperuricemia.

  Food supplements that are given as adjuvant therapy for osteoarthritis are described in Table 9.13.

TABLE 9.13: Food supplements as adjuvant therapy for osteoarthritis

Supplements	Dose and route	Special feature
Sodium hyaluronate	2 mg once a week for 5 week injected into the affected knee	Relief of pain in the knees of arthritis patients whose disease is unresponsive to conventional treatment
Chondroitin		It is a major component of cartilage that helps to retain water It can be manufactured from the cartilage of animals like cows, pigs or sharks
Glucosamine	750 mg BD orally	Like chondroitin, glucosamine is a natural compound found in healthy cartilage, particularly in the fluid around the joints

The pharmacological basis of use of these compounds is yet to be established.

ANTIPYRETICS

Paracetamol or Acetaminophen

Paracetamol (Acetaminophen) is an active metabolite of phenacetin.

- It is a nonselective COX-1 and COX-2 inhibitor.
- It also inhibits COX-3 enzyme (discovered in 2002), which is a spliced variant of COX-1. Inhibition of COX-3 is responsible for its antipyretic and analgesic effects.
- It is the most important analgesic for the management of mild to moderate pain with poor anti-inflammatory effects.
- It is available as OTC as antipyretic and analgesic.
- It differs from other NSAIDs in following respects:
  - It is the fastest acting antipyretic agent.
  - It neither produces gastric mucosal damage nor affects the platelet aggregation.
  - It neither affects acid base balance nor stimulates the respiration.
  - It does not have uricosuric action.
  - Hypersensitivity reactions and drug interactions are very rare.

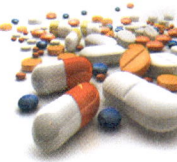

Phenacetin was banned due to its association with analgesic abuse nephropathy. It was called as Coal tar analgesic due to its involvement in the causation of analgesic nephropathy, hemolytic anemia and sometimes bladder cancer also.

Pharmacokinetics

- It is well absorbed orally, metabolized in liver and excreted through kidneys.
- The effect after an oral dose lasts for 3–5 hours.

Indications

- As antipyretic for all age groups including children, adults, elderly, pregnant, lactating women, gastric ulcer patients. It is used as suitable substitute for patients in whom aspirin is contraindicated.
- Headache, mild migraine, mild musculoskeletal pain
- Osteoarthritis
- Dysmenorrhea.

Adverse Effects

- At therapeutic doses, it is well tolerated, very rarely mild nausea may occur.
- Over dosages may cause hepatic necrosis, renal tubular necrosis and hypoglycemia, which may prove fatal if not treated timely.

Acute Paracetamol Poisoning

Causes

It is common in children at a dose more than 150 mg/kg due to their low glucoronide conjugation ability than adults. Acute or repeated supratherapeutic ingestion of paracetamol at a dose of more than 10–15 g in adults may lead to serious toxicity. The toxic effects are most commonly seen in adults with poor hepatic functions and chronic alcoholics. The fatal dose is more than 20–25 g.

Clinical features

Early manifestations are nausea, vomiting, abdominal pain and liver tenderness without sensorium alteration. After 12–18 hours, signs and symptoms of hepatic and renal tubular necrosis with hypoglycemia appear, which leads to coma. If the intake of paracetamol is not interrupted, hepatic failure and death can occur.

Mechanism of toxicity

Paracetamol is metabolized to N-acetyl-p-benzoquinine imine (NAPQI), which is detoxified by conjugation with glutathione. When a very large dose of paracetamol is taken, glucuronidation capacity of liver cells is saturated due to depletion of glutathione. This metabolite binds covalently to proteins in liver cells and renal tubules causing necrosis.

In chronic alcoholics, hepatotoxicity can occur even at a dose of 5–6 g taken in one day. Paracetamol is not recommended in premature infants due to the fear of hepatotoxicity.

Management

- Gastric lavage followed by activated charcoal to prevent further absorption.
- As an antidote, N-acetylcysteine (NAC) 150 mg/kg should be infused IV over 15 min, followed by the same dose IV over the next 20 hours. Alternatively, 75 mg/kg may be given orally every 4–6 hours for 2–3 days. It replenishes the glutathione stores of liver and prevents binding of the toxic metabolites to other cellular constituents.
- Aggressive supportive care to manage hepatic and renal failure.
- Parameters such as arterial blood gas (ABG), electrolyte analysis, plasma glucose levels, liver function tests (LFT) and renal functions tests (RFT) should be monitored closely.
- Glutathione supplementation can also be given.

Drug Interactions

- Aspirin and other NSAIDs displace many drugs (such as phenytoin, warfarin, sulfonylureas, valproate and methotrexate) from their plasma binding sites and produce their toxicity. Hence, combination should be avoided.
- Aspirin and other NSAIDs increase the risk of bleeding in patients on anticoagulants (warfarin, heparin, etc).
- Aspirin should be avoided inpatients of gout or hyperuricemia due to its anti uricosuric action. It also inhibits the action of probenacid.
- The diuretic action of furosemide, thiazides and spironolactone are inhibited by NSAIDs. NSAIDs inhibit the prostaglandin synthesis in kidneys.
- Concurrent use of corticosteroids, alcohol and NSAIDs lead to gastric mucosal damage (PGs are gastroprotective). Hence, combination should be avoided.

Nursing Implications

- **Analgesics, NSAIDs and antipyretics**
  - Assess for contraindications or cautions: history of allergy to any NSAIDs to avoid hypersensitivity reactions.
  - Nurse should also enquire about history of gastritis, peptic ulcers, bleeding disorders, renal disease, hepatic disease, chicken pox or influenza in children (to avoid the risk of Reye's syndrome with aspirin) to avoid any adverse effects.
  - Monitor the vital regularly.

Contd...

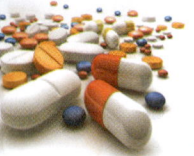

Textbook of Pharmacology for BSc Nursing Students for KUHS

 Nursing Implications

☞ Monitor for severe reactions to avoid problems and provide emergency procedures (gastric lavage, induction of vomiting, administration of charcoal) if they occur.

☞ Nurse should check the prescription and match it with the drugs before administering them.

☞ Nurse should educate the patient about the adverse effects of NSAIDs, as the patients on NSAIDs are suffering from pain; chances of selfoverdose are always there.

☞ Provide thorough patient teaching, including measures to avoid adverse effects and warning signs of problems, as well as proper administration, to increase knowledge about drug therapy and to increase compliance with the drug regimen.

TABLE 9.14: Classification of opioids

Natural opium alkaloids (opiates)	Semi-synthetic opiates	Synthetic opioids
• Morphine • Codeine	• Diacetylmorphine (Heroin) • Pholcodeine • Ethylmorphine • Hydromorphone* • Oxymorphone* • Hydrocodone* • Oxycodone*	• Pethidine (Meperidine) • Fentanyl • Methadone • Dextropropoxyphene • Tramadol • Tapentadol • Levorphanol* • Dextromoramide* • Dipipanone* • Alfentanil* • Sufentanil* • Remifentanil*

Not available in India.

OPIOID ANALGESICS AND ANTAGONISTS

All opioid analgesics act by binding to specific opioid receptors in the CNS to produce analgesic effects. Although the opioids have a broad range of effects, their primary use is to relieve intense pain, whether that pain results from surgery, injury, or chronic disease.

- The term 'opioids analgesics' literally means opium like analgesics.
- The opium word is derived from a Greek word 'opus' which means 'juice'.
- Opium is an extract of the juice of unripe seed capsule of the poppy plant (*Papaver somniferum*). This juice (milky exudate) is collected, dried and powdered. This is called opium powder, which is dark brown in color.
- Opium contains two types of alkaloids:
  - Alkaloids having *phenanthrene* group
    - ◆ Morphine (10% in opium)
    - ◆ Codeine (0.5–2.5% in opium)
    - ◆ Thebaine (0.2–0.4% in opium)
  - Alkaloids having *benzoisoquinoline* group
    - ◆ Papavarine (1% in opium)
    - ◆ Noscapine (6% in opium)
- The alkaloids derived from opium are called *opiates* and opioids like substances which are synthetic in nature are called *opioid* analgesic.

  Based upon their nature of origin, the classification of opioids is given in Table 9.14.
- Both opiates and opioids produce their pharmacological effects by acting upon certain receptors known as opioid receptors.
- These receptors are:
  - μ (mu) receptors
  - δ (delta) receptors
  - κ (kappa) receptors

These receptors are present on the neurons of CNS (brain, spinal cord) and peripheral nervous system (gastrointestinal tract, blood vessels, heart, lungs and immune cells) in different concentration.

Endogenous Opioid Peptides
- Some endogenous peptides are present in brain, pituitary, spinal cord and gastrointestinal tract, which act on opioid receptors to produce certain beneficial physiological effects (*morphine-like effects*).
- These endogenous peptides are endorphins, enkephalins and dynorphins A and B.
- These opioid peptides are released in the body in response to pain.
- In normal conditions, these endogenous opioids modulate pain perception, motor behavior, emesis, pituitary hormone release and GI motility, etc.
- The effect of these endogenous peptides is inhibited by naloxone (opioid antagonist).

NATURAL OPIUM ALKALOIDS (OPIATES)

(Morphine, Codeine)

Morphine

- The word morphine has been derived from the name of *Morpheus, the Greek God of dreams* as it used to produce sedation and dream like state.
- Morphine was isolated from pure opium alkaloid by *Sertuner* in 1806.
- All the opiates and opioids have pharmacological effects similar to morphine with slight differences only.
- This is due to difference in their affinity to the different opioid receptors.

Pharmacological Effects

- Morphine is a pure agonist at the μ opioid receptors.
- **Effects on central nervous system (CNS):** Morphine has both CNS depressant and stimulant actions depending upon the site on which it acts.
  - **CNS depressant effects of morphine are**
    - *Analgesic:* It is a potent analgesic. It is more effective in dull, unlocalized visceral pain than defined somatic pain. The pain associated reactions and the distressing symptoms like fear, anxiety and autonomic effects are controlled well.
    - It gives feeling of wellbeing and pleasurable sensation (*euphoria*).
    - It has dose dependent *drowsiness, calming and sleeping effect.* In a higher dose, it may lead to coma and death.
    - Morphine depresses both *respiratory and cough center.* Cough center is more sensitive than respiratory center to morphine. *Respiratory failure is the major cause of Morphine poisoning.*
    - Morphine also has effects on *thermoregulatory and vasomotor* center, which may cause *hypothermia and hypotension,* respectively.
  - **CNS stimulant effects of morphine**
    - Morphine induces *nausea and vomiting* by activation of chemoreceptor trigger zone (CTZ). But, it cannot be used to induce vomiting as it depresses the vomiting center in high doses.
    - Morphine causes *bradycardia* due to stimulation of *vagal center.*
    - Morphine causes *miosis* due to stimulation of *Edinger Westphal nucleus of III cranial nerve.*
- **Effects on cardiovascular system:** Morphine causes depression of vasomotor center, release of histamine and decrease in blood vessel tone. Morphine is used to treat congestive heart failure as it decreases anxiety and also reduces cardiac work by shifting the blood from pulmonary to systemic circulation by decreasing peripheral resistance.
- **Effects on GIT:** Morphine causes *constipation* by increasing the tone and reducing GI secretions and intestinal motility.
  - Morphine may *aggravate biliary colic* as it causes spasm of sphincter of Oddi.
  - Morphine *aggravates asthma* by causing bronchoconstriction due to release of histamines.
  - Morphine *increases the intracranial pressure* by increasing CO_2 retention in the brain leading to cerebral vasodilatation. Hence, it is contraindicated in intracranial hemorrhage.

Pharmacokinetics

- It is well absorbed when given by subcutaneous, intramuscular, and oral routes. The oral bioavailability of morphine is very poor as it undergoes first-pass metabolism. Hence, higher oral dose is required.
- It poorly penetrates blood-brain barrier and freely crosses placental barrier; can affect the fetus more than the mother.
- The plasma t½ is 2–3 hours.
- It is metabolized by liver and excreted through urine.

Indications

- As analgesics in trauma, myocardial infarction, renal colic and cancer related pain, etc.
- Acute congestive heart failure.
- As pre-anesthetic medication in some patients.

Dose

- **Adults:** Oral dose: 10–50 mg. IM/ SC: 10–15 mg, IV: 2–6 mg.
- **Children:** Oral dose: 0.3 mg/kg. IV: 0.1 mg/kg.

> Morphine is not commercially available in the market, while it is available in hospital setups. (Ward sister should maintain the consumption record)

Adverse Effects

The common side effects with morphine are:
- Nausea and vomiting
- Constipation
- Postural hypotension accentuated by hypovolemia
- Respiratory depression
- Urinary retention
- Increased intracranial pressure
- Itching around nose, urticaria (more frequent with parenteral and spinal administration).

Contraindications

- In patients with respiratory insufficiency (emphysema, pulmonary fibrosis, cor pulmonale) sudden death can occur.
- Bronchial asthma
- Head injury
- Hypovolemia and hypotensive states.
- Undiagnosed acute abdominal pain
- In elderly male, chances of urinary retention are high.

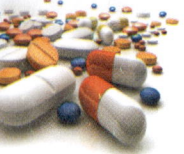

Acute Morphine Poisoning

Cause: This condition is usually seen in individuals with drug abuse, suicidal personality and even accidental overdose.

In normal individuals, 50 mg IM of morphine may produce toxic effects, while 250 mg produces lethal effects.

Clinical features: Shallow and occasional breathing, cyanosis, pinpoint pupil, flaccidity, hypotension, stupor or coma. Death occurs due to respiratory failure.

Management:
- Resuscitation consists of respiratory support (positive pressure ventilation).
- Management of hypotension (IV fluids, vasoconstrictors).
- Gastric lavage by using potassium permanganate (Lavage is indicated even when morphine has been injected as it is secreted into gastric juice and can be reabsorbed by enterohepatic circulation).
- Specific antidote: *Naloxone* 0.4–0.8 mg intravenously and repeated every 2–3 minutes until respiration is stored.

Codeine

- It is another form of natural alkaloid of opium.
- It is partial agonist at μ opioid receptor with a low ceiling effect.
- The potency and efficacy is less than morphine; 300 mg of codeine is similar to 30 mg of morphine.
- It is indicated in mild to moderate pain, diarrhea and for dry cough (in low dose of 10–30 mg).
- The oral absorption is better than morphine.
- Parenteral preparation of codeine is not available.
- The most common side effect is constipation.

SEMISYNTHETIC OPIATES

[Diacetylmorphine (Heroin), Pholcodeine, Ethylmorphine]

Diacetylmorphine (Heroin)

- This drug is not used therapeutically worldwide except in the United Kingdom.
- It is highly addictive drug and notorious for illicit drug trafficking.
- It is three times more potent and fast acting than morphine.
- Being lipid soluble, it crosses the blood-brain barrier and produces euphoria; hence having more addictive property than morphine.

Pholcodeine, Ethylmorphine

(Described in Chapter 5)

- These drugs are having similar properties as codeine.
- These drugs are mainly used as antitussives and spasmodic.
- They have low incidence of constipation as a side effect.

SYNTHETIC OPIOIDS

(Pethidine (Meperidine), Methadone, Fentanyl, Tapentadol Dextropropoxyphene, Tramadol)

Pethidine (Meperidine)

- It was synthesized as an atropine substitute in 1939, and has some actions like atropine.
- It acts on the μ opioid receptors like morphine.
- It is well absorbed orally, metabolized in liver and excreted through urine with a plasma t½ of 2–3 hours.
- It is indicated for the management of pain, as pre-anesthetic and even as post-anesthetic medication to treat shivering.
- Side effects are similar to morphine and in addition, some atropinic side effects may occur like dry mouth, tachycardia and blurred vision due to action on muscarinic receptor. Differences between pethidine and morphine are given in Table 9.15.
- Overdose of pethidine may lead to mydriasis, delirium, tremor, and convulsions. These symptoms are more common in renal failure patients who receive pethidine.
- It is given in a dose of 50–100 mg IV/IM/SC.

Fentanyl

- It is more potent synthetic opioids than morphine.
- It has potent analgesic and respiratory depressant effect.
- It is highly lipid soluble and easily crosses blood-brain barrier; produces analgesic effects within 5 minutes after IV injection. Hence, exclusively used in anesthesia.
- It has shorter duration of action (≤40 minutes) due to redistribution.

TABLE 9.15: Differences between pethidine and morphine

Properties	Pethidine	Morphine
Analgesic	Less	More
Onset of action	Rapid	Slow
Duration of action	Less	More
Action on smooth muscles	Less	More
Cough center	No effect	Depresses
Effect on biliary spasm	Less	More
Effects on asthma	Can be given [less histamine release]	Contraindicated
Effects on cardiovascular system	Tachycardia (due to antimuscarinic effects)	Bradycardia
Effects on CNS	Same	Same

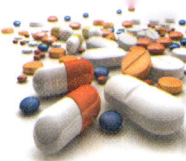

- The transdermal preparations are mostly used in patients with cancer, terminal illness or other types of chronic pain. Transdermal patch is available in a concentration of 12 µg/hour, 25–µg/hr, 50–µg/hr, 75–µg/hr or 100-µg/hr; the patch is changed after 3 days.
- At analgesic dose, it rarely causes cardiovascular side effects.
- The common side effects are mild hypotension, bradycardia.
- Patient may experience nausea, vomiting and pruritus during recovery phase.

Methadone

- It is a synthetic opioid, having similar pharmacological properties as morphine.
- It has similar analgesic, emetic, antitussive, constipating and respiratory depressant actions to morphine.
- It is metabolized in liver and excreted through urine.
- The plasma t½ is 25–52 hours with 4–6 hours duration of action after IM injection.
- The abuse potential is less than morphine; withdrawal symptoms take 1–2 days after discontinuation of therapy.
- It is used as a substitution therapy in opioids dependence: 1 mg of oral methadone can be substituted for 4 mg of morphine, 2 mg of heroin and 20 mg of pethidine.
- Methadone maintenance therapy in opioid addicts: 10–40 mg/day, given orally over long-term to produce high degree of tolerance so that pleasurable effects of IV doses of morphine or heroin are not perceived and the addicts gives up the habit.
- It is used as analgesic in a dose of 2.5–10 mg oral or IM.

Dextropropoxyphene

- It is chemically related to methadone.
- The side effects and analgesic actions are similar to codeine.
- It also has low incidence of constipation and less antitussive action.
- It is metabolized in liver with a t½ of 4–12 hours.
- It is indicated as mild analgesic and is given in a dose of 60–120 mg orally in combination with paracetamol.
- Overdose may present as delirium and convulsions.

Tramadol

- Tramadol has low affinity for µ opioid receptors and very low affinity for κ and δ receptors.
- It is an atypical opioid because, in addition to actions at opioid receptors, it also inhibits reuptake of noradrenaline and 5-hydroxytryptamine receptors (5-HT); thus inhibits the pain at spinal level also.
- Fifty mg of IM tramadol provides analgesic effects equal to five mg of morphine IM.

- It is given in a dose of 50–100 mg oral/IM/slow IV infusion (children 1–2 mg/kg) 4–6 hourly. More specifically the safer dose is 37.5 mg.
- It is metabolized in liver and excreted through kidneys with plasma t½ of 6 hours.
- It is indicated in mild to moderate short lasting pain after therapeutic or surgical procedures.
- It can also be used in chronic painful conditions such as cancer related pain but not effective in severe pain.
- It is well tolerated with few side effects such as vomiting, nausea, dry mouth, headache, dizziness and sweating.
- The abuse potential is very low; therefore, it is also used as a part of opioid de-addiction therapy.
- The side effects (respiratory depression, sedation, constipation, urinary retention) are lesser than morphine.
- Tramadol may increase the risk of '**serotonin syndrome**'; hence, concomitant therapy of tramadol and selective serotonin reuptake inhibitors (SSRI) should be avoided.

Tapentadol

- It is structurally similar to tramadol.
- It is a µ opioid receptors agonist and also blocks the re-uptake of nor-adrenaline and to some extent serotonin.
- Like tramadol, it also increases the risk of serotonin syndrome.
- It is indicated for the treatment of moderate to severe pain for both acute and chronic musculoskeletal pain.
- It is also used in diabetic neuropathic pain.
- It is given orally in a dose of 50–100 mg BD/TDS.

OPIOID ANTAGONISTS

The classification of opioid antagonists is given in Table 9.16.

Agonistic-antagonists (κ-Analgesics)

(Nalorphine, Pentazocine, Butorphanol)

Nalorphine

- It is the first opioid antagonist, introduced in 1951.
- It produces dysphoria and psychotomimetic side effects. Hence, not used nowadays.

TABLE 9.16: Classification of opioid antagonists

Agonistic-antago-nists (κ analgesics)	Partial/weak µ ago-nist + κ antagonist	Pure antagonists
• Nalorphine	• Buprenorphine	• Naloxone
• Pentazocine		• Naltrexone
• Butorphanol		• Nalmefene

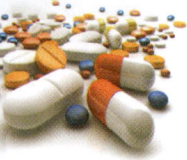

Pentazocine

- It has potent κ-agonist and weak μ-antagonistic property.
- It is metabolized in liver with plasma t½ of 3–4 hours.
- It is indicated in post-operative pain, burns and pain due to trauma.
- It is given in a dose of 30–60 mg IM/SC and 50–100 mg orally.
- The side effects are similar to opioids but lesser in severity.
- The abuse potential is lesser than morphine.
- It is contraindicated in patients with hypertension, myocardial infarction (*sympathetic stimulant action*), head injury (*increased intracranial tension*), epilepsy (*lowers seizure threshold*) and psychotic patients (*psychosomatic effects*).
- The tolerance, psychological and physical dependence of pentazocine usually develops after prolonged and repeated use.
- It differs from morphine in many aspects (Table 9.17).

Butorphanol

- It is more potent than pentazocine (1 mg butorphanol = 15 mg pentazocine).
- It has potent κ-agonist and weak or partial antagonist to μ receptors.
- It is used as analgesic; having similar action to buprenorphine.
- It is given in a dose of 1–4 mg IM/IV for post-operative and other painful conditions for short-term use only.
- The side effects are nausea, vomiting, sedation, tachycardia and should be avoided in patients with cardiac ischemia.
- The addiction with butorphanol is less; it may produce physical dependence in drug-addicted individuals.

TABLE 9.17: Differences between pentazocine and morphine

Properties	Pentazocine	Morphine
Analgesia	Spinal level (less potent)	Spinal and supraspinal level (more potent)
Sedation	Less	More
Biliary spasm	Less	More
Vomiting	Less	More
Respiratory depression	Less	More
Cardiovascular effects	Tachycardia	Bradycardia
Addictive property	Higher at low dose; low at high dose	More common (any dose)

Partial/Weak μ-Agonist + κ-Antagonist

Buprenorphine

- It is a synthetic derivative of **thebaine**.
- It is 25–50 times more potent than morphine, (0.4 mg of buprenorphine produces similar effects as 10–20 mg of morphine on IM injection).
- It is metabolized in liver and excreted through bile.
- It is well absorbed by most routes; on sublingual administration, the drug (0.4–0.8 mg) produces satisfactory analgesia in post-operative patients within 1–2 hours and by intramuscularly, it takes 5 minutes to produce same effect. The sublingual route is preferred to avoid the first pass metabolism.
- The plasma t½ is 3 hours with long duration of action.
- It is indicated in chronic pain conditions like cancer-induced pain, post-operative pain, myocardial infarction, morphine dependence and opioids with drawl.
- The side effects are usually similar to morphine, but it produces severe postural hypotension, while constipation is uncommon.
- As morphine also depresses the respiratory center; hence should be avoided during labor.
- Tolerance with buprenorphine is low, but on chronic use people may develop physical and psychological dependence, which is prevented by high dose of naloxone.
- It is given in a dose of 0.3–0.6 mg IM, SC or slow IV, and sublingual dose is 0.2–0.4 mg 6–8 hourly.

Pure Opioid Antagonists

(Naloxone, Naltrexone, Nalmefene)

Naloxone

- It is non-selective competitive antagonist of opioid receptors, but it has more affinity for μ receptors than κ or δ receptors. It immediately antagonizes all the action of opioids.
- It is orally inactive due to high first pass metabolism. It is metabolized in liver.
- It does not produce any subjective or autonomic effect on normal individuals and it does not produce any physical/psychological dependence.
- It also blocks the action of endogenous opioids such as endorphins and enkephalins.
- It is ineffective for the management of buprenorphine overdose.
- It is given in a dose of 0.1–0.4 mg IV until the desirable effects are achieved.

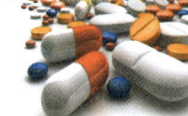

Indications and doses

- **Morphine poisoning:** Naloxone [drug of choice] given in a dose of 0.4–0.8 mg IV, inhibits all actions of morphine and stimulates respiratory center.
- **For reversal of neonatal asphyxia due to opioid use during labor:** 10 μ g/kg in the umbilical cord.
- **Opioid overdose:** Naloxone given in a dose of 4–10 mg inhibits the action of nalorphine, pentazocine, etc. It does not have any effect on dysphoria and psychomimetic symptoms produced by opioids.

It is well tolerated with few side effects such as hypertension and pulmonary edema of low intensity.

Naltrexone

- It is also a pure opioid antagonist chemically related to naloxone.
- It is more potent than naloxone.
- Due to better oral bioavailability and longer duration of action, it may be given in post-drug addict individuals as '*opioid blockade*' therapy.
- It is given in a dose of 50 mg/day in drug addict individuals to reduce craving.
- Before initiation of therapy, the patient should be opioid free for at least 7–10 days. The therapy is started orally with 25 mg initially under supervision, then 50 mg daily till the patient stabilizes. Then, 100 mg three times a week.
- The de-addiction treatment with naltrexone should ideally begin in a residential setting in order to prevent withdrawal symptoms. But, it can be prescribed in outpatient medical settings also.
- It is also used to prevent alcohol craving in chronic alcoholics.
- The common side effects are nausea, headache and hepatotoxicity (on prolong use).
- It blocks opioids from binding to their receptors and thereby prevents their euphoric and other effects.

Recently, a long-acting injectable version of naltrexone (depot form) has been approved to treat opioid addiction. It only needs to be injected once a month to improve compliance.

Methyl Naltrexone

It is a derivative of naltrexone, used to manage constipation in cancer patients, who are being given opioids for cancer pain management and taking methadone maintenance therapy.

Nalmefene

- It is another pure opioid antagonist with higher oral bioavailability and longer duration of action.
- It does not cause hepatotoxicity.

Nursing Implications

☞ **Opioid analgesics and antagonists**
- ☞ Assess for contraindications or cautions: any known allergies.
- ☞ When administering the narcotic drugs through IV route, equipment for assisted ventilation and narcotic antagonist should be readily available to provide patient support in case of severe reaction.
- ☞ Narcotics should not be given on patient demand.
- ☞ Monitor timing of analgesic doses.
- ☞ Narcotics should be kept under lock, as there are chances of abuse of these drugs by paramedical staff and others.
- ☞ Use additional measures to relieve pain (e.g., back rubs, stress reduction, hot packs, ice packs) to increase the effectiveness of the narcotic being given and reduce pain.

TRANQUILIZERS OR ANXIOLYTIC DRUGS AND HYPNOTICS

TRANQUILIZERS

The drugs, which are used to reduce anxiety, fear, tension, agitation and related state of mental disturbances, are known as tranquilizers.

Tranquilizers are of two types:
- **Minor tranquilizers:** They are also known as anxiolytic/anti-anxiety agents because they are used to treat minor state of mental disturbance such as anxiety, insomnia, etc.
- **Major tranquilizers:** They are also known as anti-psychotic/neuroleptic agents because they are used to treat major state of mental disturbance such as schizophrenia and other bipolar disorders.

The term 'tranquilizer' is non-specific and very rarely used these days in human pharmacology. It has been replaced by various specific terms such as sedatives, hypnotics, antipsychotics, antidepressants, etc.

SEDATIVES AND HYPNOTICS

- **Sedatives:** The drugs that exert a calming effect with decrease in alertness without inducing sleep are known as sedatives. They may produce drowsiness and also decrease the response to any level of stimulation.
- **Hypnotics:** The drugs that induce or maintain natural sleep-like state are known as hypnotics. The person who is under the effect of these drugs can be aroused by strong stimuli like pin prick or sound of alarm clock.

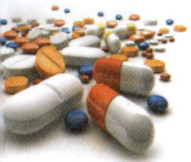

- **Hypnosis:** It is a different term from hypnotics. It is a trans-like condition in which the objective manifestations of the mind are more or less inactive and accompanied by an increased suggestibility.

SLEEP

- It is a periodic state of rest accompanied by varying degree of unconsciousness and relative inactivity.
- The duration of sleep per day is dependent upon the age. The newborns are having longest sleep-hours (≥20 hours), while average adults sleep 8–10 hours.
- The average duration of sleep decreases to <8 hours in elderly.

Sleep is classified into two types:
- Rapid eye movement (REM) sleep
- Non- rapid eye movement (NREM) sleep

REM and NREM sleep alternate during the sleep cycle; each cycle requires 90–100 minutes. The sleep cycle is composed of 75% of NREM and 25% of REM with inter-individual variations and with the advancing age, the REM sleep is further decreased.

The sleep cycle has five stages described in Table 9.18.

BENZODIAZEPINES AND BARBITURATES

- Benzodiazepines (BZDs) and barbiturates are the drugs having both sedative and hypnotic effects.
- The drugs having faster and shorter action are preferably used as *hypnotics*.
- The drugs with slow and prolonged action are preferably used as *sedatives*.

TABLE 9.18: Stages of sleep and their physiological effects

Stage	Physiological effects
0	From lying down to falling asleep. Eyes open/close, responsive to external stimuli, can hold intelligible conversation
1	It is a light sleep where you drift in and out of sleep and can be awakened easily. In this stage, the eyes move slowly and muscle activity slows. During this stage, many people experience sudden muscle contractions preceded by a sensation of falling
2	Eye movement further reduced and brain waves become slower but person can be easily aroused.
3	Deep sleep, eye movement stops and not easily aroused. Extremely slow brain waves called delta waves
4	Deepest sleep stage. The stages 3 and 4 are referred to as deep sleep or delta sleep and it is very difficult to wake someone from it. In deep sleep, there is no eye movement or muscle activity and there is increased secretion of growth hormone and decreased body metabolic rate

- Hypnotics at lower dose can act as sedatives and their effects overlap with each other depending upon dose and route employed.
- The increasing grade of CNS depression is sedation hypnosis general anesthesia.
- Hence, hypnotics are also used to produce anesthesia in higher doses.

Classification

The classification of benzodiazepines, non-benzodiazepines and barbiturates are given in Table 9.19.

Benzodiazepines

According to duration of action, BZDs are classified into short-acting, intermediate-acting and long-acting (Table 9.20).

BZDs are used both as sedatives and hypnotic and preferred over barbiturates.

TABLE 9.19: Classification of benzodiazepines, non-benzodiazepines and barbiturates

Benzodiazepines (BZDs)		
Hypnotic	**Antianxiety**	**Anticonvulsant**
• Diazepam	• Diazepam	• Diazepam
• Flurazepam	• Chlordiazepoxide	• Lorazepam
• Alprazolam	• Lorazepam	• Clobazam
• Nitrazepam	• Oxazepam	• Clonazepam
• Temazepam	• Alprazolam	
• Triazolam	• Etizolam	

Non-benzodiazepine hypnotics	
Zopiclone	Zolpidem
Eszopiclone	Zaleplon

Barbiturates		
Long-acting	**Short-acting**	**Ultra-short-acting**
• Phenobarbitone	• Butobarbitone	• Thiopentone
• Mephobarbital	• Pentobarbitone	• Methohexitone

TABLE 9.20: Classification of benzodiazepines according to duration of action

Short-acting (<8 hours)	Intermediate-acting (8–24 hours)	Long-acting (>24 hours)
• Triazolam	• Alprazolam	• Diazepam
• Oxazepam	• Etizolam	• Flurazepam
• Midazolam	• Estazolam	• Clonazepam
	• Temazepam	• Chlordiazepoxide
	• Lorazepam	• Nitrazepam

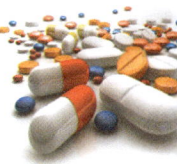

Mechanism of Action

- GABA, gamma aminobutyric acid, is a neurotransmitter involved in CNS depression and acts through GABA receptors.
- BZDs bind to specific GABA$_A$ receptors and facilitate the *frequency* of GABA-mediated Cl$^-$ channel opening (GABA mimetic action).
- This potentiates the inhibitory effect of GABA on CNS and causes depression (Fig. 9.2).

Pharmacokinetics

- All BZDs are well absorbed orally and have marked pharmacokinetic variations.
- IM/IV and rectal route(diazepam) of administration are also employed depending upon requirement.
- The plasma protein binding of BZDs is variable (flurazepam 10% to diazepam 99%).
- The more lipid soluble drugs enter brain rapidly (Triazolam).
- They are metabolized in liver and excreted in urine with variable plasma t½.
- They are widely distributed in body tissues. They cross placenta and are also secreted in milk; hence avoided during pregnancy and lactation.

Pharmacological Actions and Therapeutic uses

- **Anxiolytic and hypnotics:** BZDs are mostly used as anxiolytic and hypnotics. The widely used BZDs are alprazolam, etizolam, diazepam, chlordiazepoxide, lorazepam, and oxazepam.

These drugs in low doses act as anxiolytics and in slightly higher doses as hypnotics.

- **Insomnia** (Table 9.21).
- **As anticonvulsant:** Diazepam and clonazepam are used for the treatment of status epilepticus. These are also used in febrile seizures and tetanus. In myoclonic or petit mal seizures, clonazepam is used.
- **As muscle relaxant:** BZDs by virtue of their central action produce skeletal muscles relaxation. They are commonly used in muscle spasms and spasticity due to spinal cord injury and tetanus. The most preferred drug is diazepam.
- **For alcohol withdrawal syndrome (AWS) management:** Diazepam, oxazepam and chlordiazepoxide are used for symptomatic management of AWS.
- **As pre-anesthetic medications:** Diazepam, lorazepam and midazolam are the commonly used drugs. Intravenous midazolam has potent amnestic effect.
- **Diagnostic and minor operative procedures like endoscopy, bronchoscopy, etc:** BZDs are used intravenously for their sedative, amnesic, analgesic and muscle relaxant properties. Midazolam is most preferred.

Adverse Effects

- The BZDs are well tolerated with few side effects. At hypnotic doses, commonly seen side effects are dizziness, vertigo, disorientation, amnesia and impairment of psychomotor skills (*patients are advised not to drive or work on machinery*).

TABLE 9.21: Management of insomnia with benzodiazepines

Insomnia	Presentation	Management
Transient	Accounting 15%. Usually presented with jet lag, shift work, overnight train journey	Triazolam: 0.125–0.25 mg or Temazepam: 15–30 mg, HS Triazolam is used in patients having difficulty in sleep These drugs are used alternatively to avoid rebound insomnia
Short-term	Last for 1–3 weeks and presents with sleep difficulty and frequent nocturnal waking up	Temazepam: 15–30 mg or Flurazepam: 15–30 mg or Estazolam: 1–2 mg, HS
Long term/ chronic	Last for ≥3 weeks; usually presents with personality disorder	Nitrazepam (5–10 mg) or Flurazepam (15–30 mg), HS. These drugs should be withheld every third day. These drugs have very low incidence of rebound insomnia

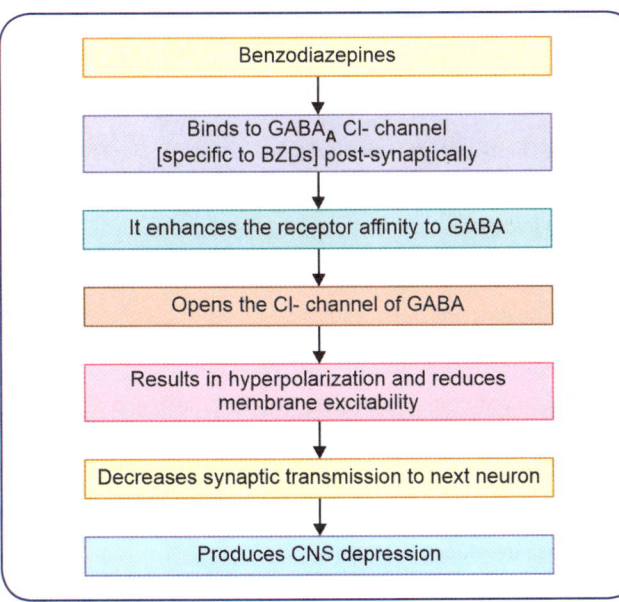

FIG. 9.2: Mechanism of action of benzodiazepines

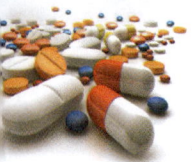

- Tolerance to sedative effects develops gradually and cross-tolerance to alcohol and other CNS depressants occurs.
- After chronic use, withdrawal a symptoms may appear due to dependence.
- Diazepam may cause flaccidity and respiratory depression in the neonate; hence, it should be avoided in pregnancy.
- *Flurazepam* and *Nitrazepam* may cause nightmares and behavioral disturbance.
- **Flunitrazepam** is also known as '*date rape drug*' due to its abusive use in sexual assaults. It is tasteless compound; misused widely and has both sedative and amnesic effects. Table 9.22 summarizes the pharmacological profile of BZDs.

Non-Benzodiazepine Hypnotics

(Zopiclone, Eszopiclone, Zolpidem, Zaleplon)
- These drugs produce near normal sleep with minimal hangover and are less likely to produce drug dependence and tolerance.
- These agents inhibit specific subset of BZDs receptors only (BZDs receptors containing α1 subunit).
- They have potent hypnotic and amnestic effects while have poor anticonvulsant, antianxiety and muscle relaxant effects.

- These agents are more useful to treat insomnia than BZDs.
- Zopiclone was the first of the non-BZD hypnotic.
- Flumazenil is a competitive inhibitor of non-BZDs hypnotics.
- Table 9.23 summarizes the pharmacological profile of non-benzodiazepine hypnotics.

Melatonin Congeners

Melatonin

- Melatonin is secreted from the pineal gland as a principal hormone at night.
- It has an important role to regulate circadian rhythm [Sleep-wake cycle].
- Melatonin acts through MT_1 and MT_2 receptors, which act through G-protein–coupled-receptors (GPCR).
- It induces sleep at high dose (80 mg), while low dose (2–10 mg) of melatonin may increase the tendency of falling asleep.
- It is indicated for the management of insomnia in elderly, jet lag and shift workers.
- The level of melatonin is reduced with the age; hence, it is recommended as supplements in a dose of 2–5 mg/day in many countries.

TABLE 9.22: Benzodiazepines: Pharmacological profile

Drugs	t½ (Hrs)	Dose and route	Special features
Triazolam	2–3	0.125–0.25 mg orally	• Used in insomnia
Oxazepam	10–20	15–30 mg TDS-QID, orally	• Used in anxiety disorders.
Midazolam	2–2.5	1–2.5 mg IV, IM	• Used in pre-anesthetic and intra-operative medication
Alprazolam	12–15	0.25–0.5 mg BD-TDS daily	• Anxiety disorders, agoraphobia. • Withdrawal amnesia may occur
Etizolam	6–8 hrs	0.5 –1 mg BD-TDS daily	• 10 times more potent than diazepam • Used in insomnia, anxiety and panic disorders
Estazolam	10–24	1–2 mg orally	• Used in insomnia
Temazepam	10–40	7.5–30 mg orally	• Used in insomnia
Lorazepam	10–20	2–4 mg, oral, IV, IM	• Used in anxiety and pre-anesthetic
Nitrazepam	30	5–10 mg OD	• Used in anxiety disorders
Diazepam	20–80	5–10 mg TDS-QID, oral, IV, IM	• Used in anxiety, status epileptics, pre-anesthetic and as muscle relaxant
Flurazepam	40–100	15–30 mg, orally	• Used in insomnia, accumulates at higher doses.
Clonazepam	23–28	Adults: 0.5–5 mg TDS Children: 0.02–0.2 mg/kg/day. Oral	• Used in seizure, acute mania and movement disorder. • Tolerance develops to anticonvulsant effects
Chlordiazepoxide	15–40	50–100, oral, IV/IM	• Used in anxiety, alcohol withdrawal syndrome and pre-anesthetic

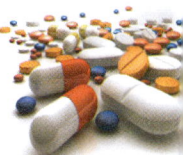

TABLE 9.23: Non-benzodiazepine hypnotics: Pharmacological profile

Properties	Zopiclone	Zolpidem	Zaleplon	Eszopiclone
Mechanism of action	It is the selective BZD receptor agonist	It is the selective BZD receptor agonist	It is the shortest acting selective BZD receptor agonist	It is recently approved active derivative (stereo-isomer) of zopiclone
Effect on sleep cycle	It does not alter REM sleep and tends to prolong stages 3 and 4	It does not interfere sleep stages	It does not prolong total sleep time and have no effect on nocturnal awakenings	The tolerance and physical dependence are very low; hence used to treat short-term even chronic insomnia
t½	5–6 hours	2 hours.	1 hour	6 hours
Indications	Short-term insomnia	Short-term (1–2 weeks) treatment sleep onset insomnia and intermittent awakenings	Sleep-onset insomnia only	To prolong sleep time in insomnia
Side effects	Alteration of taste (metallic or bitter), dry mouth, psychological disturbance, impaired alertness	Very few. Duration of effect is up to 8 hours, so day time sedation can occur if taken late night	Uncommon, tolerance and dependence not seen	Safety not established in long-term usage. Side effects are dry mouth and metallic taste
Doses	7.5 mg tab HS; but not more than 2–4 weeks (elderly 3.75 mg)	5–10 mg (max 20 mg) HS. Half dose in elderly and liver disease patients	5–10 mg (max 20 mg) should be taken late night	1–3 mg at bed time

Ramelteon

- It is a melatonin receptor agonist, and activates both MT_1 and MT_2 receptors in suprachiasmatic nuclei in the CNS.
- It is well absorbed orally, metabolized in liver and undergoes enterohepatic circulation.
- The plasma t½ is 1–3 hours.
- It is used in the treatment of sleep disorders, chronic insomnia and in persons having difficulty in falling asleep.
- It is given in a dose of 8 mg, half hour before going to bed.
- The common side effects are fatigue, dizziness and endocrine abnormalities.

Benzodiazepine Antagonists

Flumazenil

- It is a 1,4-benzodiazepine derivative and acts as competitive inhibitor at $GABA_A$ receptor.
- It inhibits both BZDs as well as non-BZDs, but does not antagonize the action of general anesthetics, ethanol, opioids and hypnotics or sedative, which act centrally; hence, used for the reversal of CNS depressant effects of BZDs toxicity.
- It is well absorbed orally but has very poor bioavailability; hence, given intravenously.
- The plasma t½ is 40–80 minutes.

Indications

Following table is showing dose of fumazenil to get the treatment results.

Conditions	To reverse BZD anesthesia	BZD overdose
Dose	0.3–1 mg, IV	0.2 mg/min IV, till the patient regains consciousness

Adverse effects

The common side effects are anxiety, nausea, agitation, dizziness and confusion.

Barbiturates

(Phenobarbitone, Mephobarbital, Butobarbitone, Pentobarbitone, Thiopentone, Methohexitone)

Barbiturates are the drugs used extensively as hypnotics and sedatives. This three classes of this drug are as written in following table:

Long-acting	Short-acting	Ultra-short-acting
• Phenobarbitone	• Butobarbitone	• Thiopentone
• Mephobarbital	• Pentobarbitone	• Methohexitone

Mechanism of Action

- They act on the $GABA_A$ Cl⁻ channels and prolong the opening time of Cl⁻ channels, and produce inhibitory actions called GABAnergic inhibition.
- At higher doses, they directly act on the Cl⁻ channels producing GABA mimetic action.

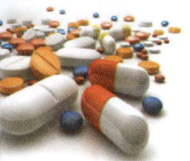

Pharmacokinetics

- They are well absorbed orally and widely distributed in the body.
- They are lipid soluble compounds; hence, the absorption, metabolism and excretion depend upon their lipid solubility.
- They are metabolized in liver and excreted through kidneys.
- These agents also cross placenta and secreted into the milk.

The systemic effects of barbiturates are enlisted in Table 9.24. The special features of various barbiturates are enlisted in Table 9.25.

Adverse Effects

- The common adverse effect of barbiturates is hangover (at higher doses only).
- Other side effects are confusion, psychomotor disturbances and hypersensitivity reactions [facial swelling, rashes and erythematous dermatitis].
- On prolonged and repeated use, tolerance and dependence [psychological and physical] may occur.

Acute Barbiturate Poisoning

- This condition is mostly seen in the individuals having habitual suicidal tendency, chronic drug abusers and rarely accidental.
- It is very serious condition that may lead to death due to cardiovascular collapse, renal shutdown and respiratory failure.
- The lethal dose of barbiturates also depends upon their lipid solubility; 2–3 g of lipid-soluble barbiturates produce sufficient toxicity while lipid insoluble barbiturates require 5–10 g to produce similar toxicity.

Management

- Gastric lavage followed by administration of activated charcoal for absorption of residual barbiturates.
- Oxygen therapy for respiratory failure.
- IV fluids and vasopressor agents for electrolyte imbalance.
- **For renal shutdown:** Dopamine is used as renal vasodilating agent.
- **Alkaline diuresis:** Sodium bicarbonate 1 mEq/kg IV with or without mannitol may be useful mainly in long-acting barbiturates, which are eliminated primarily by renal excretion.
- **Hemodialysis and hemoperfusion:** It is highly effective in removing long-acting as well as short-acting barbiturates. (No specific Antidote is available for barbiturate poisoning.)

The pharmacological differences between benzodiazepines and barbiturates are given in Table 9.26.

TABLE 9.24: Systemic effects of barbiturates

Systems	Effects
CNS	• Anticonvulsant at sub-hypnotic doses • They produce dose dependent CNS effects; these effects are sedation followed by hypnosis, anesthesia, coma and death
Cardiovascular system	• Uncommon, but at higher doses may produce hypotension and bradycardia
Gastrointestinal tract	• Some barbiturates decrease the GI tone and rhythmic contractions of GIT
Kidney	• Severe oliguria or anuria may occur in acute barbiturate poisoning due to hypotension
Respiratory system	• They depress both the respiratory drive and rhythmic character of respiration • At high dose, they also depress neurogenic drive of respiration
Skeletal system	• At higher doses, neuromuscular contraction is inhibited

TABLE 9.25: Various barbiturates and their special features

Drugs	t½ (hours)	Routes	Special features
Phenobarbitone	80–120	Oral/IM/IV	• Generalized tonic-clonic seizures, simple and complex partial seizures • In neonatal jaundice, it acts as microsomal enzyme inducer and enhances the production of glucuronyl transferase, the enzyme required for metabolism and excretion of bilirubin • Single daily dose can be used for maintenance due to long t½

Contd...

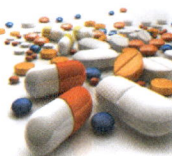

Drugs	t½ (hours)	Routes	Special features
Mephobarbital	10–70	Oral	• Used as second-line anticonvulsant • Indicated in daytime sedation and seizure disorders
Butobarbitone	35–40	Oral	• It has shorter duration of action • Indicated in pre-operative sedation and insomnia
Pentobarbitone	15–50	Oral, IV, IM, Rectal	• Used in pre-operative sedation, insomnia and as emergency management of seizure
Thiopentone	8–10	IV	• Used for the induction of anesthesia, pre-operative sedation, and as emergency management of seizure
Methohexitone	3–5	IV	• Used for the induction and maintenance of anesthesia • A single dose provides ≤7 minutes of anesthesia

TABLE 9.26: Pharmacological differences between benzodiazepines and barbiturates

Pharmacological properties	Benzodiazepines	Barbiturates
Toxicity	Uncommon, even in high dose (having high therapeutic index)	More common (having low therapeutic index)
Microsomal enzyme induction	It does not induce microsomal enzyme; hence no interaction seen	It does induce microsomal enzymes; hence interferes with many drug actions
Level of drug abuse	Uncommon	Very common, with physical and psychological dependence
Effect on sleep cycle	It does not interfere rapid eye movement sleep	It markedly decreases the REM sleep; rebound REM attack may occur as nightmare. Person may develop hangover also
Hyperalgesia	Not seen	Present, it enhances the pain sensation
Automatism	Absent	Markedly present with amnesia
Skeletal muscles	Potent muscles relaxant	Very poor relaxant activity
Respiratory system	No effect	Causes respiratory depression
Cardiovascular system	No effect	Hypotension, bradycardia
Antidotes	Flumazenil	No specific antidote (hemodialysis is only option)

Drug Interactions

- Barbiturates are strong microsomal enzyme inducers and decrease the efficacy of many drugs (tolbutamide, warfarin, griseofulvin, theophylline, steroidal contraceptives, etc.) by increasing their metabolism.
- The metabolism of phenobarbitone is inhibited by sodium valproate. Hence, phenobarbitone toxicity may occur.
- Phenobarbitone interferes with the metabolism of imipramine and phenytoin. Hence, combination should be avoided.
- Benzodiazepine in combination with valproic acid initiates psychotic symptoms.
- Benzodiazepine potentiates the effect of CNS depressants and alcohol. Hence, combination should be avoided.
- Ketoconazole and erythromycin are microsomal enzyme inhibitors; therefore slowdown the rate of metabolism of benzodiazepine.

Nursing Implications

- **Tranquilizers or hypnotics and sedatives**
  - Assess for contraindications or cautions: known allergies to barbiturates or benzodiazepines to prevent hypersensitivity reactions.
  - Assess the impaired liver or kidney function, which could alter the metabolism and excretion of a particular drug.
  - Do not administer intra-arterially because serious arteriospasm and gangrene could occur. Monitor injection sites carefully for local reactions to institute treatment as soon as possible.
  - Do not mix intravenous (IV) drugs in solution with any other drugs to avoid potential drug–drug interactions.
  - Always give IV drugs slowly because these agents have been associated with hypotension, bradycardia, and cardiac arrest.

Contd...

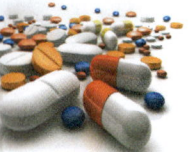

 Nursing Implications

- ☞ Observe patients who receive parenteral benzodiazepines in bed for a period of at least 3 hours.
- ☞ Monitor patient response to the drug (alleviation of signs and symptoms of anxiety; sleep; sedation).
- ☞ Provide thorough patient teaching, including drug name, prescribed dose, measures for avoidance of adverse effects, and warning signs that may indicate possible problems.

GENERAL AND LOCAL ANESTHETICS

- The term *anesthesia* is derived from two words [*an* (absence) + *aesthesia* (sensation of pain)] meaning 'absence of pain sensation'.
- The drugs which are used to produce anesthesia are known as anesthetics or anesthetic drugs.
- **General anesthesia** is defined as reversible loss of all the sensations and consciousness. It is produced by the drugs, which act at CNS level and are known as general anesthetic drugs.
- **Local anesthesia** is defined as reversible loss of all the local sensations without loss of consciousness. It is produced by the drugs, which act at peripheral level and are known as *local anesthetic drugs*.

GENERAL ANESTHETICS (GAs)

General anesthesia is the reversible loss of all the sensations and consciousness. This involves following special components:

- Analgesia (loss of pain sensations)
- Unconsciousness (Loss of consciousness)
- Amnesia
- Immobility and skeletal muscles relaxation
- Loss of all somatic and autonomic reflexes

An ideal anesthetic drug should be able to induce the unconsciousness smoothly and rapidly with prompt recovery from anesthesia whenever required. **The drug, which is unable to produce the above effects, is not considered as general anesthetic drug**.

There is no anesthetic agent, which can produce all the above effects individually without producing toxicity. Hence, in the modern day anesthetic practice, several different categories of drugs are used simultaneously to produce '**balanced anesthesia**'. The drug regimen for balanced anesthesia is made by keeping in view the advantage of the individual beneficial effects of different drugs and minimizing their individual toxic effects. This is usually made by making a combination of intravenous and inhaled drugs.

The protocol of general anesthesia for major surgical procedures includes the following steps:

Steps of general anesthesia

- Pre-anesthetic medication.
- Induction of anesthesia (IV route for adults; Inhalational for children).
- Maintenance of all phases of anesthesia.
- Reversal of anesthesia.

Stages of Anesthesia

Traditionally, the anesthetic drugs produce sequential effects as a part of increasing depth of CNS depression. These stages of anesthesia were described by Guedel in 1920 and ether was used as an anesthetic agent at that time. These are known as Guedel's signs. In modern anesthesia, all these stages may not be seen very clear and even the sequence may differ in some.

These stages are:

- **Stage of analgesia:** It remains from beginning of anesthesia to loss of consciousness. Patient remains conscious and feels a dream-like state. Very short procedures can be carried out during this stage.
- **Stage of excitement:** During this stage, patient appears delirious or may lose consciousness and sympathetic activity is increased which is manifested in the form of shouts, struggle, jerky breathing, vomiting, involuntary micturition or defecation. Heart rate and blood pressure may rise and pupils dilate due to sympathetic stimulation. No operative procedure can be carried out during this stage.
- **Stage of surgical anesthesia:** This stage begins with slowing of respiration and heart rate and extends to complete cessation of spontaneous respiration (apnea). It has been further subdivided into four planes depending upon changes in ocular movements, eye reflexes and pupil size indicating the depth of anesthesia.
  Most of the surgical procedures are performed in this stage.
- **Stage of medullary paralysis:** Due to increasing depth of CNS depression, and depression of respiration and vasomotor center, respiratory and circulatory failure occurs. Without respiratory and circulatory support, it progresses to death.

Important Factors of Anesthesia

The following factors are important for anesthesia:

Minimum Alveolar Concentration (MAC)

- It is the lowest concentration of any anesthetic that produces immobility or loss of consciousness in 50% individuals.

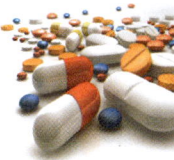

TABLE 9.27: MAC and BGS values of inhalational anesthetic

Inhalational anesthetic gases	MAC	BGS
Xenon	71	0.13–0.20
Desflurane	5.8	0.42
Nitrous oxide	105	0.45
Sevoflurane	2	0.63
Isoflurane	1.12	1.4
Halothane	0.74	2.25

- The potency of any inhalational anesthetic depends upon their MAC.
- MAC is inversely proportional to potency of drugs.
- Example: nitrous oxide has high MAC (104), and is very less potent; while methoxyflurane has very low MAC (0.13) and is the most potent inhalational anesthetic.

Blood Gas Solubility (BGS)

- It is the solubility of inhalational anesthetic gases into the blood.
- BGS determines the speed of induction and recovery by the inhalational agent.
- If the inhalational anesthetic gas is less soluble into the blood, it will induce quickly and vice-versa. Example, N_2O, sevoflurane, and desflurane are used for quick induction, as these are less blood soluble.
  The MAC and BGS values of inhalational anesthetic gases are given in Table 9.27.

Classification of Anesthetics

Classification of anesthetics is given in Table 9.28.

Inhalational Agents

Carrying Gases

(Nitrous oxide, Xenon)

Nitrous oxide (N_2O)

- It is non-inflammable, colorless, odorless and non-irritating gas.

- It is used as carrying agent for inhalational anesthetics.
- It has good analgesic with poor muscle relaxant property.
- In major surgical procedure, it is used in a mixture of 70% N_2O + 25–30% O_2 + 0.2–2% another potent anesthetic.
- The onset of action is quick and smooth with rapid recovery.
- Post-anesthetic nausea is not seen with this agent.
- It has a wide margin of safety as it has minimal effect on heart, blood pressure, respiration and is not toxic to liver, brain and kidney.
- *Second gas effect* and *diffusion hypoxia* is seen with this agent.
- It is contraindicated in air embolism, pneumothorax and intestinal obstruction as it moves very swiftly from blood into these compartments and aggravates these conditions.
- The commercially preparation of N_2O gas comes in blue colored cylinder.

Xenon gas

- It is an inert gas.
- Being least soluble in blood, it has very rapid inducing action.
- It is commercially available in white body with green-black shoulder cylinder.
- It has to be extracted from air and is very expensive than other carrying agents.
- It is rarely used.

Volatile Liquids

(Halothane, Isoflurane, Desflurane, Sevoflurane, Ether)

Halothane

- It is a non-inflammable, volatile liquid with sweet odor and non-irritant in nature.
- The induction with this agent can be achieved quickly and pleasantly due to intermediate solubility.
- 2–4% of halothane is given for induction and 0.5–1% for maintenance.
- It is delivered by the use of a special vaporizer.

TABLE 9.28: Classification of anesthetics

General anesthetic agents			
Inhalational agents		**Parenteral agents**	
Carrying gases	**Volatile liquids**	**Inducing agents**	**Short-acting agents**
• Nitrous oxide	• Halothane	• Thiopentone sodium	• Benzodiazepine (Diazepam, Midazolam, Lorazepam)
• Xenon	• Isoflurane	• Propofol	• Opioids (Fentanyl, Remifentanil, Sufentanil)
	• Desflurane	• Etomidate	• Ketamine
	• Sevoflurane		
	• Ether		

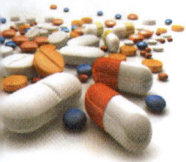

- Being highly potent, precise control of administered concentration of halothane is very important as slight deviation from the required concentration can be harmful.
- It causes hypotension to the extent of 20–30 mm Hg drop.
- It is a preferred agent for asthmatics as it dilates the bronchi but respiratory depression can also occur.
- It can prolong delivery and increase postpartum blood loss; if used during labor. It is used to facilitate external or internal podalic version during late pregnancy due its property of inhibition of uterine contractions.
- In genetically predisposed individuals, *hepatitis* and *malignant hyperthermia* can occur.
- Malignant hyperthermia is treated by:
  - Rapid external cooling
  - Bicarbonate infusion
  - 100% O_2 inhalation
  - IV dantrolene (1 mg/kg repeated as required).
- In children, it is suitable for both for induction as well as maintenance.
- In adults, it is mainly used for maintenance after IV induction.
- Practically, halothane is quite common in use.

Isoflurane

- Isoflurane is commonly used anesthetic agent as it produces relatively rapid induction and recovery as compared to halothane.
- It is administered through a special vaporizer.
- One and half to three percent of isoflurane is given for induction and one to two percent for maintenance.
- Hypotension is similar to halothane with prominent respiratory depression.
- It is not preferred for induction because of its pungent nature.
- It is a good maintenance anesthetic, and is suitable for neurosurgery.

Sevoflurane

- It has pleasant odor and it is more suitable anesthetic agent for induction in children.
- It is administered through a face mask.
- It is intermediate between isoflurane and desflurane in different pharmacological properties.
- The solubility in blood and potency are less than isoflurane but more than desflurane.
- It is good agent for induction as well as maintenance with quick recovery.
- It is suitable both for outpatient as well as inpatient surgery.
- It is very expensive; rarely used in government hospitals while commonly used in corporate hospitals.

Desflurane

- It has pungent odor and is not suitable for induction.
- It is 5 times less potent than isoflurane.
- It is administered in the vapor form along with carrier gas ($N_2O + O_2$) mixture.
- The induction and recovery is very fast due to very low solubility in blood.
- It is most commonly used as an anesthetic for outpatient surgery.

Comparative Features of Different Inhalational Agents

The comparative features of different inhalational agents are enlisted in Table 9.29.

- All inhalational anesthetics are respiratory depressants.
- **Isoflurane** causes **coronary steal phenomenon**; hence contraindicated in myocardial infarction.
- **Sevoflurane** is the inhalational agent of choice for induction of general anesthesia.
- **Desflurane** is used as maintenance of choice for GAs.

TABLE 9.29: Comparative features of different inhalational agents

Properties	Halothane	Isoflurane	Sevoflurane	Desflurane
Chemical structure	Halogenated ether	Isomer of enflurane	Halogenated ether	It is a structure analogue of isoflurane with replacement of chloride to fluoride
Boiling point	50°C	48°C	59°C	24°C (room temperature) to prevent it from boiling TEC-6 vaporizer is used
Minimum alveolar concentration	0.75	1.12	2	5.8
Blood gas solubility	2.25	1.4	0.63	0.42
Color code	Red	Purple	Yellow	Magenta blue
Muscles relaxant	Least potent	More than halothane	More than Isoflurane	Most potent
Malignant hyperthermia	More common	Less common than halothane	Less common than Isoflurane	Least common

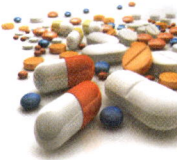

- **Desflurane** is the inhalational agent of choice for surgery in elderly patient, renal impaired and for day care surgery.
- **Halothane** is potent bronchodilator and best uterine relaxant may cause uterine atony and postpartum hemorrhage.
- **Malignant hyperthermia** is more common with halothane, which presents as fever, hypertension and tachycardia and is managed by IV injection of Dantrolene. Propofol is a drug of choice for malignant hyperthermia during anesthesia.
- **Methoxyflurane** is more potent than other inhalational anesthetics but it is not used nowadays due to severe nephrotoxicity.
- **Enflurane** is also inhalational anesthetic, obsolete nowadays due to epileptogenic effects.

Ether

- Ether is an inflammable and highly volatile liquid.
- It has potent anesthetic, analgesic and muscle relaxant properties.
- It is not used nowadays due to its potent side effects.

Advantages and disadvantages of ether are enlisted in Table 9.30

Parenteral Anesthetics

Inducing Agents

(Thiopentone sodium, Propofol, Etomidate)

Thiopentone sodium

- It is most commonly used ultra short-acting thiobarbiturate.
- The solution for injection (2.5%) should be freshly prepared.
- The solution is alkaline in nature with a pH of 10.5.
- It produces induction within 10–12 seconds after IV injection.
- It has short duration of action and the consciousness is regained within 6–8 minutes.
- It is given in a dose of 3–5 mg/kg.

TABLE 9.30: Advantages and disadvantages of ether

Advantages	Disadvantages
• It is cardiovascular stable drug	• Both induction and recovery are slow as it is highly soluble in blood
• It does not depress respiratory center; no hypoxia is seen	• It produces irritant vapors and increases the tracheobronchial secretions; prior atropine is required
• It obeys all five criteria of GAs	
• It is a good bronchodilator	• It is a highly inflammable agent
• It is quite economical	

- It decreases cerebral blood flow as well as cerebral oxygen demand; cerebral perfusion is maintained as per the requirement.
- It also causes hypotension and tachycardia due to peripheral vasodilatory effects.
- It is useful for induction of anesthesia, narcoanalysis (*used as truth serum*), management of status epilepticus, electroconvulsive therapy and brain surgery.
- Most commonly seen adverse effects are delirium and shivering during reversal of anesthesia.
- It is contraindicated in patients with asthma as it may cause laryngospasm due to increased respiratory secretions.
- It is also contraindicated in shock and porphyria.

Thiopentone sodium should be administered only into the vein; if accidentally injected into the artery, intense pain, necrosis and gangrene can occur.

The first symptom, which appears after injection into the artery, is **severe pain** and first sign is **pallor**.

Management:

Leave the cannula in situ.

Start injection of 500 unit of heparin.

1% Lignocaine 10 mL given; causes vasodilation and reduces pain.

Ganglionic block may be done by blocking stellate ganglion.

Propofol

- It is preferred over thiopentone for induction.
- It is used for both induction and maintenance purpose.
- It is oily in nature and commercially prepared from the egg extract; painful during injection.
- The patient becomes unconscious within 15–45 seconds and the effect lasts for 5–10 minutes.
- It is given in a dose of 2 mg/kg in 1–2% concentration bolus IV for induction; 100–200 µg/kg/min for maintenance.
  The recovery with propofol is pleasant; hence, it is a drug of choice for day care surgery.
- It relaxes the upper airways; it is agent of choice for endoscopy, intubation and in asthmatics. Higher doses may produce respiratory depression also.
- It also decreases cerebral metabolic O_2 demand, cerebral blood flow and intracranial tension as thiopentone.
- The incidence of post-operative nausea and vomiting is very low.
- The cardiac effects are similar to thiopentone.
- In high dose, it may lead to metabolic acidosis, lipidemia and heart failure even in adults.
- It is contraindicated in shock.
- Intermittent injection or continuous infusion of propofol with fentanyl supplementation is used to produce total IV anesthesia.

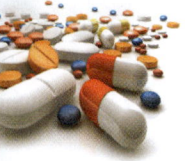

Etomidate

- It is also ultra-short-acting anesthetic with brief duration of action.
- It is given in a dose of 0.2–0.5 mg/kg.
- It produces less cardiovascular and respiratory depression.
- It is not used these days due to:
  - Pain on injection.
  - Excessive muscles movement on induction.
  - Nausea, vomiting on recovery.
  - Adrenocortical suppression if infusion is given for prolonged period.

Short-acting Agents

(Benzodiazepine, Opioids, Ketamine)

Benzodiazepines

(Diazepam, Midazolam, Lorazepam)

- These agents are used in pre-anesthetic medication, induction, maintaining and supplementing anesthesia as well as for 'conscious sedation'.
- They slightly decrease respiration, blood pressure and cardiac contractility when given in combination with opioids.
- They produce amnesia, sedation and unconsciousness within 5–10 minutes, when given in slightly higher doses.
- The side effects such as nausea or vomiting are uncommon with BZDs.
- The common indications of BZDs are endoscopies, angiography, cardiac catheterization, setting of fractures, local/regional anesthesia.
- BZDs are also an important component of balanced anesthesia.
- Flumazenil in a dose of 0.5–2 mg IV is used for the reversal of anesthetic effects of BZDs.

Diazepam

Administered in a running IV infusion in a dose of 0.2–0.5 mg/kg slowly to prevent thrombophlebitis.

Lorazepam

- It is a slow-acting, less irritant and three times more potent than diazepam.
- It is given in a dose of 2–4 mg IV.
- It has potent amnesic effect.

Midazolam

- It is short-acting, non-irritant to veins and water soluble BZD.
- It is three times more potent than diazepam.

- It is given in a dose of 1–2.5 mg IV, while the dose of 0.02–0.1 mg/kg/hour continuous IV infusion is given in the critical care anesthesia.
- It is also used for the sedation of intubated and mechanically ventilated patients, and for debridement and dressing of burn wounds.
- It is preferred over diazepam for anesthetic use.

Opioids

[Fentanyl, Remifentanil, Sufentanil]
(Described in Opioids)

Fentanyl

- It is more lipid soluble and easily crosses blood-brain barrier; produces analgesic effects within 5 minutes after IV injection.
- It is given in a dose of 2–4 µg/kg and can be used in combination with BZDs.
- It is used for endoscopic, angiographic and minor surgical procedures in low risk patients.
- It is used as adjunct in nerve block, spinal block and for the management of post-operative pain.

  Alfentanil, Sufentanil and Remifentanil are still shorter acting analogues, which can be used in place of fentanyl.

Ketamine

- It induces *'dissociative anesthesia'*, which is characterized by dissociation from the body and surroundings with profound analgesia, immobility, amnesia and light sleep.
- The primary site of action is in the cortex and subcortical areas; not in the reticular activating system, which is the site of action of barbiturates.
- It acts by inhibition of N-methyl D-aspartate (NMDA) receptor complex.
- Respiration is not depressed, bronchi dilate, airway reflexes are maintained, muscle tone increases.
- A dose of 1–2 mg/kg IV or 3–5 mg/kg IM produces the above effects within a minute, and recovery starts after 10–15 min, but patient remains amnesic for 1–2 hr.
- Ketamine has been used for operations on the head and neck, in asthmatics (relieves bronchospasm), in those who do not want to lose consciousness and for short operations.
- It is the only IV anesthetic that produces analgesic effects.
- Ketamine increases the cerebral blood flow, intraocular pressure (IOP) and intracranial tension (ICT). Therefore, it is contraindicated in patients with hypertension, ischemic heart disease, glaucoma and neurosurgical procedures but suitable for patient of hypovolemic shock.
- It is used in combination with diazepam for angiographies, cardiac catheterization and trauma surgery.
- Children tolerate this drug better than adults.

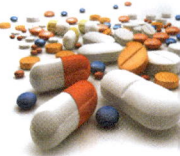

Dexmedetomidine is a centrally active selective α$_{2A}$ agonist that has been introduced for sedating critically ill/ventilated patients in intensive care units.

Pre-anesthetic Medications

- Pre-anesthetic medications are the drugs given before anesthesia to make patient calm and to make the anesthesia more pleasant and safe.
- It is given:
  - To decrease the level of anxiety and apprehension
  - To facilitate induction
  - For pre- and post-operative amnesia
  - To decrease the requirement of anesthetic drugs
  - To decrease gastric and respiratory secretions and antiemetic effect.

Conscious Sedation

'Conscious sedation' is a state of altered consciousness that is used in minor procedures (*localized surgical or therapeutic procedure*) which do not require proper anesthesia. In this condition, the patient is in conscious state but doesn't feel any pain stimulus. This is due to CNS depressant effects by the drugs without interfering the level of consciousness of patient.

Drugs used for conscious sedation are:

- **Fentanyl:** At 1–2 μg/kg every 15–30 minutes with/without combination of other drugs (Propofol, Midazolam).
- **Nitrous oxide:** 10% nitrous oxide (maximum up to 50%) in combination with 100% oxygen. The effects last only for ≤ 1 hour.
- **Propofol:** Given as continuous IV infusion till the procedure is performed. It has very short action. As soon as Propofol is withdrawn, patient recovers within minutes.
- **Diazepam:** 1–2 mg slow IV infusion in small repeated doses produces satisfactory sedative effects like slurring of speech, ptosis, muscle relaxation, etc. The further administration is stopped after this observation. The effects of diazepam persist for an hour while the psychomotor impairment persists for 6–24 hours.
- **Midazolam:** It is used as an alternative to diazepam.

- Depending upon the need of patient and type of surgery being performed, different combinations of drugs are used as pre-anesthetic medications. These are:

Sedative-antianxiety Drugs

(Discussed in Benzodiazepines)

- BZDs like diazepam, lorazepam, midazolam, and promethazine are commonly used drugs as pre-anesthetic medications for their tranquilizer and smooth induction property.

- Diazepam (5–10 mg oral) or lorazepam (2 mg oral or 0.05 mg/kg IM) are used one hour before the surgery.
- Midazolam is commonly used intravenously due to its shorter action and water solubility. It is used along with pethidine/fentanyl for a variety of minor surgical and endoscopic procedures.
- Promethazine having antihistaminic, antiemetic anticholinergic and sedative effects is used in a dose of 50 mg intramuscularly.

Anticholinergics

(Discussed in Chapters 4 and 6)

- These drugs are less frequently used nowadays due to availability of non-irritant anesthetic drugs.
- The commonly used anticholinergics for pre-anesthetics are atropine or hyoscine or glycopyrrolate.
- These drugs are used to reduce GI and bronchial secretions to prevent aspiration.
- Atropine or hyoscine is given in a dose of 0.6 mg or 10–20 μg/kg IM/IV and glycopyrrolate at 0.2–0.3 mg or 5–10 μg/kg IM/IV.
- Glycopyrrolate is more preferred than atropine due to its lesser side effects and good anti-secretory action after IM injection.
- Hyoscine having both antiemetic and amnestic effects but may lead to delirium and disorientation; hence less frequently used.

H$_2$ Blockers/Proton Pump Inhibitors

(Discussed in Chapters 4 and 5)

- These agents are mainly indicated in the individuals who are at high risk of gastric regurgitation and aspiration pneumonia usually seen after prolonged GI surgery, cesarean section and obese patients.
- The commonly prescribed drugs are pantoprazole (40 mg) or Ranitidine (150 mg) or famotidine (20 mg) or omeprazole (20 mg). These are given night before and in the morning or preferably 12 hours before any procedure.
- They reduce GI secretions as well as pH; hence routinely prescribed nowadays.
- They are also beneficial to prevent stress ulcer.

Antiemetics

(Discussed in Chapter 4)

- The commonly prescribed drugs are metoclopramide, ondansetron and domperidone.
- Table 9.31 enlists the basic information of the common antiemetics.

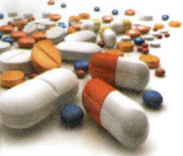

TABLE 9.31: Comparison of commonly prescribed antiemetics

Metoclopramide	Ondansetron	Domperidone
• Pre-operatively 10–20 mg IM is given to counteract post-operative vomiting • It increases lower esophageal sphincter tone and promoting gastric emptying • It can be used in combination with H_2 blockers	• Pre-operatively 4–8 mg IV is given to counteract post-operative nausea and vomiting • It selectively inhibits 5-HT$_3$ receptors. • It has very few side effects; hence most commonly used	• Domperidone is nearly as effective and does not produce extrapyramidal side effects

Opioids

(Discussed in Opioids)

- Nowadays opioids are less commonly *used* in post-operative pain; fentanyl is used only if specifically indicated.
- Opioids are used for induction, pre- and post-operative analgesia and to manage pre-operative anxiety.
- Commonly, intramuscular morphine (10 mg) or pethidine (50–100 mg) are used.
- They may cause respiratory depression, biliary spasm, hypotension and may precipitate asthma.
- Morphine may cause post-operative vomiting, urinary retention and constipation; while pethidine induces tachycardia.

Neuroleptics

- These agents have great potency to develop hypotension and respiratory depression; hence *infrequently used nowadays.*
- In children, muscle dystonia and involuntary movements may be seen.
- These agents are used as antiemetics and antianxiety for induction.
- The commonly used pre-anesthetic drugs are chlorpromazine (25 mg), triflupromazine (10 mg) or haloperidol (2–4 mg) given intramuscularly.

Drug Interactions

- MAO inhibitors increase the pharmacological actions of morphine by slowing its metabolism. Hence, combination should be avoided.
- Alcohol, barbiturates and antipsychotics when concurrently used with morphine exhibit intense sedative and antidepressant effect.
- Morphine delays the gastric emptying; therefore, slowdown the rate of absorption of many orally administered drugs.
- The effect of general anesthetic drugs is potentiated by opioids, neuroleptics and monoamine oxidase inhibitors.
- The general anesthetic drugs potentiate the effect of antihypertensive drugs and cause marked fall in blood pressure.
- Hydrocortisone 100 mg is given intravenously (during intra-operative period) to the patients who are already on steroid therapy. This prevents the acute adrenal cortical insufficiency and cardiovascular collapse in these patients.
- Adrenaline may produce cardiac arrhythmias in patients who are given halothane as anesthesia.

Nursing Implications

- **General anesthetics**
  - Evaluate the effectiveness of the teaching plan (patient can give the drug name and dosage, possible adverse effects to watch for and specific measures to prevent adverse effects, and therapeutic goals).
  - Assess for contraindications or cautions: any known allergies to general anesthetics to avoid hypersensitivity reactions.
  - Patient should be assessing for personal or family history of malignant hyperthermia, which may be triggered by the use of general anesthetics.
  - Nurse should reassure the patient and help in allaying the anxiety of patient the night before surgery and give anti-anxiety drug.
  - The drugs used in general anesthesia should only be used by trained personnel or anesthesiologist only.
  - Monitor temperature for prompt detection and treatment of malignant hyperthermia. Maintain dantrolene on standby.
  - Monitor pulse, respiration, blood pressure, ECG, and cardiac output continuously during and after the anesthesia.
  - Monitor for adverse effects (respiratory depression, hypotension, bronchospasm, slowed GI activity, malignant hyperthermia).
  - Nurse should protect herself against the effect of exhaled anesthetic gases.
  - Evaluate the effectiveness of the teaching plan.

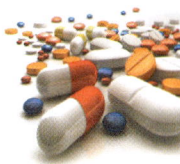

LOCAL ANESTHETICS (LAs)

Local anesthesia refers to a reversible loss of sensations in limited area of the body. The local anesthetic drugs block generation and conduction of nerve impulse at any part of the neuron with which they come in contact, without causing any structural damage to the nerve. When a local anesthesia is applied to a mixed nerve, both sensory and motor impulses are interrupted, which result in muscular paralysis and loss of autonomic control as well.

Local anesthesia can be achieved by several different methods. Topical administration, infiltration, field block, nerve block, and intravenous regional anesthesia.

Topical Administration

- Topical local anesthesia involves the application of a cream, lotion, ointment, or drop of a local anesthetic to skin or mucous membrane to relieve pain or to anesthetize the area to facilitate a medical procedure.
- Although systemic absorption is rare with topical application, it can occur if there is damage or breakdown of the tissues in the area.

Infiltration Anesthesia

- Infiltration local anesthesia involves injecting the anesthetic drug directly into the tissues to be anesthetized.
- The infiltrated anesthetic comes into contact with the nerve endings in the area and prevents them from transmitting nerve impulses to the brain.

Field Block

Field block local anesthesia involves injecting the anesthetic drug all around the area, which needs to be anesthetized for procedure or surgery. Example: block for tooth extractions.

Nerve Block

- Nerve block local anesthesia involves injecting the anesthetic drug at some point along the nerve or nerves that run to and from the region, in which the loss of pain sensation or muscle paralysis is desired.
- The blocks are given at some distance from the field to be operated.
- Several types of nerve blocks are possible:
  - **Peripheral nerve block:** For relief of pain or for diagnostic purposes.
  - **Central nerve block:** Injection of anesthetic into the roots of the nerves in the spinal cord.
  - **Epidural anesthesia:** Injection of the drug into the epidural space where the nerves emerge from the spinal cord.
  - **Caudal block:** Injection of anesthetic into the sacral canal, below the epidural area.
  - **Spinal anesthesia:** Injection of anesthetic into the spinal subarachnoid space.

Intravenous Regional Local Anesthesia

- Intravenous regional local anesthesia involves carefully draining all of the blood from the patient's arm or leg, securing a tourniquet to prevent the anesthetic from entering the general circulation, and then injecting the anesthetic into the vein of the arm or leg.
- This technique is used for very specific surgical procedures. The local anesthetic drugs are classified in Table 9.32.

The differences between ester and amide forms of local anesthetics are given in Table 9.33.

TABLE 9.32: Classification of local anesthetics

Injectable anesthetics		
Low potency and short duration	**Intermediate potency and duration**	**High potency and long duration**
• Procaine • Chloroprocaine	• Lidocaine (Lignocaine) • Prilocaine	• Tetracaine • Bupivacaine • Ropivacaine • Dibucaine
Surface anesthetics		
Soluble	**Insoluble**	
• Cocaine • Lidocaine • Tetracaine • Benoxinate	• Benzocaine • Oxethazaine • Butylaminobenzoate	

TABLE 9.33: Differences between ester and amide forms of local anesthetics

Properties	Ester	Amide
Onset of action	Slow	Fast
Duration of action	Short	Intermediate
Tissue penetration	Poor	Good
Metabolism	By cholinesterase	By liver microsomal enzyme
Allergic reactions	Common	Uncommon
Drugs	Cocaine, Procaine, Benzocaine, Tetracaine Chloroprocaine	Lidocaine, Dibucaine, Bupivacaine, Ropivacaine, Prilocaine, Articaine

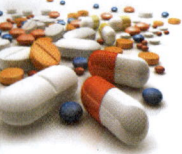

Mechanism of Action

- LAs interfere with the sodium ions entry during action potential and this leads to inhibition of nerve conduction.
- They mainly act on the voltage gated sodium channel and open it, leading to efflux of positive ions and cell become negative inside causing hyperpolarization.
- Mostly, the LAs are used for their local action, but after systemic absorption from the local site, some systemic effects may be seen.

Mechanism of action of local anesthetics is shown is Figure 9.3.

- The systemic actions are seen depending upon the concentration attained in plasma and tissues.
- All LAs produce CNS stimulation followed by depression. The LAs act as cardiac depressants if they achieve concentration 2–3 times higher than that producing CNS effects or accidently these are injected intravenously.
- They decrease automaticity, excitability, contractility, conductivity and prolong effective refractory period (ERP).
- By causing vasodilation, they cause hypotension.

Failure of LAs: Sometimes, there is a failure in induction of local anesthesia, which may be due to the reasons given in Table 9.34.

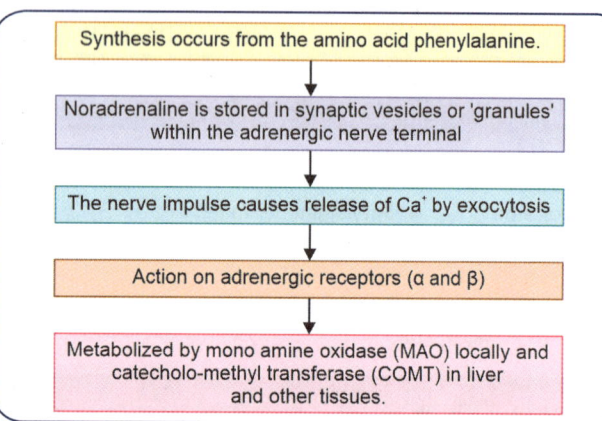

Synthesis occurs from the amino acid phenylalanine.

↓

Noradrenaline is stored in synaptic vesicles or 'granules' within the adrenergic nerve terminal

↓

The nerve impulse causes release of Ca⁺ by exocytosis

↓

Action on adrenergic receptors (α and β)

↓

Metabolized by mono amine oxidase (MAO) locally and catecholo-methyl transferase (COMT) in liver and other tissues.

FIG. 9.3: Mechanism of action of local anesthetics

✔

The local anesthetic agents are not able to provide adequate pain control in inflamed tissues.

This occurs due to following reasons:

Due to inflammation, the pH of the tissues becomes acidic, which causes ionization of greater fraction of the local anesthesia. This hinders the diffusion of LAs into the axolemma of nerve.

The LA is removed more rapidly from the site due to increased blood flow to the inflamed area.

Inflammatory mediators may oppose LA action.

Usually, adrenaline is added to the local anesthetic solutions. The adrenaline acts as vasoconstrictor in a ratio of 1:50,000 to 1:200,000 and the addition of a vasoconstrictor offers following advantages as compared to plain local anesthetic solution:

- It prolongs the duration of action of LAs by decreasing their rate of removal from the local site. It increases the intensity of nerve block.
- As the rate of absorption is reduced, the plasma concentration remains on the lower side and the systemic toxicity of LAs is reduced.
- Due to intense local vasoconstriction, the field of surgery remains bloodless.
- Simultaneously, there are disadvantages of this combination in the form of local tissue edema, necrosis, delay in wound healing due to local tissue hypoxia and rise in blood pressure and arrhythmias in the susceptible individuals.

Precautions while Using LAs

- Before injecting the LAs, aspiration test should be performed to avoid intravascular injection.
- Inject the LA slowly and take care not to exceed the maximum safe dose, especially in children.
- Propranolol (probably other β blockers also) may reduce metabolism of lidocaine and other amide LAs by reducing hepatic blood flow.
- Vasoconstrictor (adrenaline) containing LA should be avoided for patients with ischemic heart disease, cardiac arrhythmia, thyrotoxicosis, uncontrolled hypertension, and those receiving β blockers (rise in BP can occur due to unopposed α action) or tricyclic antidepressants (uptake blockade and potentiation of Adr).

TABLE 9.34: Causes of failure of local anesthesia and its management

Causes of failure of local anesthesia	Management of failed local anesthesia
• Wrong technique and anatomical variations	• Check anatomical landmarks
• Inadequate dose	• Repeat injection
• Sepsis	• Settle pain and inflammation and try again about a week later
• Injection in blood vessels	• Manage accordingly
• Anxiety (reduces patient pain threshold)	• Consider whether anxiety may be contributory

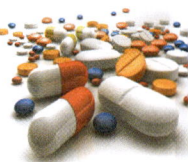

Injectable Anesthetics

The pharmacological features of injectable anesthetics are given in Table 9.35.

Surface Anesthetics

The pharmacological features of surface anesthetics are given in Table 9.36.

TABLE 9.35: Pharmacological features of injectable anesthetics

Drugs	Groups	Duration of action (minutes)	Onset of action	Special features
Procaine	Ester	15–30	Slow	• It was the first synthetic LA • It slows the absorption of penicillin making it OD dose • Presented as injection procaine penicillin fortified (PPF)
Chloroprocaine	Ester	15–30	Rapid	• Low toxicity due to rapid metabolism
Lidocaine (Lignocaine)	Amide	30–60	Rapid	• Most widely used LA • Both surface and injectable forms are available • Used for most of the surgical procedures
Prilocaine	Amide	30–90	Intermediate	• Used for infiltration, nerve block and intravenous regional anesthesia
Tetracaine	Ester	120–240	Very slow	• Use is restricted to eye, nose, throat and tracheobronchial tree
Bupivacaine	Amide	120–240	Intermediate	• Epidural injection (0.25–0.5%) provides analgesia- painless vaginal delivery • Cardiotoxic at ≥0.75% concentration
Ropivacaine	Amide	120–360	Intermediate	• Similar to bupivacaine with less cardiotoxicity, preferred over bupivacaine in post-operative pain and painless vaginal delivery
Dibucaine	Amide	180–600	Slow	• It is most potent, most toxic and longest acting LA • Used only topically

TABLE 9.36: Pharmacological features of surface anesthetics

Drugs	Onset of action	Special features
Cocaine	Fast	• Rarely used as anesthetic agent • Produces drug dependence and abuse
Benoxinate	Rapid	• 0.4% solution is used for corneal anesthesia for tonometry (intraocular pressure measurement procedure)
Tetracaine	Very slow	• 0.5% solution is used for eye, nose, throat and tracheobronchial tree
Lidocaine (Lignocaine)	Rapid	• Topical: 4%, jelly and viscous form: 2%, ointment: 5%, spray: 10% available in the market • Transdermal patch is used in post-herpetic neuralgia
Benzocaine	Intermediate	• It is not absorbed from mucous membrane • Used as lozenges for stomatitis, sore throat • As powder/ointment for wound/ulcerated surface and suppository for anorectal lesions
Butylaminobenzoate	Intermediate	• Same as above
Oxethazaine	Slow	• It is active even at low pH. Hence, used along with antacids for anesthetizing gastric mucosa

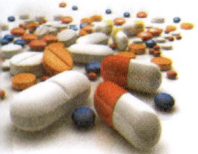

✔

EMLA (Eutectic mixture of local anesthetics lignocaine 2.5% and pilocaine 2.5%)

Eutectic mixture is made by mixing 2.5% lidocaine and 2.5% prilocaine in equal proportions at 25°C. This lowers the melting point of these two drugs. The resulting oil is emulsified into water to form a cream.

- This preparation can anesthetize intact skin after surface application.
- The method of application of this cream is unique.
- The EMLA cream is applied under occlusive dressing for 1 hour before the requirement of anesthesia in conditions such as split skin graft harvesting, painless IV cannulation and other superficial procedures.
- The part remains anesthetized for 1–2 hours after removal of occlusive dressing.
- It is used as an alternative to lidocaine infiltration.
- It should not be used on mucous membranes and abraded skin.
- It is available in 5% concentration.

Adverse Effects Of Local Anesthetics

The rapidly absorbed LAs with slow metabolism are more toxic and produce side effects when they come in circulation and reach to various organs such as CNS, cardiovascular system, etc.

These side effects are:

- CNS effects: Dizziness, mental confusion, disorientation, shivering, twitching, auditory and visual disturbances, convulsions and respiratory arrest. This is treated by diazepam.
- Cardiovascular toxicity of LAs presents as bradycardia, hypotension, cardiac arrhythmias and vascular collapse.
- Injection of LAs is painful and addition of vasoconstrictor enhances the local tissue damage. The lignocaine with adrenaline combination should not be used for infiltration in ring block of hands, feet, fingers, toes, in pinna and penis as gangrene can occur.
- Hypersensitivity reactions and rarely anaphylaxis can also occur. These reactions are more common with ester-linked LAs, but rare with lidocaine or its congeners. Cross reactivity is frequent among ester compounds, but not with amide-linked LAs. The cause of allergic reaction is methylparaben, which is added as preservative in certain LA solutions.

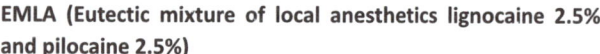

Drug Interactions

- Propranolol and other β blockers reduce the metabolism of lidocaine and other amide LAs by decreasing hepatic blood flow.
- Adrenaline containing LA should not be given to the patients of uncontrolled hypertension, cardiac arrhythmia, ischemic heart disease, thyrotoxicosis or tricyclic antidepressants. Giving adrenaline may cause worsening of these diseases.

Nursing Implications

- **Local anesthetics**
  - Assess for contraindications and cautions: any known allergies to these drugs or to parabens to avoid hypersensitivity reactions.
  - Aspiration should be performed invariably before giving LAs to avoid intravascular injection.
  - The LAs should be injected slowly and within the recommended doses.
  - Have emergency equipment readily available to maintain airway and provide mechanical ventilation if needed.
  - Ensure that drugs for managing hypotension, cardiac arrest, and central nervous system alterations are readily available in case of severe reaction and toxicity.
  - Ensure that patients receiving spinal anesthesia or epidural anesthesia are well hydrated and remain lying down for up to 12 hours after the anesthesia to minimize headache.
  - Establish safety precautions to prevent injury during the time that the patient has a loss of sensation and/or mobility.
  - Monitor for adverse effects (respiratory depression, blood pressure changes, arrhythmias, gastrointestinal upset, and CNS alterations).
  - Evaluate the effectiveness of the teaching plan.

GASES (OXYGEN, NITROUS OXIDE, CARBON DIOXIDE)

OXYGEN

- It is a colorless and odorless diatomic gas with the formula O_2.
- Oxygen (O_2) is essential to life and constitutes 20.8% of earth's atmosphere.
- Oxygen enters inside the body through the process of respiration and is essentially required for cellular respiration.

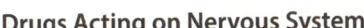

- *Hypoxia* is the term used to denote insufficient oxygenation of the tissues.
- *Hypoxemia* generally implies a failure of the respiratory system to oxygenate arterial blood.
- Hypoxia is a life-threatening condition in which oxygen delivery is inadequate to meet the metabolic demands of the tissues. An inadequate supply of oxygen ultimately results in the cessation of aerobic metabolism and oxidative phosphorylation, depletion of high-energy compounds, cellular dysfunction, and death.
- Oxygen inhalation is used therapeutically to reverse or prevent the development of hypoxia.
- Oxygen breathed in excessive amounts or for prolonged periods can produce secondary physiological changes and toxic effects too.

Commercial Availability of Oxygen

- Oxygen is supplied in the form of compressed gas in steel cylinders, and a purity of 99% is referred to as *medical grade*. Most hospitals have continuous bedside oxygen supply through pipes. This oxygen supply is delivered from either oxygen plants or insulated liquid oxygen containers. For safety, oxygen cylinders and piping are color-coded and some form of mechanical indexing of valve connections is used to prevent the connection of other gases to oxygen systems.
- The oxygen cylinders are '**black colored cylinder with white collar**'.
- Oxygen concentrators, which employ molecular sieve, membrane, or electrochemical technologies, are available for use at home. Such systems produce 30-95% oxygen depending on the flow rate.

Devices to Administer Oxygen

- **Nasal cannulae** are small, flexible prongs that are put just inside each naris and deliver oxygen at a rate of 1–6 L/min. The nasopharynx acts as a reservoir for storing the oxygen, and patients may breathe through either the mouth or nose as long as the nasal passages remain patent.
- **The simple facemask**, a clear plastic mask with side holes for clearance of expiratory gas and inspiratory air entrainment, is used when higher concentrations of oxygen delivered without tight control are desired. The maximum flow of inspired oxygen through a facemask can be increased from around 60% at 6–15 L/min to >85% by adding a 600–1000 mL reservoir bag. With this partial rebreathing mask, most of the inspired volume is drawn from the reservoir, avoiding dilution by entrainment of room air.
- **The Venturi-style mask** uses a specially designed mask insert to entrain room air reliably in a fixed ratio.
- **Oxygen nebulizers** provide patients with humidified oxygen.

Monitoring of Oxygenation

- **Invasive** approach for monitoring oxygenation is by drawing blood from either artery or vein and laboratory analysis of arterial or venous blood gases.
- **Noninvasive** monitoring of arterial oxygen saturation can be achieved using transcutaneous pulse oximetry, in which oxygen saturation is measured from the differential absorption of light by oxyhemoglobin and deoxyhemoglobin and the arterial saturation determined from the pulsatile component of this signal.

Therapeutic Uses of Oxygen

- Oxygen therapy is used to correct hypoxia in the patients of emphysema, pneumonia, and some heart disorders such as congestive heart failure and any disease that impairs the body's ability to take up and use gases.
- In situations such as bowel distension due to obstruction or ileus, intravascular air embolism, or pneumothorax, it is desirable to reduce the volume of air-filled spaces. Since nitrogen is relatively insoluble, inhalation of high concentrations of oxygen (and thus low concentrations of nitrogen) rapidly lowers the total-body partial pressure of nitrogen and provides a substantial gradient for the removal of nitrogen from gas spaces.
- Administration of oxygen for air embolism is additionally beneficial because it helps to relieve localized hypoxia distal to the vascular obstruction.
- In the case of *decompression sickness*, oxygen inhalation prior to or during a barometric decompression reduces the supersaturation that occurs after decompression so that bubbles do not form.
- Oxygen can be administered at greater than atmospheric pressure in hyperbaric chambers. Clinical uses of *hyperbaric oxygen therapy* include the treatment of trauma, burns, radiation damage, infections, non-healing ulcers, skin grafts, spasticity, and other neurological conditions. Hyperbaric oxygen may be useful in generalized hypoxia and in carbon-monoxide poisoning.

Complications of Oxygen Therapy

Administration of supplemental oxygen is not without potential complications. Common complications are:

- **Respiratory tract:** The pulmonary system is usually the first to exhibit toxicity. Exposure to the highest oxygen (100% O_2) tensions produces subtle changes in pulmonary function within 8–12 hours of exposure.
- **Nervous system:** Central nervous system problems are rare, and toxicity occurs only under hyperbaric conditions where exposure exceeds 200 kPa (2 atm). Retinopathy of prematurity (ROP) is an eye disease in premature infants involving abnormal vascularization of the developing

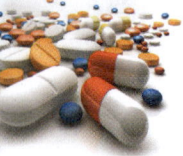

retina that can result from oxygen toxicity or relative hypoxia. Retinal changes can progress to blindness and are likely caused by fibrovascular proliferation.

NITROUS OXIDE

(Described in General Anesthetics)

CARBON DIOXIDE

- Carbon dioxide is produced by metabolism at approximately the same rate as O_2 is consumed. At rest, this value is ~3 mL/kg min, but it may increase dramatically with exercise.
- CO_2 diffuses readily from the cells into the blood, where it is carried partly as bicarbonate ion (HCO_3^-), partly in chemical combination with hemoglobin and plasma proteins, and partly in solution at a partial pressure of ~6 kPa (46 mm Hg) in mixed venous blood.
- Carbon dioxide (CO_2) is transported to the lung, where it is normally exhaled at the rate it is produced, leaving a partial pressure of ~5.2 kPa (40 mm Hg) in the alveoli and in arterial blood.
- An increase in partial pressure of carbon dioxide (PCO_2) results in a respiratory acidosis and may be due to decreased ventilation or excessive inhalation of CO_2, whereas an increase in ventilation results in decreased PCO_2 and a respiratory alkalosis.
- Since CO_2 is freely diffusible, the changes in blood PCO_2 and pH soon are reflected by intracellular changes in PCO_2 and pH.

Effects of Carbon Dioxide

- Alterations in PCO_2 and pH have widespread effects in the body, particularly on respiration, circulation, and the CNS.
- **Respiratory effects:** CO_2 is a rapid, potent stimulus to ventilation in direct proportion to the inspired CO_2. Inhalation of 10% carbon dioxide can produce minute volumes of 75 L/min in normal individuals. CO_2 stimulates breathing by acidifying central chemoreceptors and the peripheral carotid bodies.
- **Circulatory effects:** The circulatory effects of CO_2 result from the combination of its direct local effects and its centrally mediated effects on the autonomic nervous system. The direct effect of CO_2 on the heart are diminished contractility, results from pH changes and a decreased myofilament Ca^{2+} responsiveness.
- The direct effect on systemic blood vessels results in vasodilation. CO_2 causes widespread activation of the sympathetic nervous system and an increase in the plasma concentrations of epinephrine, norepinephrine, angiotensin, and other vasoactive peptides. The results of sympathetic nervous system activation generally

are opposite to the local effects of carbon dioxide. The sympathetic effects consist of increases in cardiac contractility, heart rate, and vasoconstriction. *Hypocarbia* results in opposite effects: decreased blood pressure and vasoconstriction in skin, intestine, brain, kidney, and heart. These actions are exploited clinically in the form of induced hyperventilation to diminish intracranial tension.

- **CNS effects:** Hypercarbia depresses the excitability of the cerebral cortex and increases the cutaneous pain threshold through a central action. This central depression has therapeutic importance. For example, in patients who are hypoventilating from narcotics or anesthetics, increasing PCO_2 may result in further CNS depression, which in turn may worsen the respiratory depression.

Availability and Methods of Administration

- CO_2 is marketed in gray metal cylinders as the pure gas or as CO_2 mixed with oxygen.
- It usually is administered through facemask at a concentration of 5–10% in combination with O_2.
- Another method for the temporary administration of CO_2 is by rebreathing, such as from an anesthesia breathing circuit, when the soda lime canister is by passed or from something as simple as a paper bag.

Therapeutic Uses

- CO_2 is used for insufflation during endoscopic procedures (e.g. laparoscopic surgery) because it is highly soluble and does not support combustion. Inadvertent gas emboli thus are dissolved and eliminated more easily by the respiratory system.
- CO_2 can be used to flood the surgical field during cardiac surgery. Because of its density, carbon dioxide displaces the air surrounding the open heart so that any gas bubbles trapped in the heart are carbon dioxide rather than insoluble nitrogen.
- Similarly, CO_2 is used to de-bubble cardiopulmonary by-pass and extracorporeal membrane oxygenation (ECMO) circuits. It is used to adjust pH during cardiopulmonary bypass procedures when the patient is cooled.
- Hypocarbia, with its attendant respiratory alkalosis, still has some uses in anesthesia. It constricts cerebral vessels, decreasing brain size slightly, and thus may facilitate the performance of neurosurgical operations.
- While short-term hypocarbia is effective for this purpose, sustained hypocarbia has been associated with worse outcomes in patients with head injury.
- Consequently, hypocarbia should be instituted with a clearly defined indication and normocarbia should be re-established as soon the indication for hypocarbia no longer applies.

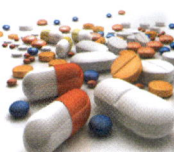

Nursing Implications

☞ **Gases**
- ☞ Nurse should be aware of the color coding of different gas cylinders.
- ☞ The empty cylinders should be kept separately from the filled cylinders and nurse should attach a sticker when the cylinder becomes empty.
- ☞ Nurse should ensure that the accessories required along with gas cylinders are readily available when required.
- ☞ Nurse should be vigilant about the leakage of gases from the cylinders.
- ☞ Nurse should ensure that nobody smokes or burns incense sticks or Dhoop near the gas cylinders.

CHOLINERGIC AND ANTICHOLINERGIC DRUGS

AUTONOMIC NERVOUS SYSTEM

The division of nervous system is given in Figure 9.4.

The autonomic nervous system (ANS) mainly controls visceral functions and acts largely below the level of consciousness. The main differences between the somatic and autonomic nervous systems are given in Table 9.37.

Like the somatic nervous system, the ANS consists of afferents, central connections and efferents.

Autonomic Afferents

- Most of the visceral nerves carry non-myelinated visceral afferent fibers. These are mostly mixed nerves.
- They mediate visceral pain, cardiovascular, respiratory and other visceral reflexes.

Central Autonomic Connections

- Integration of somatic and autonomic innervations occurs in the CNS.
- The highest seat regulating autonomic functions is hypothalamus. The posterior and lateral nuclei of hypothalamus are *primarily sympathetic* and anterior and medial nuclei are *primarily parasympathetic*.

TABLE 9.37: Differences between somatic and autonomic nervous systems

	Somatic	Autonomic
Organ innervated	Skeletal muscles	All other organs
Distal most synapse	Within CNS	Outside CNS (in ganglia)
Nerve fibers	Myelinated	Pre-ganglionic—myelinated Post-ganglionic—non-myelinated
Peripheral plexus formation	Absent	Present
Primary efferent transmitter	Acetylcholine	Acetylcholine, Noradrenaline
Effect of nerve section on organ supplied	Paralysis and atrophy	Activity maintained, no atrophy

- The location of many autonomic centers (pupillary, vagal, respiratory, etc.) is in the mid-brain and medulla.
- The lateral column in the thoracic spinal cord contains cells, which give rise to the sympathetic outflow.

Autonomic Efferents

- The motor limb of the ANS has been divided into sympathetic and parasympathetic efferents.
- Many organs receive both sympathetic and parasympathetic innervations (Fig. 9.5).
- These two systems mostly work opposite to each other physiologically.
- The organs innervated specifically by sympathetic system are blood vessels, spleen, sweat glands and hair follicles.
- The organs innervated specifically by parasympathetic system are ciliary muscles, bronchial smooth muscles, gastric and pancreatic glands, etc.

ENTERIC NERVOUS SYSTEM

- The '*enteric nervous system*' controls various activities of gastrointestinal tract and it works independently in controlling the bowel movements as well as secretion and absorption processes.

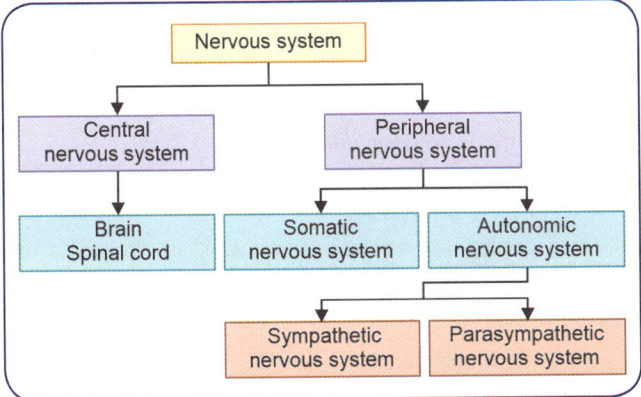

FIG. 9.4: Division of nervous system

233

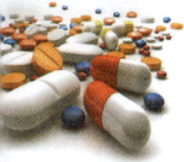

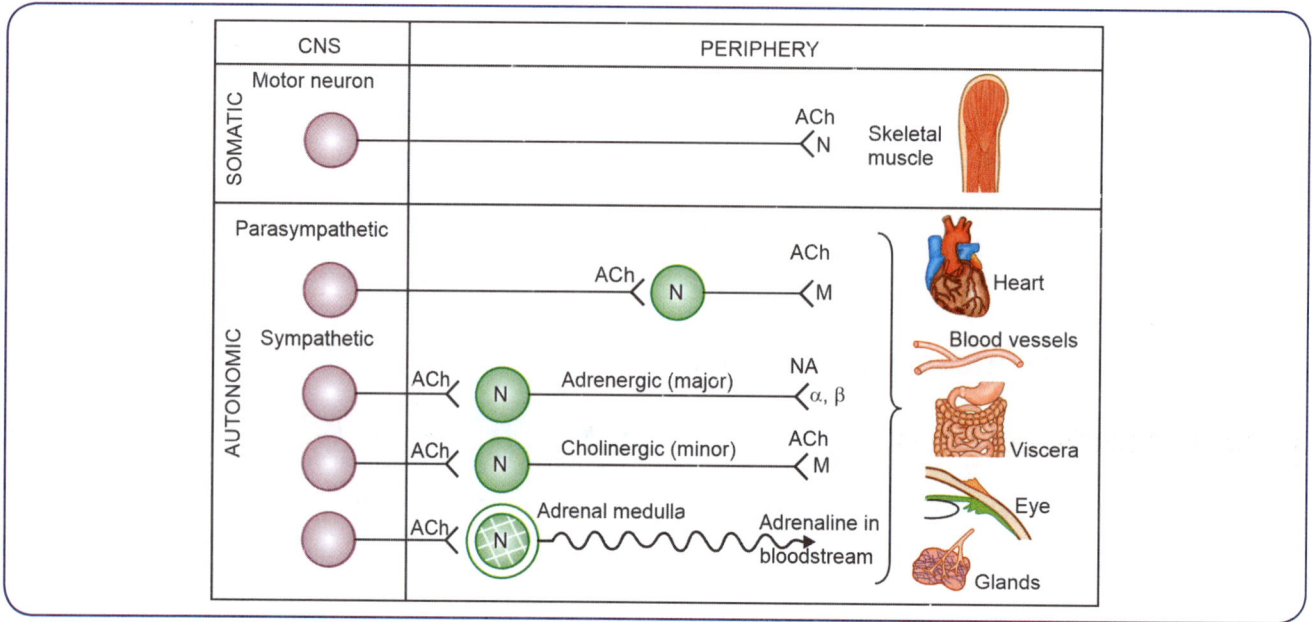

FIG. 9.5: Innervations of somatic and peripheral nervous system

- Both sympathetic and parasympathetic divisions of ANS, provide input to enteric plexus.

NEUROCHEMICAL/NEUROHUMORAL TRANSMISSION

The nerves transmit their messages to other nerves by the release of certain signal molecules or chemical messengers in the synapses and these chemical substances act on neuroeffector junctions to propagate the signal. These signal molecules are chemical messengers and are known as neurotransmitters. Although over 50 different types of neurotransmitters have been identified in the nervous system. Norepinephrine (and the closely related epinephrine), acetylcholine, dopamine, serotonin, histamine, glutamate, and γ-aminobutyric acid are most commonly involved in the actions of therapeutically useful drugs. Each of these neurotransmitter binds to a specific family of receptors. Acetylcholine and norepinephrine are the primary neurotransmitters in the ANS, whereas a wide variety of neurotransmitters function in the CNS.

The various steps involved in neurohumoral transmission are:

- Impulse conduction
- Transmitter release
- Transmitter action on post-junctional membrane
- Post-junctional activity
- Termination of transmitter action

The autonomic nervous system has been broadly divided into sympathetic and parasympathetic system, their differences are given in Table 9.38.

The autonomic nerve fibers can be divided into two groups based on the type of neurotransmitter released. These are cholinergic and adrenergic nerve fibers.

- If transmission is mediated by acetylcholine, the neuron is termed **cholinergic**. Acetylcholine mediates the transmission of nerve impulses across autonomic ganglia in both the sympathetic and parasympathetic nervous systems. It is the neurotransmitter at the adrenal medulla.
- In the somatic nervous system, transmission at the neuromuscular junction (the junction of nerve fibers and voluntary muscles) is also cholinergic.
- When norepinephrine and epinephrine are the neurotransmitters, the fiber is termed **adrenergic**. In the sympathetic system, norepinephrine mediates the transmission of nerve impulses from autonomic Post-ganglionic nerves to effector organs.
- The actions of sympathetic and parasympathetic nervous systems are given in Figure 9.6.
- The major neurotransmitter at autonomic, somatic and central sites is *acetylcholine* (ACh).
- It is synthesized locally in the cholinergic nerve endings and stored in the vesicles.
- After getting appropriate stimulus, it is released from the pre-synaptic membrane into the synapse, acts on the cholinoceptors present on the post-synaptic membrane, produces effects and is hydrolyzed by the enzyme acetyl cholinesterase (AChE).

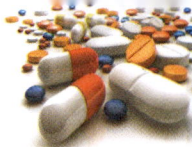

TABLE 9.38: Differences between sympathetic and parasympathetic nervous system

Features	Sympathetic nervous system	Parasympathetic nervous system
Sites of origin	Thoracic and lumbar region of the spinal cord (thoracolumbar)	Brain and sacral area of the spinal cord (craniosacral)
Length of fibers	Short Pre-ganglionic Long Post-ganglionic	Long Pre-ganglionic Short Post-ganglionic
Location of ganglia	Close to the spinal cord	Within or near effector organs
Pre-ganglionic fiber branching	Extensive	Minimal
Distribution	Wide	Limited
Type of response	Diffuse	Discrete
Stimulus required for activation		

"Flight-or-fight" stimulus

Sympathetic output
(Diffuse because postganglionic neurons may innervate more than one organ)

"Rest-and-digest" stimulus

Parasympathetic output
(Discrete because postganglionic neurons are not branched, but are directed to a specific organ)

Sympathetic and parasympathetic action often oppose each other

Acetylcholine

$$Acetylcholine \xrightarrow{\text{Cholinesterase}} Choline + Acetate$$

- There are two types of enzymes, which are responsible for the hydrolysis of acetylcholine. These are:
  1. *Acetylcholinesterase* (AChE or true cholinesterase).
  2. *Butyrylcholinesterase* (BuChE or pseudocholinesterase).

Acetylcholinesterase is involved in the termination of ACh action at cholinergic sites, whereas, Butyrylcholinesterase plays a role in the hydrolysis of ingested esters in plasma, liver and intestines.

Cholinoceptors

- ACh produces it effects after acting on acetylcholine receptors, which are known as *cholinoceptors*. Receptors are essential for the action of acetylcholine.
- There are two types of cholinoceptors through which ACh acts; they are muscarinic (M) receptors and nicotinic (N) receptors.
- Muscarinic receptors are mainly G protein coupled receptors, while nicotinic receptors are ligand gated cation channels.
- Both muscarinic and nicotinic receptors have their subtypes and the net parasympathetic effects produced by ACh are dependent upon the subtype of receptors stimulated.

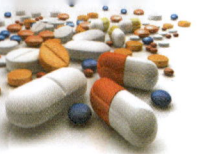

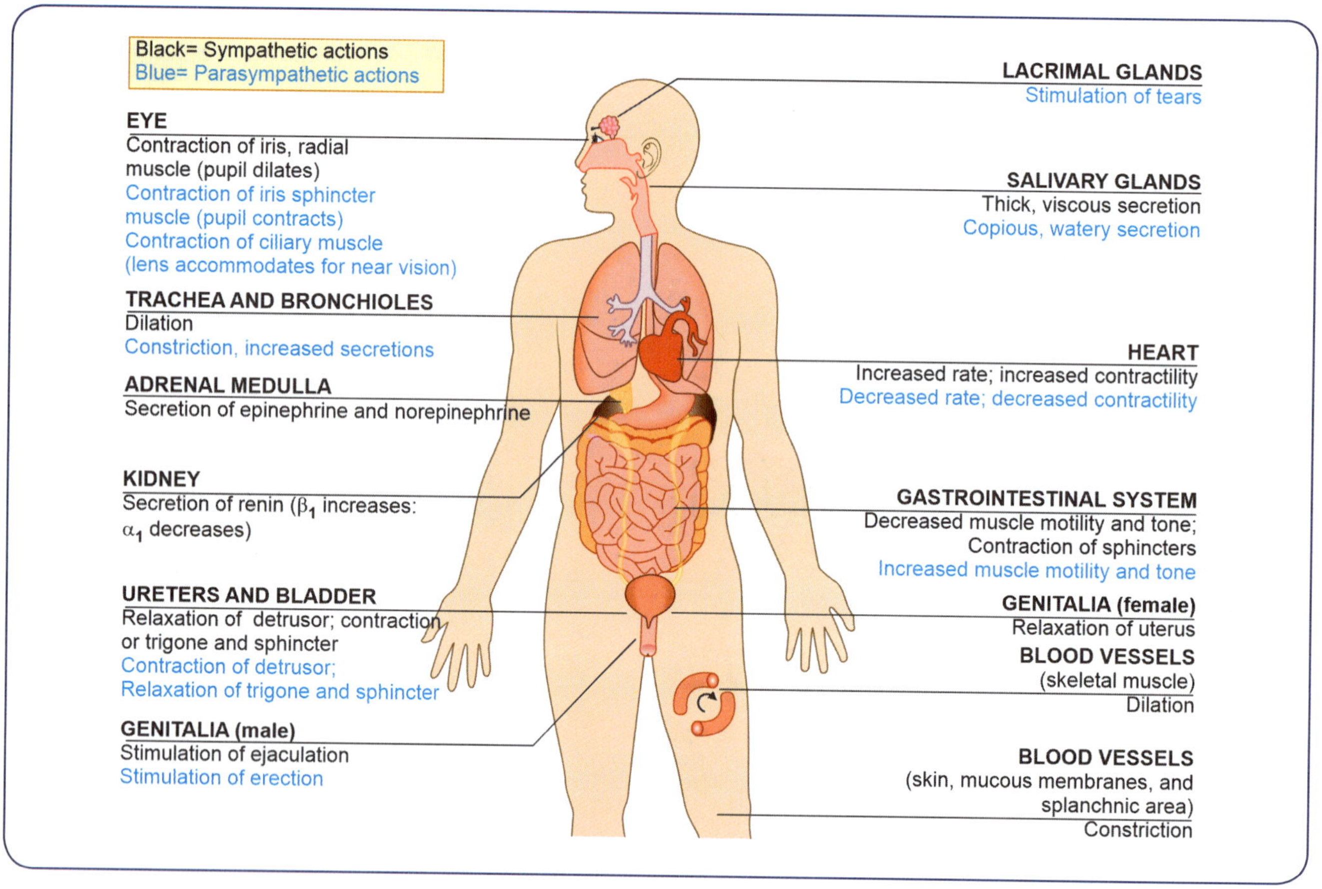

Black= Sympathetic actions
Blue= Parasympathetic actions

EYE
Contraction of iris, radial
muscle (pupil dilates)
Contraction of iris sphincter
muscle (pupil contracts)
Contraction of ciliary muscle
(lens accommodates for near vision)

TRACHEA AND BRONCHIOLES
Dilation
Constriction, increased secretions

ADRENAL MEDULLA
Secretion of epinephrine and norepinephrine

KIDNEY
Secretion of renin (β_1 increases:
α_1 decreases)

URETERS AND BLADDER
Relaxation of detrusor; contraction
or trigone and sphincter
Contraction of detrusor;
Relaxation of trigone and sphincter

GENITALIA (male)
Stimulation of ejaculation
Stimulation of erection

LACRIMAL GLANDS
Stimulation of tears

SALIVARY GLANDS
Thick, viscous secretion
Copious, watery secretion

HEART
Increased rate; increased contractility
Decreased rate; decreased contractility

GASTROINTESTINAL SYSTEM
Decreased muscle motility and tone;
Contraction of sphincters
Increased muscle motility and tone

GENITALIA (female)
Relaxation of uterus
BLOOD VESSELS
(skeletal muscle)
Dilation

BLOOD VESSELS
(skin, mucous membranes, and
splanchnic area)
Constriction

FIG. 9.6: Actions of sympathetic and parasympathetic nervous systems on effector organs

Muscarinic Receptors (M)

- These receptors are located primarily on autonomic effector cells in heart, blood vessels, eye, smooth muscles and glands of gastrointestinal tracts, respiratory and urinary tract, sweat glands, CNS, etc.
- These receptors are selectively stimulated by muscarine and blocked by atropine.
- The muscarinic receptors have been divided into five subtypes M_1, M_2, M_3, M_4 and M_5.
- M_1, M_2, and M_3 are the major subtypes responsible for majority of parasympathetic activities.
- The M_4 and M_5 receptors are present mainly on nerve endings in certain areas of the brain and regulate the release of other neurotransmitters.

Nicotinic Receptors (N)

- There are two subtypes of nicotinic receptors known as NM and NN.
  - **N_M:** These receptors are present at skeletal muscle endplate.

- **N_N:** These receptors are present on the sympathetic as well as parasympathetic ganglionic cells, adrenal medullary cells, in spinal cord and certain areas of brain.
- These receptors are selectively activated by nicotine and blocked by tubocurarine or hexamethonium.

Cholinergic Drugs

(Cholinomimetics, Parasympathomimetics)

Table 9.39 enlists the names of the cholinergic agonists and anticholinesterases.

Most of the actions of cholinergic drugs simulate the actions of ACh on different cholinoceptors.

The actions of ACh are classified as muscarinic or nicotinic.

ACh produces systemic effects depending upon the type of receptor through which these are mediated (Table 9.40).

Acetylcholine is not used clinically. Bethanechol and pilocarpine are in clinical use.

Bethanechol is used in post-operative/postpartum non-obstructive urinary retention and in neurogenic bladder to promote evacuation of bladder.

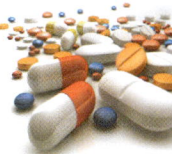

TABLE 9.39: Cholinomimetics, agonists, anticholinesterases

Cholinergic drugs agonists	
Choline esters	**Alkaloids**
• Acetylcholine • Methacholine • Carbachol • Bethanechol	• Muscarine • Pilocarpine • Arecoline

Anticholinesterases (anti-ChEs)	
Reversible anti-ChEs	**Irreversible anti-ChEs**
• Physostigmine • Neostigmine • Pyridostigmine • Edrophonium • Rivastigmine • Donepezil • Galantamine • Tacrine	• Organophosphates • Dyflos • Echothiophate • Malathion (insecticide) • Diazinon (insecticide) • Tabun, Sarin, Soman (nerve gases) • *Carbamates* • Carbaryl (insecticide) • Propoxur (insecticide)

TABLE 9.40: Muscarinic and nicotinic action of ACh

Muscarinic actions	
Site and receptors involved	**Effects produced**
Heart (M_2)	Bradycardia, slowing in conduction, reduction in force of atrial contraction, cardiac arrest in higher doses
Blood vessels (M_3)	Hypotension and flushing due to vasodilatory action
Smooth muscle (M_3)	• GIT: Abdominal cramps and evacuation of bowel due to increased tone and peristalsis in the gastrointestinal tract and sphincters relaxation. • Urinary system: Emptying of bladder occurs due to contraction of detrusor muscles and relaxation bladder trigone and sphincter • Respiratory system: Bronchospasm, dyspnea, precipitation of an attack of bronchial asthma due to constriction of bronchial smooth muscles
Glands (M_2, M_3)	• Secretion from all glands is increased such as sweating, salivation, lacrimation, increased tracheobronchial and gastric secretions
Eye	• Miosis due to contraction of circular muscle of iris • Decrease in intraocular pressure

Contd…

Nicotinic actions	
Sites	**Effects**
Autonomic ganglia (NN)	Both sympathetic and parasympathetic ganglia are stimulated
Skeletal muscles (NM)	Twitching, fasciculations and muscles contraction
CNS (NN)	No central effects seen as ACh does not cross blood-brain barrier

Pilocarpine causes marked sweating, salivation and increase in other secretions. Pilocarpine is used only in the eye as 0.5–4% drops. It is a third-line drug in open angle glaucoma.

Mushroom Poisoning

It occurs due to accidental consumption of poisonous mushrooms Amanita muscaria and Inocybe species. Due to the presence of *muscarine alkaloid in these species*, the muscarinic actions are seen.

Three types of mushroom poisonings are known. The symptoms depend upon the toxic principle present in the particular species.

- **Early mushroom poisoning (Muscarine type):** It occurs due to consumption of Inocybe and related species. Symptoms appear within an hour of eating the mushroom, and are promptly reversed by atropine.
- **Hallucinogenic type:** It occurs due to consumption of A. muscaria and related mushrooms. These compounds produce hallucinogenic symptoms due to muscarinic receptors blockade in the brain. There is no specific treatment and atropine is contraindicated.
- **Late mushroom poisoning (Phalloidin type):** It occurs due to consumption of A. phalloides, galerina and related species. Symptoms are due to damage to the gastrointestinal mucosa, liver and kidney and appear after many hours of consumption of poisonous mushrooms. Supportive measures need to be given and in some cases thioctic acid may be given as antidote.

Cholinesterase Inhibitors or Anticholinesterases or Indirectly-acting Cholinergic Drugs

All cholinesterase inhibitors increase the concentration of endogenous acetylcholine at cholinoceptors by inhibiting acetylcholinesterase. The acetylcholinesterase is the primary target of these drugs and the hydrolysis of acetylcholine is prevented due to inhibition of this enzyme. In addition, some anticholinesterases also act on nicotinic cholinoceptors and produce the cholinergic effects.

Mechanism of Action

- The anti-ChEs react with the cholinesterase enzyme in the same way as the ACh acts.

The carbamates and phosphates respectively carbamylate and phosphorylate the enzyme and prevent its action on acetylcholine.

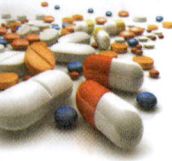

- The actions of anti-ChEs are due to amplification of the actions of endogenous ACh.

Pharmacological actions of these agents are the extension of cholinergic effects of acetylcholine.

- **Lipid-soluble agents** (physostigmine and organophosphates) have more marked muscarinic and CNS effects and less prominent on skeletal muscles.
- **Lipid-insoluble agents** (neostigmine and other quaternary ammonium compounds) produce more marked effect on the skeletal muscles and less prominent muscarinic effects. They do not penetrate CNS and have no central effects.
- **Organophosphates:** These are absorbed from all sites including intact skin and lungs. They are hydrolyzed as well as oxidized in the body and little is excreted unchanged.

Individual Compounds

- **Physostigmine:** It is rapidly absorbed from GIT and parenteral sites. Applied to the eye, it penetrates cornea freely. It crosses blood-brain barrier and is disposed after hydrolysis by ChE. *Physostigmine* eye drops are usually prepared freshly by ophthalmology departments.
- **Neostigmine and congeners:** These are poorly absorbed orally; oral dose is 20–30 times higher than parenteral dose. They do not effectively penetrate cornea or cross blood-brain barrier. They are partially hydrolyzed and partially excreted unchanged in urine.
- The pharmacological differences between physostigmine and neostigmine are given in Table 9.41.
- **Pyridostigmine:** It is similar to neostigmine in all features except duration of action. It is a longer acting agent; hence preferred over neostigmine in myasthenia gravis. It is available as 60 mg tab and given as 1–3 tablets TDS.
- **Ambenonium** is another long-acting congener used in myasthenia gravis.
- **Edrophonium:** It resembles neostigmine. It has a brief duration of action of 10–30 minutes It is used as a diagnostic agent for myasthenia gravis. It is given in a dose of 2–10 mg IV.
- **Tacrine:** It was used for symptomatic improvement in Alzheimer's disease, but not used nowadays due to hepatotoxicity.

- **Rivastigmine, Donepezil and Galantamine** are used in the treatment of Alzheimer's disease.
- **Dyflos** and **Echothiophate** were used as miotics in the past, but not used nowadays due to their toxic effects.

Therapeutic Indications of Reversible Anti-cholinesterase

- **Eye**
  - In glaucoma: Pilocarpine is used due to its miotic effect. The action is rapid and lasts for 4–6 hours. Physostigmine (0.1%) is used only to supplement pilocarpine.
  - To reverse the effect of mydriatics after refraction testing.
  - The formation of adhesions between iris and lens or iris and cornea are prevented due to miotic effects of pilocarpine and physostigmine. A miotic drug is alternated with a mydriatic to break the already formed adhesions.
- **Myasthenia gravis:** Neostigmine 15 mg orally QID. Dose and frequency needs to be adjusted to obtain optimum relief from weakness. Pyridostigmine is an alternative. Other drugs useful in treatment of myasthenia gravis are corticosteroids (Prednisolone 30–60 mg OD), immunosuppressants (azathioprine and cyclosporine). Plasmaphresis and thymectomy are also part of treatment in severe cases.
- **Post-operative paralytic ileus/urinary retention:** Neostigmine in a dose of 0.5–1 mg SC, provides relief.
- **Post-operative decurarization:** Neostigmine 0.5–2.0 mg (30–50 µg/kg) IV, preceded by atropine or glycopyrrolate 10 µg/kg to block muscarinic effects, rapidly reverses muscle paralysis induced by competitive neuromuscular blockers.
- **Cobra bite:** Neostigmine + atropine are helpful to prevent respiratory paralysis.
- **Belladonna poisoning:** Physostigmine is given in a dose of 0.5–2 mg IV as specific antidote. Neostigmine being lipid insoluble does not cross blood-brain barrier and is unable to block the CNS effects.

TABLE 9.41: Pharmacological differences between physostigmine and neostigmine

Physostigmine	Neostigmine
It is a natural alkaloid obtained from Physostigma venenosum	It is synthetic in nature
It has good oral absorption	Poor oral absorption
Both central and peripheral effects are seen	Only peripheral effects seen
It crosses blood-brain barrier	It doesn't cross blood-brain barrier
It is given in a dose of 0.5–1 mg oral/ parenteral, 0.1–1.0% eye drops	It is given in a dose of 0.5–2.5 mg IM/SC and 15–30 mg orally
The duration of action is 4–6 hours when given systemically and 6–24 hours when applied topically in the eye	The duration of action is 3–4 hours
It is useful in glaucoma and atropine poisoning	It is useful in myasthenia gravis, post-operative urinary retention and paralytic ileus

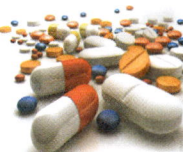

- **Alzheimer's disease:** It is a neurodegenerative disorder, primarily affecting cholinergic neurons in the brain and manifest clinically as progressive dementia. *Rivastigmine, donepezil* and *galantamine* are cerebroselective cholinomimetic drugs and are useful in the treatment of Alzheimer's disease.

Anticholinesterase Poisoning

The various agricultural and household insecticides are cholinomimetic agents, as these are anticholinesterases. The poisoning with these agents can be accidental, suicidal or homicidal. The symptoms observed are due to persistence action of acetylcholine on the cholinomimetic receptors. The various symptoms observed are:

- **Eye:** Irritation of eye, lacrimation, salivation, sweating, copious tracheobronchial secretions, miosis, blurring of vision
- **CVS:** Fall in blood pressure, bradycardia or tachycardia, cardiac arrhythmias, vascular collapse
- **Respiratory, GIT and urinary system:** Bronchospasm, breathlessness, colic, involuntary defecation and urination.
- **Skeletal system:** Muscular fasciculations, weakness, respiratory paralysis (central as well as peripheral).
- **CNS:** Irritability, disorientation, unsteadiness, tremors, ataxia, convulsions, coma and death.
- **Death is generally due to respiratory failure.**

Treatment

Treatment should be started as early as possible (within few hours). The patients are managed by following general management and specific management guidelines.

- **General management**
    - Prevention of further exposure to the poison: Area of contact should be cleaned with soap and water. The further absorption is prevented by gastric lavage.
    - Maintenance of airway patency and oxygenation.
    - Supportive measures: To maintain BP and prevention/ treatment convulsions.

- **Specific management**
- Atropine (Dose: 2 mg IV, repeat every 10 minutes until signs of atropinization such as mydriasis and tachycardia appear.)
- Cholinesterase reactivators: Pralidoxime, obidoxime and diacetyl-monoxime (DAM). These drugs reactivate the cholinesterase enzyme by blocking the action of anticholinesterase.

Chronic Organophosphate Poisoning

- Repeated exposure to certain organophosphates manifest as polyneuritis and demyelination after a latent period of days to weeks.
- Clinically, sensory disturbances, muscle weakness, tenderness and depressed tendon reflexes occur due to lower motor neurone paralysis.
- Later on, spasticity and upper motor neurone paralysis occur gradually.
- There is no specific treatment. Avoidance of further exposure to organophosphates along with symptomatic management are the only measures which can be taken.
- Recovery may take quite a long time.

Summary of important cholinergic drugs is given in Table 9.42.

Anticholinergic Drugs

(Muscarinic Receptor Antagonists, Atropinic Drugs, Parasympatholytics)

The drugs which block the actions of acetylcholine at muscarinic receptors are known as 'anticholinergic drugs' and those which block the actions of acetylcholine at nicotinic receptors are known as 'ganglion blockers' or 'neuromuscular blockers'.

All anticholinergics drugs are competitive antagonists of ACh at cholinoceptors.

TABLE 9.42: Summary of various cholinergic/cholinomimetic drugs

Bethanechol	Physostigmine	Rivastigmine, galantamine, donepezil
• Used in treatment of urinary retention • Binds preferentially at muscarinic receptors	• Increases intestinal and bladder motility • Reverses CNS and cardiac effects of tricyclic antidepressants • Reverse CNS effects of atropine • Uncharged, tertiary, amine that can penetrate the CNS	• Used as first-line treatments for Alzheimer's disease, though confers modest benefit • Have not been shown to reduce healthcare costs or delay institutionalization • Can be used with *memantine* (N-methyl-D-aspartate antagonsist) with moderate to severe disease
Carbachol	**Neostigmine**	**Echothiphate**
• Produces miosis during ocular surgery • Used topically to reduce intraocular pressure in open-angle or narrow-angle glaucoma, particularly in patients who have become tolerant to *pilocarpine*	• Prevents post-operative abdominal distention and urinary retention • Used in treatment of myasthenia gravis • Used as an antidote for competitive neuromuscular blockers • Has intermediate duration of action (0.5–2 hours)	• Used in treatment of open-angle glaucoma • Has long duration of action (100 hours)

Contd...

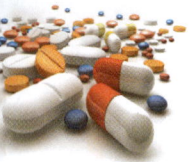

Pilocarpine

- Reduce intraocular pressure in open-angle and narrow-angle glaucoma
- Binds preferentially at muscarinic receptors
- Uncharged, tertiary amine that can penetrate the CNS

Edrophonium

- Used for diagnosis of myasthenia gravis
- Used as an antidote for competitive neuromuscular blockers
- Has short duration of action (10–20 minutes)

Acetylcholine

- Used to produce miosis in ophthalmic surgery

Classification

- **Natural alkaloids:** Atropine, Hyoscine (Scopolamine)
- **Semisynthetic derivatives:** Homatropine, atropine methonitrate, hyoscine butyl bromide, ipratropium bromide, tiotropium bromide
- **Synthetic compounds**
  - **Mydriatics:** Cyclopentolate, tropicamide
  - **Antisecretory-antispasmodics**
  - **Quaternary compounds:** Propantheline, oxyphenonium, clidinium, pipenzolate methyl bromide, isopropamide, glycopyrrolate
  - **Tertiary amines:** Dicyclomine, valethamate, pirenzepine
- **Vasicoselective:** Oxybutynin, flavoxate, tolterodine
- **Antiparkinsonian:** Trihexyphenidyl, procyclidine, biperiden

Atropine

Atropine is the representative of anticholinergics and is an alkaloid obtained from plant of *Atropa belladonna*. It is highly selective for muscarinic receptors, whereas, some of its synthetic derivatives possess significant nicotinic blocking properties.

Pharmacological actions of atropine are:

Atropine blocks all subtypes of muscarinic receptors and the actions are just opposite to the muscarinic effects seen with ACh. The effects are prominent in organs receiving strong parasympathetic tone.

- **Glands:** Atropine markedly decreases sweat, salivary, tracheobronchial and lacrimal secretions. Skin and eyes become dry, talking and swallowing may become difficult.
- **Eye:** Topical instillation of atropine causes mydriasis, abolition of light reflex and cycloplegia which lasts for 7–10 days. This causes photophobia and blurring of near vision.
- **Smooth muscles:** It causes constipation due to decrease in tone and motility of the gut and increase in sphincter tone. It also causes urinary retention due to relaxation effect on detrusor muscles. It leads to bronchodilatation and reduction in bronchial secretions.
- **CVS:** Tachycardia is the most prominent effect seen with atropine.

- **Body temperature:** Rise in body temperature occurs at higher doses.
- **CNS effects** are seen at higher doses only due to restricted entry of atropine into the brain. Hyoscine produces central depressant effects even at low doses.

Stimulation of vagal, respiratory and vasomotor centers and depression of vestibular excitation occurs with atropine. At therapeutic doses, antiparkinsonian effect is seen due to blocking of cholinergic overactivity in basal ganglia.

The sensitivity of different organs and tissues to atropine varies and can be graded as:

Saliva, sweat, bronchial secretion > eye, bronchial muscle, heart > smooth muscle of intestine, bladder > gastric glands and smooth muscle

Hyoscine

This is a natural anticholinergic alkaloid. It differs from atropine in many respects (Table 9.43).

Hyoscine hydrobromide is given in a dose of 0.3–0.5 mg oral/IM and available as transdermal patch.

Common Indications of Individual Anticholinergic Drugs

- **As mydriatic and cycloplegic:** Homatropine, Tropicamide, Cyclopentolate and Atropine ointment are used.

TABLE 9.43: Comparative features of atropine and hyoscine

Features	Atropine	Hyoscine
Chief source	Atropa belladonna, Datura stramonium	Hyoscyamus niger
CNS effects	Excitatory	Depressant
Anticholinergic property	More potent on heart, bronchial muscle and intestines	More potent on eye and secretory glands
Duration of action	Longer	Shorter
Anti-motion sickness property	Mild- moderate	Moderate to high

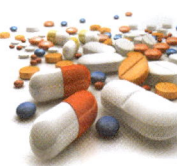

- **As antispasmodic:** Dicyclomine and Hyoscine are used in intestinal and renal colic, abdominal cramps, drug induced diarrhea, spastic constipation, irritable bowel syndrome, nervous dyspepsia, dysmenorrhea, urinary frequency and urgency.
- **As antisecretory** with pre-anesthetic medication to check increased salivary and tracheobronchial secretions (atropine, hyoscine, glycopyrrolate). To **prevent laryngospasm and vasovagal attack** during anesthesia.
- **In bronchial asthma, asthmatic bronchitis, chronic obstructive pulmonary disease:** Ipratropium bromide, Tiotropium bromide are used.
- **As cardiac vagolytic action:** Atropine is used.

- **In motion sickness:** Hyoscine is used. It is given prophylactically (0.2 mg oral), because administration after the onset of symptoms is less effective.
- **In Parkinsonism:** Trihexyphenidyl, Procyclidine, Biperiden are used.
- **To antagonize muscarinic effects of drugs and poisons:** Atropine is the specific antidote for organophosphates and early mushroom poisoning. Atropine or glycopyrrolate is also given to block muscarinic actions of neostigmine used for myasthenia gravis, decurarization or cobra envenomation.
- Description of individual anticholinergic drugs are given in Table 9.44.

TABLE 9.44: Description of individual anticholinergic drugs

Drugs	Dose	Indications
Semisynthetic derivatives		
Homatropine	1%, 2% eye drops	For inducing mydriasis
Atropine methonitrate	2.5–10 mg oral, IM	Abdominal colics and hyperacidity
Hyoscine butyl bromide	20–40 mg oral, IM, SC, IV	For esophageal and gastrointestinal spasm and motion sickness
Ipratropium bromide	40–80 µg by inhalation	For bronchial asthma and COPD
Tiotropium bromide	18 µg by inhalation OD	
Synthetic compounds		
Mydriatics		
Cyclopentolate	0.5%, 1% eye drops	For cycloplegic refraction, iritis and uveitis
Tropicamide	0.5%, 1.0% eye drops	For refraction testing and mydriatic for fundoscopy
Antisecretory-antispasmodics		
Quaternary compounds		
Propantheline	15–30 mg oral	Peptic ulcer and gastritis. (H$_2$ blockers and PPIs are preferred)
Oxyphenonium	5–10 mg (children 3–5 mg) oral	Same as above
Clidinium	2.5–5 mg oral	For nervous dyspepsia, gastritis, irritable bowel syndrome, colic, peptic ulcer, etc.
Pipenzolate methyl bromide	5–10 mg (children 2–3 mg) oral	For flatulent dyspepsia, infantile colics and abdominal cramps
Isopropamide	5 mg oral	For hyperacidity, nervous dyspepsia, irritable bowel and other gastrointestinal problems
Glycopyrrolate	0.1–0.3 mg IM (5–10 µg/kg)	For pre-anesthetic medication and during anesthesia
Tertiary amines		
Dicyclomine	20 mg oral/IM, children 5–10 mg	For morning sickness, motion sickness, dysmenorrhea and irritable bowel syndrome.
Valethamate	8 mg IM, 10 mg oral	For hastening the cervix during labor, urinary, biliary and intestinal colic
Pirenzepine	100–150 mg/day oral	To reduce gastric secretions (H$_2$ blockers and proton pump inhibitions are preferred)

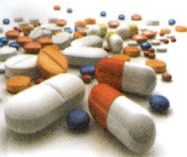

Vasicoselective		
Oxybutynin	5 mg BD/TDS oral; children above 5 years 2.5 mg BD	For detrusor instability, urge incontinence, nocturnal enuresis, neurogenic bladder
Flavoxate	200 mg tab, 1 tab TDS	For urinary frequency, urgency and dysuria associated with lower urinary tract infection
Tolterodine	1–2 mg BD or 2–4 mg OD of sustained release tab. oral	For overactive bladder with urinary frequency and urgency
Antiparkinsonian		
Trihexyphenidyl	2-10 mg /day	Parkinson's disease
Procyclidine	5–20 mg/day	Parkinson's disease
Biperiden	2-10 mg/day oral/IM/IV	Parkinson's disease

Common Adverse Effects and Toxicity of Anti-Cholinergic Drugs

Manifestations of anticholinergic drugs toxicity or overdose are due to exaggerated pharmacological actions. These are:

- Dry mouth, difficulty in swallowing and talking.
- Dry, flushed and hot skin, fever, scarlet rash.
- Difficulty in micturition, decreased bowel sounds.
- Dilated pupil, photophobia, blurring of near vision.
- Hypotension, palpitation, weak pulse, cardiovascular collapse with respiratory depression.
- In severe poisoning, convulsions and coma may occur.

Management of Belladonna Poisoning or Acute Anticholinergic Drugs Overdose

- Patient should be kept in a dark and quiet room.
- Gastric lavage should be performed (if poison has been ingested).
- The cold sponging or ice bags are applied to reduce body temperature.
- Physostigmine 1–3 mg SC/IV; antagonizes both central and peripheral effects.
- Other general measures (maintenance of blood volume, assisted respiration, diazepam to control convulsions) should be taken as appropriate.

 ## Drug Interactions

- The action of acetylcholine is potentiated by anticholinesterases.
- Adrenaline acts as physiological antagonist of acetylcholine.
- Atropine increases the absorption of tetracycline and digoxin by delaying gastric emptying.
- Atropine delays the absorption of levodopa by slowing down the absorption process.
- The absorption of anticholinergic drugs is interfered by antacids.
- The effect of anticholinergic drugs is potentiated by TCAs, antihistaminics, pethidine, phenothiazines due to their additional anticholinergic property.

 ## Nursing Implications

☞ **Cholinergic and anticholinergic drugs**
- ☞ Assess for contraindications or cautions: known allergies to these drugs to avoid hypersensitivity reactions.
- ☞ Nurse should be aware of the possible side effects of cholinergic/anticholinergic drugs to rightly identify the patients in whom these drugs are not to be administrated.
- ☞ Ensure proper administration of ophthalmic preparations to increase the effectiveness of drug therapy and minimize the risk of systemic absorption.
- ☞ Administer oral drug on an empty stomach to decrease nausea and vomiting.
- ☞ Maintain a cholinergic-blocking drug on standby such as atropine to use as an antidote for excessive doses of cholinergic drugs.
- ☞ Monitor patient response closely, including blood pressure, ECG, urine output, and cardiac output, and arrange to adjust dose accordingly to ensure the most benefit with the least amount of toxicity.
- ☞ Monitor urinary output to evaluate effects on the bladder; ensure ready access to bathroom facilities as needed with GI stimulation.
- ☞ Monitor for adverse effects (cardiovascular changes, GI stimulation, urinary urgency, respiratory distress).
- ☞ Evaluate the effectiveness of the teaching plan.

ADRENERGIC SYSTEM AND DRUGS

- The sympathetic nervous system is synonymous with the adrenergic system. Adrenaline (Adr) and noradrenaline (NA) are the major neurotransmitters involved in its functioning. Dopamine (DA) also acts as neurotransmitter at CNS level.
- The Adr, NA and DA are synthesized endogenously from the amino acid phenylalanine and all contain catechol ring in their structure. Hence, the combined term used for all these compounds is '*catecholamines*' (CAs).

- This system is an important regulator of *'fight and flight response'* during acute stressful conditions.
- The nerve fibers that synthesize, store and release noradrenaline are termed as adrenergic nerves.
- In the sympathetic system, noradrenaline (norepinephrine) mediates the transmission of nerve impulses from autonomic Post-ganglionic nerves to effector organs.

✓
- *Noradrenaline* (NA) acts as transmitter at Post-ganglionic sympathetic sites (except sweat glands, hair follicles and some vasodilator fibers) and in certain areas of brain.
- *Adrenaline* (Ad) is secreted by adrenal medulla and acts as a hormone as well as a neurotransmitter in the brain.
- *Dopamine* (DA) is a major transmitter in basal ganglia, limbic system, CTZ, anterior pituitary, etc. and in a limited manner in the periphery.

Synthesis action and degradation of catecholamines is given in Figure 9.7.

ADRENERGIC RECEPTORS

The adrenergic receptors (adrenoceptors) were broadly classified into two types α and β by Ahlquist in 1948.

The α receptors have been further subdivided into α_1 and α_2 receptors.

The β receptors have been further subdivided into β_1, β_2 and β_3 receptors.

Locations of α and β receptors are given in Table 9.45.

In some tissues, both types of receptors are present. In normal physiological conditions, there is a balance between both type of receptor actions and the net effects depend upon the predominant receptor type present in a particular tissue.

ADRENERGIC DRUGS OR SYMPATHOMIMETICS

The drugs having actions similar to that of Adr or of sympathetic stimulation are known as adrenergic drugs or sympathomimetics drugs. The action of these drugs mimics the natural sympathetic activity.

The adrenergic actions on various tissues are tabulated in Table 9.46.

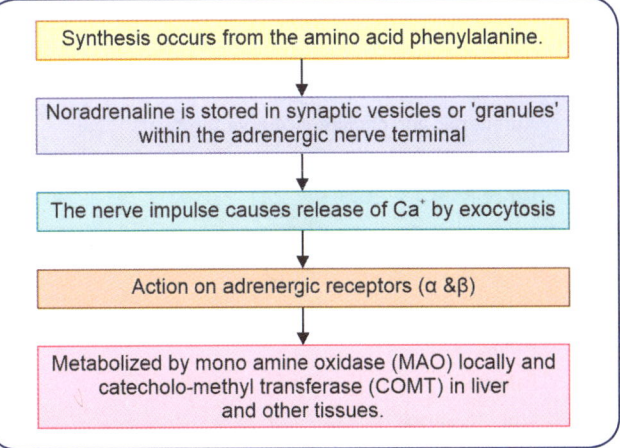

FIG. 9.7: Synthesis action and degradation of catecholamines

TABLE 9.45: Locations of α and β receptors

Receptors	Locations
α_1	Post-junctional on effector organs
α_2	Pre-junctional on nerve ending (α_{2A}), also post-junctional in brain, pancreatic β cells and extra-junctional in certain blood vessels, platelets.
β_1	Heart, juxtaglomerular cells in kidney
β_2	Bronchi, blood vessels, uterus, liver, GIT, urinary tract, eye
β_3	Adipose tissue

Adrenaline and noradrenaline act on both α and β receptors with slight variation in their preference to different subtypes of these receptors.

✓
- Adrenaline: $\alpha_1 + \alpha_2 + \beta_1 + \beta_2$ and weak β_3 action
- Nor-adrenaline: $\alpha_1 + \alpha_2 + \beta_1 + \beta_2$ but no β_2 action
- Isoprenaline: $\beta_1 + \beta_2 + \beta_3$ but no α action

Adrenergic responses mediated through α and β receptors are given in Table 9.47. Classification of adrenergic drugs based on therapeutic uses and mechanism of action are given in Tables 9.48 and 9.49, respectively. Commonly used sympathomimetic drugs are described in Table 9.50.

TABLE 9.46: Adrenergic drug actions on various tissues

Type	Tissue	Actions
α_1	Most vascular smooth muscle (innervated)	Contraction
	Pupillary dilator muscle	Contraction (dilates pupil)
	Pilomotor smooth muscle	Erects hair
	Prostate	Contraction
	Heart	Increases force of contraction

243

Contd...

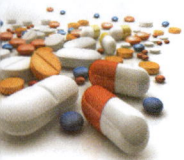

Type	Tissue	Actions
α_2	Post-synaptic CNS neurons	Probably multiple
	Platelets	Aggregation
	Adrenergic and cholinergic nerve terminals	Inhibits transmitter release
	Some vascular smooth muscle	Contraction
	Fat cells	Inhibits lipolysis
β_1	Heart, juxtaglomerular cells	Increases force and rate of contraction; increases renin release
β_2	Respiratory, uterine, and vascular smooth muscle	Promotes smooth muscle relaxation
	Skeletal muscle	Promotes potassium uptake
	Human liver	Activates glycogenolysis
β_3	Fat cells	Activates lipolysis
D_1	Smooth muscle	Dilates renal blood vessels
D_2	Nerve endings	Modulates transmitter release

TABLE 9.47: Adrenergic responses medicated through α and β receptors

Site	Effects
Heart (β_1)	• Positive inotropic effect: Increase in myocardial contractility • Positive chronotropic effect: Increase in heart rate • Positive dromotropic effects: Increase in conduction velocity • The overall effect seen is increased cardiac output
Blood vessels (α_2, β_2)	• Constriction of arterioles and veins: Rise in BP ($\alpha_1 + \alpha_2$) • Dilatation of arterioles and veins: Fall in BP (β_2)
Respiratory system (β_2)	• Bronchodilatation
Eye (α_1)	• Contraction of radial muscles of iris, mydriasis
GIT (α_2, β_2)	• Decreased peristalsis and constriction of sphincters causing constipation
Bladder (β_2) trigone (α_1)	• Retention of urine due to detrusor relaxation (β) and trigone • Constriction (α)
Uterus (β_2)	• Relaxation at term of pregnancy
Skeletal muscles (α, β_2)	• α-receptor activation on motor nerve endings augments ACh release causing contraction of muscles fibers • Direct stimulation of muscle fibers (β_2) causing tremors
CNS (α_1, α_2)	• Activation of α_2 receptors in the brainstem (by selective α_2 agonists) results in decreased sympathetic outflow → fall in BP and bradycardia
Metabolism (α_2, β_2, β_3)	• Glycogenolysis: Hyperglycemia, hyperlactacidemia (β_2) • Lipolysis: Rise in plasma free fatty acid (FFA) and calorigenesis ($\beta_2 + \beta_3$) • Reduction of insulin (α_2) and augmentation of glucagon (β_2) secretion
Endocrine system (β_1)	• Renin release from kidney (β_1) • ADH secretion from posterior pituitary (β_1)
Reproductive system (α_1)	• Male sex organs: Ejaculation
Glands	• Salivary gland: Increased secretion of potassium and water by α_1 • Apocrine sweat gland: Increased sweating on palm of hand

TABLE 9.48: Classification of adrenergic drugs based upon therapeutic uses

Gropus	Drugs
Pressor agents	Noradrenaline, phenylephrine, ephedrine methoxamine, dopamine, mephentermine
Cardiac stimulants	Adrenaline, dobutamine, isoprenaline

Contd...

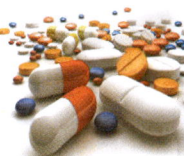

Gropus	Drugs
Bronchodilators	Isoprenaline, salmeterol, salbutamol, formoterol, bambuterol, terbutaline
Nasal decongestants	Phenylephrine, naphazoline, xylometazoline, pseudoephedrine, oxymetazoline, phenyl propanolamine
CNS stimulants	Amphetamine, methamphetamine, dexamphetamine
Anorectics	Fenfluramine, sibutramine, dexfenfluramine
Uterine relaxant and vasodilators	Ritodrine, salbutamol, isoxsuprine, terbutaline

TABLE 9.49: Classification of adrenergic drugs based upon mechanism of action

Class	Mode of action	Drugs
Direct acting sympathomimetics	They act by direct stimulation of adrenergic receptor	Adrenaline, noradrenaline, dobutamine, isoprenaline, phenylephrine, almeterol, salbutamol, formoterol, bambuterol, terbutaline, naphazoline, xylometazoline, oxymetazoline, phenylpropanolamine, ritodrine
Indirect acting sympathomimetics	They act by releasing NA from Adr nerve endings	Amphetamine, methamphetamine, methylphenidate, modafinil, tyramine
Mixed acting sympathomimetics	They act by both direct and indirect mechanisms	Ephedrine, pseudoephedrine, dopamine

TABLE 9.50: Commonly used sympathomimetic drugs

Drugs	Dose	Special features
Dopamine	0.2–1.0 mg/min IV infusion	• It acts on D_1 receptors located in renal and mesenteric blood vessels • Causes rise in systolic BP. • Uses: cardiogenic shock, septic shock, severe congestive heart failure (it increases and urine outflow) • Concomitant BP and urine output monitoring is required for regulation of infusion rate
Dobutamine	2.5–10 µg/kg/min IV infusion	• Use: Congestive heart failure with myocardial infarction, cardiac surgery, and severe congestive heart failure (for short-term management only)
Ephedrine	15–60 mg oral, 15–30 mg IM/IV 0.5–0.75% topically in nose	• Uses: Mild chronic bronchial asthma, hypotension during spinal anesthesia
Phenylephrine	5–10 mg oral, 2–5 mg IM, 0.1–0.5 mg slow IV inj, 30–60 µg/min IV infusion, 0.25% topically in nose, 5–10% topically in eye	• Uses: As nasal decongestant, mydriatic (when cycloplegia is not required. • Nasal decongestant oral and topical both
Amphetamines	Amphetamine: 5–15 mg oral Dexamphetamine: 5–10 mg (children 2.5–5 mg) oral Methamphetamine: 5–10 mg oral	• Potent CNS stimulant and induces alertness, increased concentration and attention span, euphoria, talkativeness, increased work capacity • It is drug of abuse and one of the drugs included in the 'dope test' for athletes • Also used in attention deficit hyperkinetic disorder
Mephentramine	10–20 mg oral/IM, also by IV infusion	• For prevention and treatment of hypotension due to spinal anesthesia and surgical procedures, shock in myocardial infarction and other hypotensive states
Isoxsuprine	5–10 mg oral, IM 4–6 hourly	• It is used as uterine relaxant for threatened abortion and dysmenorrhea
Xylometazoline	0.05–0.1% topically in nose	• Used as topical nasal decongestant • On prolonged use, atrophic rhinitis and anosmia can occur
Oxymetazoline	0.025–0.05% topically in nose	
Naphazoline	0.1% topically in nose	

245

Contd...

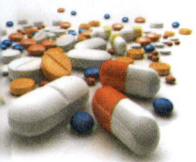

Drugs	Dose	Special features
Pseudoephedrine	30–60 mg oral TDS	• Used as antitussive and decongestant for symptomatic relief in common cold, allergic rhinitis, blocked eustachian tubes and upper respiratory tract infections • In hypertensives, BP can rise
Phenylpropanolamine	25–50 mg TDS	• Banned due to adverse effects such as hemorrhagic stroke and psychiatric disturbances
Sibutramine	Start with 10 mg OD, increase to 15 mg OD if needed	• It was used as appetite suppressant, now banned since March 2011
Fenfluramine	—	• It was used as appetite suppressant, now banned

Therapeutic Indications of Sympathomimetic Drugs

- **Cardiovascular applications:**
  - *Treatment of acute hypotension*: Dopamine, Dobutamine or NA are used for the treatment of shock (hypovolemic, septic and cardiogenic shock) associated with oliguria.
  - *Treatment of chronic orthostatic hypotension*: Midodrine (orally active α_1 agonist), oral ephedrine are used to treat this condition. *Droxidopa (A prodrug of Dopamine)* is used to treat neurogentic orthostatic hypotension. It is converted to NA and then to DA.
  - *Cardiac applications:* Adr is used in cardiac arrest, Isoprenaline is used in partial and complete A-V block and DA/Dobutamine infusion is used in congestive heart failure.
  - **Inducing local vasoconstriction**
    - Along with local anesthetics: Adr in a dilution of 1 in 100,000 to 1 in 200,000 is used for infiltration, nerve block and spinal anesthesia.
    - Control of local bleeding: In control of epistaxis, compresses *(Adr 1 in 10,000, phenylephrine/ephedrine 1% soaked in cotton)* can be used to control arteriolar and capillary bleeding.
    - Nasal decongestant: In cold, rhinitis, sinusitis, etc. pseudoephedrine and phenylephrine can be used orally as decongestants.
- **Pulmonary applications:** Sympathomimetic drugs (β_2 selective agonists) are very useful in the treatment of asthma and chronic obstructive pulmonary disease.
- **Ophthalmic applications:** Phenylephrine is used to facilitate fundus examination where cycloplegia is not required. It tends to reduce intraocular tension in wide angle glaucoma.
- **Allergic disorders:** Adrenaline is a physiological antagonist of histamine, which is an important mediator of many acute hypersensitivity reactions. It is life saving in laryngeal edema and anaphylaxis and provides quick relief in urticaria and angioedema. It is not effective in delayed types of allergies because histamine does not play any role there.

- **Genitourinary applications** in suppression of premature labor. Amphetamine provides relief in the patient of nocturnal enuresis both by its central action as well as by increasing tone of vesical sphincter.
- **Central applications:**
  - In patients with attention deficit hyperactivity disorder (Amphetamines).
  - Narcolepsy (Modafinil)
  - Obesity

ANTIADRENERGIC DRUGS

(Adrenergic Receptor Antagonists)

The drugs which antagonize the action of adrenaline and related drugs at receptor level are known as anti-adrenergic drugs. These drugs are competitive antagonists at α or β or both α and β adrenergic receptors.

The anti-adrenergic drugs are of two types depending upon the adrenoceptors they block. These are:
- α adrenergic blocking drug or α-blockers.
- β adrenergic blocking drugs or β-blockers.

α-Adrenergic Blockers

These drugs block the α receptors and inhibit the α receptor mediated response of the sympathetic stimulation and adrenergic agonist. Classification of α-adrenergic blockers is given in Table 9.51.

Common Pharmacological Effects of α-Blockers

- Hypotension occurs due to decrease in both preload and afterload. Preload decreases due to vasodilation of veins, peripheral pooling and decreased venous return to right ventricle (α_1-blocking action). Afterload decreases due to decrease in the peripheral arterial resistance (α_1-blocking action). Reflex tachycardia is usually seen.
- Miosis due to blockade of radial muscles of iris (α-blocking action).
- Diarrhea due to increased GI motility and relaxation of sphincters (α-blocking action).

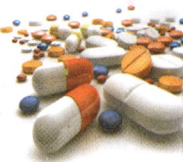

TABLE 9.51: Classification of α-adrenergic blockers

Non-selective α-blockers		Selective α- blockers	
Reversible	**Irreversible**	**α₁- selective**	**α₂- selective**
• Phentolamine • Tolazoline (priscoline) • Ergot alkaloid: • Ergotamine, • Ergotoxine, • Dihydroergotamine (DHE) • Dihydroergotoxine	• Phenoxy-benzamine	• Prazosin • Terazosin • Doxazosin • Alfuzosin • Tamsulosin • Silodosin	• Yohimbine • Idazoxan

- Urine flow improves in patients with benign prostatic hyperplasia (relaxes trigone sphincter).
- Impotence and impaired ejaculation due to inhibition of contraction of organs involved in ejaculation.
- Nasal stuffiness.
- Individual α-blockers are described in Table 9.52.

Clinical Uses of α-Blockers

- **Pheochromocytoma**
- **Benign prostate hypertrophy (BPH)**
- **Hypertension:** Phentolamine or phenoxybenzamine are used in hypertensive emergencies due to pheochromocytoma,

overdose of sympathomimetic drug, clonidine withdrawal and hypertensive crisis due to cheese reaction.

- **Erectile dysfunction:** Papaverine/Phentolamine or both are injected directly into the penis in the patients with erectile dysfunction. *Papaverine/Phentolamine induced penile erection (PIPE) therapy for impotence* is rarely used nowadays. Sildenafil and alternative therapies are preferred these days.
- **Peripheral vascular diseases:** Prazosin or Phenoxybenzamine are used.
- **Congestive heart failure (CHF):** The vasodilator action of prazosin provides symptomatic relief in patients of CHF. This is used for short-term management only.

TABLE 9.52: Individual α-blockers

Drugs	Dose	Special features
Phenoxybenzamine	20–60 mg/day oral, 1 mg/kg slow IV infusion over 1 hour	• Used in the pre-operative management of Pheochromocytoma • It causes postural hypotension and impotence
Phentolamine	5 mg IV repeated as required	• Used in diagnosis and intra-operative management of pheochromocytoma and cheese reaction
Prazosin	Start with 0.5–1 mg at bedtime; usual dose 1–4 mg BD or TDS	• Used as an antihypertensive, Raynaud's disease and benign prostatic hyperplasia • 'First dose effect' in the form of postural hypotension and syncope attack occurs on the initiation of therapy and decreases with time due to tolerance
Terazosin	Usual maintenance dose 2–10 mg OD	• Same as prazosin • It has longer duration of action; hence, single daily dose is sufficient
Doxazosin	1 mg OD initially, increase up to 8 mg BD	• Used as an antihypertensive and benign prostatic hyperplasia
Tamsulosin	0.4 mg, 1 cap (max 2) in the morning with meals	• It is uroselective (α₁A), bladder and prostate specific
Alfuzosin	2.5 BD-QID or 10 mg OD as modified release tab	• Short-acting and used for symptomatic treatment of benign prostatic hyperplasia
Silodosin	4-8 mg/day	• α₁A- antagonist (uroselective) for prostate • No orthostatic hypotension is seen • Loss of seminal emission
Yohimbine	2 mg oral	• No valid indications for its use are there • Previously it was used as aphrodisiac

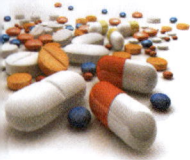

β-Adrenergic Blocking Drugs or beta-Blockers or Beta Receptor Antagonists

- These drugs block the β-receptors and inhibit the β receptors mediated response of the sympathetic stimulation (catecholamines) and adrenergic agonists. All β-blockers are competitive antagonists and reduce receptor occupancy by catecholamines and other β agonists.
- Propranolol was the first β-blocker, which was found clinically useful.
- Propranolol antagonizes both β_1 and β_2 receptors, and has poor action on β_3 receptors.
- Most β-blocking drugs in clinical use are *pure antagonists* as the occupancy of a β receptor by such a drug causes no activation of the receptor.
- Some β-blocking drugs are *partial agonists* as they cause partial activation of the receptor, albeit less than that caused by the *full agonists* epinephrine and isoproterenol. Partial agonists moderately activate the receptors in the absence of endogenous agonists and inhibit the activation of β receptors.
- Some β blockers (e.g., betaxolol, metoprolol) are *inverse agonists* as these drugs reduce constitutive activity of β receptors in some tissues.
- The β-receptor–blocking drugs differ amongst each other in their
  - Relative affinities for β_1 and β_2 receptors. Some have a higher affinity for β_1 than for β_2 receptors, and this selectivity may have important clinical implications.
  - Pharmacokinetic characteristics and local anesthetic membrane- stabilizing effects.

TABLE 9.53: Pharmacological classification of β-blockers

Nonselective (β_1 and β_2)	Cardioselective (β_1)
- With intrinsic sympathomimetic activity: - Pindolol - Without intrinsic sympathomimetic activity: - Propranolol - Sotalol - Timolol - With additional α blocking property: - Labetalol - Carvedilol	- Metoprolol - Atenolol - Acebutolol - Bisoprolol - Esmolol - Betaxolol - Celiprolol - Nebivolol

- Pharmacological classification of β-blockers are given in Table 9.53. Classification of β-blockers according to their development is given in Table. 9.54.

Pharmacological Actions of β-Blockers

The pharmacological actions of most of the β-blockers are similar to that of propranolol with some differences due to receptor subtype specificity.

Some of the pharmacological actions of propranolol are given in Table 9.55.

Pharmacokinetics

- Propranolol is well absorbed orally.
- It has low oral bioavailability due to high first pass metabolism in liver.

TABLE 9.54: Classification of β-blockers according to their development (generation-wise)

Generation	Special feature	Drugs
First Generation	Older, nonselective	Propranolol, Timolol, Sotalol, Pindolol
Second Generation	β1 selective	Metoprolol, Atenolol, Acebutolol, Bisoprolol, Esmolol
Third Generation	With additional α blocking and/or vasodilator property	Labetalol, Carvedilol, Celiprolol, Nebivolol, Betaxolol

TABLE 9.55: Pharmacological actions of propranolol

Site	Effects
Cardiovascular system	- They act as a cardiac depressant such as: - Negative inotropic effect: Decreases myocardial contractility - Negative chronotropic effect: Decreases heart rate - Negative dromotropic effect: Decreases A-V conduction - Decreases cardiac output and myocardial oxygen demand
Blood vessels	Both systolic and diastolic BP fall on continuous treatment with beta-blockers due to reduced cardiac output, total peripheral resistance and decreased renin release (β_1 mediated)
Respiratory system	It antagonizes the bronchodilatory effect of β_2 receptors and causes bronchoconstriction. Hence contraindicated in asthmatic individuals
CNS	Long-term therapy may result in forgetfulness, increased dreaming and nightmares. Propranolol is used as short-term anti-anxiety medication

Contd...

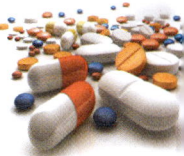

Site	Effects
Skeletal	Propranolol inhibits the β_2 receptor mediated tremors by blocking β_2 receptor and acting directly on the muscle fibers
Eye	β-blocker decreases the aqueous humor secretion and lowers the intraocular tension
Metabolism and endocrine	Causes rise in plasma free fatty acid and triglyceride levels due to inhibition of lipolysis Propranolol also masks the features of hypoglycemia. Hence, propranolol should be used cautiously in diabetic individuals

- It is a highly lipid soluble drug and easily crosses blood-brain barrier.
- The metabolism takes place in liver and excreted through urine.
- Individual β-blockers along with their special features are given in Table 9.56.

Common Indications of β-Blockers

- **Cardiovascular system**
  - **Hypertension:** β-blockers are the first line drugs for the management of mild to moderate hypertension. They are usually used alone or in combination with other antihypertensives which produce tachycardia.
  - **Angina pectoris and ischemic heart disease**: All β-blockers are beneficial in angina. They reduce the frequency of attacks and increase the exercise capacity of patients. They decrease both cardiac work and myocardial oxygen demand.
  - **Cardiac arrhythmia:** Beta-blockers are useful both in ventricular and supraventricular arrhythmias. Esmolol is also used in paroxysmal supraventricular tachycardia (PSVT).
  - **Myocardial infarction:** Beta-blockers are useful both during and after the myocardial infarction (MI).
    - During attack of MI, beta-blockers limit the infarct size and prevent ventricular arrhythmias and are given by IV infusion within 4–6 hours of an attack followed by oral therapy. These are given only if the patient is not in shock or cardiac failure or heart rate is not below than 50 beats per minute.
    - After the attack of MI, beta-blockers are used as secondary prophylaxis for MI to prevent reinfarction and post MI ventricular fibrillations.
  - **Congestive heart failure (CHF):** Metoprolol, bisoprolol, nebivolol and carvedilol have beneficial effects in patients with CHF. They reduce the risk of sudden death and prolong survival.
- **Pheochromocytoma:** β-blockers are useful to treat pheochromocytoma induced tachycardia and arrhythmia. Propranolol is given with α-blocker before surgery to control hypertension.
- **Hyperthyroidism:** Propranolol inhibits the peripheral conversion of T_4 to T_3. It is used to control palpitations, nervousness, tremors, sweating and severe myopathy associated with hyperthyroidism.
- **Migraine:** Propranolol, atenolol and metoprolol are used for prophylaxis of migraine.
- **Glaucoma:** These drugs reduce aqueous humor and decrease the intraocular pressure; hence used for the treatment of glaucoma.
- **Anxiety:** These drugs are used to treat anxiety induced palpitations, tachycardia and tremors. Propranolol is beneficial to control performance anxiety or '*stage fright*'.
- **Essential tremors:** Propranolol is useful for the treatment of tremors.

Common Adverse Effects and Contraindications of β-Blockers

The adverse effects are mostly seen with non-selective beta-blockers and rarely with cardio-selective Beta-blockers.

- **Cardiovascular effects:** β-blockers may precipitate CHF due to inhibition of sympathetic stimulation of heart.
  - β-blockers produce bradycardia; hence contraindicated in patients with sick sinus syndrome.
  - β-blockade cause unopposed action at α-receptors, which lead to coronary constriction and exacerbate the variant angina due to vasospasm. Hence, these are contraindicated in variant or prinzmetal's angina.
  - β-blockers are contraindicated in partial or complete heart block.
- **Pulmonary effects:** β-blockers cause broncho-constriction by inhibiting β_2 receptors and may exacerbate the features of chronic obstructive pulmonary disease (COPD) and asthma. Hence, use of beta-blockers is contraindicated in these conditions.
- **Central nervous systems (CNS):** These may cause confusion, sleep disturbance and hallucinations.
- **Metabolic effects:** Non-selective β-blockers may derange the lipid profile and may promote the progression of coronary heart disease. The cardio-selective β-blockers have little/minimal effects.
- **Withdrawal effects:** Sudden withdrawal of β-blockers after chronic use should be avoided because it may lead to rebound hypertension, may induce angina attack and even sudden cardiac death.
- Worsening of peripheral vascular disease occurs and presents as cold hands and feet due to blockade of vasodilatory β_2 receptors.

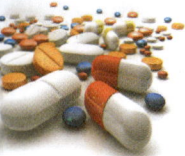

TABLE 9.56: Individual β-blockers

Nonselective (β$_1$ and β$_2$) Beta blockers		
Drug	Dose	• Special features
Pindolol	5–15 mg BD	• Used primarily as antihypertensive • Low incidence of rebound hypertension on withdrawal
Propranolol	Oral: 10 mg BD to 160 mg TDS.	• Used in thyrotoxicosis, portal hypertension, pheochromocytoma, migraine headache and patients non-responsive to other antihypertensive medications
Timolol	Start with 0.25% eye drops BD 0.5% OD as gel forming solution Orally: 10-40 mg OD	• Used topically for glaucoma • Orally used in hypertension, angina and prophylaxis of myocardial infarction
Sotalol	80 mg BD–160 mg TDS oral	• It has low lipid solubility • It also blocks the K$^+$ channel and used as class III antiarrhythmic drug
Cardioselective (β$_1$ and β$_2$) Beta blockers		
Metoprolol	25 mg BD–100 mg QID oral 5–15 mg slow IV inj	• Used in hypertension, angina and congestive heart failure • IV metoprolol used in myocardial infarction • Low bronchoconstriction effect; can be given safely to asthmatic • Preferred in diabetic individuals
Atenolol	25 mg OD–50 mg BD	• It is most commonly used in hypertension and angina • It has longer duration of action; hence, once daily regimen is sufficient
Acebutolol	200 mg BD–400 mg TDS oral 20–40 mg slow IV injection	• It is a β$_1$ selective drug with significant partial agonistic and membrane stabilizing properties • Used in cardiac arrhythmia and hypertension as single daily dose
Bisoprolol	2.5–10 mg OD	• Used in angina, hypertension and congestive heart failure
Esmolol	0.5 mg/kg IV injection followed by 0.05–0.2 mg/kg/min IV infusion	• It is an ultrashort-acting β$_1$ blocker with partial agonistic or membrane stabilizing properties • It is used in supraventricular tachycardia, episodic atrial fibrillation or flutter, arrhythmia during anesthesia and to reduce heart rate and blood pressure during and after cardiac surgery
Celiprolol	100 mg OD–300 mg BD	• Used as antihypertensive drug • Has additional weak β$_2$ agonistic action; safe in asthmatic individuals • Produces vasodilatation by acting as nitric oxide donor
Nebivolol	5 mg OD (start with 2.5 mg OD in elderly)	• Highly selective β$_1$ blocker also acts as a nitric oxide donor, produces vasodilatation • Used in hypertension and congestive heart failure
Betaxolol	0.5% topically in eye BD	• Used in chronic open angle glaucoma
Both α and β blocking agents		
Labetalol	Start with 50 mg BD, increase to 100–200 mg TDS oral In hypertensive emergencies, 20–40 mg slow IV injection every 10 minutes till desired response is obtained	• Used in pheochromocytoma, clonidine withdrawal and can also be given in essential hypertension • It blocks both α and β receptors • It is 5 times more potent in blocking β than α receptors • It causes hypotension (both fall in systolic and diastolic BP), which is due to blocking of both α$_1$ and β$_1$ receptor and β$_2$ agonistic (vasodilatation) action • Postural hypotension and failure of ejaculation are the important side effects of labetalol
Carvedilol	• In congestive heart failure: Start with 3.125 mg BD for 2 weeks, if well tolerated, gradually increase to maximum up to 25 mg BD • In hypertension/angina: 6.25 mg BD initially, titrate to maximum up to 25 mg BD	• It is used in hypertension and in congestive heart failure • It blocks the β$_1$ + β$_2$ + α$_1$ adrenoceptor • It produces vasodilatation by blocking α$_1$ and calcium channel • It also has antioxidant property

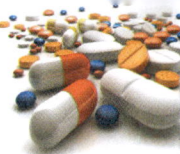

Drug Interactions

- Adrenaline can produce arrhythmias in patients who have been given halothane anesthesia. Hence, should be avoided.
- Adrenaline can produce marked rise in blood pressure in the patients who are taking β blockers. This occurs due to unopposed action of adrenaline on α adrenergic receptors.
- Propranolol should not be given to the patients of diabetes on hypoglycemic drugs/insulin. Because the warning sign of hypoglycemia and sympathetic stimulation like tachycardia and tremors are suppressed and this can be fatal.
- The anti cold preparations containing ephedrine or phenylephrine should be avoided in hypertensive patients as these may cause marked hypertension.
- The antihypertensive effect of β blockers is reduced by NSAIDs.
- Propranolol decreases the metabolism of many drugs such as lignocaine, etc. by decreasing hepatic blood flow.

Nursing Implications

- **Adrenergic and antiadrenergic drugs**
  - Assess for contraindications or cautions: known allergies to these drugs to avoid hypersensitivity reactions.
  - Adrenaline tends to be oxidized and turn pink. Any solution of adrenaline, i.e., pink, should not be administered.
  - The adrenergic drugs should not be given intravenously.
  - If the eye drops containing adrenergic drugs are to be given to hypertensive patients, nurse should teach the patient to press the medial canthus to stop the drug from entering into the nose.
  - The beta-blockers should not be withdrawn suddenly as this may produce serious cardiac arrhythmias.
  - Monitor patient response closely, including blood pressure, ECG, urine output, and cardiac output, and arrange to adjust dose accordingly to ensure the most benefit with the least amount of toxicity.
  - Monitor for adverse effects (cardiovascular changes, GI stimulation, urinary urgency, respiratory distress).
  - Evaluate the effectiveness of the teaching plan.

SKELETAL MUSCLE RELAXANTS

Skeletal muscle relaxants are the drugs, which produce the relaxation of skeletal muscles either by reducing the muscle tone or by causing reversible muscular paralysis. This group of drugs is very important to carry out the various surgical procedures smoothly as well as in providing relief from painful muscle spasms.

There are two groups of skeletal muscle relaxants:

1. The drugs, which act peripherally at neuromuscular junction or muscle fibers and interfere with the transmission at neuromuscular end-plate to produce reversible muscle paralysis, are known as **neuromuscular blockers or peripherally-acting muscles relaxants**. These drugs are primarily used in combination with general anesthetic drugs to provide muscle relaxation during surgical and other invasive procedures.

2. The drugs, which act centrally at cerebrospinal axis or directly on the contractile mechanism of the muscle to reduce the muscular spasm in various painful conditions, are known as a **spasmolytics or centrally-acting muscles relaxants**.

On the basis of their site of action as well as mechanism of action, the skeletal muscle relaxant drugs have been classified into peripherally-acting and centrally-acting muscle relaxants (Table 9.57).

PERIPHERALLY-ACTING MUSCLE RELAXANTS

Neuromuscular Blocking Agents

Non-depolarizing Blockers or Competitive Blockers

Mechanism of Action

- The site of action of competitive blockers is the end plate of skeletal muscle fibers.
- In normal conditions, *acetylcholine* is responsible for muscular contractions by acting at the nicotinic cholinoceptors (N_M) at neuromuscular junction.
- The *competitive blocker drugs* block the N_M receptors competitively and prevent the action of ACh on these receptors. These drugs have an affinity for the N_M receptors without any intrinsic activity over them, i.e., they prevent the end plate depolarization by ACh. It causes paralysis of the skeletal muscles.
- This competitive antagonism can be easily reversed by anti-cholinesterase drugs like *neostigmine*, which are used for the purpose of reversal.

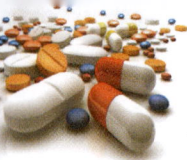

TABLE 9.57: Classification of skeletal muscle relaxants

Peripherally-acting muscle relaxants		
Neuromuscular blocking agents		**Directly-acting agents**
A. Non-depolarizing (Competitive) blockers		• Dantrolene sodium
Long-acting agents	d-Tubocurarine, Pancuronium, Doxacurium, Pipecuronium	• Quinine
Intermediate-acting agents	Vecuronium, Atracurium, Cisatracurium, Rocuronium, Rapacuronium	
Short-acting agents	Mivacurium	
B. Depolarizing blockers		
• Succinylcholine (SCh., Suxamethonium), Decamethonium*		

Centrally-acting Muscle Relaxants		
Class		**Drugs**
Mephenesin congeners	–	Mephenesin, Carisoprodol, Chlorzoxazone, Chlormezanone, Methocarbamol.
Benzodiazepines	–	Diazepam and others.
GABA mimetic	–	Baclofen, Thiocolchicoside
Central α_2 agonist	–	Tizanidine, Tolperisone
Miscellaneous		Gabapentin, pregabalin, Riluzole, Metaxolone

* Not used clinically.

Depolarizing Blockers

Mechanism of action

- The site of action of depolarizing blockers is also the end plate of skeletal muscle fibers.
- As stated above, in normal conditions, *acetylcholine* is responsible for muscular contractions by acting at the nicotinic cholinoceptors (N_M) at neuromuscular junction.
- These drugs have affinity as well as submaximal intrinsic activity at the N_M cholinoceptors.
- Due to the intrinsic activity, these drugs depolarize muscle end plates by opening Na^+ channels like acetylcholine and initially produce twitching and fasciculations.
- The ACh released during the action potential and the drug present at N_M junction binds to the already depolarized motor end plate and prevent the repolarization. This causes flaccid paralysis.
- Neostigmine does not reverse this type of paralysis rather augment it.

Pharmacokinetics

- The neuromuscular blockers are not absorbed orally as they are quaternary compounds and remain ionized at physiological pH.
- They are always given by intravenous route.
- They do not cross placental and blood-brain barrier.
- They are metabolized in liver and some are excreted unchanged in urine.
- Atracurium and cisatracurium are metabolized by spontaneous degradation (Hoffman elimination).

Pharmacological Actions of Non-Depolarizing Blockers

d-Tubocurarine (d-TC)

Curare was used by South American tribes as arrow poison for hunting wild animals because it was used to paralyze animals. The natural sources of curare are *Strychnos toxifera*, *Chondrodendron tomentosum* and related plants. The active principles responsible for action of curare were identified as tubocurarine, toxiferins, etc.

- Tubocurarine is a natural compound whereas many synthetic compounds were introduced subsequently.
- The recent additions are *doxacurium, pipecuronium, rocuronium, mivacurium, rapacuronium* and *cisatracurium*.
- These synthetic compounds have pharmacological actions similar to d-TC with slight variations.

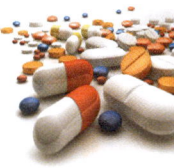

The systemic actions of d-tubocurarine are as follows:

- **Skeletal muscles paralysis:** Non-depolarizing blockers when given by intravenous injection produce muscle weakness followed by flaccid paralysis. The sequence of paralysis is specific. The fast moving small muscles of eye, fingers, jaw and larynx are affected first followed by large muscles of arm, leg, neck, face, trunk, intercostal muscle and finally diaphragm. The respiration stops finally.

The rate of attainment of peak effect and the duration for which it is maintained depends on the drug. Apnea generally occurs within 45–90 sec, but lasts only 2–5 minutes. The recovery of muscles occurs in reverse order.

As evident from their mechanism of action, the depolarizing blockers typically produce fasciculations lasting a few seconds before inducing flaccid paralysis. The sequence of muscle involvement is neck → limbs → face → jaw → eyes → pharynx → trunk → respiratory muscles. This sequence is somewhat different from that of competitive blockers. This sequence of actions develops so rapidly that it is difficult to appreciate these.

- **Effects on autonomic ganglia:** Competitive neuromuscular blockers produce some degree of ganglionic blockade whereas, depolarizing blockers produce ganglionic stimulation by their agonistic action on nicotinic receptors.
- **Histamine release:** Hypotension, flushing, bronchospasm and increased respiratory secretions are some of the effects seen due to histamine release by d-TC. Other derivatives also release histamine, but to a lesser extent.
- **Effects on cardiovascular system:** Hypotension occurs with d-TC due to ganglionic blockade, histamine release and reduction in venous return due to paralysis of various muscles. Other agents do not produce this effect very frequently.
- **Effects on gastrointestinal tract (GIT):** Post-operative paralytic ileus is a commonly seen after effect of competitive blockers.

Individual Drugs

Table 9.58 enlists the features of non-depolarizing blockers.

TABLE 9.58: Non-depolarizing blockers

Drugs	Onset of action	Duration of action	Special features
Long-acting non-depolarizing blockers			
d-Tubocurarine	4–5 minutes	30–60 minutes	• Due to side effect profile, not used these days
Doxacurium	4–8 minutes	60–120 minutes	• Suitable for long duration surgery • Very good cardiovascular stability
Pipecuronium	2–4 minutes	50–100 minutes	• Steroidal derivative • Suitable for long duration surgery • Very good cardiovascular stability
Pancuronium	4–6 minutes	60–120 minutes	• Steroidal derivative • Suitable for long duration surgery (especially in neurosurgery) • May cause rise in BP tachycardia due to vagal block • It is economical and most commonly used
Intermediate-acting non-depolarizing blockers			
Atracurium	2–4 minutes	20–40 minutes	• Elimination occurs by Hoffman's elimination; hence, preferred in neonates, elderly and patients with hepatic and renal insufficiency • Reversal mostly not required
Cisatracurium	3–6 minutes	20–40 minutes	• R-Cis- enantiomer of atracurium and four times more potent • Reversal mostly not required
Rocuronium	1–2 minutes	25–40 minutes	• Reversal not required • Popular due to précised time of onset of action • Used in tracheal intubation and in intensive care unit to facilitate mechanical ventilation
Rapacuronium	1–2 minutes	15–30 minutes	• It has been withdrawn due to life threatening complication like bronchospasm

253

Contd...

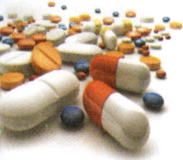

Vecuronium	2–4 minutes	30–60 minutes	• Better cardiovascular stability due to lack of histamine release and ganglionic blockade • Used routinely in surgery and intensive care unit
Short-acting non-depolarizing blockers			
Mivacurium	2–4 minutes	15–30 minutes	• Shortest-acting and does not need reversal • Hypotension can occur • Prolonged paralysis can occur in pseudocholinesterase deficient patients, which is easily reversed by giving neostigmine
Depolarizing blockers			
Succinylcholine (SCh., Suxamethonium)	1–1.5 minutes	5–8 minutes	• Most commonly used muscles relaxant for tracheal intubation as induction is rapid, complete and with predictable paralysis and spontaneous recovery • Used by continuous IV infusion for producing controlled muscle relaxation of longer duration • Causes muscle fasciculations and soreness

Decamethonium is not used *clinically*

Adverse Effects

The most common adverse effects seen are:
- Respiratory paralysis and prolonged apnea, hypotension, flushing and precipitation of asthma (by histamine releasing neuromuscular blockers) and sometime aspiration of gastric contents.
- Succinyl choline (SCh) can cause malignant hyperthermia in patients anesthetized with fluorinated anesthetic agents, cardiac arrhythmia and arrest due to K+ release from muscles.

Common Uses of Peripherally-acting Muscle Relaxants

- **As adjutants to general anesthesia:**
  - *Short-acting agents (SCh and mivacurium)* are used for brief procedures like endotracheal intubation, bronchoscopy, esophagoscopy, endoscopy and laryngoscopy.
  - *Intermediate and long-acting agents* are used for longer duration surgeries. *Vecuronium* and *rocuronium* are the most frequently selected non-depolarizing blockers.
  - *Pancuronium* is routinely used in developing countries due to better cost-benefit ratio.
- **To facilitate assisted ventilation in intensive care unit (ICU):** *Vecuronium* is the most commonly used. It is given as continuous infusion in sub-anesthetic doses.
- In severe cases of **tetanus and status epilepticus,** to maintain intermittent positive pressure respiration till the disease subsides
- SCh is used during **electroconvulsive therapy (ECT)** to prevent trauma due to convulsions. Mivacurium can also be used as an alternative.

DIRECTLY-ACTING MUSCLE RELAXANTS

Dantrolene

- Dantrolene resembles to centrally-acting muscle relaxants but acts directly at the muscles fibers. It acts on the *Ryanodine* receptor (RyR1) in the sarcoplasmic reticulum of the skeletal muscles and produces muscle relaxation by interfering with excitation-contraction coupling.
- The cardiac and smooth muscles are not affected as the sarcoplasmic reticulum of these muscles contains different subtype of ryanodine receptors (RyR2).

Pharmacokinetics

Dantrolene is slowly absorbed from the GIT and crosses blood-brain barrier and produces some sedation. It is metabolized in liver and excreted by kidney with a t½ of 8–12 hours.

Indications

- To reduce spasticity in upper motor neurone disorders, hemiplegia, paraplegia, cerebral palsy and multiple sclerosis. It is given orally in a dose of 25–100 mg QID.
- To treat malignant hyperthermia, it is given in a dose of 1 mg/kg by IV route till required.

Adverse Effects

Sedation, light-headedness, diarrhea, hepatotoxicity (on long-term use) and muscular weakness.

Quinine

- It decreases excitability of motor end plates by increasing the refractoriness.

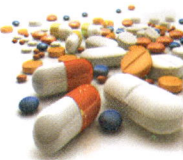

- It is used to decrease muscle tone in myotonia congenita.
- It also abolishes nocturnal leg cramps when given in a dose of 200–300 mg at bedtime.

Drug used for reversal of non-depolarizing neuromuscular blockade
- Neostigmine
- Pyridostigmine
- Edrophonium
- Sugamadex

Special Precautions while using Neuromuscular Blocking Agents
Patients of myasthenia gravis and patients on aminoglycoside antibiotics, calcium channel blockers, diuretics and fluorinated anesthetics show potentiated and prolonged effect of neuromuscular blockers due to synergism. Hence, necessary precautions should be taken before hand.

CENTRALLY-ACTING MUSCLE RELAXANTS (SPASMOLYTICS)

- These drugs reduce skeletal muscle tone by a selective action in the cerebrospinal axis, without altering consciousness.
- All centrally-acting muscle relaxants have some sedative property also.
- They decrease muscle tone without reducing voluntary power.
- They are given orally and sometimes parenterally.
- These drugs are used in chronic spastic conditions, acute muscle spasms and tetanus, etc.
- These drugs can be used for longer durations also.

These drugs have been classified as given in Table 9.59.

Mephenesin Congeners

(Mephenesin, carisoprodol, chlorzoxazone, chlormezanone, methocarbamol)

TABLE 9.59: Centrally-acting muscle relaxants

Class	Drugs
Mephenesin congeners	Mephenesin, carisoprodol, chlorzoxazone, chlormezanone, methocarbamol
Benzodiazepines	Diazepam and others
Gamma aminobutyric acid mimetic	Baclofen, thiocolchicoside
Central α₂ agonist	Tizanidine, tolperisone
Miscellaneous	Gabapentin, pregabalin, riluzole

These drugs inhibit the polysynaptic reflexes and act at the level of brain stem.

These drugs are used to treat muscle spasm of local origin resulting from spondylosis, sprains and low backache.

- **Mephenesin** was the first drug found to cause muscle relaxation but not used clinically these days, due to marked gastritis by oral route and thrombophlebitis, hemolysis and hypotension by IV route. It is used as a part of counter irritant ointments only.

Capsaicin
- It is an active substance found in chilli peppers.
- It produces intense irritation by binding to a receptor called Transient Receptor Potential Vanilloid receptor-1 (TRPV-1).
- It is used topically for relieving neuropathic pain and for muscle relaxation.
- The topical capsaicin should be applied softly without any vigorous massage because it causes intense local irritation and serious contact dermatitis.

- **Carisoprodol** has medium duration of action of 4–6 hours and is converted to an active metabolite meprobamate. It has good muscle relaxant property with low sedation and weak analgesic, antipyretic and anticholinergic properties. It is used in musculoskeletal disorders associated with muscle spasm in a dose of 350 mg TDS orally.
- **Chlorzoxazone** is better tolerated orally and longer duration of action (8–12 hours). It is given in a dose of 250 mg TDS orally. It is mostly available in combination with some analgesic agents (NSAIDs).
- **Chlormezanone** is used for tension states associated with increased muscle tone due to its additional antianxiety and hypnotic actions. It is given in a dose of 100 mg TDS orally in combination with NSAIDs.
- **Methocarbamol** is preferred as an intravenous spasmolytic for orthopedic procedures and tetanus as it does not produce thrombophlebitis and hemolysis. It can also be given orally in a dose of 500 mg TDS for reflex muscle spasms and chronic neurological diseases. It produces gastric irritation and sedation as side effects.

Benzodiazepines (BZDs) Group

Diazepam and *Clonazepam* are the most commonly used BZDs as spasmolytic agents.

- These drugs reduce spasticity by enhancing the gamma aminobutyric acid (GABA) ergic transmission in the brain. Muscle tone is reduced by supraspinal rather than spinal action.
- These drugs produce marked sedation and have low muscle relaxant: sedative activity ratio.

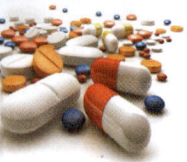

- These drugs are well tolerated with little gastric irritation.
- These drugs are useful in spasm of any origin, spinal injuries, tetanus and rheumatic disorders associated with muscle spasm.
- These drugs are more effective when given in combination with analgesics.
- Diazepam is given in a dose of 2 mg TDS, orally and 10–40 mg IV in tetanus.
- Clonazepam is given in a dose of 0.5–2 mg TDS, orally.

GABA Mimetic Agents

Baclofen

- Baclofen acts at spinal cord level where it depresses both polysynaptic and monosynaptic reflexes.
- This is an analogue of GABA and acts as a selective $GABA_B$ receptor agonist.
- It has less sedative action than diazepam.
- It is a preferred drug to provide symptomatic relief in reducing the spasticity of neurological disorders due to spinal injuries, multiple sclerosis, amyotropic lateral sclerosis (ALS) and flexor spasms.
- It is relatively ineffective in stroke, cerebral palsy, rheumatic and traumatic muscle spasms and parkinsonism.
- It is well absorbed orally and primarily excreted unchanged in urine with a t½ of 3–4 hours.
- It is given in a dose of 10–25 mg twice or thrice daily.
- The main adverse effects seen with its use are drowsiness, confusion, ataxia; and sudden withdrawal may precipitate anxiety, hallucinations and tachycardia.
- It is teratogenic in nature.

Thiocolchicoside

- It is related to colchicines.
- It produces the muscle relaxation by the GABA mimetic and glycinergic action.
- It is usually given in combination with NSAIDs.
- It is indicated in various painful muscle spasm conditions such as torticollis, sprains, backache, etc.
- It is given in a dose of 4 mg TDS/QID orally.
- Gastritis and photosensitivity are the major side effects.

Central α₂ Agonists

Tizanidine

- It is a α_2 adrenergic agonist and acts at the level of spinal cord.
- It inhibits the pre-synaptic and post-synaptic muscle output.
- It decreases muscle tone and frequency of muscle spasms without reducing muscle strength.
- It is similar in efficacy to baclofen and diazepam.

- It is absorbed orally and undergoes first pass metabolism and is excreted by the kidney with a t½ of 2–3 hours.
- It is indicated in spasm due to multiple sclerosis, stroke, amyotrophic lateral sclerosis and painful muscle spasm of spinal origin.
- It is given in a dose of 2 mg TDS to a maximum dose of 24 mg/day, orally.
- The major side effects seen with its use are drowsiness, dry mouth, insomnia and hallucinations.
- As it is a clonidine congener, it should be avoided in hypertensive patients on clonidine treatment.

Tolperisone

- It is a piperidine derivative.
- It is indicated in the treatment of spastic paralysis and muscular dystonia.
- It acts on the reticular formation in the brainstem by blocking voltage gated Na^+ and Ca^+.
- It is absorbed orally and metabolized in liver and kidney.
- It is also useful in spondylosis, cervical and lumbar syndrome, diabetic angiopathy and Raynaud's syndrome.
- The common side effects seen are nausea, vomiting, dry mouth, muscle weakness and headache.

Miscellaneous Group

(Gabapentin, Pregabalin, Riluzole, Metaxolone)

Gabapentin and Pregabalin

Gabapentin and Pregabalin are GABA analogue, which readily cross blood brain barrier and increase the synthesis and release of GABA to increase the GABA concentration in the brain.

- These drugs are used as adjuvants in treating drug resistance partial seizures and generalized tonic clonic seizures.
- These are useful in treating diabetic neuropathy, post herpetic neuralgia and pain associated with multiple sclerosis.
- These are given in a dose of 200–600 mg TDS, orally.

Riluzole

- It is recommended for the treatment of amyotrophic lateral sclerosis (ALS).
- It decreases glutaminergic transmission in CNS and blocks post-synaptic N-methyl-D-aspartate (NMDA) type glutamate receptor.
- It is given in a dose of 50 mg BD, orally.
- Nausea and diarrhea are the prominent side effects.

Metaxalone

- It is used for the treatment of acute local muscular spasms.
- It produces less dizziness and drowsiness.

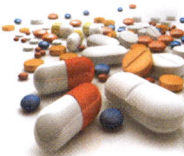

- It should be used with caution in liver failure patients and not recommended below 12 years of age.

   Other drugs used for acute localized muscle spasms are chlorphenesin, cyclobenzaprine and orphenadrine.

Common Uses of Centrally-acting Spasmolytic Drugs

- Torticollis, low backache (lumbago), neuralgias, etc.
- Acute muscular spasms associate with sprains, tearing of ligaments and tendons, dislocation, fibrositis, bursitis, rheumatic disorders, etc.
- Spastic neurological conditions such as hemiplegia, paraplegia, spinal injuries, multiple sclerosis, amyotrophic lateral sclerosis and cerebral palsy are treated with baclofen, diazepam, tizanidine and dantrolene.
- Orthopedic manipulations may be performed under the influence of diazepam or methocarbamol given intravenously.
- Muscular spasms associated with anxiety and tension: Diazepam group of drugs and chlormezanone are effective due to their antianxiety and muscle relaxant properties.
- Electroconvulsive therapy

Drug Interactions

- Thiopentone and succinylcholine react chemically; hence should not be mixed in same syringe.
- Antibiotics such as aminoglycoside, clindamycin, tetracyclines, lincomycin and calcium channel blockers potentiate the effect of competitive blockers by acting at neuromuscular junction.
- The diuretic drugs also potentiate the effect of competitive blockers by producing hypokalemia.
- Diazepam and other benzodiazepines also potentiate the effect of competitive blockers.
- The high dose of corticosteroids attenuates the effect of competitive blockers.

Nursing Implications

- **Muscle relaxants**
   - Assess for contraindications or cautions for the use of the drug including any known allergies to prevent hypersensitivity reactions.
   - Nurse must ensure that, the correct muscle relaxant drug is handed to the anesthetist.
   - Antagonist of these drugs should be kept ready in emergency tray.
   - Institute other supportive measures (e.g., ventilation, anticonvulsants as needed and cooling blankets) for the treatment of malignant hyperthermia to support the patient through the reaction.
   - Monitor for adverse effects (CNS changes, diarrhea, liver toxicity, urinary urgency).

Contd...

Nursing Implications

- Evaluate the effectiveness of the teaching plan (patient can give the drug name and dosage, possible adverse effects to watch for and specific measures to prevent adverse effects, and therapeutic goals).
- Assess for contraindications or cautions for the use of drug, including any known allergies to the drug to be used.
- Monitor patient response to the drug and the possible side effects (CNS stimulation, CV effects, rash, physical or psychological dependence, gastrointestinal dysfunction).

ANTIPSYCHOTICS OR MAJOR TRANQUILIZERS OR NEUROLEPTIC DRUGS

- The *antipsychotic drugs* are broadly defined as the drugs, which are used to treat the psychiatric disorders.
- In earlier times, these drugs were also known as *major tranquilizers* due to their calming effect; but this term has been abandoned now.
- These drugs are also called **neuroleptic agents** as they reduce the agitation and disturbed behavior associated with delusions and hallucinations in schizophrenia (antipsychotic effect) as well as produce a high incidence of extrapyramidal side effects (EPS) at clinically effective doses.
- The various types of psychiatric illnesses, which are treated with these drugs are, cognitive disorders such as delirium and dementia with psychotic features and functional disorders such as schizophrenia, paranoid state and mood disorders such as mania, depression, bipolar and unipolar disorders.
- The probable cause of mental illnesses involving mania and schizophernia is dopaminergic overactivity in the limbic system, whereas, depression involves monoaminergic (NA, 5-HT) deficiency.
- The **"atypical"** antipsychotic drugs are most widely used nowadays due to their better antipsychotic and minimal extrapyramidal side effect profile.

The antipsychotic or neuroleptic drugs are classified as follows:

- Typical antipsychotic drugs
   - **Phenothiazines:** Chlorpromazine (CPZ), Triflupromazine, Thioridazine, Trifluoperazine, Fluphenazine
   - **Butyrophenones:** Haloperidol, Trifluperidol, Penfluridol
   - **Thioxanthenes:** Flupenthixol
   - **Other heterocyclics:** Pimozide, Loxapine

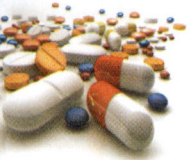

- **Atypical antipsychotics:** Clozapine, risperidone, olanzapine, quetiapine, aripiprazole, ziprasidone, amisulpiride, zotepine

MECHANISM OF ACTION OF ANTIPSYCHOTIC DRUGS

- All antipsychotics (except atypical antipsychotics) have common mechanism of action.
- These drugs have potent dopaminergic D_2 receptor blocking action in the 'limbic system' and in mesocortical region, which is responsible for their antipsychotic action.
- The atypical antipsychotic drugs block dopaminergic as well as other monoamine receptors especially $5HT_{2A}$.
- The pharmacological actions of all antipsychotics (except atypical antipsychotics) are similar to chlorpromazine (CPZ) with slight variation in their potency and profile of actions.
- The CPZ shows pharmacological effects on various body systems (Table 9.60).

PHARMACOKINETICS

- Antipsychotic drugs are erratically absorbed from the GIT; whereas, intramuscular and intravenous doses produce consistent effects.
- These drugs are widely distributed in the tissues and often accumulate after repeated administrations.
- These drugs crosses blood-brain barrier and attain higher concentrations in brain than in plasma. These drugs cross placental barrier and also enter the breast milk.
- They are metabolized in the liver and excreted through the bile and urine with an average $t_{1/2}$ of 18–30 hours.
- The excretion remains continued for months even after discontinuation of the drug due to cumulative effect.
- The dose adjustment of antipsychotic drugs is advocated according to age as metabolism of these drugs is faster in children and slow in elderly individuals.
- The patients should be informed/counseled regarding long duration of treatment as the clinical effects of these drugs appear after few weeks only.
- Individual typical anti-psychotic drugs are enlisted in Table 9.61.

TABLE 9.60: Pharmacological effects of chlorpromazine

Site	Effects
CNS (by blocking Dopaminergic receptors)	
- **Limbic system** - **Mesocortical area**	Decrease in spontaneous motor activity, Induction of sleep and improvement of cognitive and intellectual function
- **Basal ganglia**	Extrapyramidal symptoms, reduces spasticity
- **Pituitary**	Prolactin release (gynecomastia in male; galactorrhea in females)
- **Chemoreceptor trigger zone**	Antiemetic effects
Cardiovascular system (α_1 adrenergic receptor)	Postural hypotension, tachycardia, palpitations and Q-Tc prolongation (at higher doses)
Skin (H_1 receptor)	Antipruritic effects
GIT (M_3 receptor)	Dry mouth, constipation
Eye (M_3 receptor)	Blurred vision
Urinary bladder (M_3 receptor)	Urinary retention

ATYPICAL ANTIPSYCHOTIC DRUGS

(Clozapine, Risperidone, Olanzapine, Quetiapine, Aripiprazole, Ziprasidone, Amisulpiride, Zotepine)

- These are also called 2nd generation antipsychotic drugs.
- They differ from typical or classic antipsychotic drugs as follows:
  - They have weak D_2 receptor blocking activity along with potent $5-HT_2$ antagonistic activity. The antipsychotic effect is attributed to a combination of dopaminergic and $5-HT_2$ receptor blockade.
  - They are effective in the patients refractory to typical antipsychotic drugs.
  - The incidence of extrapyramidal side effects is very low than typical antipsychotics as their affinity towards D_1 and D_2 receptors is very low.
- Atypical anti-psychotic drugs have been enlisted in Table 9.62.

TABLE 9.61: Individual typical anti-psychotic drugs

Drug	Dose (mg/day)	Common pharmacological effects			Special features
		Extrapyramidal	Sedative	Hypotension	
Triflupromazine	50–200	High	High	Moderate	- More potent than CPZ - Used as antiemetic - On IV injection, it produces acute muscle dystonias (especially in children)

Contd...

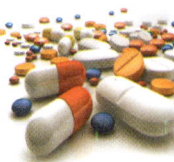

Drug	Dose (mg/day)	Common pharmacological effects			Special features
		Extrapyramidal	**Sedative**	**Hypotension**	
Thioridazine	100–400	Very low	High	High	• Has marked central anticholinergic action • Cardiotoxic and causes inhibition of ejaculation • It also damages eye; hence long-term therapy should be avoided
Trifluoperazine	2–20	High	Low	Low	• They have minimum autonomic actions • The incidence of loss of glycemic control, hepatotoxicity and hypersensitivity reactions are little
Fluphenazine	1–10				
Haloperidol	2–20	High	Low	Low	• It is a potent antipsychotic • Used in acute schizophrenia, Huntington's disease and Gilles de la Tourette's syndrome • Fewer incidences of seizure, weight gain and hepatotoxicity
Trifluperidol	1–8	High	Low	Low	• Same as above • The potency is greater than haloperidol
Flupenthixol	3–15	High	Low	Low	• Less sedative than CPZ • Used in schizophrenia and other psychotic disorders such as in withdrawn and apathetic patients • Rarely used nowadays
Pimozide	2–6	High	Low	Low	• Selective DA antagonist with little α-adrenergic or cholinergic blocking activity • Used for the treatment of Gilles de la Tourett's syndrome and in ticks • It has long duration of action; hence, used for maintenance therapy • Causes cardiac arrhythmia as a side effect
Loxapine	20–50	Moderate	Low	Moderate	• It is the shortest and fastest acting antipsychotic drug

TABLE 9.62: Atypical antipsychotic drugs (2nd generation antipsychotics)

Drugs	Dose (mg/day)	Common side effects			Special features
		Extrapyramidal	**Sedation**	**Hypotension**	
Clozapine	100–300	No	High	High	• It is the first atypical antipsychotic • It blocks D1, D4 5-HT$_2$, α-adrenergic and H$_1$ receptor with relatively weak D$_2$ selectivity • Most effective in both positive and negative symptoms of schizophrenia and in refractory schizophrenia • Low sedation and low incidence of extra pyramidal side effects is there • The common side effects are weight gain, hyperlipidemia, loss of glycemic control, seizure (in high dose), tachycardia and urinary incontinence • It causes agranulocytosis and other blood dyscrasias: hence, weekly monitoring of leukocyte count is advocated
Risperidone	2–8	Moderate	Moderate	Moderate	• D$_2$ + 5-HT$_2$ receptor antagonist with high affinity for α$_1$, α$_2$ and H$_1$ receptors • More potent than clozapine • Weight gain and the incidence of diabetes is less prominent than clozapine • It increases the level of prolactin • Should be avoided in elderly patients with stroke

Contd...

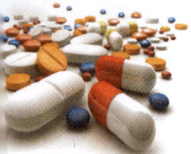

Drugs	Dose (mg/day)	Common side effects			Special features
		Extrapyramidal	Sedation	Hypotension	
Olanzapine	2.5–20	Low	Low	Moderate	• Blocks D_2, 5-HT$_2$, α_1, α_2, H$_1$ and muscarinic receptors • Used for both positive and negative symptoms of schizophrenia and mania • The common side effects are weight gain, loss of diabetic control and increased incidence of seizure
Quetiapine	50–400	Very low	High	Moderate	• Short-acting atypical antipsychotic • It blocks the 5-HT$_{1A}$, 5-HT$_2$, D_2, α_1, α_2 and H$_1$ receptors in the brain • Used in mania and bipolar depressive disorder as maintenance therapy • Not effective in schizophrenia
Aripiprazole	5–30	Very low	Very low	Very low	• It is partial agonist at D_2, 5-HT$_{1}$A with 5-HT$_2$ receptors antagonist • Used in schizophrenia, mania and bipolar disorders • The common side effects are nausea, dyspepsia, constipation, light-headedness and prolongation of Q-Tc (at higher doses)
Ziprasidone	40–160	Low	Low	Low	• It blocks D_2 + 5-HT$_{2A/2C}$+ H$_1$+ α_1 for antipsychotic action. • It also blocks the 5-HT$_{1D}$ and agonist at 5-HT$_{1A}$ receptors with inhibition of 5-HT and noradrenaline reuptake resulting its antianxiety and antidepressant actions • The common side effects are nausea, vomiting and dose related prolongations of Q-Tc
Amisulpiride	Schizophrenia 50–300 mg/day BD Acute psychosis 200–400 mg BD	Low	No	Low	• It has high affinity for D_2 and D_3 and has low-affinity for 5-HT$_2$ receptors • Used in the treatment for negative symptoms associated with schizophrenia • The common side effects are anxiety, insomnia, agitation, Q-Tc (in elderly) and hyperprolactinemia • It has low incidence of weight gain
Zotepine	25–100 mg TDS	Low	Low	Low	• Blocks D_2+D_1, 5-HT$_2$, α_1, H$_1$ receptors and noradrenaline reuptake • Used for positive and negative symptoms of schizophrenia • The common side effects are headache, postural hypotension, weight gain, hyperglycemia and dyslipidemia

Lurasidone
- It is a novel 5-HT/DA antagonist.
- It possesses potent activity at 5-HT$_7$ receptor sites, actions that, based on preclinical and early clinical studies, may be associated with cognitive benefits.
- It is devoid of most of the side effects associated with atypical antipsychotics.

COMMON INDICATIONS OF ANTIPSYCHOTIC/NEUROLEPTIC DRUGS

- **Psychiatric illness**
  - Schizophrenia
  - Control of acute mania and also for long-term treatment.
  - Organic brain syndromes (dementia and delirium).
  - Anxiety (BZDs preferred).

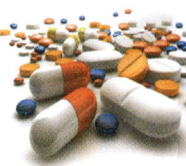

- **Non-psychiatric illness**
  - As antiemetic (at doses much lower than needed as antipsychotic).
  - Intractable hiccough (parenteral chlorpromazine is used).
  - As pre-anesthetic medication (promethazine).
- **Neuro-psychiatric illness**
  - Alcoholic hallucinations.
  - Huntington's disease.
  - Gilles de la Tourette's.

COMMON SIDE EFFECTS OF ANTIPSYCHOTIC/ NEUROLEPTIC DRUGS

Antipsychotic or neuroleptic drugs cause side effects which are given in Table 9.63.

Extrapyramidal side effects (EPS) seen with Antipsychotic Drugs are:

- The extrapyramidal side effects are mostly seen with potent typical antipsychotic drugs and rarely with atypical antipsychotics.
- Parkinsonism, acute muscular dystonias, akathisia and malignant neuroleptic syndrome appear early during the treatment, whereas *Rabbit syndrome* and *Tardive dyskinesia* appear nearly a year after initiating the treatment.
- The extrapyramidal effects of these drugs are categorized as given in Table 9.64.
- Comparative side effects of atypical antipsychotics are given in Table 9.65.

TABLE 9.63: Common side effects of antipsychotic drugs

System	Adverse effects
CNS	Drowsiness, lethargy, mental confusion and agitation, extrapyramidal side effects
CVS	Postural hypotension, palpitations, Q-Tc prolongation and cardiac arrhythmias
Endocrine	Hyperprolactinemia Amenorrhea, infertility, galactorrhea in females and gynecomastia in males also occur, but infrequently after prolonged treatment
Metabolic	Increase in appetite, weight gain, loss of diabetic control and dyslipidemia
Eye	Blurring of vision
Gastrointestinal tract	Constipation, dry mouth
Urinary system	Urinary hesitancy in elderly males

TABLE 9.64: Extrapyramidal side effects of antipsychotic drugs and their management

Types	Clinical features	Management
Parkinsonism	• Presents as rigidity, tremors, hypokinesia, mask like facies, shuffling gait • Appears between 1 and 4 weeks of therapy and persists unless dose is reduced • Perioral tremors 'rabbit syndrome' seen after a few years of therapy.	• Changing from typical to atypical antipsychotic reduces these symptoms • Central anticholinergic drugs are used to treat Perioral tremors
Acute muscular dystonias	• Presents as muscle spasms with involvement of linguo-facial muscles (tongue thrusting, torticollis, locked jaw are seen) • It occurs within a few hours of a single dose or within first week of therapy • Most common seen in children ≤10 years and in girls, particularly after parenteral administration	• Central anticholinergics, promethazine or hydroxyzine injected IM, provide relief within 10–15 minutes
Akathisia	• It is the most common extrapyramidal side effects of antipsychotic medications • Patient presents as feeling of discomfort, restlessness and agitation • It occurs between 1–8 weeks of therapy	• Changing of antipsychotic from typical to atypical reduces these symptoms • Benzodiazepine like clonazepam or diazepam is used as the first choice of treatment • In non-responsive individuals, propranolol is used

Contd...

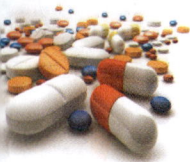
Types	Clinical features	Management
Malignant neuroleptic syndrome	• It is rare condition and seen at higher dose of potent typical antipsychotics • It presents as marked rigidity, immobility, tremor, hyperthermia, semi-consciousness, fluctuating BP and heart rate • It is a fatal condition; death occurs due to cardio-pulmonary collapse	• Symptomatic management is advocated first • Intravenous dantrolene may benefit • Bromocriptine in large doses has been found useful
Tardive dyskinesia	• It presents as purposeless involuntary facial and limb movements such as chewing, puffing of cheeks and choreoathetoid movements • It is more common in elderly women	• Changing of antipsychotic from typical to atypical ones may reduce these symptoms

TABLE 9.65: Comparative adverse effects profile of atypical antipsychotic drugs

Drugs	Weight Gain	Hyperlipidemia	New-Onset Diabetes Mellitus	QTc Prolongation
Clozapine	High	High	High	Negligible
Risperidone	Moderate	Moderate	Moderate	Low
Olanzapine	High	High	High	Negligible
Quetiapine	Moderate	Moderate	Moderate	High
Aripiprazole	Negligible	No	No	Moderate
Ziprasidone	Negligible	No	No	High
Lurasidone	No	No	No	No

Drug Interactions

⌕ **Anti-psychotics**

☞ The effect of nearly all CNS depressants is enhanced by antipsychotic drugs.

☞ The antipsychotic drugs exacerbate the symptoms of parkinsonism by blocking the action of levodopa and dopamine agonist.

☞ Barbiturates and phenothiazines are enzyme inducers that can reduce the effect of antipsychotic drugs.

ANTICONVULSANTS

• Anticonvulsants are the drugs, which are used for prophylaxis and control of convulsions. '*Antiepileptics*' is a more precise term in this regard.

• Epilepsy is a Greek word, which means '*convulsions*'.

• The convulsions are '*repeated, involuntary and violent muscular contraction and relaxation*' resulting in an uncontrolled shaking of the body. The convulsion is often a symptom of an epileptic seizure.

• Convulsion word is sometimes used as a synonym for '*seizure*'.

• Seizure is a sudden discharge of excessive electrical energy from nerve cells located within the brain.

• The recurrent episodes of such seizures are called '*epilepsy*'.

• However, **not all-epileptic seizures lead to convulsions and not all convulsions are caused by epileptic seizures.**

• Epilepsy is the most prevalent neurological disorder and affects about 1% of world population. It is not a single disease but a collection of different syndromes characterized by the same feature. The episodes of epilepsy are highly unpredictable and the frequency is also variable.

• The word '*fit/fits*' is often used in common language to describe epileptic seizure.

CLASSIFICATION OF SEIZURES

• Seizures are classified on the basis of case history, clinical manifestations and the findings of electroencephalogram (EEG).

• Accurate diagnosis of the type of seizure is very important for deciding the treatment line for the disease and to prevent future episodes of seizures.

Seizures have been classified into various types as given in Figure 9.8. The characteristic features of seizures are summarized in Table 9.66.

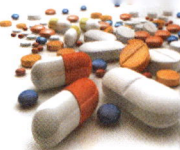

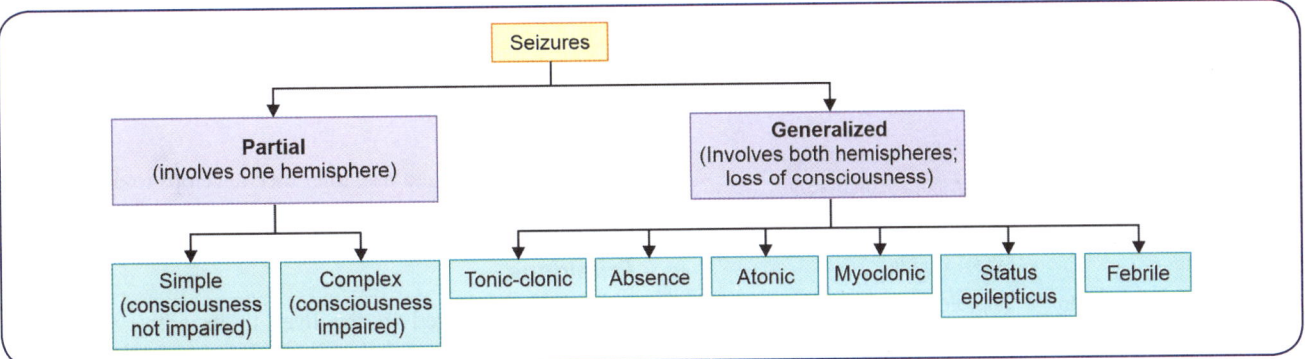

FIG. 9.8: Classification of seizures

TABLE 9.66: Characteristic features of seizures

Seizure Type	Key Features
Focal seizures or partial seizure	• It has focal origin in the brain and the manifestations depend upon the location/site of the focus. It may evolve to a bilateral or generalized convulsive seizure • These may occur with or without impairment of consciousness
Generalized seizures	The involvement of brain is diffuse at the onset of seizure
Tonic-clonic (grand mal) seizures	• Tonic phase: Sudden loss of consciousness, with rigidity and arrest of respiration, lasting < 1 minute • Clonic phase: Jerking occurs, usually for < 2–3 minutes • Flaccid coma: Variable duration • May be accompanied by tongue biting, incontinence, or aspiration; commonly followed by postictal confusion(variable in duration)
Absence (petit mal) seizures	• Consciousness impaired briefly; patient often unaware of attacks • May have clonic, tonic, or atonic (i.e., loss of postural tone) components; autonomic components (e.g., enuresis); or accompanying automatisms • Almost always begin in childhood and frequently cease by age 20
Atypical absence seizures	• May be more gradual in onset and termination than typical absence seizures. • More marked changes in tone may occur
Myoclonic seizures	• Single or multiple myoclonic jerks of a limb or whole body
Status epilepticus	• Repeated seizures without recovery between them; a fixed and enduring epileptic condition lasting≥ 30 minutes

ANTIEPILEPTIC DRUGS

- Antiepileptic drugs are given to control the seizures but, they do not cure the disease.
- The goals of antiepileptic therapy are both short-term and long-term goals.
  - Short-term goal is to provide immediate neuro-protection by minimizing deleterious effects from seizure attacks.
  - Long-term goal is to provide the prophylactic therapy to prevent the future seizure attacks.
- The antiepileptic therapy is usually continued for three years after the last seizure episode, i.e., 3 years seizure free period is mandatory for stopping the treatment.

Classification

Classification of antiepileptic drugs is given in Table 9.67.

The mechanism of action of all the above drugs have been categorized into three types as given in Table 9.68.

Barbiturates

Phenobarbitone

- This was the first efficacious antiepileptic drug, which was introduced in 1912.
- It is still in use due to cost-effectiveness and least toxicity.

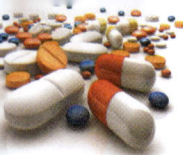

TABLE 9.67: Classification of antiepileptic durgs

Class	Drugs
Barbiturates	Phenobarbitone
Deoxybarbiturate	Primidone
Hydantoin	Phenytoin, Fosphenytoin
Iminostilbene	Carbamazepine, Oxcarbazepine
Succinimide	Ethosuximide
Aliphatic carboxylic acid	Valproic acid (sodium valproate), Divalproex
Benzodiazepines	Clonazepam, Diazepam, Lorazepam
Phenyltriazine	Lamotrigine
Cyclic GABA analogues	Gabapentin, Pregabalin
Newer drugs	Topiramate, Zonisamide, Levetiracetam, Vigabatrin, Tiagabine, Lacosamide

TABLE 9.68: Various mechanism of action according to respective drug classes

Mechanism of action	Drug/drug classes
Potentiation of GABA mediated chloride channel opening leading to inhibitory effects in the brain and control of convulsions	Barbiturates, Benzodiazepines, Sodium valproate, Gabapentin, Vigabatrin, Tiagabine
Prolongation of inactivated state of sodium channels	Phenytoin, Sodium valproate, Fosphenytoin, Carbamazepine, Oxcarbazepine, Lamotrigine, Topiramate, Zonisamide, Lacosamide
Inhibition of T-type calcium current	Ethosuximide, Sodium valproate, Zonisamide

- It acts by potentiation of GABA mediated chloride channel opening, which leads to inhibitory effects in the brain and control of convulsions.
- It is slowly but completely absorbed by oral route with 50% plasma protein binding.
- It is a microsomal enzyme inducer and can cause drug interactions.
- It is indicated in generalized tonic-clonic (GTCS) and partial seizures.
- It is also indicated for the treatment of hyperbilirubinemia in neonates. It increases the activity of glucuronyl tranferase enzyme and causes fast conjugation of bilirubin; thereby helping its excretion through bile.
- It is given in a dose of 60 mg OD–TDS orally and 100–200 mg IM/IV in adults and 3–6 mg/ kg/day in children.

- The major side effects are:
  - CNS: Ataxia, drowsiness, learning difficulties, hyperactivity in children.
  - Eye: Nystagmus
  - Skin: Rashes.
  - After prolonged use, tolerance develops to drowsiness.

Deoxybarbiturate
Primidone

- It is metabolized in the liver to its active metabolites phenobarbitone and phenyl-ethyl-melonamide (PEMA).
- It is converted to phenobarbitone but the action simulates phenytoin.
- It is indicated in generalized tonic-clonic and partial seizures.
- It is given in a dose of 250–500 mg BD for adult and 10–20 mg/kg/day in children.
- The major side effects are:
  - CNS: Sedation, ataxia, irritability.
  - Eyes and nose and throat (ENT): Nystagmus, vertigo.
  - GIT: Nausea, vomiting.
  - Skin: Rashes

Hydantoin
Phenytoin

- It is the oldest non-sedative antiepileptic drug.
- Its antiepileptic activity is due to stabilization of the neuronal membrane by following three mechanisms:
  1. It delays the recovery of inactivated sodium channels.
  2. It blocks the activated sodium channel also.
  3. It blocks the high frequency firing in neurons.
- It is absorbed slowly but completely when given by oral route with approximately 90% plasma protein binding.
- It is also a potent microsomal enzyme inducer.
- It is never given by intramuscular route as the drug precipitates in the muscles, causes pain and makes the absorption unpredictable. It causes thrombophlebitis and hypotension when given by IV route. *Fosphenytoin can be given by both IV and IM routes.*
- It is indicated in generalized tonic-clonic, partial seizures and status epilepticus.
- The other uses are in the treatment of trigeminal neuralgia (the first choice is carbamazepine) and ventricular arrhythmia due to digitalis toxicity.
- It is given in a dose of 100–200 mg BD oral and 25 mg/min slow IV injection (max 1.0 g) in adults and 5–8 mg/kg/day in children (fosphenytoin is preferred for parenteral use).
- Phenytoin has dose dependent adverse effects.
- The adverse effects seen after prolonged use even when the plasma levels of drug are maintained within therapeutic range (10–20 µg/mL).

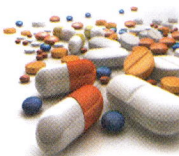

- Gum hypertrophy
- Hirsutism (in females) and acne
- Hyperglycemia
- Osteomalacia and hypocalcemia
- Megaloblastic anemia
- If used during pregnancy *'fetal hydantoin syndrome'* is produced, which is characterized by cleft palate, cleft lip, digital hypoplasia, microcephaly and congenital heart disease.
- The adverse effects seen when the plasma levels of drug exceed >30 μg/mL are:
  - CNS: Ataxia, metal confusion and disorientation.
  - Eye and ENT: Vertigo, diplopia, nystagmus
  - Cardiovascular system: Hypotension and cardiac arrhythmia, when given by IV route in higher dose or at a very fast rate.
  - GIT: Nausea, vomiting and dyspepsia.

Fosphenytoin

- It is a prodrug of phenytoin and is rapidly converted to phenytoin after IV administration. It is given in a dose of 25–100 mg/min IV injection (max 1.0 g) for status epilepticus.
- It has following advantages over phenytoin:
  - It is more potent and less cardiotoxic.
  - It is safe on the GIT.
  - It can be given by both IV and IM routes and damage to intima of vessels is very less.
  - It can be injected with both saline and glucose. The slightly faster infusion rate is tolerable.
  - It can be safely used in emergency such as status epilepticus.

Iminostilbenes

Carbamazepine

- It is one of the most commonly used antiepileptic drugs.
- It acts like phenytoin by blocking the sodium channels and inhibiting the high frequency firing of the neurons in the brain.
- It is given by oral route and is a powerful microsomal enzyme inducer.
- **Auto-induction** is special phenomenon seen with carbamazepine, in which it reduces its own half-life from 30–36 hours to 8–12 hours due to enzyme induction.
- It is indicated in:
  - GTCS
  - Simple and complex partial seizure
  - Trigeminal neuralgia (drug of choice)
  - Chronic neuropathic pain
  - Bipolar mood disorder (as an alternative to lithium)

- It is given in a dose of 200–400 mg TDS in adults and 15–30 mg/kg/day in children.
- The major adverse effects are:
  - CNS: Ataxia, drowsiness and may exacerbate myoclonic seizure.
  - GIT: Nausea, blood dyscrasias.
  - Skin: Stevens-Johnson syndrome
  - Eye: Nystagmus, diplopia.

Oxcarbazepine

- It is similar to carbamazepine in actions and uses with following advantages over it.
  - Few hypersensitivity reactions.
  - Weak microsomal enzyme induction and low auto-induction phenomenon
  - Low hepatotoxicity.
  - Better tolerated
- It is given in a dose of 300–600 mg BD.

Succinimide

Ethosuximide

- It acts differently from other antiepileptic drugs by reducing the low threshold calcium currents (T-current) in thalamocortical system.
- These T calcium-currents are responsible for the generation of absence seizure.
- It is completely absorbed when given by oral route.
- Absence seizures is the only indication of this drug. Valproic acid is preferred.
- It is given in a dose of 20–30 mg/kg/day.
- The major adverse effects are:
  - GIT: Nausea, vomiting and blood dyscrasias.
  - CNS: Headache, lethargy, unsteadiness.
  - Skin: Systemic lupus erythematosus, urticaria, pruritus.

Aliphatic Carboxylic Acid

(Valproic acid [sodium valproate], Divalproex)

Valproic acid (Sodium Valproate)

- Valproic acid is a very effective and most widely used antiepileptic agent.
- It is also known as broad spectrum antiepileptic due to its effectiveness in many types of epileptic disorders.
- It acts at multiple sites and its action resembles both ethosuximide and phenytoin.
- It inhibits the T type Ca^+ current, delays the recovery of inactivated Na^+ channels and increases the GABA activity.
- It has rapid and nearly complete oral absorption. 80–95% is plasma protein bound. It is metabolized in liver and excreted in urine.

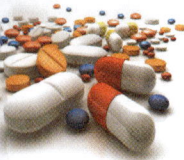

- It is used therapeutically in following conditions:
  - Myoclonic and atonic seizures
  - Absence seizures
  - Combined grand mal and petit mal epilepsy
  - Focal epilepsy
  - Manic depressive psychosis
  - Prophylactically in febrile convulsions and migraine.
  - As an alternative to carbamazepine in trigeminal neuralgia.
- Its main side effects are:
  - GIT: Nausea, vomiting, gastritis and occasionally loose motions.
  - CNS: Ataxia, sedation.
  - Increase in appetite, weight gain and curling of hair can be seen.
  - Idiosyncratic hepatotoxicity can also occur in children; monitoring of liver functions should be done regularly.
  - It is teratogenic and can cause neural tube defects like spina bifida.
- **To begin the treatment**, it is given in a dose of 10 mg/kg/day in 2–3 divided doses and **gradually increased** by 5–10 mg/kg/day at weekly intervals up to a maximum dose of 20–30 mg/kg/day.
- It is an inhibitor of hepatic microsomal enzymes and can increase plasma levels of phenobarbitone, phenytoin, carbamazepine and lamotrigine.

Divalproex

- It is a chemically compounded form of valproic acid with sodium valproate having actions and therapeutic uses similar to valproic acid.
- It has following advantages over sodium valproate:
  - It has slow rate of absorption.
  - Better gastric tolerance.
  - Better bioavailability.

Benzodiazepines

(Clonazepam, Diazepam, Lorazepam)

Benzodiazepines (BZDs) are used for short-term control of epilepsy such as status epilepticus and are not a good choice for the long-term treatment of epilepsies.

Diazepam, clonazepam and lorazepam are some of the BZDs used as anticonvulsants in status epilepticus.

Diazepam is given by both IV route and rectally. Rectal route is preferred in febrile convulsions.

It is given in a dose of 0.2–0.3 mg/kg by slow IV injection in status epilepticus and 0.5 mg/kg rectal route in febrile convulsions.

Lorazepam can also be used in status epilepticus in a dose of 0.1 mg/kg IV (slow injection).

Phenyltriazines

Lamotrigine

- It is a new broad spectrum antiepileptic drug.
- Its actions resemble carbamazepine.
- It is completely absorbed orally and metabolized in liver.
- It is can be used either alone or in combination with other drugs in partial seizures, generalized seizure, absence seizure and myoclonic seizures.
- The treatment is started with a dose of 50 mg/day. The dose can be increased up to a maximum of 300 mg/day.
- The major side effects are:
  - CNS: Sedation, ataxia.
  - Eye: Visual disturbances.
  - Skin: Rashes
  - GIT: Dyspepsia
- It should not be used in children.

Cyclic GABA Analogues

(Gabapentin, Pregabalin)

Gabapentin

- It is a lipid soluble analogue of GABA, which easily crosses blood-brain barrier.
- It enhances the release of GABA and decreases the calcium entry by binding to the L-type voltage gated calcium channels.
- The oral absorption is good.
- It is used in combination with other antiepileptic drugs in GTCS, partial seizures.
- Other uses:
  - Migraine
  - Neuropathic pain (diabetic neuropathy, post-herpetic neuralgia)
  - Bipolar mood disorders.
- The major side effects are fatigue, weight loss, ataxia, sedation, nystagmus. The tolerance usually develops to these side effects within 1–2 weeks.

Pregabalin

- It is a prodrug of gabapentin, which is more potent than gabapentin with less side effects.
- The pharmacokinetic profile and therapeutic uses are similar to gabapentin.
- It is given in a dose of 75–150 mg BD.
- The major side effects are:
  - CNS: Poor concentration, dizziness, somnolence (less prominent).
  - Skin: Rashes, anaphylactoid reactions.
  - Others: Weight gain, thrombocytopenia.

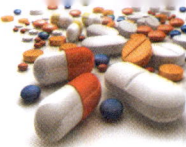

NEWER DRUGS

(Topiramate, Zonisamide, Levetiracetam, Vigabatrin, Tiagabine, Lacosamide)

- These newer drugs are used as add-on drugs to other antiepileptic agents.
- These are useful both in focal and generalized seizures.
- Some special features of these drugs are given in Table 9.69.
- Types of epilepsy and their indicated drugs are given in Table 9.70.

TABLE 9.69: Characteristic features of newer antiepileptic drugs

Drug	Dose	Special features
Topiramate	Adult: Initially 25 mg OD, increase weekly up to 100–200 mg BD as required Children: 5–10 mg/kg/day	• Its action is similar to phenytoin with some GABA receptor enhancing and glutamate receptor inhibiting activity • Used in refractory focal seizure, absence seizure and migraine headache. • Also useful as anticraving drug in chronic alcoholics • The major side effects are nausea, dyspepsia, sedation, confusion, fatigue, parasthesias, renal calculi, weight loss, and hyperthermia
Zonisamide	25–100 mg BD (it should not to be given in children)	• It is a sulfonamide derivative and should not be used in patients with sulfonamide allergy • Used as add-on drug in refractory partial seizures • The major side effects are ataxia, anorexia, nausea, rash, confusion
Levetiracetam	Adult: 500–1000 mg BD Children: 10–30 mg/kg/ day	• It is similar to drug piracetam • Used in generalized tonic clonic seizure, complex partial seizure (CPS) as add-on therapy • The major side effects are drowsiness, headache, and behavioral changes
Vigabatrin	Adult: 2–4 g/day Children: 40–100 mg/kg/ day	• It acts as irreversible inhibitor of GABA transaminase • Used in infantile spasm • It worsens absence seizure and myoclonic seizure • The major side effects are anorexia, nausea, vomiting, visual field defects, confusion
Tiagabine	4–12 mg TDS	• Used in partial seizures • The major side effects are somnolence, anxiety, dizziness, poor concentration, tremor, diarrhea
Lacosamide	100–400 mg in two divided doses	• Used in partial seizures as add-on therapy • The major side effects are fatigue, diplopia, vertigo, headache, tremors, etc.

TABLE 9.70: Types of epilepsy and indicated drugs

Types of Epilepsy	Drugs of 1st choice	Drugs of 2nd choice	Add-on drugs
Generalized tonic choice spasms	Carbamazepine, Phenytoin	• Valproic acid • Phenobarbitone	• Topiramate • Lamotrigine • Levetiracetam • Gabapentin
Absence seizures	Valproic acid	• Ethosuximide • Lamotrigine	• Clonazepam
Myoclonic seizures	Valproic acid	• Topiramate • Lamotrigine	• Clonazepam • Levetiracetam
Atonic seizures	Valproic acid	• Clonazepam	• Lamotrigine
Febrile seizure	Diazepam	• Lorazepam	—

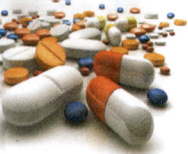

STATUS EPILEPTICUS

- It is an emergency condition, which can prove fatal if not treated timely.
- It is defined as the condition when the seizures occur repeatedly without any evidence of recovery in between the seizures.
- The period of seizure activity is mostly more than 30 minutes. If proper and timely intervention is not done, it can lead to permanent brain damage and death.
- The management of patients suffering from status epilepticus is as follows.
- Initial general management includes:
  - Hospitalization
  - Maintenance of the airways.
  - Maintenance of fluid and electrolytes.
  - Monitoring of cardiac rhythm and BP.
- Drug management:
  - Diazepam in a dose of 0.2–0.3 mg/kg or 10 mg IV is given.
  - Alternatively, lorazepam can be given in a dose of 0.1 mg/kg or 4 mg injected IV slowly.
  - If available, fosphenytoin can be given in a dose of 15–20 mg/kg in the form of IV infusion.
  - Alternatively, phenytoin sodium is given in a loading dose of 500–1000 mg followed by IV infusion at the rate of 25–50 mg/min.
  - Phenobarbitone sodium can be given in a dose of 10–15 mg/kg IV, if previous mentioned drugs do not control the seizure activity. Respiratory depression is the major side effect; hence, should be watched carefully.
  - If the seizures are not controlled with above mentioned management or drugs, the last resort is giving general anesthesia with propofol or thiopentone sodium.

After the control of seizures, long-term antiepileptic therapy is mandatory.

ANTIDEPRESSANTS

- *Antidepressants* are the drugs, which are used to elevate mood in depressive illnesses such as depression.
- *Depression* is a very common affective disorder, which manifests as feelings of sadness, listlessness, loss of interest in surroundings, sleep disturbances, lack of appetite, limited libido, inability to perform activities of daily living and suicidal thoughts in severe cases.
- The depression interferes with a person's family life, job, and social interactions and in majority of cases remains undiagnosed.
- If left untreated, it can produce multiple physical problems that can lead to further depression or, in extreme cases, even suicide.

- Depression results due to deficiency of monoamines in cortical and limbic area of the brain; these biogenic amines include serotonin (5HT), norepinephrine (NE) and dopamine. Both serotonin and norepinephrine are known to regulate arousal, alertness, attention, moods, appetite and central sensory processing functions.
- This deficiency of neurotransmitters in the intra-synaptic areas of brain can be overcome by:
  - Inhibiting the reuptake of these amines by *reuptake inhibitors*.
  - Inhibiting the amine metabolism by enzyme inhibitors such as *monoamine oxidase inhibitors (MAOIs)*. Monoamine oxidase-A (MAO-A) enzyme is responsible for degradation of these amines.
  - *Receptor blockade*

Based upon their mode of action the antidepressant drugs have been classified into following types:

CLASSIFICATION

The classification of antidepressants is given in Table 9.71.

TRICYCLIC ANTIDEPRESSANTS (TCAs)

(Imipramine, Amitriptyline, Trimipramine, Doxepin, Dothiepin, Clomipramine, Desipramine, Nortriptyline, Amoxapine, Reboxetine)

- Normally, a large proportion of 5-HT and norepinephrine liberated in the nerve endings is inactivated by their reabsorption into their storage sites.

TABLE 9.71: Classification of antidepressants

Class	Drugs
Tricyclic antidepressants (TCAs)	
NA+ 5-HT reuptake inhibitors	Imipramine, amitriptyline, trimipramine, doxepin, dothiepin, clomipramine
Predominantly NA reuptake inhibitors	Desipramine, nortriptyline, amoxapine, reboxetine
Selective serotonin reuptake inhibitors (SSRIs)	Fluoxetine, fluvoxamine, paroxetine, sertraline, citalopram, escitalopram, dapoxetine
Serotonin and noradrenaline reuptake inhibitors (SNRIs)	Venlafaxine, desvenlafaxine, duloxetine, milnacipran
Monoamine oxidase inhibitors (MAOIs)	Moclobemide, clorgyline
Atypical antidepressants	Trazodone, mianserin, mirtazapine, bupropion, tianeptine, amineptine, atomoxetine

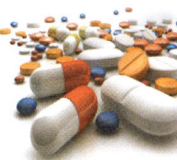

- The **tricyclic antidepressants (TCAs)** reduce the reuptake of NE and 5-HT by inhibiting norepinephrine transporter (NET) and serotonin transporter (SERT) located at neuronal/platelet membrane at low and therapeutically attained concentrations. This keeps the concentration of these amines elevated at intra-synaptic sites for a longer duration and causes prolonged action. This helps in elevation of the mood.
- Some studies show that in addition to above mechanism, TCAs also elevate the mood by facilitating dopaminergic transmission.
- TCAs also interact with a variety of receptors such as muscarinic, α adrenergic, histamine H_1, 5-HT$_1$, 5-HT$_2$ and occasionally dopamine D_2.
- All TCAs show similar actions except their relative potency, which differs among different compounds.
- The choice of TCA depends on individual response to the drug and tolerance of adverse effects. Patient not responding to one TCA, may respond to another drug from the same class.

Pharmacokinetics

- The TCAs are well absorbed from the GIT.
- They are lipid soluble and highly bound to plasma proteins and tissue; distributed widely in the tissues, including the brain. They cross the placenta and enter breast milk.
- They are metabolized in liver and excreted through urine with relatively long plasma half-lives (8–46 hours).
- The individual dose titration is advocated as the plasma concentration attained by different individuals is different even when given in the same dose.
- Common pharmacological actions of TCAs are given in Tables 9.72. Table 9.73 enlists the features of individual TCAs. Common adverse effects of TCAs are given in Table 9.74.

TABLE 9.72: Common pharmacological actions of tricyclic anti-depressants

Systems	Actions of TCAs
CNS	Drowsiness in normal individuals while elevation of mood in depressed individuals They lower the seizure thresholds may cause seizures
Gastrointestinal tract	Dry mouth, constipation, increased appetite, weight gain
Cardiovascular system	Postural hypotension, tachycardia and arrhythmias
Eye	Blurring of vision, may precipitate glaucoma

TABLE 9.73: Individual tricyclic anti-depressant drugs

Drug	Dose (mg/day)	Relative pharmacological effects			
		Cardiac arrhythmia	*Sedative*	*Hypotension*	*Anti-cholinergic*
Imipramine	50–200	High	Low	Moderate	Moderate
Amitriptyline	50–200	High	High	Moderate	High
Trimipramine	50–150	High	High	Moderate	High
Doxepin	50–150	High	High	Moderate	Moderate
Dothiepin	50–150	Moderate	Moderate	Moderate	Moderate
Clomipramine	50–150	High	Moderate	Moderate	High
Nortriptyline	50-150	Moderate	Low	Low	Moderate
Amoxapine	100–300	Moderate	Low	Moderate	Low
Reboxetine	8	Low	Very low	Low	Very low

TABLE 9.74: Common adverse effects of tricyclic antidepressants

Systems	Adverse effects
CNS	• They lower the seizure threshold and may cause seizures (especially in children) • Tiredness, sedation, confusion, sweating, fine tremors
Gastrointestinal tract	Taste alteration, dry mouth, constipation, increased appetite, weight gain, epigastric disturbance
Cardiovascular system	Postural hypotension (especially in elderly individuals), tachycardia and arrhythmias

269

Contd...

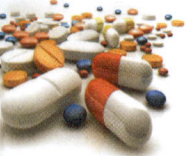

Systems	Adverse effects
EYE	Blurring of vision, may precipitate glaucoma
Bladder	Urinary retention especially in elderly individuals
Endocrine	Delayed ejaculation
Liver	Jaundice
Skin	Rashes

SELECTIVE SEROTONIN REUPTAKE INHIBITORS (SSRIs)

(Fluoxetine, Fluvoxamine, Paroxetine, Sertraline, Citalopram, Escitalopram, Dapoxetine)

- These are relatively newer class of antidepressant drugs and preferred over TCAs and MAOIs due to better tolerance and lesser side effects.
- **Mechanism of action:**
  These drugs specifically block the reuptake of 5-HT by inhibiting the serotonin transporters (SERT) and enhance the serotonin levels in the synapses which produces the prolonged antidepressant effect.
- **Pharmacokinetics:**
  SSRIS are well absorbed when given orally. Most of the drugs are plasma protein bound. SSRIs are microsomal enzyme inhibitors.

- **Common uses:**
  The SSRIs are first line drugs in depression and extensively used in anxiety, phobias, obsessive compulsive disorder (OCD) and related disorders due to their safety and better acceptability.
- **Advantages of SSRIs over TCAs:**
  - Less sedation
  - Low cardiovascular side effects
  - Safer in overdose (safer in patients with suicidal tendencies)
  - Low anticholinergic side effects (safer in elderly)
  - Individual SSRI drug profiles are given in Table 9.75.

Common Adverse Effects of SSRIs

Nausea, headache, anorexia, diarrhea, interference with ejaculation and orgasm, restlessness, insomnia, epistaxis, and ecchymosis (due to interference with platelets function) are common side effects.

Serotonin Syndrome

Serotonin syndrome is a major side effect seen when patient on SSRIs takes another serotonergic drug such as MAOIs, tramadol, pethidine, cocaine, buspirone, tryptophan, sumatriptan (5-HT agonist), etc. It occurs due to excessive serotonergic activity at synapse. It manifests as agitation, restlessness, variable BP, rigidity, hyperthermia, delirium, sweating, twitching followed by convulsions. It can be life threatening.

The treatment includes:
- Hospitalization for observation and treatment of symptoms.
- Stopping the SSRIs or alleged drug to avoid further exposure.
- IV fluids to maintain hydration and external cooling to treat hyperthermia.
- BZDs to treat agitation or seizures.
- In severe cases, cyproheptadine in a dose of 4 mg orally or by gastric tube hourly for 3–4 doses is given. It blocks the serotonin production.

TABLE 9.75: Individual SSRI drug profile

Drug	Dose (mg/day)	Special features
Fluoxetine	20–40	• It is the first SSRI with longest action (7–10 days) • Used to treat depression, bulimia, obsessive compulsive disorder, panic disorders • Agitation and dermatological reactions are the prominent side effects
Fluvoxamine	50–200	• Shorter-acting SSRI • Used in generalized anxiety disorder and obsessive compulsive disorder • Dyspepsia, flatulence, nervousness are the prominent side effects
Paroxetine	20–50	• Short-acting SSRI • Sexual distress, agitation and GIT adverse effects are common

Contd...

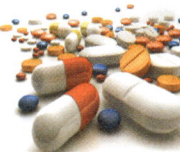

Drug	Dose (mg/day)	Special features
Sertraline	50–150	• Longer acting SSRI • Used for anxiety and post-traumatic stress disorder (PTSD)
Citalopram	20–40	• Used in depression, panic disorders, premenstrual dysphoric disorder (PMDD), obsessive compulsive disorder, PTSD, social phobias and trichotillomania
Escitalopram	10–20	• It is an enantiomer of citalopram which is more potent and safer than it • Used for maintenance of patients with major depressive disorder and generalized anxiety disorder
Dapoxetine	30–60	• It used to treat premature ejaculation • Nausea, vomiting, loose motions, headache, dizziness and occasionally insomnia are the common side effects

SEROTONIN AND NOREPINEPHRINE INHIBITORS (SNRIs)

(Venlafaxine, Desvenlafaxine, Duloxetine, Milnacipran)

- SNRIs inhibit the uptake of both serotonin (5-HT) and the norepinephrine (NE) by binding to SERT and NET like the TCAs.
- The SNRIs lack the antihistamine, α-adrenergic blocking, and anticholinergic effects.
- Venlafaxine is a weak inhibitor of norepinephrine transporter (NET), whereas desvenlafaxine, duloxetine, and milnacipran are more balanced inhibitors of both SERT and NET.
- The SNRIs are favored over the TCAs in the treatment of major depressive disorders (MDD) and pain syndromes because of their better tolerability profile.
- **Individual drugs profiles are given in Table 9.76.**

MONOAMINE OXIDASE INHIBITORS (MAOIs)

(Moclobemide, Clorgyline)

- Monoamine oxidase (MAO) is a mitochondrial enzyme found in nerves and other tissues.
- It is involved in metabolism of the biogenic amines NE, dopamine, 5-HT and tyramine.
- MAO is available in two isoforms; MAO-A and MAO- B.
  - MAO-A is predominantly found in intestinal mucosa, human placenta and peripheral adrenergic nerve endings.
  - MAO-B predominates found in brain and in platelets.
  - Liver is an exception, which contains both MAO-A and MAO-B.
- Monoamine oxidase inhibitor (MAOIs) inhibits MAO, thereby increases biogenic amines in the brain and relieves the symptoms of depression.

TABLE 9.76: SNRI drug profiles

Drugs	Dose (mg/day)	Special features
Venlafaxine	75–150	• It is a fast acting drug • Useful in patients not responding to other antidepressants • Used for the treatment and prevention of depression in generalized anxiety disorder; social anxiety disorder; decreases addictive behavior • Withdrawal symptoms may occur if the doses are missed
Desvenlafaxine	50–100	• It is a metabolite of venlafaxine • Used in treatment of major depressive disorder in adults • Contraindicated in nursing mothers
Duloxetine	30–80	• Similar to venlafaxine • Used for the treatment of major depressive disorders, diabetic neuropathic pain, panic attacks, stress induced urinary incontinence in females and fibromyalgia • Patients should be monitored for liver toxicity. • It should be avoided during pregnancy and lactation
Milnacipran	12.5–100	• It is only approved for use in the treatment of fibromyalgia in adults • It should be avoided during pregnancy and lactation • It increases the suicidal tendency; hence, patients should be monitored during therapy

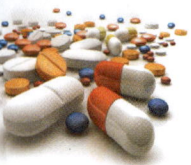

- MAOIs are divided into two classes:
  - **Selective inhibitors or reversible inhibitors:** Selective MAO-A inhibitors have antidepressant property, while MAO-B selective inhibitors like selegiline does not have antidepressant property.
  - **Non-selective or irreversible inhibitors:** The non-selective MAO inhibitors are not in clinical practice because they interact with many food ingredients, alcohol and drugs such as barbiturates, opioids, antihistamines, tricyclic antidepressants, cough and cold therapy and reserpine. They are responsible for a notorious reaction, known as *cheese reaction*.
- The antidepressant effect develops slowly over weeks of treatment and the recovery time after stopping the drug is also 1–2 weeks due to long-acting nature of these drugs.
- Abruptly stopping the drug causes withdrawl symptoms with confusion, excitement and even psychosis.
- Due to their side effects and drug interactions, MAOIs are not preferred antidepressants.

Pharmacokinetics

- The MAOIs are well absorbed from the GI tract.
- They are metabolized in the liver and excreted in the urine.
- They also cross the placenta and enter breast milk.

Reversible Inhibitors of MAO-A (RIMAs)

Moclobemide

- Moclobemide is a reversible and selective competitive inhibitor of MAO-A.
- It has short duration of action.

- It does not have anticholinergic effects; hence, the incidence of sedation, psychomotor and cardiovascular side effects is lower than typical TCAs.
- It is more suitable in elderly patients and patients with heart disease.
- It is well tolerated as an alternative to TCAs for mild to moderate depression and for social phobias.
- It is given in a dose of 150 mg BD–TDS.
- The common adverse effects are nausea, headache, dizziness, insomnia, and hepatotoxicity.

Cheese Reaction
- If the patients on MAOIs consume tyramine containing foods such as cheese, beer, red wines, pickled meat and fish, yeast extract, butter milk, over-ripe banana, stale food, avocados, figs, soy sauce, salami, sausage, etc., they develop severe hypertension known as Cheese reaction.
- Tyramine is normally metabolized by MAO in the gut wall and liver. On inhibition of MAO by MAOIs, tyramine escapes metabolism and displaces large amounts of NE from transmitter loaded adrenergic nerve endings.
- This reaction can lead to hypertensive crisis and cerebrovascular accidents.
- The treatment of this reaction is done by IV injection of a rapidly acting α-blocker, e.g., phentolamine, prazosin or chlorpromazines are alternatives.

ATYPICAL ANTIDEPRESSANTS

(Trazodone, Mianserin, Mirtazapine, Bupropion, Tianeptine, Amineptine, Atomoxetine)

Drug antidepressants are given in Table 9.77

TABLE 9.77: Typical antidepressants drugs profile

Drugs	Dose (mg/day)	Special features
Trazodone	100–300	• It has prominent α adrenergic and weak $5HT_2$ antagonistic action • It is short-acting, well tolerated and safe even in over dosages • Suited for the elderly as arrhythmia incidence is less • Useful in obsessive compulsive disorder due to mild anxiolytic effect • Nausea at beginning of therapy, priapism and impotence are major side effects
Mianserin	30–100	• It blocks pre-synaptic α 2 receptors and increases the release and turnover of norepinephrine in brain • Relieves anxiety and suppresses panic attacks due to sedative actions • Major side effects are liver dysfunction and blood dyscrasias
Mirtazapine	15–45, OD at bed time	• It blocks α 2 as well as H_1 receptor blocker • It is sedative drug but without anticholinergic or antidopaminergic effects • Efficacious in mild as well as severe depression and insomnia • Increased appetite and weight gain are some of the side effects • No sexual dysfunction occurs with its use
Bupropion	150–300	• It is inhibitor of dopamine and norepinephrine uptake and has excitant property • Used for smoking cessation • It is contraindicated in eating disorders and in bipolar illness

Contd...

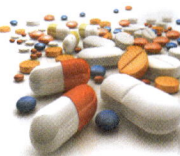

Drugs	Dose (mg/day)	Special features
Tianeptine	12.5–40	• It increases the 5-HT uptake, and is neither sedative nor stimulant • It is effective in anxiodepressive states, particularly with psychosomatic symptoms, as well as in endogenous depression • Side effects are dry mouth, epigastric pain, flatulence, drowsiness, insomnia, tremors and bodyache
Amineptine	200	• It enhances 5-HT uptake like tianeptine • It has antidepressant properties • The side effects are tachycardia, confusion and delirium
Atomoxetine	40–100	• It is selective norepinephrine reuptake inhibitor • It is approved only for treatment of attention deficit hyperactivity disorder

COMMON USES OF ANTIDEPRESSANTS

- **Endogenous depression**
  - The SSRIs are currently used as first choice. SNRIs and newer atypical agents also used.
  - The TCAs are mostly used as alternatives in non-responsive cases.
  - Electro-convulsive-thera (ECT) is given in the patient with severe depression.
- **Panic attacks and anxiety disorders:** SSRIs are preferred.
- **Obsessive-compulsive disorders (OCDs):** The SSRIs are the most preferred agents along with psychotherapy.
- **Neuropathic pain:** SNRI (duloxetine), is now a first line drug for diabetic neuropathy, fibromyalgia. Other drugs such as pregabalin or gabapentin are also useful.
- **Attention deficit-hyperactivity disorder (ADHD) in children**: TCAs such as imipramine, nortriptyline and amoxapine used as first-line therapy.
- **Premature ejaculation:** Depoxetine is used.
- **Enuresis:** Imipramine in a dose of 25 mg is used at bedtime.

DRUG THERAPY FOR ANXIETY

Common drugs used for treatment of anxiety given in Table 9.78.

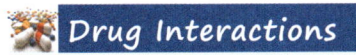

Drug Interactions

☞ **Antidepressants**
☞ TCAs potentiate the effect of nearly all CNS depressants such as antihistaminics and alcohol.
- ☞ Some drugs (such as aspirin, phenylbutazone, phenytoin) displace tricyclic antidepressant from their protein binding sites and produce toxicity.
- ☞ Carbamazepine, phenobarbitone and other enzyme inducers increase the metabolism of TCAs and decrease their effects.
- ☞ SSRIs and TCAs should not be given together as dangerous toxicity may be seen.
- ☞ Concurrent use of MAO inhibitors with TCAs can produce hypertensive crisis with excitement and hallucinations.

TABLE 9.78: Drug therapy for anxiety

A. Benzodiazepines	
Drugs	**Doses (As daily regimen)**
Alprazolam	0.5 mg
Chlordiazepoxide	10–20 mg
Clonazepam	1–2 mg
Clorazepate	15–30 mg
Diazepam	5–15 mg
Lorazepam	2–4 mg
Oxazepam	10–30 mg
B. Miscellaneous	
Buspirone	10–30 mg
Phenobarbital	15–30 mg

CENTRAL NERVOUS SYSTEM STIMULANTS

- Central nervous system stimulants are the drugs, which have predominantly stimulant effects on the central nervous system.
- These drugs can produce convulsions if given in higher doses.
- Psychomotor stimulants and hallucinogens are two groups of drugs that act primarily to stimulate the CNS.
- The psychomotor stimulants cause excitement and euphoria, decrease feelings of fatigue, and increase motor activity.
- The hallucinogens produce profound changes in thought patterns and mood, with little effect on the brainstem and spinal cord.
- Table 9.79 gives the classification of CNS stimulants

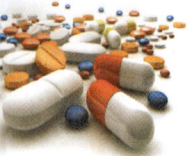

TABLE 9.79: Classification of CNS stimulants according to their site of action

Drugs that direct acting on the CNS	
Class	**Drugs**
Cortical or psychomotor stimulants	Xanthine alkaloids (theophylline, caffeine, theobromine), amphetamine, methylamphetamine, methylphenidate, modafinil.
Medullary or respiratory stimulants	Nikethamide, doxapram.
Spinal stimulants or convulsants	Strychnine, picrotoxin, pentylenetetrazol (PTZ)
Drugs that stimulate CNS reflexly	

Lobeline, Ammonia, Veratrum and Nicotine.

CORTICAL OR PSYCHOMOTOR STIMULANTS

Xanthine Alkaloids (Theophylline, Caffeine, Theobromine)

- The beverages such as tea contains theophylline, coffee contains caffeine and cocoa contains caffeine and theobromine.
- These alkaloids produce a sense of well-being and increase the mental alertness.
- Caffeine also stimulates the respiratory center.
- Methylxanthines increase the myocardial contractility, heart rate, urinary output and power of muscle contraction.
- These are well absorbed orally and metabolized in liver.
- These are mainly used in migraine, headache, bronchial asthma and apnea in premature infants.

Amphetamine and Methylamphetamine

These are sympathomimetic drugs having central actions more than peripheral actions.

Methylphenidate

- It is similar to amphetamine and acts by releasing norepinephrine (NE) and dopamine (DA).
- It is useful in attention deficit hyperkinetic disorders in a dose of 0.25 mg/kg/day up to a maximum of 1mg/kg/day.
- It is also used in narcolepsy and in poor concentration in adults in a dose of 5–10 mg BD.

Modafinil

- It is useful drug in the treatment of narcolepsy.
- It increases the attention span.

MEDULLARY OR RESPIRATORY STIMULANTS

(Nikethamide, Doxapram)

- These are respiratory stimulants and useful in resuscitation.
- Situations in which they may be employed are:
  - As an expedient measure in hypnotic drug poisoning until mechanical ventilation is instituted.

- Suffocation on drowning, acute respiratory insufficiency.
- Apnea in premature infant.
- Failure to ventilate spontaneously after general anesthesia. However, the overall utility of analeptics is dubious.

SPINAL STIMULANTS OR CONVULSANTS

(Strychnine, Picrotoxin, Pentylenetetrazol)

- **Strychnine** is a potent spinal convulsant as it causes stimulation of whole cerebrospinal axis and causes tonic-clonic and symmetrical convulsions. It is not clinically used nowadays.
- **Picrotoxin** is also a potent convulsant and does not have any therapeutic use.
- **Pentylenetetrazol** is also a potent CNS stimulant and used in laboratory animals to check the anticonvulsant effects of newer drugs.

Cerebroactive Drugs or Cognition Enhancer Drugs
- This group of drugs are useful in the treatment of memory related disorders such as dementia, Alzheimer's disease, mental retardation in children, organic psychosyndrome and following stroke and other cerebrovascular accidents.

- The various drugs used for these disorders act by providing direct support to neurons or enhancing neurotransmission or by increasing the cerebral blood flow and improve the cerebral functions.
- The commonly used drugs are:
  - Rivastigmine
  - Donepezil
  - Galantamine
  - Memantine
  - Piracetam
  - Citicoline
  - Ginkgo-biloba

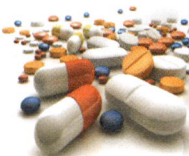

MOOD STABILIZERS

- Mood stabilizers are the drugs that are used to control the mood swings. Mood swings are often seen in **bipolar mood disorder**. These drugs are also known as **anti-maniac drugs**.
- Bipolar disorder is a psychiatric illness, which is characterized by a period of depression followed by a period of mania.
- The cause of mania is not understood, but it is thought to be due to overstimulation of certain neurons in the brain that manifests as hyperactivity, agitation, uncontrolled thought and speech disorder, etc.
- The mainstay for treatment of mania has always been lithium.
- Nowadays, many other drugs are also used for the treatment of bipolar disorders, which include antipsychotic drugs such as aripiprazole, olanzapine, quetiapine, ziprasidone (described in antipsychotics) and antiepileptic drugs such as lamotrigine (described in antiepileptics).

Lithium

- Lithium was first used in patients with gout in 19th century.
- In 1949, Cade discovered that lithium was an effective treatment for bipolar disorders.
- It reduces episodes and phases of maniac-depressive disorder by reduction of mood swings, motor activity of brain, euphoria and insomnia.

Mechanism of Action

- The exact mechanism is still unknown. It is a monovalent cation which mimics the role of sodium ions at many sites.
- The proposed hypothesis is as follows:
  - Lithium competes and replaces sodium at many sites including neurons. It alters sodium transport in nerve and muscle cells and results in mood stabilizing effects.
  - It also inhibits the release of norepinephrine and dopamine, but not serotonin, from stimulated neurons.
  - It increases the intraneuronal stores of norepinephrine and dopamine slightly; and decreases intraneuronal content of second messengers.
  - It selectively modulates the responsiveness of hyperactive neurons that might contribute to the manic state.

Pharmacokinetics

- The oral absorption of lithium is virtually complete within 6–8 hours.
- It is not metabolized in the body and handled by the kidneys in the same way as sodium ions.
- Lithium is excreted from the kidneys within 10–12 hours, although about 80% is reabsorbed.
- The plasma t½ is 20 hours.
- It slowly crosses the bloodbrain barrier. It also crosses the placenta and enters breast milk; hence contraindicated in pregnancy and lactation.
- Sodium depletion reduces the rate of excretion of lithium, thus increases the lithium toxicity. Therefore, patients must be encouraged to maintain hydration while taking this drug.
- It has low therapeutic index; therefore, continuous monitoring (by salivary concentration of lithium) is required for optimal therapy.

Dose

Initial dose: 600 mg/day followed by 600–1200 mg/day till the optimal therapeutic concentration achieved.

The therapeutically effective serum level is 0.6–1.2 mEq/L (0.5–1.5 mmol/L).

Indications

- Prophylaxis for bipolar disorder.
- Acute mania.
- Chemotherapy induced leucopenia.
- Syndrome of inappropriate anti-diuretic hormone (SIADH).
- Cluster headache.

Adverse Effects

The side effects of lithium are directly associated with the serum levels of drug.

- **Serum levels of <1.5 mEq/L:** CNS problems, including lethargy, slurred speech, muscle weakness, and fine tremor; polyuria, which relates to renal toxicity; and beginning of gastric toxicity, with nausea, vomiting, and diarrhea.
- **Serum levels of 1.5–2 mEq/L:** Intensification of all of the foregoing reactions, with electrocardiogram (ECG) changes.
- **Serum levels of 2–2.5 mEq/L:** Possible progression of CNS effects to ataxia, clonic movements, hyperreflexia, and seizures; possible cardiovascular effects such as severe ECG changes and hypotension; large output of dilute urine secondary to renal toxicity; fatalities secondary to pulmonary toxicity.
- **Serum levels >2.5 mEq/L:** Complex multi-organ toxicity, with a significant risk of death.
- Other side effects include hypothyroidism, weight gain, and diabetes insipidus.

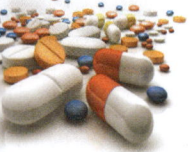

Management of Lithium Overdose

- Lithium should be stopped immediately.
- The serum level of lithium should be monitored regularly.
- IV administration of normal saline restores sodium levels and promotes lithium excretion.
- IV infusion of mannitol increases lithium excretion.
- If serum level is >4 mEq/L; hemodialysis is required.
- Other diuretics, which increase sodium loss can cause the reabsorption of lithium from the kidney tubules and enhance the toxicity; hence, contraindicated.

 Nursing Implications

☞ **Mood stabilizers**
- ☞ Nurse should teach the relatives of the epileptic patient to note the frequency of attack and spot management of convulsions.
- ☞ Establish safety precautions, including side rails, lighting, and noise control for the patients of convulsion admitted indoors.
- ☞ Nurse should also stress upon the importance of completion of antiepileptic treatment and warn against the sudden stoppage of drugs.
- ☞ Evaluate effectiveness of the teaching plan (patient can give the drug name and dosage, name possible adverse effects to watch for and specific measures to help avoid adverse effects, and describe the need for follow-up and evaluation).

Assess Yourself

Long and Short Answer Questions

1. What are NSAIDs? Describe mode of action, contraindications and uses of aspirin.
2. What are benzodiazepines? Describe alprazolam and its uses.
3. Describe the role of nurses in the management of opioid toxicity.
4. Describe the stages of general anesthesia.
5. Classify inhalational anesthetics and describe sevoflurane.
6. Describe the therapeutic uses of oxygen therapy.
7. Classify the anticholinesterase drugs. Write their clinical uses.
8. Describe the management of organophosphate poisoning.
9. Describe the management of belladonna poisoning.
10. Describe the mechanism of cheese reaction and its management.
11. Describe treatment and management of status epilepticus.
12. Why adrenaline is used with lignocaine in local anesthetic preparation?
13. Describe the therapeutic use of dopamine/dobutamine.
14. Write short notes on:
    a. Antipyretics
    b. Hypnotics
    c. Opioids analgesics
    d. Lignocaine
    e. Propofol
    f. Thiopentone sodium
    g. Ketamine
    h. Diazepam
    i. Phenytoin
    j. Succinylcholine
    k. Indication and adverse effect of anticholinergic drugs
    l. Antipsychotics
    m. Lithium
    n. Management of migraine

Multiple Choice Questions

1. **Drug of choice for myoclonic seizures:**
   a. Vigabatrin
   b. Phenytoin
   c. Valporate
   d. Carbamazepine

2. **Fosphenytoin is given:**
   a. Oral
   b. IM
   c. IV
   d. SC

Contd...

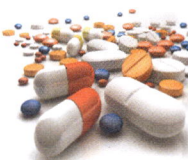

3. **IV diazepam has which of the following effect which is not seen by other routes:**
   a. Analgesia
   b. Diazepam
   c. Hypotension
   d. Coronary dilatation

4. **Buprenorphine is:**
   a. Partial agonist at µ receptor
   b. Partial agonist at k receptor
   c. Full agonist at µ receptor
   d. Full agonist at κ receptor

5. **Naltrexone is used in opioid dependence:**
   a. To treat withdrawal symptoms
   b. To prevent relapse
   c. To treat overdose
   d. For opioid rotation therapy

6. **Dextromethorphan should not be given with which drug?**
   a. SSRIs
   b. MAO inhibitors
   c. Atropine
   d. Paracetamol

Answer Key

| 1. | c. | 2. | c. | 3. | d. | 4. | a. | 5. | b. | 6. | b. |

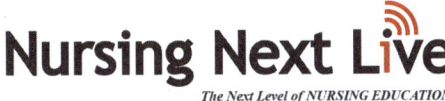

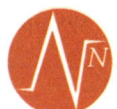

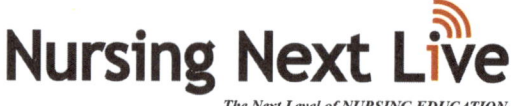

Nursing Next Live
The Next Level of NURSING EDUCATION

PREPARE ANYTIME, ANYWHERE FOR
Nursing Officer/Staff Nurse/CHO/ Nursing Undergraduate & Postgraduate Exams

AIIMS NORCET 2020

Rank **3**

Rahul Dahiya
Roll No. 9016060

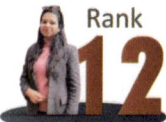

Rank **12**

Nisha Singla
Roll No. 9101820

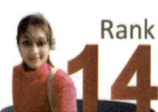

Rank **14**

Arushi Mittal
Roll No. 9079646

Rank **51**

Komal Dhull
Roll No. 9024458

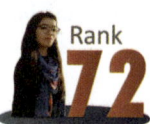

Rank **72**

Shivani Bourai
Roll No. 9092877

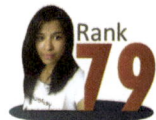

Rank **79**

Nivedita Saini
Roll No. 9004587

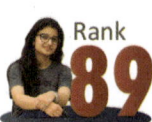

Rank **89**

Rupali Garg
Roll No. 9054544

CHO 2020

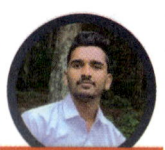

Suresh Kumsr
Rank- 1
Roll No. 12090
MP

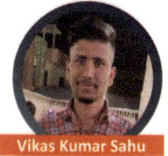

Vikas Kumar Sahu
Rank- 14
Roll No. 10011
MP

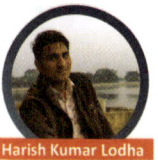

Harish Kumar Lodha
Rank- 18
Roll No. 7930
MP

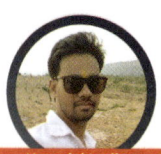

Heeralal Lodha
Rank- 33
Roll No. 10009
MP

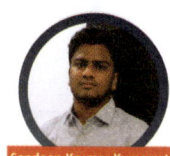

Sandeep Krumar Kumawat
Rank- 44
Roll No. 12585
MP

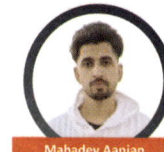

Mahadev Aanjan
Rank- 50
Roll No. 10130
MP

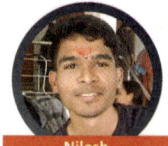

Nilesh
Rank- 81
Roll No. 10572
MP

BFUHS 2021

Rank **1**

Harjeet Singh
Roll No- 472478

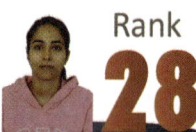

Rank **28**

Kuljit Kaur
Roll No. 473956

Rank **32**

Karan Sharma
Roll No. 469134

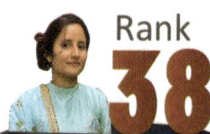

Rank **38**

Smriti Rana
Roll No. 463342

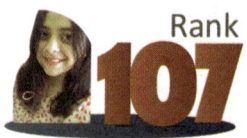

Rank **107**

Harpreet Kaur
Roll No. 474125

AIIMS MSc ENTRANCE EXAM 2021

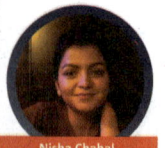

Nisha Chahal
AIIMS AIR-18

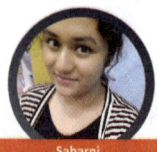

Sabarni
AIIMS AIR-21

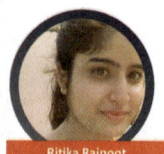

Ritika Rajpoot
AIIMS AIR-23

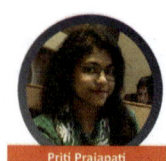

Priti Prajapati
AIIMS AIR-39

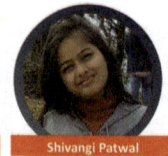

Shivangi Patwal
AIIMS AIR-64

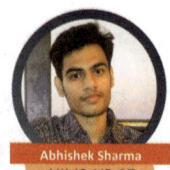

Abhishek Sharma
AIIMS AIR-97

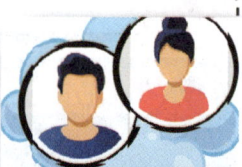

You Will Be The Next...

Follow us:

CALL US +91- 999-911-7411
www.nursingnextlive.com

Scan the QR Code
to download the app

Cardiovascular Drugs

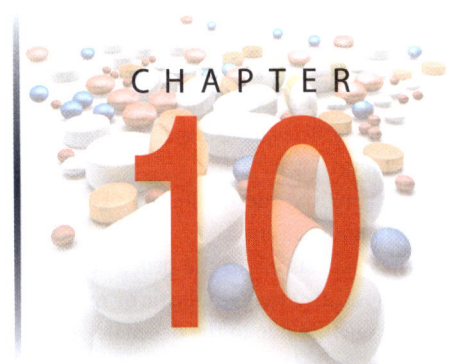

10

 CHAPTER OUTLINE

HEMATINICS

- Hematinics are the nutrients/compounds, which are required for the synthesis of blood cells in the process of hematopoiesis.
- Major hematinics are:
  - **Iron**
  - **Folic acid or vitamin B$_9$**
  - **Vitamin B$_{12}$**
- All the above-mentioned hematinics are essential for normal hematopoiesis process.
- Clinically, hematinics are used for the prevention and treatment of anemias.

- **Anemia** occurs due to imbalance between the rate of destruction and production of RBCs. There are many causes and varieties of anemias.
- **The various causes of anemia are:**
  - **Decreased RBCs production** due to deficiency of iron, folic acid and vitamin B$_{12}$.
  - **Increased RBCs destruction** due to hemolytic anemia and sickle cell anemia.
  - **Acute/chronic blood loss** due to GI bleeding and worm infestations.
  - **Anemia due to chronic systemic diseases** such as chronic inflammatory diseases and autoimmune diseases.

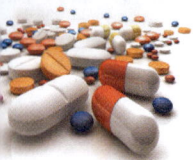

- ▪ **Anemia due to adverse effects of various drugs** such as cancer chemotherapy and radiotherapy.
    - ▪ **There are still many more causes of anemia**.
- The hematinics are prescribed invariably in all types of anemias. They have a specific site of action which is shown in Figure 10.1.
- The anemia due to the deficiency of iron is called **iron deficiency anemia**.
- The anemia due to the deficiency of vitamin B$_{12}$ and folic acid is called **megaloblastic or macrocytic anemia**.
- The anemia due to the deficiency of both iron and vitamin B$_{12}$ is called **dimorphic anemia**, in which RBCs of two different morphologies are seen in the blood.

IRON

- Iron is essential for the production of hemoglobin, which is the oxygen-carrying component of RBCs.
- Iron is an important constituent of *hemoglobin, ferritin, myoglobin, cytochromes* and *other enzymes*.
- The total body iron content is about 3.5–4 g in adult male and about 2.5 g in adult females, out of which 70% iron is present in **hemoglobin**.
- Fifteen to twenty percent of iron is stored in **liver, spleen** and **bone marrow**.
- Ten to fifteen percent of iron is present in **myoglobin, cytochromes** and **other enzymes**.

Dietary Sources

Liver, egg yolk, meat, fish, chicken, spinach, jaggery, dry fruits, wheat germ, apple, banana, pulses, root vegetables, etc. Milk and milk products are poor sources of iron.

Daily Requirement of Iron

- Adult male: 0.5–1 mg of iron
- Adult female: 1–2 mg (non-pregnant)
- 3–5 mg (pregnancy and lactation)
- Children: 25 µg/kg of iron

Pharmacokinetics

- Only 10% of dietary iron is absorbed.
- The iron is absorbed in ferrous form (Fe^{2+}) whereas the dietary iron exists in ferric form (Fe^{3+}).
- The ferric form needs to be converted to ferrous form before absorption. The heme form of dietary iron (from non-vegetarian sources) is in the form of ferrous ions and absorbed better than the inorganic ferric (Fe^{3+}) form of iron (from vegetarian sources).
- The maximum absorption of iron takes place in the duodenum and upper jejunum.
- The iron absorption is better in the presence of reducing substances such as vitamin C, amino acids, acidic pH of stomach as these substances facilitate the conversion of ferric to absorbable ferrous form.

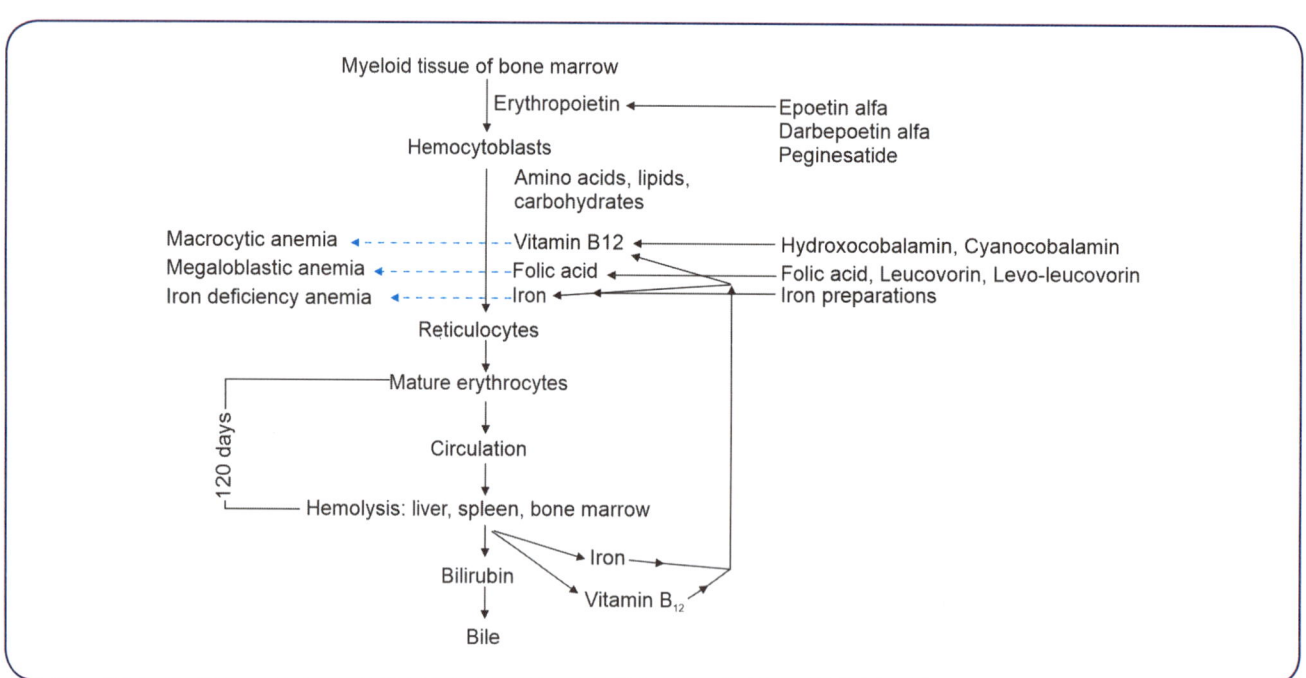

FIG. 10.1: Sites of action of hematinics

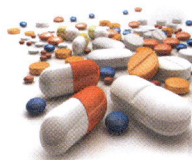

- The iron absorption is decreased by excess of phosphates (in egg yolk), phytates (in wheat and maize), food in stomach, alkaline pH of stomach, antacids and tetracyclines as these substances form insoluble complexes with iron, and render iron unabsorbable.

Preparations of Iron

Iron is available both in oral and parenteral forms.

Oral Preparations of Iron

- Following are the oral preparations:
  - **Ferrous sulfate** (contains 20% of iron) is the oldest and most economical form of iron. It is available commercially as well as in government supplies for prevention as well as therapeutic purpose. Metallic taste in mouth is a disadvantage with this form of iron.
  - **Ferrous gluconate** (contains 12% of iron) has better gastric tolerance.
  - **Ferrous fumarate** (contains 33% of iron) is tasteless form of iron.
  - **Colloidal ferric hydroxide** (contains 50% of iron)
  - **Ferrous succinate** (contains 35% of iron)
  - **Ferric ammonium citrate** (contains 20% of iron)
  - **Carbonyl iron** has better gastric tolerance due to micro-fine powder form.
  - **Iron choline citrate**
  - **Ferric hydroxy polymaltose.**
- Oral forms of iron cause gastric irritation and constipation, which depends upon the iron content of preparation.
- The gastric tolerance is better with latest formulations.
- Liquid formulations of iron may stain the teeth. For the prevention of this, smaller doses of iron are advocated in between the meals.
- The oral administration of iron is indicated for long-term treatment of iron deficiency.
- The long-term treatment should be such that it should recover deficiency state as well as replenish the iron stores.

Parenteral Preparations of Iron

- Parenteral iron releases inorganic ferric form of iron. The preparations in use are:
  - **Iron-dextran:** It is a colloidal solution, which can be given both by IM and IV route.
  - **Iron-sorbitol citric acid:** It can be given only by IM route.
  - **Ferrous sucrose:** It can be given only by IM route with less antigenicity than iron-dextran.

- **Ferric carboxymaltose:** This is the recently introduced form of iron having very low incidence of anaphylactic reactions.
- **The parenteral route of administering iron is indicated in following conditions:**
  - When oral iron is not tolerated by patients
  - Malabsorption and intestinal disorders
  - Poor compliance to oral iron
  - When fast replenishment of iron stores is required
  - Post-gastrectomy patients.

The total iron requirement is calculated by the following formula:
Iron requirement (mg) = 4.4 × body weight (kg) × Hb deficit (g/dL)

Once the total iron requirement has been calculated it can be administered either by IM or by IV route by following special procedure as follows:

- **Intramuscular therapy:** Iron-dextran in a dose of 100 mg/day or on alternate days can be given. It is given deep intramuscularly in the gluteal region using 'Z' technique to avoid discoloration of skin.
- **Intravenous therapy:** Iron-dextran complex is administered after performing a sensitivity test. The total calculated dose is diluted in 500 mL of normal saline or glucose and infused intravenously over a period of 6–8 hours keeping a vigil on any adverse reaction. The risk of anaphylactic reaction is less with ferric carboxymaltose and ferric sucrose.

Indications of Iron

- To treat iron-deficiency anemia in nutritional iron deficiency, during pregnancy, due to blood loss and poor iron absorption from gut.
- For prophylaxis of iron deficiency anemia in pregnancy, lactation, chronic illnesses and blood loss.

Adverse Reactions of Iron

Oral iron therapy has following side effects:

Epigastric pain, nausea, vomiting, metallic taste in mouth, abdominal colic, constipation or diarrhea and staining of teeth with liquid preparations.

Parenteral iron therapy can have both local and systemic side effects as follows:

- **Local:** Pain at the site of injection, pigmentation of skin and formation of sterile abscess at the injection site.
- **Systemic:** Headache, nausea, vomiting, urticaria, fever, lymphnode enlargement, joints pain, and rarely anaphylactic reaction.

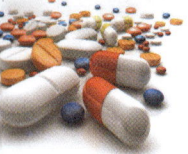

Iron Poisoning

It is common in infants and children and occurs due to accidental ingestion of large number of iron tablets.

It is manifested as nausea, vomiting, epigastric pain, bloody diarrhea, hematemesis, dehydration, convulsions and cardiovascular collapse.

Diagnosis and immediate treatment is nessesary as death may occur within 6–12 hours.

Treatment

- Gastric lavage with sodium bicarbonate solution and administration of milk or egg yolk. (*It makes iron complexes and render it unabsorbable.*)
- **Desferrioxamine** is given by IM/IV route, which acts as an antidote and reduces serum iron levels by helping early excretion of iron.
- Other iron chelating agents are **deferiprone** and **deferasirox**. These are given by oral route and given in chronic iron overload cases.
- General supportive measures should be instituted simultaneously.

FOLIC ACID AND VITAMIN-B$_{12}$

- These vitamins are essentially required for the maturation of the RBCs in the bone marrow; hence also known as maturation factors.
- The deficiency of these vitamins causes maturation defects in RBCs. The large size RBCs are seen in peripheral blood smear. The condition is known as megaloblastic anemia.
- The details have been described in chapter vitamins and minerals.

ERYTHROPOIESIS-STIMULATING AGENTS

- Erythropoiesis stimulating agents are beneficial for the patients who are no longer able to produce enough erythropoietin in the kidneys.
- Erythropoietin is essential for erythropoiesis and is produced naturally in the body by peritubular cells of the kidneys and act on erythropoietin-receptors in the bone marrow and stimulate red cell production.
- Erythropoiesis stimulating agents are recombinant human erythropoietin such as Epoetin alfa and Darbepoetin alfa, which are nearly identical to the endogenous erythropoietin. These are non-immunogenic in nature.
- Adequate supplementation of hematinics is mandatory along with these agents.
- **Epoetin alfa** is given thrice weekly in a dose of 25–100 units/kg by IV/SC route.
- **Darbepoetin alfa** is a modified recombinant human erythropoietin with longer half life and similar pharmacological properties and indications. It can be given

once weekly or once every 2–4 weeks depending upon the indication. It is given in a dose of 0.45 mcg/kg, IV/SC once per week, and 2.25 mcg/kg/wk, SC (with chemotherapy).

Indications

- Anemia associated with chronic renal failure and patients on dialysis.
- Anemia associated with AIDS therapy.
- Anemia associated with cancer chemotherapy.
- Aplastic anemia.
- Multiple myeloma.
- *It should not be used to treat other anemias and is not a replacement for whole blood in the emergency treatment of anemia.*

Adverse Reactions

- Increased risk of clot formation (most commonly seen with patients on dialysis).
- Increased risk of thromboembolism.
- Hypertension.
- Flu-like symptoms.
- Seizures (rare).

Drug Interactions

- Iron is better absorbed in the presence of reducing substances such as ascorbic acid (vit-C). These substances convert the ferric form of iron to ferrous form and make it more absorbable. Hence, concurrent administration of vitamin-C should be done for better absorption of inorganic iron.
- The absorption of iron is decreased in the presence of alkalies, phosphates, phytates, food and drugs such as tetracyclines. Hence, concurrent consumption of these items should be avoided

Nursing Implications

- **Hematinics**
  - Assess for contraindications or cautions and any known allergies to the drug to be administered to avoid hypersensitivity reactions.
  - Ensure that iron deficiency anemia is confirmed before administering drugs to ensure proper use of the drug.
  - Administer the oral form of iron with meals that do not include eggs, milk, coffee, and tea to prevent GI irritation.
  - Nurse should educate the patient, to take iron with citrus juices to enhance its absorption.
  - Patient should be educated regarding good dietary habits and importance of taking balanced diet.
  - Take measures to help alleviate constipation to prevent discomfort and the adverse effects of severe constipation.
  - IV infusion of iron should be given slowly to prevent hypersensitivity.

Contd...

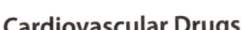

Nursing Implications

☞ Administer iron intramuscularly only by Z-track technique to ensure proper administration and to avoid brown staining of the tissues. Warn the patient that the injection can be painful.

☞ Monitor for adverse effects (GI upset and reaction, CNS toxicity, coma).

CARDIOTONICS

- Cardiotonic agents are the drugs, which increase the contractility of the cardiac muscles.
- These drugs are most commonly used in patients suffering from heart failure (HF).
- HF is a clinical condition in which the heart is unable to maintain effective circulation due to the failure in pumping action.
- The cardiac cycle normally involves a balance between the pumping of the right and left sides of the heart.
- Due to failure in pumping action of heart, pooling of blood occurs, which causes congestion of blood vessels of various body tissues and appearance of pedal and pulmonary edema.
- The congested body tissues become deprived of oxygen and nutrients leading to various systemic symptoms.
- The cardiotonic agents help the heart muscles to contract more efficiently to restore the normal circulation.

CARDIOTONIC AGENTS

- Cardiotonic agents are also known as inotropic drugs.
- These drugs increase the contractile strength of the heart and cardiac output without increase in the myocardial oxygen demand.
- Sympathomimetic drugs such as adrenaline, etc. are not cardiotonic agents, but they are cardiac stimulants: (*These drugs increase the cardiac contractility, but also increase the myocardial oxygen demand; overall, cardiac efficiency is decreased.*)
- **The cardiotonic drugs are of two types:**
  - Classic cardiac glycosides: **Digoxin, Digitoxin, Ouabain**.
  - Newer phosphodiesterase-3 inhibitors: **Inamrinone, Milrinone, Levosimendan, Enoximone**.

CARDIAC GLYCOSIDES

(Digoxin, Digitoxin, Ouabain)

The cardiac glycosides were obtained from the foxglove or digitalis plant.

Clinically, digoxin is the only cardiac glycoside in use and is obtained from *Digitalis lanata*.

Digitoxin and Ouabain are not in use these days.

Mechanism of Action

- Digoxin inhibits the Na⁺K⁺ATPase present on the cardiac cell membrane. This results in increase of intracellular calcium ions and triggers the contractile mechanism of failing heart.
- This increases the force of myocardial contraction producing a positive inotropic effect.
- This produces following effects in addition:
  - Increased cardiac output.
  - Improved renal perfusion occurs, which produces diuretic effect and decreases the renin release.
  - The heart rate is decreased due to slowing of the rate of cellular repolarization. This produces a negative chronotropic effect.
  - The conduction velocity through the atrioventricular (AV) node is also decreased.
  - The higher doses of digoxin can produce CNS effects in the form of nausea, vomiting, increased respiration rate, mental confusion and disorientation.

Pharmacokinetics

- Digoxin can be given by both oral and parenteral routes.
- The oral absorption is good (60–80%).
- It has a rapid onset of action within 30–120 minutes (orally) and 5–30 minutes when given intravenously.
- It is widely distributed throughout the body and gets concentrated in heart, skeletal muscles, liver and kidney.
- The plasma t½ is 40 hours.
- It is primarily excreted unchanged in the urine and precautions should be taken in the patients of renal impairment as the drug may accumulate due to poor excretion and toxicity may occur.
- **Dose:** As digoxin accumulates in the body and produces toxic effects, sometimes the treatment is started with maintenance doses and therapeutic effect is produced after 6–7 days, when steady state levels are attained. The loading dose is 0.75–1.25 mg orally or 0.125–0.25 mg IV, followed by the maintenance dose of 0.125–0.25 mg/day, orally.

Indications

- Congestive heart failure
- Atrial flutter and atrial fibrillations
- Paroxysmal atrial tachycardia.

Adverse Effects

Cardiac glycoside has low safety margin due to narrow therapeutic index (1.3–2).

The adverse effects are of two types.

- **Extra-cardiac**
  - GIT: Anorexia, nausea, vomiting, abdominal cramps, diarrhea.

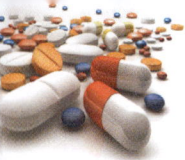

- **CNS:** Headache, drowsiness, vision changes (a yellow halo around objects is seen), restlessness, etc.
- **Endocrine:** Gynecomastia in males.

Management of these adverse effects is done by reducing the dose of digoxin.

- **Cardiac:** Many types of arrhythmias (literally all types) can be produced by digoxin. Some of these are pulsus bigeminus, ventricular tachycardia and bradycardia, ventricular extra systoles, A-V block, atrial flutter, atrial fibrillations and ventricular fibrillations.

Management of cardiac adverse effects is done in following ways:

- Stop digoxin immediately.
- Stop diuretics, if being given concurrently.
- Measure plasma potassium levels and if low start KCl infusion.
- For supraventricular arrhythmias, IV propranolol is given.
- For ventricular arrhythmia, IV lidocaine is given.
- For bradycardia and A-V block, IM/IV atropine is given.
- In severe digoxin toxicity, IV infusion of anti-digoxin specific antibody (digoxin-Fab) is given.

Contraindications

- In the presence of allergy
- Ventricular tachycardia or fibrillations
- Heart block or sick sinus syndrome
- Idiopathic hypertrophic subaortic stenosis (IHSS)
- Acute MI
- Hypokalemia
- Pregnant or lactating mother (*teratogenicity and secretion in breast milk occurs*). It should be given during pregnancy only if the benefit to the mother clearly outweighs the risk to the fetus.

PHOSPHODIESTERASE-3 INHIBITORS

(Inamrinone, Milrinone, Levosimendan, Enoximone)
Phosphodiesterase-3 inhibitors act as cardiotonic (inotropic) agents.

Mechanism of Action

- These drugs specifically block phosphodiesterase-3 isoenzyme (PDE-3).
- PDE-3 isoenzyme degrades cyclic adenosine monophosphate (cAMP) in heart, blood vessels and bronchial smooth muscles.
- Blockade of PDE-3 leads to an increase in myocardial cell cAMP, which increases calcium levels in the myocardial cells. It triggers the myocardial contraction and improves cardiac output.

- These drugs are indicated for the short-term management of heart failure in non-responsive patients or those having poor response to other drugs.

Pharmacokinetics

- These are given only by intravenous route.
- Milrinone is more potent, selective for PDE-3 and short lasting with fewer side effects as compared to inamrinone.
- They are metabolized in the liver and excreted primarily in the urine.

Dosage Schedule

Inamrinone

- Loading dose: 0.5 mg/kg IV bolus
- Maintenance dose: 5–10 µg/kg/min IV infusion (max. 10 mg/kg in 24 hours).

Milrinone

- Loading dose: 50 mcg/kg IV bolus over 10 minutes.
- Maintenance dose: 0.375–0.75 mcg/kg/min IV infusion.

Indications

Short-term management of severe heart failure or heart failure refractory to other treatments.

Adverse Effects

- GIT: Nausea, vomiting, anorexia, and abdominal pain.
- CVS: Ventricular arrhythmias, hypotension, and chest pain.
- Blood: Thrombocytopenia occurs frequently with inamrinone and rarely with milrinone.
- Hypersensitivity reactions such as vasculitis, pleuritis, pericarditis and ascites.

Drug Interactions

- Concurrent use of digitalis with diuretics increases the risk of digitalis toxicity (arrhythmias) due to hypokalemia; hence, prophylactically, K+ supplements should be given.
- Calcium supplements precipitate digitalis toxicity. Hence, concurrent use should be avoided.
- Concurrent use of digitalis with adrenergic drugs increases the risk of cardiac arrhythmias as both increase the ectopic automaticity.
- Metoclopramide and antacids decrease the absorption of digoxin.
- Tricyclic antidepressants and atropine increase the absorption of digoxin.

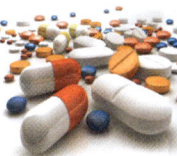

Nursing Implications

☞ **Cardiotonics**

☞ Assess for contraindications or cautions and known allergies to any digitalis or phosphodiesterase inhibitors to avoid hypersensitivity reactions.

☞ Monitor apical pulse for 1 full minute before administering the drug to monitor for adverse effects. Check for bradycardia or tachycardia before administering digoxin.

☞ Check the dose and preparation carefully because digoxin has a very small margin of safety, and inadvertent drug errors can cause serious problems.

☞ Follow dilution instructions carefully for intravenous use; use promptly to avoid drug degradation.

☞ Administer intravenous doses very slowly over at least 5 minutes to avoid cardiac arrhythmias and adverse effects.

☞ Avoid intramuscular administration of digoxin, which could be quite painful.

☞ Monitoring for fluid retention and heart failure should be done by taking the weight of the patient in the same clothes at the same time each day. Assess dependent areas for edema and note the amount and degree of pitting to evaluate the severity of fluid retention.

☞ Maintain emergency equipment on standby: potassium salts, lidocaine (for treatment of arrhythmias), phenytoin (for treatment of seizures), atropine (to increase heart rate), and a cardiac monitor, in case severe toxicity should occur.

☞ Monitor for adverse effects of digoxin (vision changes, arrhythmias, heart failure, headache, dizziness, drowsiness, GI upset, and nausea).

ANTIANGINAL AGENTS

- The drugs, which are used for prophylactic or therapeutic treatment of angina pectoris, are called as antianginal drugs.
- The angina pectoris is manifested clinically in the form of severe suffocating pain in the chest usually in the substernal region.
- It occurs due to imbalance between oxygen requirement and oxygen supply in the ischemic area of myocardium. Basically, it is the '*cry of dying myocardial muscles for oxygen and nutrition*'.
- The antianginal drugs provide relief by either or both of the following mechanisms:
  - Increasing the supply of oxygen to myocardium by dilating the coronary blood vessels.
  - Decreasing the myocardial demand for oxygen by decreasing the work of the heart.
- Angina pectoris is of following types:
  - **Stable angina or classical angina or angina on effort:** The chest pain is commonly associated with exercise, emotions or meals. It occurs due to fixed atheromatous stenosis in the coronary vessels.
  - **Unstable angina:** Recurrent attack of angina, which occurs with minimal exertion or even at rest. Risk of impending MI is always there. It occurs due to progressive atheromatous narrowing of coronary vessels or due to rupture of plaque associated with vasospasm.
  - **Prinzmetal or variant angina:** Pain appears at rest and even during sleep and is not associated with exertion. It occurs due to localized coronary spasm.

On the basis of their use in acute and chronic case of angina pectoris, the antianginal drugs are classified as given in Table 10.1.

NITRATES

[Glyceryl trinitrate (GTN), Isosorbide dinitrate, Isosorbide mononitrate, Erythrityl tetranitrate, Pentaerythritol tetranitrate]

Both short and long acting nitrates have similar pharmacological actions, but the onset and duration of action differs. Nitrates act directly on smooth muscles and produce relaxation effect. All the nitrates are vasodilators. The dose and duration of action of individual drugs are given in Table 10.2.

Mechanism of Action

- The nitrates act as prodrugs and they are denitrated in the smooth muscles to their active form '*nitric oxide*' by certain enzymes. This nitric oxide is a potent vasodilator and produces both venodilatation as well as arteriodilatory effects.
- The **venodilatation** effects are more pronounced than the **arteriolar-dilatation**.
- The venodilatation causes blood to pool in veins and capillaries, thus decreasing preload.
- The relaxation effect on the arteries decreases the total peripheral resistance, thus decreasing the afterload.
- Therefore, they reduce both **preload** and **afterload**.
- This reduces the myocardial workload as well as myocardial oxygen demand and provide relief in the patients of angina.

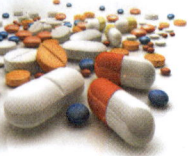

TABLE 10.1: Classification of anti-anginal drugs

Class of drugs	Drugs
For treatment of acute anginal attack	• **Nitrates (short acting):** Glyceryl trinitrate (GTN) • **Nitrates (long acting):** Isosorbide dinitrate(short acting by sublingual route)
For chronic prophylaxis of anginal attack	• **Nitrates** (*long acting):* Isosorbide dinitrate, Isosorbide mononitrate, Erythrityl tetranitrate, Pentaerythritol tetranitrate • **β Blockers:** Propranolol, Metoprolol, Atenolol and others. • **Calcium channel blockers** 　▪ *Phenyl alkylamine*: Verapamil 　▪ *Benzothiazepine*: Diltiazem 　▪ *Dihydropyridines:* Nifedipine, Felodipine, Amlodipine, Nitrendipine, Nimodipine, Lacidipine, Lercanidipine, Benidipine • **Potassium channel opener:** Nicorandil • **Others:** Dipyridamole, Trimetazidine, Ranolazine, Ivabradine,

TABLE 10.2: Individual anti anginal drugs, dose and their duration of action

Drugs	Dose	Time of Onset of action	Duration of action
GTN (Nitroglycerine)	0.5 mg sublingual 0.4–0.8 mg sublingual spray 5–15 mg oral One patch for 14–16 hr/day 5–20 µg/min IV	2–5 minutes 1–2 minutes 20–30 minutes 30–40 minutes 1–2 minutes	10–30 minutes 10–30 minutes 4–8 hours Till applied, max 24 hours Till infusion
Isosorbide dinitrate	5–10 mg sublingual 10–20 mg oral 20–40 mg oral	5–15 minutes 30–50 minutes 20–50 minutes	20–40 minutes 2–3 hours 6–10 hours
Isosorbide–5– mononitrate	20–40 mg oral	15–30 minutes	6–10 hours
Erythrityl–tetranitrate	15–60 mg oral	20–30 minutes	4–6 hours
Pentaerythritol– tetranitrate	10–40 mg oral 80 mg oral	30–40 minutes 30–40 minutes	3–5 hours 8–12 hours

- To summarize, the nitrates provide relief in anginal pain by following effects:
  - ▪ *Reduction in preload*
  - ▪ *Reduction in afterload*
  - ▪ *Coronary dilatation*.

The combination of these effects greatly reduces the cardiac workload and the demand for oxygen, thus bringing the supply and demand ratio back into balance.

Pharmacokinetics

- Nitrates are well absorbed by oral route but they undergo extensive first pass metabolism. Hence, the oral bioavailability of these drugs is very poor. The sublingual route is preferred in emergencies for early effects and better bioavailability.
- All the nitrates have good lipid solubility.
- Nitrates are available as oral, sublingual, spray form, parenteral, ointment and as transdermal patches.

Special Features

- **Nitroglycerine (GTN):** It is the most commonly used nitrate in emergencies. Sublingual tablets acts within

1–2 minutes whereas spray acts faster than tablets. IV infusion is helpful in reducing the myocardial infract size if instituted early.

- **Isosorbide dinitrate:** Also useful in emergencies. The onset of action is slower than GTN.
- **Isosorbide-5-mononitrate:** It's a longer acting active metabolite of isosorbide dinitrate.
- **Erythrityl-tetranitrate and Pentaerythritol- tetranitrate:** They are also longer acting nitrates and used for chronic prophylaxis.

Therapeutic Uses of Nitrates

- **Angina pectoris and acute coronary syndromes (ACS):** Short acting nitrates are used in emergencies and long acting ones are used for the prophylaxis purpose or long-term treatment. These are effective in both classical as well as variant angina.

Any one drug out of sublingual GTN tablet or spray, or isosorbide dinitrate can be taken on 'as and when required' basis.

For an acute attack of angina, GTN sublingual tablet (0.5 mg) provides relief within 2–3 minutes in most of the patients. Patient is advised to spit off the remaining tablet or swallow it to avoid the side effect of acute hypotension and headache.

GTN sublingual tablet can also be used for prophylactic purpose before exercise or any stressful condition.

For chronic prophylaxis purpose, longer-acting nitrates (long acting formulation of nitroglycerine also) are used. 6–8 drug free hours daily are advisable to prevent the development of tolerance and dependence.

Revascularization by thrombolytics or coronary angioplasty with stents or coronary bypass surgery is considered in high risk patients of acute coronary syndrome.

- **Myocardial infarction (MI):** During evolving phase of MI, nitroglycerine IV infusion helps in relieving chest pain and pulmonary congestion as well as limiting the size of infarct area.
- **Chronic heart failure and acute left ventricular failure:** Nitrates provide relief by decreasing both preload and afterload. Intravenous GTN is the preparation of choice in emergency conditions.
- **Cyanide poisoning:** Nitrates are life saving in cyanide poisoning (Fig. 10.2).
  Sod. nitrite: 10ml of 3% sol. IV then, Sod. Thiosulfate: 50 mL 25% sol. IV
  Sod. nitrite forms methemoglobin, which binds to cyanide and forms cyano-methemoglobin, which is converted to easily excretable form sod. thiocyanate by sod. thiosulfate.
- **GIT uses:** Nitrates are helpful in biliary; colic and esophageal spasm. Sublingual GTN or isosorbide dinitrates provide prompt relief by causing smooth muscle relaxation.

Adverse Effects

These are related to vasodilatation effects. These include nausea and vomiting, throbbing headache, flushing of face, hypotension, reflex tachycardia, dizziness and increased

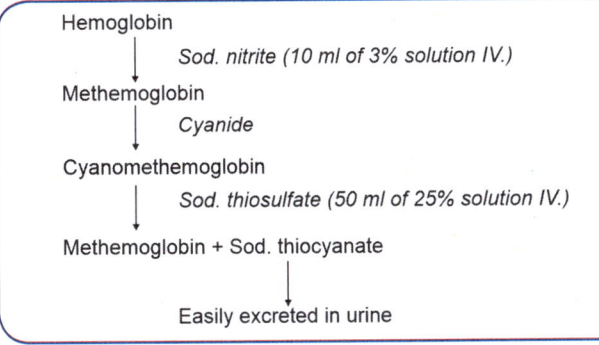

FIG. 10.2: Role of nitrates in cyanide poisoning

perspiration. With the transdermal preparations, there is a risk of contact dermatitis and local hypersensitivity reactions.

β-BLOCKERS

(Propranolol, Metoprolol, Atenolol and others.)

- β blockers have a slow action and are used on a long-term basis for the purpose of chronic prophylaxis.
- The β blockers act on β_1 receptors and decrease the heart rate and force of myocardial contraction. These effects reduce the cardiac work and oxygen demand. Due to these effects, frequency of anginal attacks is decreased and exercise tolerance is improved.
- Cardioselective β blockers such as metoprolol and atenolol are preferred over non-selective β blockers.
- In angina pectoris, β-blockers have to be taken on a regular basis and not on '*as and when required*' basis.
- Patients are advised to take these drugs regularly as abrupt discontinuation after chronic use may precipitate severe angina attacks and even myocardial infarction may occur.

CALCIUM CHANNEL BLOCKERS

[Verapamil, Diltiazem, Dihydropyridines (Nifedipine, Felodipine, Amlodipine, Nitrendipine, Nimodipine, Lacidipine, Lercanidipine, Benidipine)]

- The calcium channel blockers (CCBs) are very useful for the prophylaxis of exertional angina. These agents are preferred over nitrates in vasospastic angina.
- They inhibit the voltage sensitive calcium channels in heart and vascular smooth muscles and decrease the cardiac work load as well as peripheral vascular resistance (afterload).

Verapamil

- Verapamil has prominent cardiodepressant effects such as
  - Decrease in heart rate (negative chronotropic effect)
  - Decrease in the force of contraction (negative inotropic effect)
  - Decrease in A-V conduction.
- In addition, it also decreases total peripheral resistance by dilating arterioles as well as improves the coronary flow.
- The blood pressure is not lowered much.
- It is given in a dose of 40–160 mg TDS orally and 5 mg by slow IV injection.
- It is used mainly in arrhythmia and angina due to hypertension.
- The major adverse effects are nausea, constipation and bradycardia and occasional hypotension. It should not be given with β blockers and other cardiac depressants like quinidine and disopyramide due to additive cardiodepressant effects.

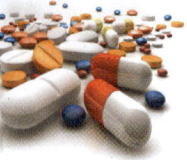

Diltiazem

- It dilates peripheral and coronary arteries with less potency as compared to DHPs.
- It has negative inotropic and chronotropic action.
- It is used in angina due to coronary dilating effect.
- It is given orally in a dose of 30–60 mg TDS or QID.

Dihydropyridines (DHPs)

(Nifedipine, Felodipine, Amlodipine, Nitrendipine, Nimodipine, Lacidipine, Lercanidipine, Benidipine)

- CCBs inhibit the movement of calcium ions across the membranes of myocardial and arterial muscle cells, altering the action potential and blocking muscle cell contraction.
- A loss of smooth muscle tone, vasodilation, and decreased peripheral resistance occur. Subsequently, preload and afterload are decreased, which in turn decreases cardiac workload and oxygen consumption.
- Short acting DHPs like nifedipine causes reflex tachycardia and palpitations, which can be controlled and minimized by addition of a beta blocker or giving sustained release preparations.

Pharmacokinetics

- All the CCBs are well absorbed by oral route.
- These drugs are metabolized in liver and excreted through kidney.

Indications of Calcium Channel Blockers

- Angina pectoris
- Hypertension
- Supraventricular arrhythmia (verapamil and diltiazem)
- Migraine (verapamil).

POTASSIUM CHANNEL OPENERS

These agents cause arterial and venodilatation by opening the potassium channels, thereby reduce both preload and afterload.

Nicorandil

- It opens the ATP sensitive potassium channels.
- It also acts as nitric oxide donor and causes relaxation of vascular smooth muscles and decreases preload and afterload.
- It also increases the coronary blood flow.
- It has variable plasma t½ ranging from 1–12 hours.
- It is indicated in resistant angina in combination with other drugs.

- It does not cause tolerance.
- It is given orally in a dose of 5–20 mg BD.
- The major side effects are headache, nausea, palpitations, flushing, weakness and dizziness.

OTHERS

Dipyridamole, Trimetazidine, Ranolazine, Ivabradine

Dipyridamole

- It is a good coronary dilator.
- It is not used in angina due '*coronary steal phenomenon*', i.e., it diverts blood from the ischemic region of the myocardium to non-ischemic zone.
- It is used for the prophylaxis of coronary and cerebral thrombosis in a dose of 25–100 mg TDS.

Trimetazidine

- It is a pFox (partial inhibitor of fatty acid oxidation) inhibitor, limits intracellular acidosis and protects the myocardial cells from free-radical (superoxide) injury.
- It is used as add-on therapy in angina and post MI patients in a dose of 20 mg TDS.

Ranolazine

- It is congener of trimetazidine.
- It has cardio-protective effects and prolongs the duration of exercise in patient of angina pectoris.
- It prolongs Q-T interval, so it should never be used with other Q-T interval prolonging drugs.
- It is given orally in a dose of 0.5–1 g BD.

Ivabradine

- It blocks the sodium channel in SA node and has potent anti-anginal heart-rate lowering effect.
- The heart rate reduction leads to decreased myocardial oxygen demand.
- It is helpful in improving the exercise tolerance and reducing the frequency of angina attack.
- It is given orally in a dose of 2.5–7.5 mg BD.

Drug Interactions

- Sildenafil potentiates the action of nitrates by causing synergistic vasodilatory effect and this may cause severe hypotension and myocardial infarction which could be fatal. Hence, the concurrent use of these drugs should be avoided.
- Concurrent use of verapamil with beta-blockers produces conduction defects and sinus depression.
- Verapamil potentiates digoxin toxicity by reducing its excretion.

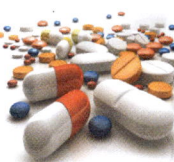

 Nursing Implications

➤ **Antianginals agents**

☞ Assess for contraindications or cautions and known allergies to any of these drugs to avoid hypersensitivity reactions.
☞ Nurse should monitor the pulse, blood pressure, electrocardiogram (ECG), respiratory rate before, during and after the therapy.
☞ Nurse should be able to handle and interpret the findings on cardiac monitors.
☞ Nurses should know about the proper way of administration of different forms of drugs such as oral, sublingual, topical, etc.
☞ Nitroglycerine is sensitive to air, light, heat and moisture; it should be stored in tightly closed amber colored glass bottles.
☞ Nitroglycerine IV preparation should be mixed with 5% dextrose or normal saline in a glass bottle with the tubing supplied by manufacturer.
☞ Give sublingual preparations under the tongue or in the buccal pouch, and encourage the patient not to swallow, to ensure that therapeutic effectiveness is achieved.
☞ Nurse should educate the patient to spit out the sublingual preparation after relief from anginal pain.
☞ Instruct the patient that a sublingual dose may be repeated in 5 minutes if relief is not felt, for a total of three doses; if pain persists, the patient should be hospitalized.
☞ Have emergency life support equipment readily available in case of severe reaction to the drug or myocardial infarction.
☞ Monitor for adverse effects (hypotension, cardiac arrhythmias, GI upset, skin reactions, and headache).
☞ Evaluate the effectiveness of the teaching plan (patient can name drug, dosage, proper administration, adverse effects to watch for, specific measures to avoid them, and the importance of continued follow-up).

ANTI-HYPERTENSIVES AND VASODILATORS

- Hypertension can be defined as the elevated level of systolic and diastolic blood pressure above that expected as normal for a particular age group.
- Hypertension is the most common cause for cardiovascular diseases.
- The prevalence of hypertension increases with age and has become a major cause of morbidity and mortality worldwide in both developed and developing countries. This is predicted to become 1.56 billion worldwide by 2025.
- The Seventh Joint National Committee report (JNC-VII) on the prevention, detection, evaluation and treatment of BP has introduced a new classification (definition) viz. normal, pre-hypertensive and hypertensive population as given in Table 10.3.
- JNC-VII recommends treating SBP and DBP to targets of <140/90 mm Hg to reduce cardiovascular complications.
- In patients with risk factors like diabetes or renal disease, the guidelines recommend a BP goal of <130/80 mm Hg.
- Most of the current guidelines recommend antihypertensive drug therapy with blood pressure >140/90 mm Hg in all and between 130–140/80–90 mm Hg if patients have a high overall risk factor or identifiable target organ damage, e.g., diabetes mellitus or renal insufficiency.
- Patients with systolic BP >140 mm Hg and above the age of 50 years of age must be treated. It should be remembered that reaching target BP is generally more difficult in geriatric Isolated Systolic Hypertension (ISH) than in younger persons with systolic-diastolic hypertension.
- The aim of antihypertensive therapy is mainly to interrupt the progress of hypertension and lower the same below the threshold.

Most efforts to control BP involve both non-pharmacological measures and pharmacological therapy.

- **Non-pharmacological measures**: Lifestyle modifications that are likely to help decrease in BP are reduced intake of salt, saturated fat, alcohol, cessation of smoking, reduction in obesity, avoidance of stress, reduction of other co-existing risk factors and increased intake of fruits, dietary fibers and physical activity. All available guidelines recommend lifestyle modifications as the most effective approach to prevent hypertension and indeed as the first-line treatment for mild hypertension.
- **Pharmacological measures (drug therapy)**: Most commonly used drugs are diuretics, beta blockers, angiotensin receptor blockers, angiotensin converting enzyme inhibitors and calcium channel blockers. These drugs are used either as monotherapy or as fixed low-dose combination therapy.

TABLE 10.3: Classification of hypertension

BP classification	SBP (mm Hg)		DBP (mm Hg)
Normal	<120	and	<80
Pre-hypertension	120-139	or	80–89
Stage-1 Hypertension	140–159	or	90–99
Stage-II Hypertension	> 160	or	>100

289

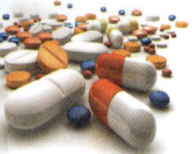

- The antihypertensive drugs are defined as the class of drugs used to control hypertension on short-term and long-term basis.
- These drugs are life saving in hypertensive emergencies and prevent long–term complications of hypertension when used regularly.

The antihypertensive drugs have been classified as follows:
- **Diuretics**
  - **Thiazides:** Hydrochlorothiazide, chlorthalidone, Indapamide
  - **High ceiling diuretics:** Furosemide, etc.
  - **K⁺ Sparing diuretics:** Spironolactone, Amiloride
- **Drugs acting on RAAS**
  - **ACE inhibitors:** Captopril, enalapril, lisinopril, Perindopril, Ramipril, Fosinopril, etc.
  - **Angiotensin (AT₁ receptor) blockers:** Losartan, candesartan, irbesartan, valsartan, telmisartan
  - **Direct renin inhibitor:** Aliskiren, ramikiren
- **Calcium channel blockers:**
  - **Dihydropyridines (DHPs):** Nifedipine, amlodipine, felodipine, nitrendipine, nimodipine, lacidipine, lercanidipine, benidipine
  - **Others:** Verapamil, diltiazem.
- **Sympatholytics drugs**
  - **β Adrenergic blockers:** Propranolol, metoprolol, atenolol, etc.
  - **β + α Adrenergic blockers:** Labetalol, carvedilol
  - **α Adrenergic blocker:** Prazosin, terazosin, doxazosin, phentolamine, phenoxybenzamine
  - **Central sympatholytics:** Clonidine, methyldopa
- **Vasodilators:**
  - **Arteriolar dilator:** Hydralazine, minoxidil, diazoxide
  - **Arteriolar and venous dilator:** Sodium nitroprusside

DIURETICS

(Hydrochlorothiazide, Chlorthalidone, Indapamide, Furosemide, Spironolactone, Amiloride)

- Diuretics are being used for the treatment of hypertension since many years.
- Initially, diuretics bring about a fall in plasma volume by enhancing the excretion of sodium and water and thus, reduce the cardiac output.
- After a continued treatment of 6–8 weeks, cardiac output becomes normal due to compensatory mechanisms and then the anti-hypertensive effect is obtained by a fall in peripheral vascular resistance.
- Restriction of dietary salt intake reduces the dose of diuretics to control the blood pressure.
- Thiazides are first–line antihypertensives.
- Hydrochlorthiazide or chlorthalidone is given in a dose of 12.5 mg daily and the dose may be increased to 25 mg daily if optimum response is not obtained.

- Thiazides are used either alone or in combination with other antihypertensive drugs to get the synergistic antihypertensive actions.
- Sometimes these are given in combination with K⁺ sparing diuretics to prevent associated hypokalemia.
- The loop diuretics have low antihypertensive effect as compared to thiazides when given on long-term basis.
- The loop diuretics are very potent diuretics and cause loss of electrolytes to a great extent and uneven fall in blood pressure. These can be used in hypertension associated with congestive heart failure, chronic renal failure and for emergency lowering of hypertension in hypertensive crisis.
- **The complete pharmacological details of diuretics have been described in Chapter 6 Drugs used in Urinary System.**

DRUGS ACTING ON RENIN-ANGIOTENSIN-ALDOSTERONE SYSTEM (RAAS)

Refer to Figure 10.3 for sites of action of drugs acting on RAAS.

Angiotensin Converting Enzyme (ACE) Inhibitors

(Captopril, Enalapril, Lisinopril, Perindopril, Ramipril, Fosinopril)

Mechanism of Action

- In most of the hypertensive patients, angiotensin-II overproduction is responsible for hypertension.

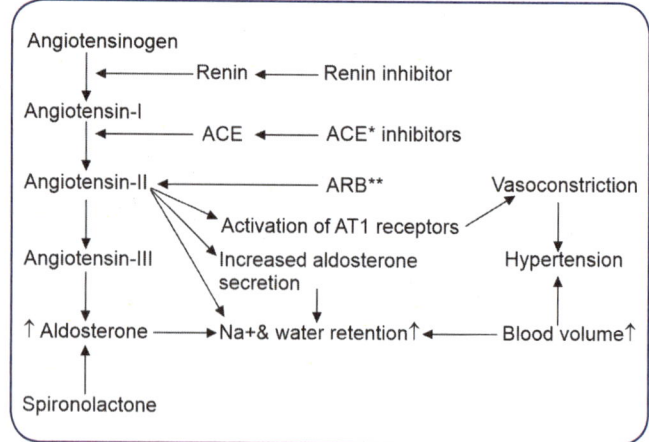

FIG. 10.3: Sites of action of drugs acting on RAAS

Inhibitors., ACE: Angiotensin converting enzyme, **ARB:** Angiotensin-2 receptor blockers.

Angiotensin-III is degraded to inactive fragments by angiotensinase enzymes.

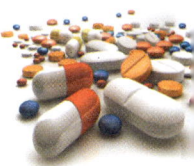

- ACE inhibitors inhibit the conversion of Angiotensin-I to angiotensin-II by inhibiting the enzyme angiotensin converting enzyme (ACE). The production of angiotensin-III is decreased which causes following effects:
  - Decrease in peripheral vascular resistance
  - Decrease in aldosterone production
  - Increase the blood supply to vital organs like kidney, brain and heart.
- The net effect of the above actions is seen in the form of decrease in blood pressure.
  ACEIs are given in Table 10.4.

Pharmacokinetics

- All ACE inhibitors are prodrugs except lisinopril and captopril.
- They are mainly given by oral route and bioavailability of different drugs varies from 25% to 70%.
- These drugs are metabolized in liver and excreted in urine.

Therapeutic Uses of ACE Inhibitors

- **Hypertension:** ACE inhibitors are agents of choice in hypertension associated with left ventricular hypertrophy, diabetes mellitus, ischemic heart disease and renal disease(except renal artery stenosis). Addition of a diuretic agent (thiazides and thiazide-like) potentiates their antihypertensive efficacy.

- **Congestive cardiac failure**: These drugs retard and reverse cardiac remodeling and hypertrophy.
- **Myocardial infarction**: These drugs decrease early and long-term mortality.
- **Diabetic nephropathy:** These drugs prevent progression of renal complications and decrease proteinuria.

Adverse Effects

- **Dry cough:** It is a major disadvantage associated with the use of ACE inhibitors. Due to inhibition of ACE present in the lungs, the levels of bradykinins rise and produce cough. Normally, ACE is involved in degradation of bradykinins also.
- Angiedema
- Rashes and urticaria
- Hypotension
- Alteration of taste
- Teratogenicity
- Precipitation of Acute renal failure in renal artery stenosis patients
- Nausea, headache, dizziness are some other side effects.

Angiotensin (AT₁) Receptor Blockers (ARBs)

Angiotensin (AT$_1$) Receptor Blockers (ARBs)

(Losartan, Telmisartan, Olmesartan, Candesartan, Irbesartan, Valsartan,)

TABLE 10.4: ACE Inhibitors (ACEIs)

Drug	Dose (mg/day)	Special features
Captopril	25–150	• It is the first ACEI • It is an active metabolite not a prodrug • It is administered 1 hour prior to meals because food interferes with its absorption • It has high incidence of adverse effects than other ACEIs
Enalapril	2.5–40	• It is a prodrug • 'Enalaprilat' is the active metabolite of enalapril and it is available as such also for IV use in emergency control of hypertension • It is more potent than captopril and food does not interfere its absorption • It has longer duration of action than captopril • The adverse reactions are less prominent than captopril
Lisinopril	5–40	• It is an active metabolite not a prodrug • It is a longer acting derivative of enalapril • Causes decrease in cardiac output, cardiac and venous return
Fosinopril	10–40	• It is a prodrug • Metabolized by both renal and hepatic system. Hence, can be given in the patient with renal impairment • The incidence of 1st dose hypotension is more
Perindopril	2–8	• It is a prodrug • Another long acting ACEI • It has slow onset of action • The incidence of 1st dose hypotension is low
Ramipril	1.25–10	• It is a prodrug • It has wide volume of distribution with triphasic elimination

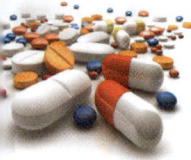

- Angiotensin-II exerts its various actions/effects through angiotensin receptors.
- There are two subtypes of Angiotensin-II receptors: AT_1 and AT_2. In normal conditions, there is a balance in the activity of AT_1 and AT_2 receptors.
- AT_1 receptors are present in myocardial tissues, vascular tissues, brain and adrenal cells.
- The main advantage of ARBs over ACE inhibitors is low incidence of dry cough with ARBs. This is because the levels of bradykinins in the lungs do not increase with ARBs.

Mechanism of Action of ARBs

- ARBs competitively antagonize the action of Angiotensin-II on the AT_1 receptors and the consequent effects to be produced by A-II are blocked.
- Therefore, ARBs help in relaxation of vascular smooth muscles, promote salt and water excretion, decrease plasma volume and overall produce a fall in blood pressure.
- The ARBs have high affinity towards AT_1 receptors as compared to AT_2 receptors.
- Stimulation or blockade of AT_2 receptors produces opposite effects to AT_1 receptors.

Pharmacokinetics

- All ARBs are mainly given by oral route and bioavailability of different drugs varies from 30 to 50%.
- These drugs are extensively protein bound.
- These are metabolized in liver and excreted via gut and urine.
- All the ARBs have nearly similar chemical structure with minor pharmacokinetic variations in relation to their affinity to AT_1 receptors.
- Individual ARBs are described in Table 10.5.

TABLE 10.5: Drug profile of individual ARBs

Drug	Dose	Special features
Losartan	25–50 mg OD	• It was the first AT_1 receptor antagonist • 10,000 times more selective for AT_1 than for AT_2 receptors
Telmisartan	20–80 mgOD	• Action starts in 3 hours and lasts for more than 24 hours • In liver diseases, dose adjustment is required
Olmesartan	20–40 mg OD	• More potent ARB • It is a prodrug • No dose adjustment is required in kidney or liver disease

Contd...

Drug	Dose	Special features
Candesartan	8 mg OD	• Dissociation from AT_1 receptors is very slow and acts for a very longer time
Irbesartan	150–300 mg OD	• It has best oral bioavailability amongst all ARBs
Valsartan	80–160 mg OD	• It has poor oral bioavailability (23%) and food interferes with its absorption

Therapeutic Uses of ARBs

- The common indications of ARBs are as follows:
  - **Hypertension:** ARBs are preferred over ACE inhibitors and are used in combination with a diuretic as first choice drug.
  - **Congestive cardiac failure:** Used as an alternative in patients not tolerating ACE inhibitors.
  - **Myocardial infarction**: Improve the long-term survival in myocardial infarction patients.
  - **Diabetic nephropathy:** The renoprotection provided by these agents is independent of their antihypertensive effects.

Adverse Effects

The common adverse effects associated with ARBs are as follows:

- **GIT:** Diarrhea, abdominal pain, nausea and dry mouth.
- **CNS:** Headache, dizziness and syncope.
- **CVS:** Hypotension.
- **Others:** Upper respiratory tract infections and mild cough, rash, dry skin, mild angiedema, teratogenicity and alopecia.

Direct Renin Inhibitors

(Aliskiren, Ramikiren)

- Renin acts in the initial steps of RAAS and converts angiotensinogen to angiotensin-I. When we interfere this step by blocking the renin (*renin is essential for the formation of angiotensin-1*), the levels of angiotensin-1 and II fall, which causes fall in BP.
- The hypotensive effects can be equated with that of ACEIs or ARBs.
- These are recommended as alternative drugs for the patients not tolerating the other antihypertensive drugs.
- These drugs are given orally and have poor bioavailability.
- Aliskerin is given in a dose of 150–300 mg OD.
- The hypotensive effect is long lasting and persists for many days after discontinuation of therapy.
- The main side effects produced are, headache, dyspepsia, loose motions, etc.
- These agents should be avoided in pregnancy.

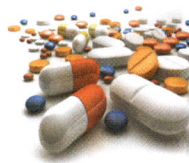

CALCIUM CHANNEL BLOCKERS (CCBs)

(Nifedipine, Amlodipine, Felodipine Nitrendipine, Nimodipine, Lacidipine, Lercanidipine, Benidipine, Verapamil, Diltiazem).

- Dihydropyridines are the most commonly used calcium channel blockers (CCBs).
- The cardiac and smooth muscles cell contraction depends upon the activation of calcium channels in the cardiac myocytes. For depolarization of cardiac and other smooth muscles cells, entry of calcium into the cells occurs through these calcium channels.
- CCBs inhibit the movement of calcium ions across the membranes of myocardial and arterial muscle cells, altering the action potential and blocking muscle cell contraction.
- A loss of smooth muscle tone, vasodilation, and decreased peripheral resistance occurs. Subsequently, preload and afterload are decreased, which in turn decreases cardiac workload and oxygen consumption.
- Short acting DHPs like nifedipine causes reflex tachycardia and palpitations, which can be controlled and minimized by addition of a beta-blocker or giving sustained release preparations.

Mechanism of Action of Calcium Channel Blockers

The mechanism of action of CCBs is elaborated in Figure 10.4. The comparative actions of DHPs and non-DHPs are shown in Figure 10.5.

Pharmacokinetics

- All the CCBs are well absorbed by oral route and have 90–100% absorption.
- All CCBs are highly protein bound.
- These drugs are metabolized in liver and excreted through kidney.
- Doses and special features of individual CCBs are given in Table 10.6.

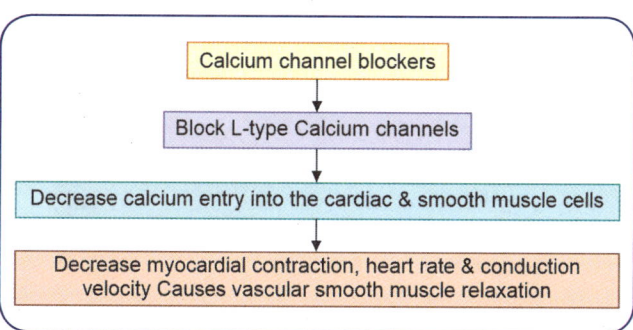

FIG. 10.4: Mechanism of action of CCBs

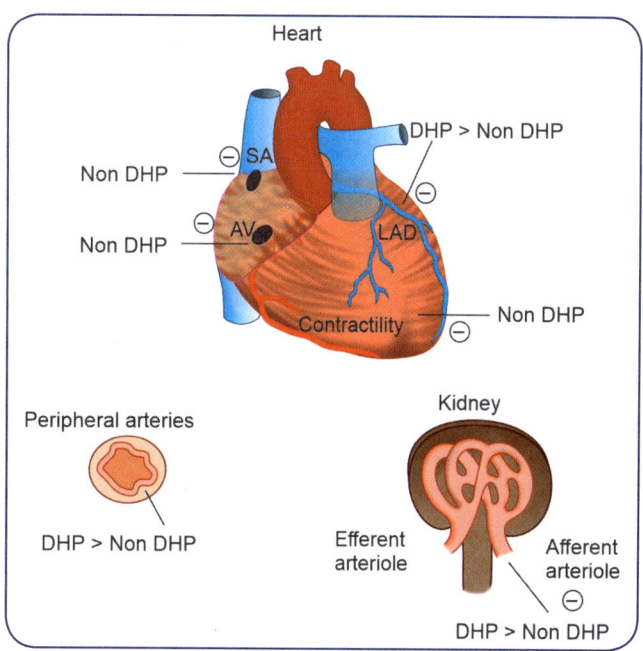

FIG. 10.5: Comparative action of CCBs (DHPs and non-DHPs)

TABLE 10.6: Drug profile of individual CCBs

Drug	Dose	Special features
Nifedipine	5-20 mg BD	• Has fast onset of action with short duration • Causes reflex tachycardia as a prominent side effect • May increase frequency of angina attack
Amlodipine	5–10 mg OD	• Has got consistent and good oral bioavailability • Diurnal fluctuation of BP are least • S-amlodipine is its enantiomer and equally effective at half the dose with less ankle edema
Felodipine	5–10 mg OD	• Has higher vascular selectivity
Nitrendipine	5–20 mg OD	• Has only 10–30% of bioavailabilty • Additionally also releases nitric oxide from the endothelium • Useful in hypertension with angina
Nimodipine	30–60 mg QID	• It is cerebrovascular selective due to high lipid solubility and blood-brain barrier penetration • Used in patients with hemorrhagic stroke and subarachnoid hemorrhage

293

Contd...

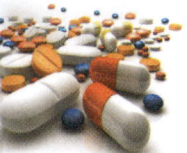

Drug	Dose	Special features
Lacidipine	4–6 mg OD	• Has vasoselective activity and useful in hypertension only
Lercanidipine	10–20 mg OD	• Long acting DHP • Useful in hypertension
Benidipine	4–8 mg OD	• Long acting DHP • Has very slow dissociation from DHP receptors • Useful in hypertension and angina

Verapamil

- Verapamil has prominent cardiodepressant effects such as
  - Decrease in heart rate (negative chronotropic effect)
  - Decrease in the force of contraction (negative inotropic effect)
  - Decrease in A-V conduction.
- In addition, it also decreases total peripheral resistance by dilating arterioles as well as improves the coronary flow. The blood pressure is not lowered much.
- It is given in a dose of 40–160 mg TDS orally and 5 mg by slow IV injection.
- It is used in *arrhythmia and angina due to hypertension* mainly.
- The major adverse effects are nausea, constipation, bradycardia and occasional hypotension. It should not be given with β blockers and other cardiac depressants like quinidine and disopyramide due to additive cardiodepressant effects.

Diltiazem

- It dilates peripheral and coronary arteries with less potency as compared to DHPs.
- It has negative inotropic and chronotropic action. It is used in angina due to coronary dilating effect. It is given orally in a dose of 30–60 mg TDS or QID.

Therapeutic Uses of CCBs

- **Hypertension:** Long acting CCBs are used for the long-term treatment of hypertension. Amlodipine is the most preferred drug.
- **Ischemic heart disease:**
  - **Angina pectoris:** DHPs like amlodipine with beta-blocker are used for long-term management. Verapamil and diltiazem are used for prophylaxis.
  - **Vasospastic angina:** Verapamil and amlodipine are the preferred agents.
- **Unstable angina:** Verapamil is used.
- **Supraventricular arrhythmia:** Verapamil and diltiazem are used due to their antiarrhythmic properties.

- **Peripheral vascular disease:** Nifedipine, Felodipine and Diltiazem are used for this purpose. Nifedipine patches are also useful.
- **Migraine prophylaxis:** Verapamil is useful.
- **Nocturnal leg cramps:** Verapamil is useful.

Adverse Effects

- Verapamil causes nausea, constipation, bradycardia, aggravation of conduction defects.
- Diltiazem also has similar side effect profile but slightly to lesser extent.
- DHPs show side effects like nausea, headache, drowsiness, palpitation, hypotension, flushing and ankle edema.
- Difficulty in micturition and worsening of gastroesophageal reflux is seen in elderly patients.

SYMPATHOLYTIC DRUGS

- β **adrenergic blockers:** Propranolol, Metoprolol, Atenolol.
- β + α **adrenergic blockers:** Labetalol, Carvedilol.
- α **adrenergic blocker:** Prazosin, Terazosin, Doxazosin, Phentolamine, Phenoxybenzamine
- **Central sympatholytics:** Clonidine, Methyldopa.

β-Blockers

(The details have been given in Chapter Anti-Adrenergics)
- The β-blockers are useful in mild to moderate hypertension.
- The antihypertensive effect of these agents is due to sum of following mechanisms (Fig. 10.6):

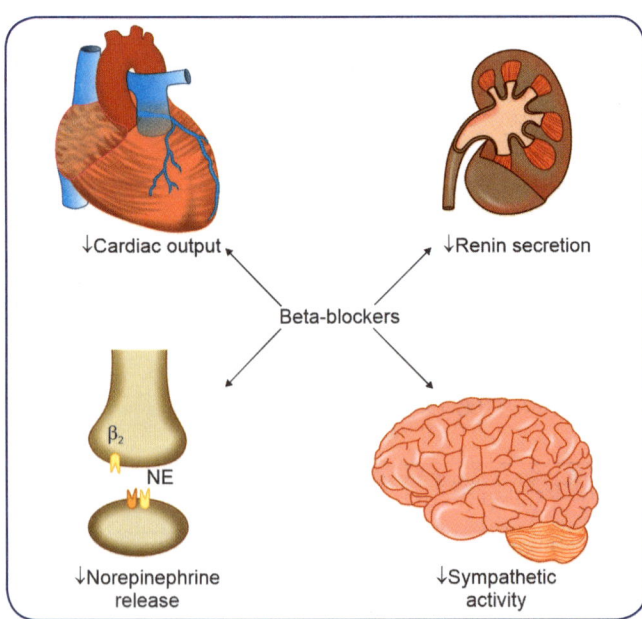

FIG. 10.6: Mechanism for antihypertensive effect of beta-blockers.

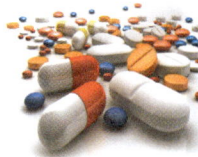

- Blockade of cardiac beta 1 receptors, which leads to decreased myocardial contractility and decreased cardiac output.
    - Lowering of plasma renin activity.
- Decrease in central sympathetic flow.
- β-blockers can be used alone or in combination with other antihypertensive drugs.
- These are specially used with the drugs which cause tachycardia as their side effect (vasodilators). These drugs should be tapered and not withdrawn abruptly as sudden stoppage can cause rebound hypertension and precipitation of angina.
- These drugs are useful in patients of hypertension with angina or arrhythmias.
- They may precipitate bronchospasm and congestive cardiac failure.
- They should be used with caution in diabetic patients as the hypoglycemic symptoms are masked.
- Atenolol is preferred antihypertensive agent due to absence of CNS side effects and once a day dosing schedule.
- Metoprolol is preferred in hypertensive patients with associated coronary artery disease and heart failure.
- Esmolol is used in hypertensive emergencies.

β + α Adrenergic Blockers

(Labetalol, Carvedilol)
The details have been described in Chapter 9.

α-Adrenergic Blockers

(Prazosin, Terazosin, Doxazosin, Phentolamine, Phenoxybenzamine)
The details have been described in Chapter 9.

Central Sympatholytics

(Clonidine, Methyldopa)

Clonidine

- Clonidine is a moderately potent antihypertensive drug.
- It acts at α_2 receptors in brainstem mainly in vasomotor center in medulla. This causes decrease in sympathetic outflow and fall in BP with bradycardia.
- It is well absorbed orally , and peak effect occurs within 2–4 hours.
- It is given in a dose of 100 µg once daily to a maximum of 300 µg thrice daily.
- Sudden withdrawal may cause rebound symptoms. Other side effects are sedation, sleep disturbances, constipation, impotence and bradycardia.

- It is occasionally used in combination with a diuretic, to treat withdrawal symptoms of opioids and also used to control the vasomotor symptoms of menopause.

Methyldopa

- Methyldopa is a precursor of dopamine and nor-adrenaline.
- It decreases the central sympathetic activity.
- It is preferred as antihypertensive drug in pregnancy as it is found to be safe for both mother and fetus.
- It is given in a dose of 250 and 500 mg in BD to QID doses depending upon the requirement.
- Main adverse effects seen with its use are lethargy, sedative effects, dryness of mouth, weight gain and nasal stuffiness.

VASODILATORS

- **Arteriolar dilators:** Hydralazine, Minoxidil, Diazoxide
- **Arteriolar and venous dilators:** Sodium nitroprusside

Arteriolar Dilator

(Hydralazine, Minoxidil, Diazoxide)
The vasodilators relax the vascular smooth muscles, decrease the peripheral vascular resistance and thus, play a role in lowering the BP.

Hydralazine

- It is given orally in a dose of 25–50 mg once to thrice daily depending upon requirement.
- It is given along with a diuretic or a beta blocker in cases where first line drugs show poor BP control.
- It is useful in hypertensive emergencies.
- It can be used safely in pregnancy.
- It should not be used in patients of ischemic heart disease and geriatric patients.

Minoxidil

- It is a powerful vasodilator and is used as antihypertensive in resistant cases only.
- It is a prodrug and the active metabolite opens the K^+ channels in smooth muscles and causes relaxation effect.
- Commonly, it is used as 2% topical solution in male baldness (alopecia) to promote hair growth.

Diazoxide

- It is related to thiazide diuretics.
- It is used in hypertensive emergencies.
- It is administered by IV route and has a long duration of action of about 24 hours.

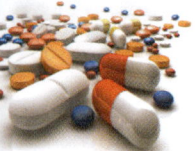

Adverse effects

- Adverse effects of the above drugs are more or less common.
- These are reflex tachycardia, sodium and water retention, throbbing headache, postural hypotension, etc.

Sodium Nitroprusside

- Sodium nitroprusside acts as a balanced vasodilator as it relaxes both arterioles and venules. Thus, both preload and afterload are decreased. It acts through the release of nitric oxide which is a potent vasodilator.
- It acts within 30 seconds and the action is short lived for 3–4 minutes only.
- It is used in hypertensive emergencies.
- It is given in the form of infusion in a dose of 0.5–10 µg/kg/min in 5% dextrose. The dose is titrated according to the response which can be recorded by regular BP monitoring.
- The solution is photosensitive and should be prepared fresh as well as the infusion bottle should be covered properly to prevent exposure to light.
- Some of the side effects seen with its use are tachycardia, vomiting, perspiration, pain in abdomen, weakness, disorientation, lactic acidosis and psychosis like symptoms due to accumulation of excess of thiocyanates.

  Fenoldopam is another vasodilator useful in hypertensive emergencies with efficacy similar to sodium nitroprusside but devoid of thiocyanate related complications.

Drug Interactions

- The antihypertensive effect of clonidine is antagonized by tricyclic antidepressants. Hence, concurrent use should be avoided.
- The antihypertensive effect of β blockers is reduced by non-steroidal anti-inflammatory drugs (NSAIDs).
- β-blockers should not be given along with verapamil as additive sinus depression can occur.
- β-blockers and slow acting dihydropyridines (DHPs) is a useful antihypertensive combination as tachycardia caused by DHPs is countered by β-blockers.
- Thiazides and thiazide like diuretics have synergistic antihypertensive effect when given along with angiotensin receptor blockers (ARBs) or (angiotensin-converting enzyme inhibitors (ACEIs).

Nursing Implications

- Anti-hypertensives and vasodilators
  - Assess for cautions or contraindications to use of the drug to be administered.
  - Encourage patient to implement lifestyle changes, including weight loss, smoking cessation, decreased alcohol and salt in the diet, and increased exercise, to increase the effectiveness of antihypertensive therapy.

Nursing Implications

- Nurse should monitor the pulse, blood pressure, ECG, respiratory rate before, during and after the therapy and enter it immediately in the record file of patient.
- The treating physician should be informed immediately about any abnormal deviation (low/high) of the blood pressure.
- Never leave the patient unattended when the IV drip is going-on.
- Monitor for adverse effects (hypotension, cardiac arrhythmias, renal dysfunction, skin reactions, cough, pancytopenia, heart failure).
- Evaluate the effectiveness of the teaching plan (patient can name drug, dosage, adverse effects to watch for, specific measures to avoid them, and the importance of continued follow-up).

ANTIARRHYTHMICS

- Any change or disturbance in the cardiac rhythm, i.e., rate, conduction, regularity, automaticity is known as arrhythmia. These abnormalities may be at the site of origin or conduction of impulse.
- Arrhythmias occur in the heart because all of the cells of the heart possess the property of automaticity and therefore, can generate an excitatory impulse.
- Disruptions in the normal rhythm of the heart can interfere with myocardial contractions and affect the cardiac output, the amount of blood pumped with each beat. Arrhythmias that seriously disrupt cardiac output can be fatal.
- Several factors are responsible for arrhythmias. These include:
  - Electrolyte and pH imbalances that alter the action potential.
  - Decreased oxygen delivery to cells due to ischemia, etc.
  - Mechanical injury and stretching, which cause structural damage changes the conduction pathways.
  - Neurogenic causes.
  - Drugs, including antiarrhythmic drugs that alters the action potential.
- **Drugs used to prevent or treat irregularities of cardiac rhythm (arrhythmias) are known as antiarrhythmics. These drugs suppress automaticity or alter the conductivity of the heart.**
- The important cardiac arrhythmias are given in Figure 10.7.
- Drug induced arrhythmias are also very commonly seen in clinical practice, e.g., digitalis induced cardiac arrhythmias.

Contd...

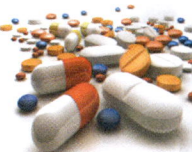

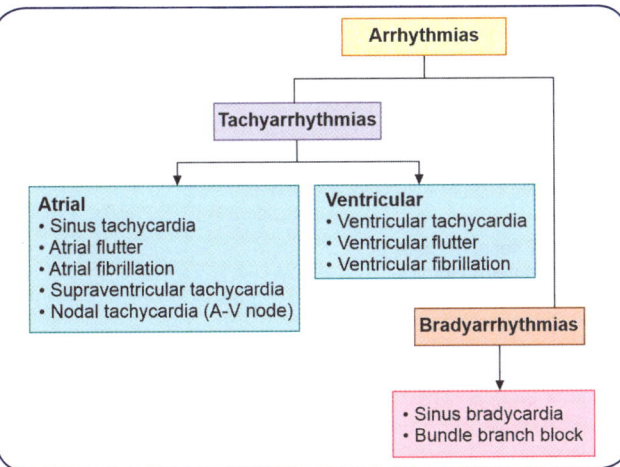

FIG. 10.7: Types of arrhythmias

TABLE 10.7: Classification of antiarrhythmic drugs

Class of anti-arrhythmics	Mechanism of action		Drugs
I (Na⁺ channel blockers)	Act on phase- 0, depolarization. Subdivided into :IA		Quinidine, Procainamide, Disopyramide
		:IB	Lignocaine, Mexiletine
		:IC	Propafenone, Flecainide
II (β blockers)	Act on phase –II and IV		Propranolol, Esmolol, Sotalol
III (K⁺ channel blockers)	Act on phase –III and prolong repolarization		Amiodarone, Dronedarone, Dofetilide, Ibutilide
IV (Ca²⁺ channel blockers)	Act on phase –II		Verapamil, Diltiazem
Others	• PSVT: Adenosine, Digoxin are used. • A-V block: Sympathomimetics (isoprenaline, etc), anticholinergics (atropine) are used. • In atrial flutter and fibrillation and paroxysmal supraventricular tachycardia (PSVT) digitalis is used to control ventricular rate.		

Normal Cardiac Cycle

The action potential of the cardiac muscle cell consists of five phases:

- **Phase 0** occurs when the cell reaches a point of stimulation. The sodium gates open and sodium rushes into the cell; this positive flow of electrons into the cell results in an electrical potential. This is called depolarization.
- **Phase 1** is a very short period during which the sodium ion concentration equalizes inside and outside of the cell.
- **Phase 2** or the plateau stage, occurs as the cell membrane becomes less permeable to sodium, calcium slowly enters the cell, and potassium begins to leave the cell. The cell membrane tries to return to its resting state, a process called repolarization or returning of the charge differences to the membrane.
- **Phase 3** is a time of rapid repolarization as the sodium gates are closed and potassium flows out of the cell.
- **Phase 4** occurs when the cell comes to rest; the sodium–potassium pump returns the membrane to its resting membrane potential, and spontaneous depolarization begins again.

- The antiarrhythmic drugs act mainly by blocking the various types of channels in the myocardial cells such as sodium, potassium and calcium channels.
- The antiarrhythmic drugs have been classified by *Vaughan Williams* and *Singh* on the basis of their action on different phases of cardiac cycle and are mentioned in Table 10.7.

CLASS-I ANTIARRYTHMIC DRUGS (Na⁺ CHANNEL BLOCKERS)

Refer to Figure 10.8 for effects of class 1A, 1B and 1C antiarrythmic

All drugs in these class block sodium channels just like anesthetics and reduce the depolarization during phase-I.

These drugs bind to the activated channels more strongly than the resting ones; hence, effective in the control of tachyarrhythmias.

The cardiac action potentials, showing the effects of class Ia, Ib, and Ic antiarrhythmics.

These have been subdivided as follows:

- **Class-IA drugs:** Quinidine, Procainamide, Disopyramide (Table 10.8).
- **Class-IB drugs:** Lignocaine, Mexiletine (Table 10.9)
- **Class-IC drugs:** Propafenone, Flecainide (Table 10.10).
  - These drugs are most potent sodium channel blockers and can cause cardiac arrest and even sudden death. Therefore not commonly used.

CLASS-II ANTIARRYTHMIC DRUGS (β-BLOCKERS)

Refer to Figure 10.9 for effects of class II, III and IV antiarrythmic on the cardiace cycle.
(Propranolol, Esmolol, Sotalol)

The beta-blockers suppress the myocardial contractility, automaticity and conduction velocity by acting on phase-IV depolarization in SA node and purkinje fibers. These drugs act on both phase-II and IV of the cardiac cycle.

These drugs suppress ectopic activity, which is mediated by adrenergic over activity.

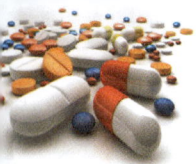

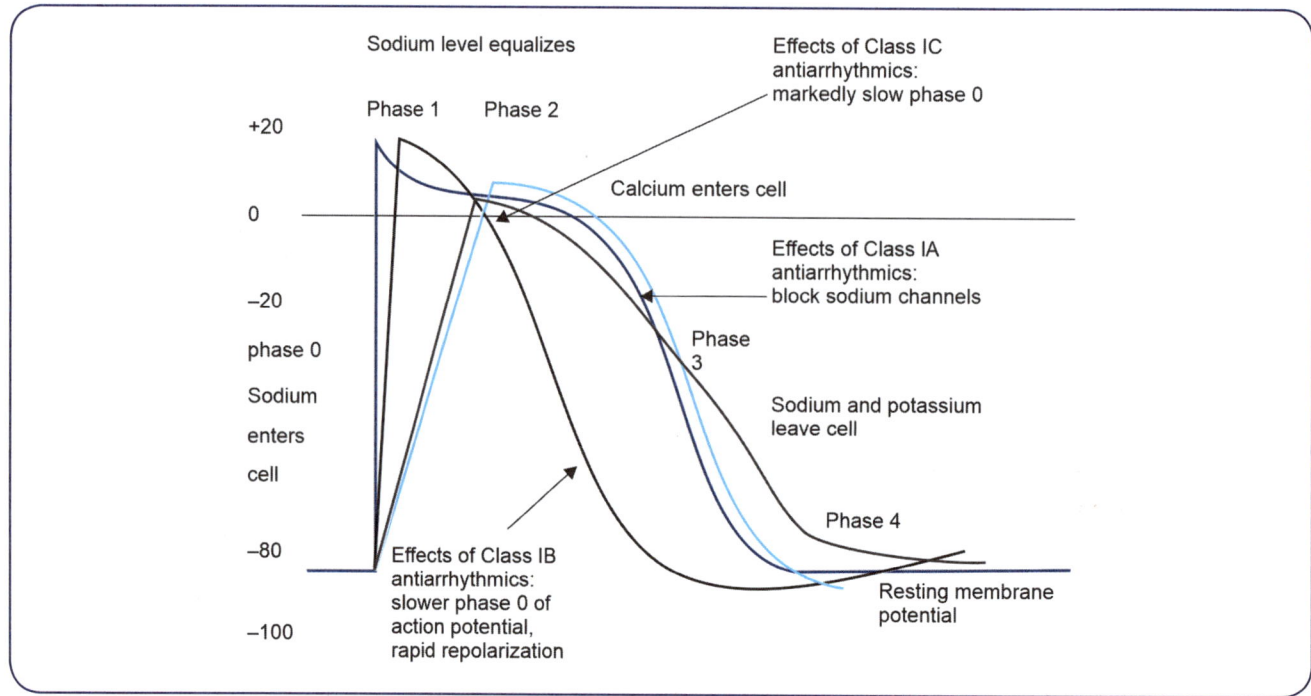

Fig. 10.8: Effects of class Ia, Ib and Ic antiarrhythmics

TABLE 10.8: Characteristics of class-Ia antiarrhythmic drugs

Drug	Dose	Special features
Quinidine	100–200 mg TDS oral	• It reduces the conduction velocity by depressing the excitability of myocardial cells • It is less commonly used these days due to adverse effects • It is effective in atrial and ventricular arrhythmias such as atrial flutter and fibrillation and ventricular tachycardia
Procainamide	0.5–1 g oral or IM followed by 0.25–0.5 g every 2 hours Maintenance dose—0.5 g every 4–6 hours	• It is amide derivative of procaine • Better tolerated than quinidine • Effective in ventricular tachycardia • Higher dose can lead to hypotension, flushing and heart block
Disopyramide	100–150 mg TDS oral.	• Better than quinidine • Has prominent anticholinergic side effects • It can cause myocardial depression also • It prevents ventricular arrhythmias

TABLE 10.9: Characteristics of class-Ib antiarrhythmic drugs

Drug	Dose	Special features
Lignocaine	50–100 mg IV bolus followed by 20–40 mg	• It is a local anesthetic with antiarrhythmic activity • Not effective by oral route due to first pass metabolism • It decreases the action potential in ventricles and purkinje fibers. Hence, not effective in atrial arrhythmias • Indicated in ventricular arrhythmias • It may cause hypotension drowsiness, confusion and convulsions
Mexiletine	100–250 mg IV over 10 minutes, 1 mg/min IV infusion. Oral: 150–200 mg TDS with meals	• It can be used orally as an alternative to lignocaine • Minor adverse effects such as nausea, blurred vision and tremors

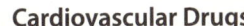
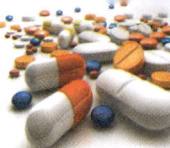

TABLE 10.10: Characteristics of class-Ic antiarrhythmic drugs

Drug	Dose	Special features
Propafenone	150–300 mg BD/TDS, orally	• Used for prophylaxis for ventricular arrhythmia, re-entrant tachycardia
Flecainide	100–200 mg BD, oral	• Has proarrhythmogenic potential • Reserved drug for resistant cases of paroxysmal atrial fibrillation

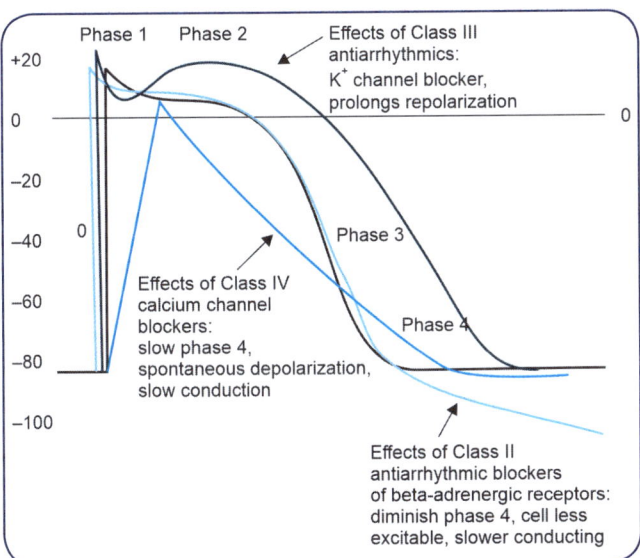

FIG. 10.9: Effects of class II, III, and IV antiarrhythmics on the cardiac cycle

Propranolol

- It is used for the treatment and prevention of supraventricular tachyarrhythmia, which is associated with emotion, exercise and hyperthyroidism.
- It is also used to suppress halothane and catecholamine (in pheochromocytoma) induced arrhythmia.
- It is used as drug of choice in-patient with congenital long QT syndrome.

Esmolol

- It is used for arrhythmias during surgery to control ventricular rate in atrial fibrillation.
- It is fast and short acting.
  Sotalol has potent antiarrhythmic activity.

CLASS-III ANTI-ARRHYTHMIC DRUGS (K⁺ CHANNEL OPENERS)

(Amiodarone, Dronedarone, Dofetilide, Ibutilide)
These drugs act on phase-III of the cardiac cycle and delay the repolarization by blocking the K⁺ channels. These drugs prolong the action potential duration (APD) and refractory period of cardiac tissue.

Amiodarone

- Amiodarone contains iodine and is a long acting drug with complex effects, showing class I, II, III, and IV actions, as well as α-blocking activity. It blocks the K⁺ channels and prolongs the action potential duration and the refractory period.
- It is the most commonly employed antiarrhythmic drug as it is the least proarrhythmic of the class I and III antiarrhythmic drugs.
- It is effective in the treatment of severe refractory supraventricular and ventricular tachyarrhythmias and atrial fibrillation or flutter.
- The most important indications are resistant ventricular tachycardia and recurrent ventricular fibrillations.
- It is incompletely absorbed after oral administration and distributed extensively in adipose tissue and has a half-life of several weeks (3–8 weeks). It is metabolized in liver.
- Its main side effects are hepatotoxicity, pulmonary fibrosis, neuropathy, corneal deposits, optic neuritis, blue-gray skin discoloration, and hypo- or hyperthyroidism. These side effects can be reduced by use of low doses and close monitoring.

Dronedarone

- Dronedarone has a shorter serum half-life than amiodarone. Due to less lipophilic nature, the tissue accumulation of this drug is also lower.
- Thyroid dysfunction is not seen as it does not have the iodine moieties like amiodarone.
- It has class I, II, III, and IV actions like amiodarone.
- It is less effective than amiodarone.
- Dronedarone has a better adverse effect profile than amiodarone except hepatotoxicity.
- It is used in a dose of 400 mg BD for maintaining sinus rhythm in atrial fibrillations or flutter.

Dofetilide

- Dofetilide is a pure potassium channel blocker.
- It can be used as a first-line antiarrhythmic agent in patients with persistent atrial fibrillation and heart failure or in those with coronary artery disease.
- The half-life of this oral drug is 10 hours.
- The side effects are very less.

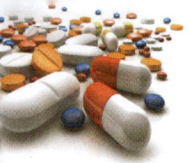

- The drug is mainly excreted unchanged in the urine, therefore, drugs which inhibit active tubular secretion should not be co-prescribed.

Ibutilide

- Ibutilide is the drug of choice for chemical conversion of atrial flutter to normal sinus rhythm.
- Ibutilide undergoes extensive first-pass metabolism and is not used orally.
- It is used by IV route only.
- The treatment initiation with Ibutilide is limited to the inpatient settings only because of the risk of QT prolongation and proarrhythmic potential.

CLASS-IV ANTI-ARRHYTHMIC DRUGS

- Class IV drugs are the non-dihydropyridine calcium channel blockers verapamil and diltiazem.
- In the heart, verapamil and diltiazem bind only to open depolarized voltage-sensitive channels, thus decreasing the inward current carried by calcium.
- They decrease the rate of phase IV spontaneous depolarization and also slow atrioventricular (AV) and sinoatrial (SA) nodal conduction (Fig. 10.9).
- They are useful in treating reentrant supraventricular tachycardia and in reducing the ventricular rate in atrial flutter and fibrillation.
- Verapamil is given in a dose of 80–120 mg TDS orally and 5 mg slowly over 2–3 minutes intravenously.
- Diltiazem is used intravenously as an alternative to verapamil in a dose of 0.25 mg/kg over 10 minutesfollowed by 5 mg/hr.

OTHER ANTIARRHYTHMIC DRUGS

Adenosine

- Intravenous adenosine is the drug of choice for abolishing acute supraventricular tachycardia (PSVT).

- Adenosine is a naturally occurring nucleoside having rapid and short antiarrythmic action.
- It decreases conduction velocity, prolongs the refractory period, decreases automaticity in the AV node and dilates coronaries.
- It is given by rapid IV injection in a dose of 6–12 mg and over a period of 1–3 seconds.
- It has an extremely short t½ of about 10 seconds and the action is also rapidly terminated in about 15–30 seconds as it is rapidly taken up by erythrocytes and endothelial cells.
- It has low toxicity but causes flushing, chest pain, and hypotension.

Atropine

- It is used in the treatment of sinus bradycardia.
- It blocks the M_2 muscarinic receptors and produces increase in heart rate.

Magnesium Sulfate

- Magnesium is necessary for the transport of sodium, calcium, and potassium across cell membranes.
- It slows the rate of SA node impulse formation and prolongs conduction time along the myocardial tissue.
- Intravenous magnesium sulfate is used to treat digitalis induced arrhythmias and torsades de pointes.

Digitalis

- Digoxin is used in the treatment of atrial fibrillations to control the ventricular rate.
- It increases the myocardial contractile force and decreases the Heart rate and A-V conduction.

CHOICE OF ANTIARRHYTHMICS FOR CARDIAC ARRHYTHMIAS

Refer to Table 10.11 for choice of antiarrhythmics for cardiac arrhythmias.

TABLE 10.11: Arrhythmias and their drugs of choice

Arrhythmias	Drugs
Atrial extrasystoles	No drug if asymptomatic or non-disturbing Propranolol (only if symptomatic)
Paroxysmal supraventricular tachycardia (PSVT)	**Therapeutic:** IV adenosine/verapamil/diltiazem/esmolol **Prophylaxis:** Oral, verapamil/diltiazem/propranolol/sotalol
Atrial fibrillation (AF)	**For reversal of sinus rhythm:** Cardioversion **For persistence AF:** IV amiodarone **Maintenance of sinus rhythm:** Sotalol/propafenone/amiodarone/dronedarone/disopyramide

Contd...

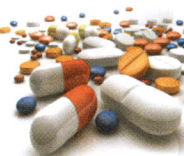

Arrhythmias	Drugs
Atrial flutter (AFl)	**For reversal of sinus rhythm:** Cardioversion, radiofrequency ablation **For control of ventricular rate:** Propranolol/verapamil/diltiazem + digoxinor Amiodarone
Wolff-Parkinson-White syndrome (WPW) tachycardia	**For termination:** Radiofrequency ablation, cardioversion **For maintenance:** Propafenone/procainamide
Acute-MI arrhythmia	**For MI induced bradycardia:** IV atropine **For prevention of ventricular extrasystol or tachycardia:** IV lidocaine/procainamide/amiodarone **For serious arrhythmias:** Cardioversion
Chronic ventricular tachycardia	**For management:** Propranolol/amiodarone (oral) **For maintenance:** Amiodarone/sotalol
Ventricular fibrillation (VF)	**For termination:** Defibrillation + amiodarone (IV) **For prevention:** Amiodarone (oral)/propranolol

 ## Drug Interactions

- The levels of digoxin and warfarin are increased by amiodarone by reducing their renal clearance.
- Amiodarone can produce additive A-V block, if given along with calcium channel blockers or β blockers.
- Lignocaine should not be given to the patient on β blockers, quinidine or other antiarrhythmic drugs as it can cause excessive bradycardia, cardiac depression and precipitation of arrhythmias.

 ## Nursing Implications

- **Antiarrhythmics**
  - Assess for contraindications or cautions and any known allergies to the drugs to be administered to avoid hypersensitivity reactions.
  - The schedule prescribed should be strictly followed.
  - Nurse should monitor the pulse, blood pressure, ECG, respiratory rate before, during and after the therapy and enter it immediately in the record file of patient.
  - The treating physician should be informed immediately about any abnormal deviation (low/high) of the blood pressure and cardiac rhythm.
  - Ensure that emergency life support equipment is readily available to treat severe adverse reactions that might occur.
  - Consult with the prescriber to reduce the dose in patients with renal or hepatic dysfunction; reduced dose may be needed to ensure therapeutic effects without increased risk of toxic effects.
  - Arrange for periodic monitoring of cardiac rhythm when the patient is receiving long-term therapy to evaluate effects on cardiac status.
  - Monitor for adverse effects (sedation, hypotension, cardiac arrhythmias, respiratory depression, and CNS effects).
  - Evaluate the effectiveness of the teaching plan (patient can name drug, dosage, adverse effects to watch for, specific measures to avoid them, and the importance of continued follow-up).

PLASMA EXPANDERS

- The plasma volume expanders are the solutions used for immediate maintenance of blood volume in case of emergency hypovolemic situations.
- These are high molecular weight substances which retain fluid in the vascular compartment when infused intravenously.
- These solutions are used to correct hypovolemia due to loss of blood or plasma.
- In emergency conditions, immediate volume replacement is essential to maintain blood pressure and tissue perfusion.

PROPERTIES OF AN IDEAL PLASMA EXPANDER

- An ideal plasma expander should be easily affordable and available.
- It should remain stable for longer duration at room temperature.
- The pH, viscosity and oncotic pressure of the solution should be comparable to plasma.

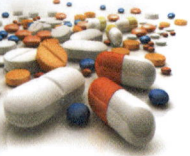

- It should be longer acting, i.e., it should remain in circulation for an adequate period.
- It should be non-pyrogenic and non-antigenic.
- It should not interfere with blood grouping and cross matching.

The commonly used plasma expanders are:

- Human albumin
- Dextran
- Degraded gelatin polymer or polygeline
- Hydroxyethyl starch or hetastarch
- Polyvinyl pyrrolidone (PVP).

HUMAN ALBUMIN

- Human albumin is prepared from pooled human plasma.
- 100 mL of 20% human albumin solution is osmotically equivalent to about 400 mL of fresh frozen plasma or to 800 mL of whole blood.
- It can be used irrespective of patient's blood group.
- As the process of its preparation involves heat treatment, the risk of transmitting serum hepatitis is not there.
- It is used in patients of hypovolemia, burns, shock, hypoproteinemia, acute liver failure and dialysis.
- It can cause hypersensitivity and overloading of intravascular fluid volume. Fever can occur sometimes with its use. Affordability is also a matter of concern with its use.
- It is available as 5% and 20% 100 mL infusion.

DEXTRAN

- It is a polysaccharide and is available in two forms, Dextran-70 and Dextran-40. It is obtained from sugar beet. Dextran-70 (MW 70,000).
- It is commonly used preparation with a prolonged effect for nearly 24 hours as its excretion occurs over week's time.
- It is infused as 6% solution and is preferred when small volumes of fluids are required.
- The major disadvantage is its propensity to interfere with blood grouping and cross matching, cross-reaction with dextran and interference with coagulation and platelet function.
- It can cause anaphylactic reaction, urticaria, itching, bronchospasm and prolongation of bleeding time. Dextran-40 (MW 40,000)
- It is given by IV infusion as 10% solution and acts more rapidly than dextran-70.
- It reduces blood viscosity, inhibits sludging of RBC and improves microcirculation.
- It acts for a shorter duration than dextran 70 due to early excretion.
- Its dose should not exceed 20 mL/kg in 24 hours.

Dextrans are the most commonly used plasma expanders due to their easy affordability and long shelf life up to 10 years.

DEGRADED GELATIN POLYMER OR POLYGELINE

- It is a polypeptide obtained from ox collagen and has molecular weight of 30,000.
- It has a shelf life of three years and is expensive than dextran.
- The plasma volume expansion lasts for up to 12 hours as it is excreted very slowly by the renals.
- It exerts oncotic pressure similar to albumin.
- It is neither antigenic nor show any interference with blood grouping and cross-matching.
- It is used as hemostatic in surgical procedures and as a priming agent in heart-lung and dialysis machines.
- It can cause hypersensitivity reactions like flushing, urticaria, wheezing and lowering of blood pressure.
- It is available as 3.5% solution in balanced electrolyte medium in 500 mL vac.

HYDROXYETHYL STARCH OR HETASTARCH

- It is derived from starch and is lesser in use due to side effects.
- It acts by increasing the osmotic effect similar to albumin.
- It is stable at room temperature and acts for more than 24 hours.
- It does not show any interference with blood grouping and cross matching.
- It is used to improve granulocyte harvesting during leukophoresis procedures.
- The main side effects with its use are vomiting, mild fever, itching, flu like symptoms, swelling of salivary glands and anaphylactoid reactions, which include urticaria, periorbital edema and bronchospasm.

POLYVINYL PYRROLIDONE (PVP)

- It is a synthetic polymer and interferes with blood grouping and cross matching.
- It is rarely used these days due to antigenicity and histamine releasing property.
- It binds to drugs like insulin and penicillins and reduces their effects.

THERAPEUTIC USES OF PLASMA EXPANDERS

Plasma expanders are used primarily as substitutes for plasma in acute phase of burns, hypovolemic shock, septic shock, severe trauma, surgical procedures, dialysis and extensive fluid loss.

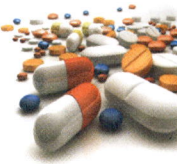

CONTRAINDICATIONS

Plasma expanders are contraindicated in congestive cardiac failure, renal failure, hepatic failure, severe anemia and pulmonary edema.

COAGULANTS AND ANTICOAGULANTS

Coagulation: The process of changing of blood from a fluid state to a solid state is known as coagulation. Normally, this is a natural process in the body to prevent blood loss by plugging the injured site.

- The vascular system must maintain an intricate balance between the tendency to clot or form a solid state, and the need to "unclot," or reverse coagulation, to keep the vessels open and the blood flowing.
- After an injury to the body tissues, there is a natural mechanism, which helps to stop the blood loss by involvement of a complex hemostatic mechanism. This mechanism is described in Figure 10.10.

BLOOD CLOTTING FACTORS

Blood clotting factors are given in Table 10.12.
The coagulation cascade along with various factors are given in Figure 10.11.

COAGULANTS

- Coagulants are the drugs that promote coagulation and control bleeding.
- They are also called hemostatic agents.

These drugs are of two types (Table 10.13):
- Systemic coagulants.
- Local coagulants (styptics).

TABLE 10.12: Blood clotting factors

Component or Factor	Common Synonym
I	Fibrinogen
II	Prothrombin
III	Tissue thromboplastin
IV	Calcium
V	Proaccelerin
VI	Accerin, supposed to be active form of factor V
VII	Proconvertin
VIII	Antihemophilic factor (AHF)
IX	Christmas factor, plasma thromboplastin component (PTC)
X	Stuart-Prower factor
XI	Plasma thromboplastin antecedent (PTA)
XII	Hageman factor
XIII	Fibrin-stabilizing factor
XIV	Prekallikrein
XV	kallikrein
XVI	Platelet factor

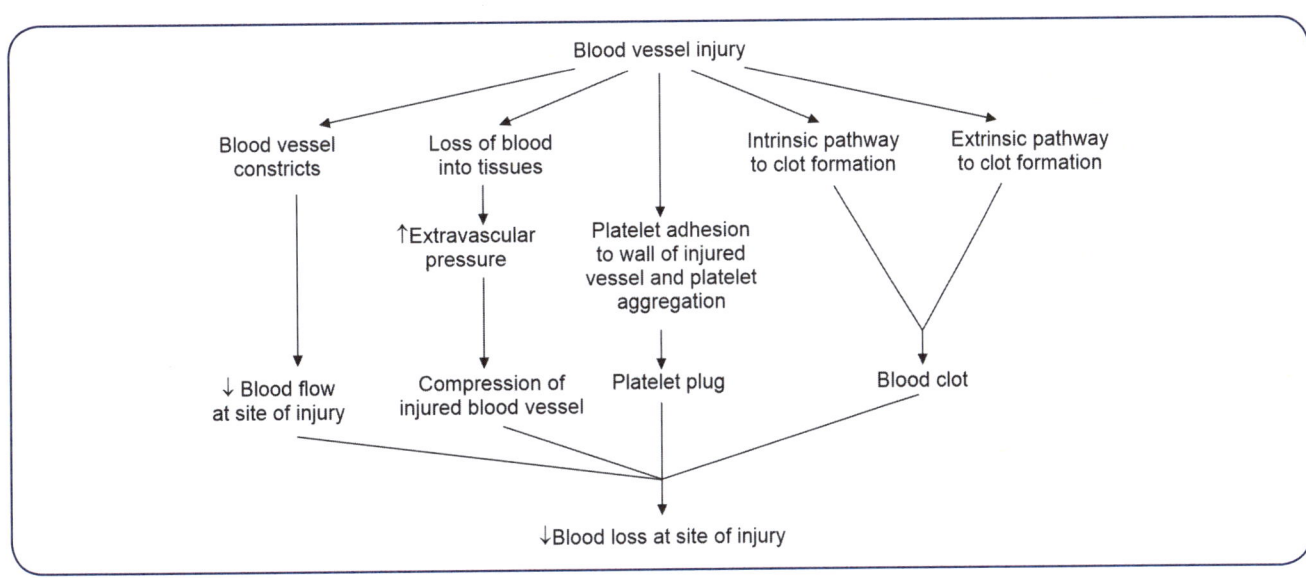

FIG. 10.10: Process of blood coagulation after injury

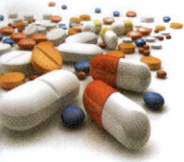

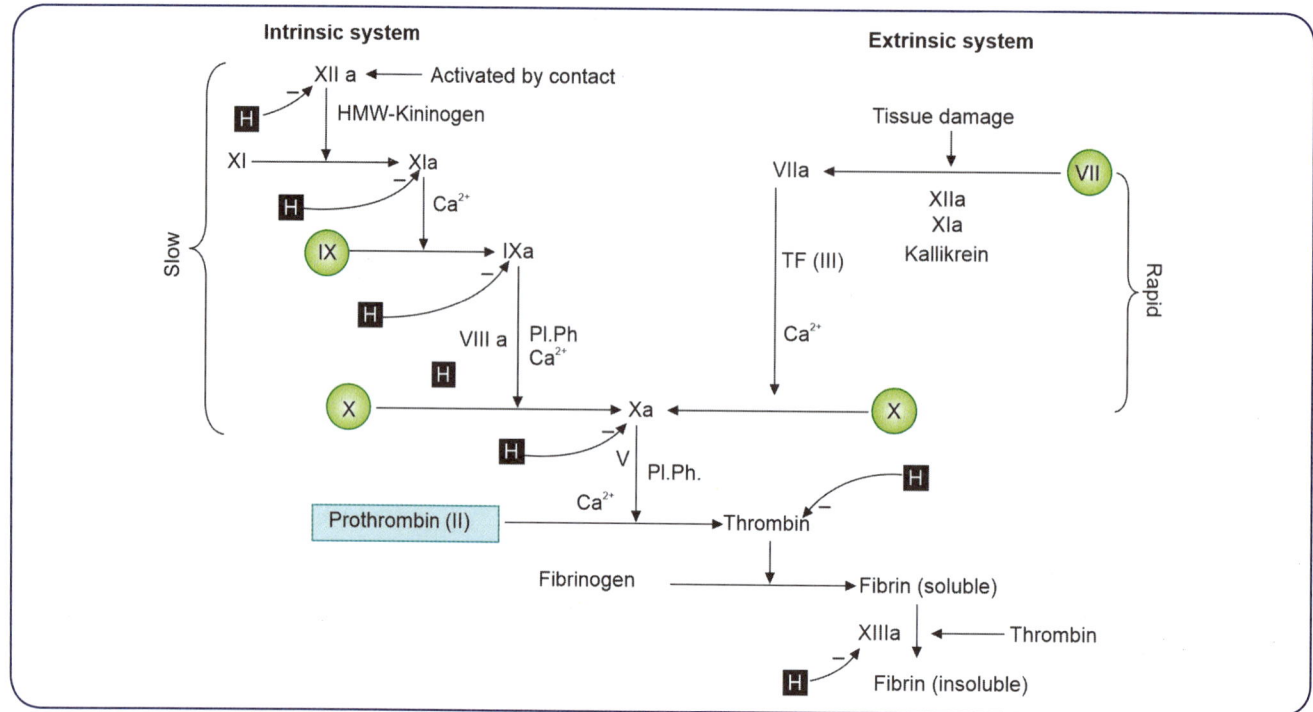

FIG. 10.11: The coagulation cascade

The vitamin K dependent factors have been encircled, Factors inactivated by heparin (H) are in red; the more important inhibited steps are highlighted by thick arrow. a—activated form; Pl.Ph.—Platelet phospholipid; HMW—High molecular weight; TF—Tissue factor (factor III)

TABLE 10.13: Systemic and local coagulants

Systemic coagulants	Local coagulants (styptics)
Vitamin K	Adrenaline
Ethamsylate	Fibrin glue
Desmopressin	Gelatin
Fibrinogen	Thrombin
Anti-hemophillic factor	Oxidized cellulose
Tranexamic acid	Hemocoagulase
Epsilon aminocaproic acid	Tranexamic acid

Systemic Coagulants Vitamin K

Vitamin K

- Vitamin K (coagulation vitamin) is essential for the coagulation process. It is not directly involved in the clotting process but required for the synthesis of four clotting factors in the liver: Factor II, VII, IX and X.
- It occurs naturally in two forms: Phylloquinone (K_1) from plant source and menaquinone (K_2) which is synthesized by colonic bacteria (*E. coli*) in the colon.
- K_3 is the synthetic form and is available as Fat-soluble forms (menadione, acetomenaphthone) and water-soluble forms (Menadione sodium bisulfate and menadione sod. diphosphate).

Dietary sources

Green leafy vegetables such as cabbage, spinach and liver, cheese, cereals, nuts, and egg yolk, etc. Wheat germ oil is the richest source.

Physiological functions

Vitamin K is essential for formation of clotting factor-II, VII, IX, X, protein-C and S.

Deficiency symptoms

- Vitamin K is only temporarily concentrated in liver and this store can be exhausted within one week.
- The deficiency of Vitamin K occurs due to liver disease, obstructive jaundice, malabsorption, long-term antimicrobial therapy, which alters intestinal flora.
- The most important manifestation is bleeding tendency due to lowering of the levels of prothrombin and other clotting factors in blood. Hematuria is usually first to occur; other common sites of bleeding are gastrointestinal tract, nose and under the skin where it presents in the form of hemorrhagic spots.

Recommended dietary allowance (RDA)

- Normal adult requirement is 50–100 µg/day.
- As it can be synthesized in the colon, even 3–10 µg/day may be sufficient.

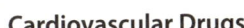

Some conditions where Vitamin K is useful are:

- For prevention of hemorrhagic disease of the newborn: All newborns especially premature infants have low levels of prothrombin and other clotting factors. Vitamin K 1 mg IM soon after birth has been recommended routinely.
- Alternatively, 5–10 mg IM to the mother 4–12 hours before delivery can be given. Hemorrhagic disease of the newborn can be effectively prevented/treated by such medication.
- Menadione (K3) should not be used for this purpose as patients with G-6-PD deficiency and neonates are especially susceptible. In the newborn menadione or its salts can precipitate kernicterus.
- As an antidote in overdose of oral anticoagulants.
- In patients suffering from liver disease (cirrhosis, viral hepatitis).
- Patients on prolonged antimicrobial therapy.
- Patients with obstructive jaundice or malabsorption syndromes (sprue, regional ileitis, steatorrhea, etc). The therapy given is Vitamin K 10 mg IM/day, or orally along with bile salts for better absorption.

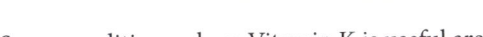

Hypervitaminosis K
- It has not been reported.
- Only severe allergic or anaphylactoid reactions can occur with IV injection of vitamin K formulations.

Ethamsylate

- It increases capillary wall stability by antihyaluronidase action. It decreases PGI_2 synthesis, and corrects abnormalities of platelet adhesion and promotes platelet aggregation.
- It is used in the prevention and treatment of capillary bleeding.
- Its common indications are menorrhagia, postpartum hemorrhage, after abortion, epistaxis, after tooth extraction and hematuria.
- Main side effects observed are nausea, rash, headache, and acute hypotension if given by fast IV injection.
- It is given in a dose of 250–500 mg TDS orally or IV.

Desmopressin

- It is an analog to vasopressin and increases the plasma concentration of factor-VIII, von Willebrand factor and directly activates platelets.
- It is a selective V_2 agonist, 12 times more potent than AVP.
- Desmopressin is useful for the treatment of hemophilia-A and von-Willebrand disease.

Fibrinogen

- It is obtained from human plasma and is a promising hemostatic agent.
- It is used to control bleeding in hemophilia, hypofibrinogenemia and in antihemophilic globulin deficiency.
- It is available as IV infusion 0.5 per bottle.

Antihemophillic Factor

- It contains coagulation factor VIII and is concentrated human AHG obtained from pooled human plasma. It is also synthesized by DNA recombinant technology.
- It is therapeutically used in hemophilia and AHG deficiency.
- It is given in a dose of 10–20 IU/kg by IV infusion, repeated 6–12 hourly.

Tranexamic Acid and Epsilon Aminocaproic Acid (EACA)

- These are antifibronolytic agents.
- They inhibit the activation of plasminogen and dissolution of clot.
- They are available as oral and IV form.
- They are indicated in:
  - To counteract the effect of fibrinolytic drugs.
  - For controlling the bleeding in tonsillectomy, prostatic surgery, tooth extraction in hemophiliacs.
  - Menorrhagia, menometrorrhagia and dysfunctional uterine bleeding (DUB).
  - Recurrent epistaxis.
- The major side effects are nausea, vomiting, thromboembolic states, allergic reactions, disturbed color vision, etc.
- Tranaxemic acid is given in a dose of 500–1000 mg TDS, orally and IV.

Local Coagulants (Styptics)

- Local coagulants are also known as styptics or **hemostatics (hemo-blood and statics to stop)**.
- These substances are used locally to stop the bleeding from the oozing surfaces such as abrasions, bleeding tooth socket after tooth extraction, etc.
- **Normal hemostasis involves three steps:**
  - **Vasoconstriction or contraction of injured vessel wall for a few minutes.**
  - **Adhesion and aggregation of platelets to form a plug.**
  - **Formation of a blood clot.**
- This is followed by dissolution of the clot by the process of fibrinolysis and maintenance of normal circulation.
- The most preferred and effective method of stopping the external bleeding is manual pressure, cotton-gauze pressure pack or by suturing.

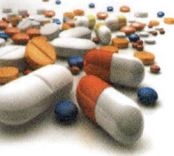

- Control of bleeding may be aided by applying *adrenaline locally* as it causes local vasoconstriction.
- A cotton pad soaked with 0.1% adrenaline is used to control capillary bleeding such as epistaxis and after tooth extraction, etc.
- Adrenaline is available in combination with lignocaine to provide better surgical field, but should be avoided in patients suffering from hypertension or cardiovascular disease.
- *Thrombin* obtained from bovine plasma is used topically to control capillary bleeding. It may cause hypersensitivity reactions also.
- **Gelatin foam, oxidized cellulose** are absorbable materials, available as film or sponge and are used in surgical procedures to control the bleeding of capillaries or arterioles. After applied dry, they swell up and form meshwork, which helps in the clotting mechanism and stops bleeding. These materials are absorbed within 4 weeks. The main adverse effects seen with these are tissue necrosis, vascular stenosis and nerve damage.
- **Astringents** such as tannic acid or metallic salts (alum) are occasionally applied for bleeding gums, cuts during shaving, bleeding piles, etc.

ANTICOAGULANTS

- These drugs reduce the coagulability of blood by interfering with the normal coagulation process. These drugs act in the clotting cascade and interfere either in the thrombin formation or inhibit the action of thrombin.
- Drugs in this class are as follows:

- **Used *in vivo***
  - **Parenteral anticoagulants**
    - **Indirect thrombin inhibitors**: Heparin, low molecular weight heparins, Fondaparinux, Danaparoid
    - **Direct thrombin inhibitors**: Lepirudin, bivalirudin, argatroban
  - **Oral anticoagulants**
    - **Coumarin derivatives:** Dicumarol, warfarin sodium Acenocoumarol
    - **Indandione derivative:** Phenindione
    - **Direct factor Xa inhibitors**: Rivaroxaban
    - **Oral direct thrombin inhibitor:** Dabigatran etexilate
- **Used *in vitro***
  - **Heparin**
  - **Calcium complexing agents**
    - Sodium citrate
    - Sodium oxalate
    - Sodium edetate

Indirect Thrombin Inhibitors

(Heparin, Low molecular weight heparins, Fondaparinux, Danaparoid)

Heparin

- In 1916, McLean discovered an anticoagulant substance in liver.
- In 1918, Howell and Holt named it heparin (due to its extraction from liver).
- In 1937, heparin was used in clinical practice after extracting the purified form.
- It is a strong organic acid having molecular weight of 10,000–30,000 *Da*.
- As it is present in the mast cells, it is normally present in all body tissues, which contain mast cells.
- Commercially, it is obtained from pig intestinal mucosa and ox lung.
- It acts as anticoagulant both in vivo and in vitro.
- It is also known as unfractionated heparin (UFH).

Mechanism of action

- Heparin binds to antithrombin III (natural endogenous anticoagulant) and heparin-antithrombin-III complex is formed.
- This heparin-antithrombin-III complex inactivates the clotting factors of both intrinsic and common pathway. (XIIa, XIa, IX, Xa, XIIIa, II) by binding to them.
- Thus, the anticoagulant effect is exerted mainly by inhibition of factor Xa and thrombin mediated conversion of fibrinogen to fibrin (refer coagulation cascade).
- To summarize, heparin speeds up the antithrombin III activity against factor IIa and factor Xa by 1000 times.

Pharmacological effects of heparin

- As anticoagulant
- As antiplatelet agent: By inhibiting the platelet aggregation.
- By activating lipoprotein lipase from the vessels wall and tissues, it acts as lipemia clearing agent.

Different effects of heparin are shown in Figure 10.12.

Pharmacokinetics

- It is not absorbed by oral route due to its large size and highly ionized nature.
- Therefore, it is given by IV route (acts immediately) and subcutaneous route (acts within an hour).
- It does not cross blood-brain barrier and placenta. Hence, can be given safely in pregnancy.
- It is metabolized in liver *by heparinase enzyme* and excreted through kidneys.
- The plasma t½ is 1–2 hours and is dose dependent.

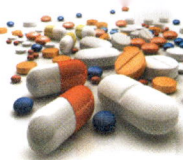

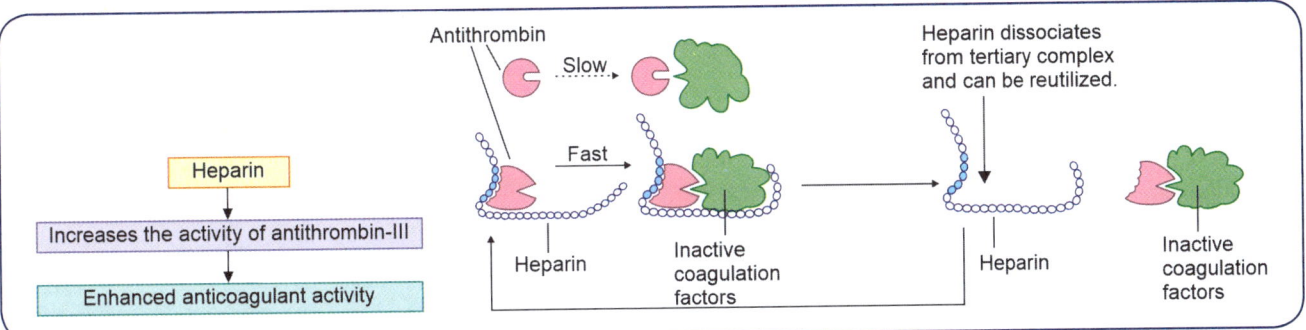

FIG. 10.12: Effects of heparin. Heparin accelerates inactivation of coagulation factors by antithrombin

- It is prolonged in kidney and liver diseases and shortened in pulmonary embolism.

Dose

- Adult: 5000–10,000 IU, IV bolus dose followed by 750–1000 IU/hr IV infusion.
- Children: 50–100 IU/kg.

Indications

- Prophylaxis of post-operative venous thrombosis.
- Post myocardial infarction.
- Pulmonary embolism.
- Deep venous thrombosis.
- Heparinization of central line and chemopods.

Adverse effects

- First clinical sign of adverse effect of heparin is, hematuria.
- The other side effects are bleeding, thrombocytopenia, reversible alopecia, osteoporosis, hepatotoxicity, and rarely hypersensitivity reaction.
- Heparin induced thrombocytopenia is a common entity and was generally manifested as decreased platelet count. In this condition, withdrawal of drug is helpful.
- On intramuscular injection, it may cause hematomas.
- The monitoring of activated partial thromboplastin time (aPTT) ratio is mandatory, if the ratio of aPTT is greater than three, there is an increased risk of bleeding.

Protamine Sulfate (Heparin Antagonist)

- It is a strong base and obtained from fish sperm.
- *Protamine sulfate* acts as an antidote for heparin overdose and is given in a dose of 1 mg IV for every 100 IU of heparin.
- It is used after cardiovascular surgeries when it has been administered in higher doses and the action needs to be terminated rapidly.

Low Molecular Weight Heparins (LMWHs)

(Enoxaparin, Deltaparin, Parnaparin, Reviparin, Ardeparin, Nadroparin, Tinzaparin)

- LMWHs have molecular weight lower than heparin (3,000–7,000 Da).
- These are obtained by the enzymatic treatment of unfractionated heparin and are also known as fractionated heparins (FHs).
- LMWHs make a complex with antithrombin III and inactivate factor Xa.
- The advantages of LMWHs over heparin are:
  - Less antigenic due to low molecular weight.
  - Better subcutaneous bioavailability.
  - Longer duration of action.
  - Low incidence of thrombocytopenia and osteoporosis.
  - aPTT monitoring is generally not required.

Various low molecular weight heparins (LMWHs) are given in Table 10.14.

TABLE 10.14: Various LMWHs with dosage schedules

Drug	Therapeutic dose	Prophylactic dose
Enoxaparin	1 mg/kg, SC, twice daily.	20-40 mg, SC, once daily.
Deltaparin	200 IU/kg SC, once daily.	2500 IU SC, once daily.
Parnaparin	6400 IU SC, once daily.	3200 IU SC, once daily.
Reviparin	3436 IU SC, once daily.	0.25 mL (1432 IU) SC, once daily.

Contd...

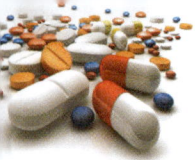

Drug	Therapeutic dose	Prophylactic dose
Ardeparin	2500-5000 IU SC, once daily.	2500 IU SC, once daily.
Nadroparin	4000-6000 IU SC, once daily/twice daily.	3000 IU SC, once daily/twice daily.
Tinzaparin	3500 IU SC, once daily.	1700 IU SC, once daily.
Note: All are available in prefilled syringes forms.		

Abbreviation: SC, subcutaneous

Indications of LMWHs

- Prophylaxis of deep venous thrombosis (DVT) in immobilized patients such as post-surgical or coma patients.
- Post myocardial infarction.
- Prophylaxis of pulmonary embolism.
- Treatment of deep venous thrombosis.
- For the maintenance of patency of cannula in dialysis patient, center line and chemopods.

Adverse effects

The adverse effects like thrombocytopenia and interference with hemostatis are seen very rarely.

Fondaparinux

- It is a synthetic derivative of heparin.
- It has pharmacological similarity to LMWHs with longer plasma half-life (17–21 hours).
- It has 100% bioavailability.
- It is given in a dose of 5–10 mg SC, OD.
- The adverse effects like thrombocytopenia and osteoporosis are even lesser than LMWHs.
- *Idraparinux* is an ultra long acting derivative of fondaparinux with t½ of 5–6 days.

Danaparoid

- It is a mixture of heparin like natural substances (84% heparin sulfate +12% dermatan sulfate + 4% chondroitin sulfate).
- It is obtained from pig intestinal mucosa.
- It has longer plasma t½ of 24 hours.
- It is used in patients with heparin induced thrombocytopenia as an alternative therapy.

Direct Thrombin Inhibitors

(Lepirudin, Bivalirudin, Argatroban)

Lepirudin

- It is a recombinant preparation of hirudin.
- It inhibits thrombin directly.
- Indicated in heparin induced thrombocytopenia.

- It cannot be given repeatedly due to formation of anti-hirudin antibodies and higher risk of anaphylaxis.
- There is no antidote available against lepirudin.

Bivalirudin

- Synthetic analog of hirudin with pharmacological actions similar to lepirudin.
- It has fast onset and offset of action due to its reversible binding nature.
- It does not form anti-hirudin antibodies.

Argatroban

- It is a reversible direct thrombin inhibitor given by IV infusion.
- It is used in patients with heparin-induced thrombocytopenia as an alternative therapy.

Oral Anticoagulants

Coumarin Derivatives

(Dicumarol, Warfarin sodium, Acenocoumarol)
- These anticoagulants act as competitive antagonists of vitamin K and interfere with the synthesis of vitamin K dependent clotting factors (II, VII, IX, X).
- Therefore, these agents are active only *in vivo* and not *in vitro*.
- They block the γ-carboxylation of glutamate residues in these factors, which is necessary to their action.
- It takes 1–3 days for the action to start as the oral anticoagulants do not destroy the already circulating clotting factors and the effect weans off after 5–7 days of stopping the drug.

Warfarin sodium

- It is the most commonly used anticoagulant.
- It is well absorbed orally and excreted through kidneys.
- It undergoes enterohepatic circulation.
- It crosses placental barrier and can affect the fetus and causes fetal warfarin syndrome. Hence, contraindicated during pregnancy.
- It is given in a dose of 1–5 mg OD and the dose is regulated according to the International Normalized Ratio (INR).

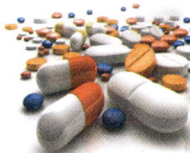

Dicumarol

- Dicumarol has unpredictable and slow oral absorption.
- It is not preferred due to GI disturbances as major side effects.
- It is given in a dose of 50 mg OD.

Acenocoumarol

- It acts more rapidly and acts for a longer time due to active metabolites.
- It causes stomatitis, gastritis, and dermatitis as major side effects.
- It is given in a dose of 8–10 mg as loading dose and then 2–8 mg as maintenance dose.

Indandione Derivative

(Phenindione, Anisindione)
- They have mechanism of action similar to coumarine derivatives.
- These agents are rarely used therapeutically due to high incidence of toxicities.

Direct Factor X Inhibitors

(Rivaroxaban, Apixaban)
- The anticoagulant action of these agents is due to binding to factor Xa and directly inactivating it immediately.
- These are given by oral route and action starts within 3–4 hours of administration of drug.
- Rivaroxaban is given in a fixed dose of 10 mg OD.
- They are indicated for the prophylaxis of embolism and stroke in-patient of atrial fibrillations and deep vein thrombosis in patient with coma and major surgeries.
- Its major advantage is:
  - Very rapid onset of action
  - No laboratory monitoring is required
- They have mild side effects such as nausea, hypotension, tachycardia and rarely bleeding episodes.

Oral Direct Thrombin Inhibitor

(Dabigatran etexilate)

Dabigatran etexilate

- It is a prodrug and converted to active metabolite dabigatran.
- It exerts a rapid anticoagulant action by reversibly inhibiting the thrombin (IIa).
- It is given in a dose of 110 mg OD (*75 mg OD in the geriatric patients more than 75 year of age*).
- It is indicated for the prophylaxis of embolism and stroke in-patient of atrial fibrillations and DVT in patients with coma and major surgeries.
- Its major advantage is:
  - Very rapid onset of action
  - No laboratory monitoring is required.

Common Indications of Oral Anticoagulants

- For prevention and treatment of DVT.
- For prevention of thromboembobolism in vascular and valvular surgeries.
- For prophylaxis in the patient of stroke, major surgeries and coma.
- For unstable angina.
- Rheumatic valvular disease to prevent embolism as atrial fibrillation is quite common in-patient with rheumatic heart disease.

Common Adverse Effects of Oral Anticoagulants

- The commonest side effect of anticoagulant is hemorrhage, which can occur from any site of the body such as epistaxis, hematuria, GI bleed, intracranial bleed, etc. Other side effects include GI disturbance, allergic reactions and teratogenicity.

  These side effects occur only when the recommended dose is exceeded and therapy is not monitored properly.

  Management of adverse effects:
- Stop the further administration of the responsible drug.
- Fresh blood transfusion is given because it is the best source of clotting factors. Alternatively, fresh frozen plasma (FFP) is preferred, if available.
- Vitamin-K_1 can be administered as an antidote.

Drug Interactions

- The anticoagulant action of oral anticoagulants is enhanced by the broad-spectrum antibiotics. These drugs decrease the production of vitamin-K by inhibiting the GI flora.
- Aspirin synergizes the anticoagulant effect of warfarin by displacing it from the protein binding site. Hence, concurrent use should be avoided.
- Ceftriaxone/cefoperazone and warfarin cause hypoprothrombinemia. Hence, concurrent use should be avoided.
- The metabolism of warfarin is inhibited by phenytoin, allopurinol metronidazole, erythromycin, and amiodarone. Hence, the dose of warfarin should be adjusted accordingly.
- The metabolism of oral anticoagulants is induced by griseofulvin, rifampin, carbamazepine and barbiturates. Hence, the dose of oral anticoagulants should be adjusted accordingly.
- Oral contraceptives induce the synthesis of clotting factors (II, VII, IX, X) and antagonize the action of oral anticoagulants.

Nursing Implications

☞ **Coagulants and anticoagulants**

☛ Assess for any known allergies to these drugs to avoid potential hypersensitivity reactions.

☛ Evaluate the effectiveness of drug therapy and monitor the patient regularly for any sign of blood loss (petechiae, bleeding gums, bruises, dark-colored stools, dark-colored urine) to evaluate the effectiveness of the drug dose and to determine the need to consult with the prescriber if bleeding becomes apparent.

☛ Establish safety precautions to protect the patient from injury.

☛ Maintain antidotes on standby (protamine sulfate for heparin, vitamin K for warfarin) in case of overdose.

☛ Monitor the patient carefully whenever any change in drug regimen is made to look for possible drug-drug interactions.

☛ Monitor patient response to the drug by regular monitoring of bleeding time, clotting time, international normalized ratio (INR), activated partial thromboplastin time (APTT), etc. and one should be aware of the importance of their different levels.

☛ Educate the patient about the importance of continued follow-up.

☛ Evaluate the effectiveness of the teaching plan (patient can name drug, dosage, adverse effects to watch for, and specific measures to avoid them.)

ANTIPLATELETS AND FIBRINOLYTICS

ANTIPLATELETS

The drugs which inhibit the platelets aggregation are known as antiplatelet drugs. Platelets aggregation is an essential step in the formation of hemostatic plug at the site of vascular injury (Fig. 10.13). These drugs have their role in some pathologic conditions where formation of this hemostatic plug is to be prevented.

The various types of antiplatelet drugs are as follows:

- **PG synthesis inhibitors:** Aspirin
- **Phosphodiesterase inhibitor:** Dipyridamole
- **ADP antagonist:** Ticlopidine, Clopidogrel, Prasugrel
- **Glycoprotein IIb/IIIa receptor antagonist:** Abciximab, Eptifibatide, Tirofiban

Prostaglandin Synthesis Inhibitors

Aspirin

- Aspirin inactivates the platelet cyclooxygenase enzyme irreversibly.
- It inhibits the synthesis of both TXA_2 and PGI_2 at high doses and only TXA_2 at low doses. Hence, it is used in low doses for the prophylaxis purpose.

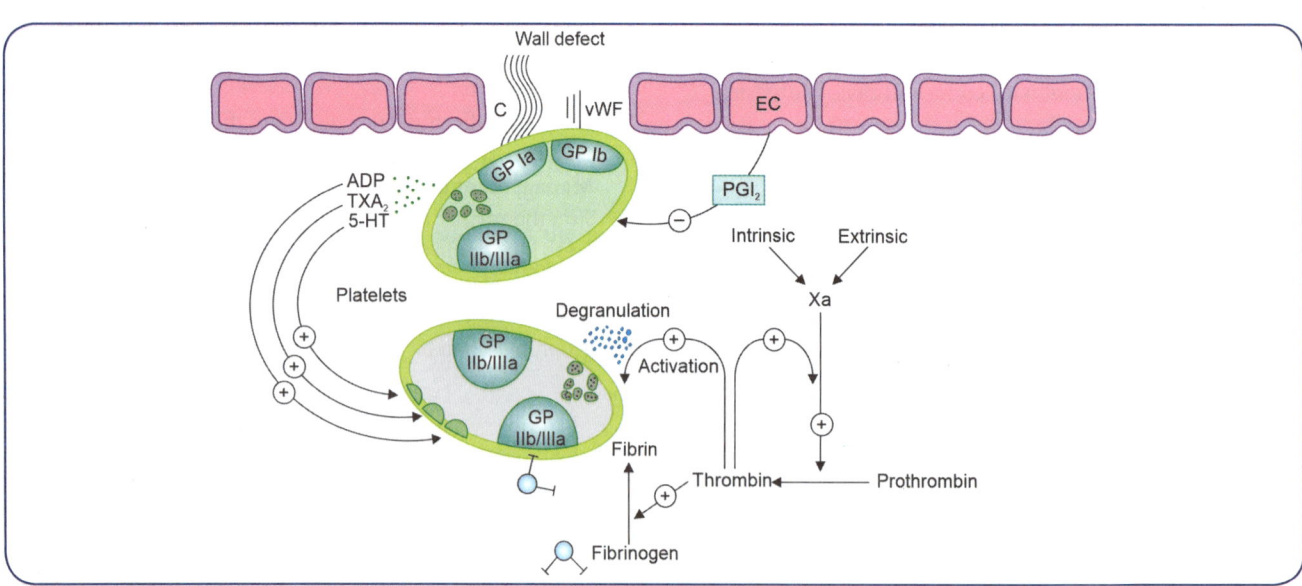

FIG. 10.13: Thrombus formation at the site of the damaged vascular wall (EC, endothelial cell) and the role of platelets and clotting factors. Platelet membrane receptors include the glycoprotein (GP) Ia receptor, binding to collagen (C); GP Ib receptor, binding von Willebrand factor (vWF); and GP IIb/IIIa, which binds fibrinogen and other macromolecules. Antiplatelet prostacyclin (PGI 2) is released from the endothelium. Aggregating substances released from the degranulating platelet include adenosine diphosphate (ADP), thromboxane A 2 (TXA 2 , and serotonin (5-HT).

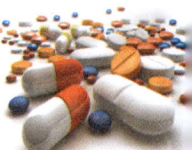

- The COX inhibition effect on the platelets last for 7–10 days (normal life span of platelets).
- It is given in a dose of 75–150 mg OD or 300 mg twice weekly.
- It is indicated for prophylaxis of stroke and myocardial infarction in susceptible individuals.

Phosphodiesterase Inhibitors

Dipyridamole

- It is a phosphodiesterase enzyme inhibitor and acts by interfering in the platelets function by increasing platelet adenosine monophosphate (AMP) levels.
- It is used in combination with aspirin or warfarin in the patients of prosthetic heart valves as a prophylactic measure to decrease the incidence of thromboembolism.
- It is given orally in a dose of 25–100 mg, TDS.
- Headache is the only and mild side effect.

ADP Antagonists

Ticlopidine, Clopidogrel, Prasugrel

- These are prodrugs and the active metabolites bind to the adenosine diphosphate (ADP) receptors ($P2Y_{12}$) on platelets and block them.
- **Platelet aggregation requires stimulation of ADP receptors. Blockade of these receptors leads to anti-aggregatory effect.**
- The effect of these drugs last for 5–7 days.
- **Ticlopidine** is given orally in a dose of 250 mg BD.
- **Clopidogrel** is given orally in a dose of 75 mg OD (300 mg as loading dose in suspected MI).
- **Prasugrel** is given orally in a dose of 10 mg OD (60 mg as loading dose).
- They are indicated for the prophylaxis of myocardial infarction, stroke, TIA, unstable angina, coronary artery bypass graft, etc. Prasugrel is specifically used in ST-elevation myocardial infarction (STEMI).
- The major side effects are increase in bleeding tendencies, GI disturbance, rashes, headache, etc.

Glycoprotein IIb/IIIa Receptor Antagonists

(Abciximab, Eptifibatide, Tirofiban)

- The glycoprotein IIB/IIIa (GP-IIb/IIIa) receptors are present on the platelet surface and have a role in platelet aggregation.
- Drugs such as *Abciximab, Eptifibatide, Tirofiban* block these receptors and inhibit the platelet agonists induced platelet aggregation.

Abciximab

- It is a monoclonal antibody and bind to the GP-IIb/IIIa receptor complex and inhibits platelets aggregation with high affinity and slow dissociation rate.
- It is given in a dose of 0.25 mg/kg IV bolus followed by 0.125 µg/kg/min IV infusion for 12 hours.
- It is indicated in acute coronary syndrome and patients undergoing coronary angioplasty and other percutaneous coronary interventions.
- It is given along with aspirin or heparin.
- It is non-antigenic, but expensive.
- The common side effects are hemorrhage, thrombocytopenia, arrhythmias and constipation.

Eptifibatide and Tirofiban

The pharmacological properties are similar to abciximab but due to quicker dissociation from the receptor site, the effect reverses in a shorter time of 6–10 hours.

Eptifibatide

- It is given in a dose of 180 µg/kg IV bolus, then 2 µg/kg/min IV infusion up to 72 hours for the management unstable angina.
- It is given in a dose of 180 µg/kg IV bolus, just before the procedure then 2 µg/kg/min IV infusion for 12–24 hours for coronary angioplasty.

Tirofiban

It is given in a dose of 0.4 µg/kg/minute for 30 minutes, then 0.1 µg/kg/minute for up to 48 hours for management of acute coronary syndromes.

Common Indications of Antiplatelets Drugs

- **Ischemic heart disease:**
  - Myocardial infarction: Aspirin in a dose of 300 mg stat is given in suspected myocardial infarction patient. Then 75–150 mg/day is given on long-term basis. Clopidogrel in addition is given to proven coronary artery disease (CAD) patients.
  - Unstable angina: Aspirin alone or in combination with clopidogrel reduces the risk of progression of angina to myocardial infarction and sudden death.
  - Angina pectoris: Aspirin daily in a dose of 75 mg/day prevents occurance of myocardial infarction.
- **Cardiac and other vascular procedures:**
  - Coronary angioplasty, stenting, coronary bypass graft: Aspirin alone or in combination with clopidogrel or abciximab reduces the risk of reocclusion.

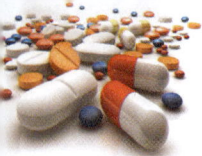

- Atrial fibrillation: Antiplatelet drugs prevent the thrombo-embolic events.
- Prosthetic heart valve: Antiplatelet drugs prevent the formation of microthrombi in these patients.
- Vascular grafts: These drugs help to maintain patency of grafts and prevent the reocclusion.
- Peripheral vascular disease.
- **Cerebrovascular accidents:** These drugs prevent the reccurence of stroke due to transient ischemic attacks. Aspirin or dipyridamole is given either alone or in combination.
- **Deep vein thrombosis and pulmonary thromboembolism:** These drugs have a prophylactic value in these disorders also.

FIBRINOLYTICS (THROMBOLYTICS)

- Fibrinolytics or thrombolytics are the drugs, which cause lysis of thrombus by activating natural fibrinolytic system. These drugs act as therapeutic agents to recanalize the vessels occluded by thrombus.
- In human body, tissue plasminogen activator, activates plasminogen, which generates plasmin. This plasmin breaks the insoluble fibrin to soluble fibrin fragments and thereby dissolves the clot.
- The various thrombolytics in use are *Streptokinase, Urokinase, Alteplase, Reteplase, Tenecteplase, etc.*

Mechanism of Action

- These agents bring about conversion of plasminogen to plasmin directly or indirectly. It causes breakdown of fibrin and thereby lysis of thrombus (Fig. 10.14).
- *Streptokinase* is obtained from β-hemolytic streptococci and is one of the first approved fibrinolytic agents. Streptokinase also catalyzes the degradation of clotting factors V and VII. Streptokinase is antigenic in nature and the antibodies formed after a single exposure of this agent persist in the body for at least five years. Repeated exposure within this period can cause anaphylactic reactions. An alternative thrombolytic agent like urokinase or tPA is used for subsequent thrombolysis, if required.

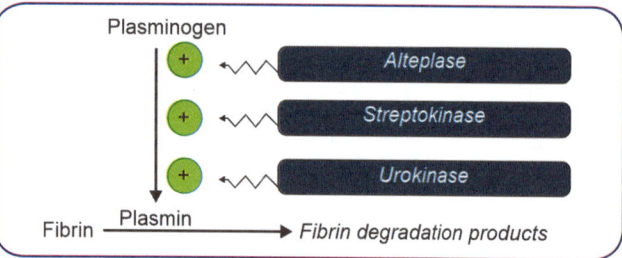

FIG. 10.14: Activation of plasminogen by thrombolytic drugs

- For myocardial infarction patients, it is given as IV infusion over 1 hour in a dose of 7.5–15 lac IU.
- **For deep vein thrombosis and pulmonary embolism:** Loading dose of 2.5 lac IU over ½–1 hour is followed by 1 lac IU/hr infusion for 24 hrs.
- **Urokinase** is an enzyme naturally obtained from human urine. For commercial preparation, human kidney cells are cultured for its extraction. It directly converts plasminogen into active plasmin and is approved for lysis of pulmonary emboli. Other uses of urokinase include treatment of acute myocardial infarction, arterial thromboembolism, coronary artery thrombosis, and severe deep vein thrombosis. Its use has decreased these days due to availability of better agents.
  - **For myocardial infarction patients** 2.5 lac IU is given intravenously over 10 minutes and it is followed by 5 lac IU over next one hour. The infusion can be stopped in between if evidence of recanalization is there. Alternatively, continuous infusion for up to two hours in a dose of 6000 IU/min can also be given.
  - **For deep vein thrombosis and pulmonary embolism:** 4400 IU/kg are given intravenously over 10 minutes and followed by 4400 IU/kg/hr for 12 hours.
- **Alteplase (recombinant tissue plasminogen activator or rt-PA):** In earlier times, it was known as tissue plasminogen activator (tPA). These days it is prepared by recombinant DNA technology using human tissue culture cells. Alteplase is "fibrin selective" at low doses, i.e., it rapidly activates the fibrin bound plasminigen present in the thrombus. It is non-antigenic.
  - **For the patient of myocardial infarction:** IV bolus dose of 15 mg, followed by infusion of 50 mg over 30 minutes and then 35 mg over the next 1 hour is given. A total 90 minutes treatment period is there.
  - **For pulmonary embolism:** 100 mg IV infusion is given in a period of over 2 hours.
  - **For ischemic stroke:** A total dose of 0.9 mg/kg is given. Out of this, 10% of the dose is injected in the first minute and the remaining 90% is infused intravenously by IV infusion over 60 minutes period.
- **Reteplase** is a genetically modified, small molecular derivative of recombinant tPA with a longer half life. It is given in a dose of 10 mg slowly in 10 minutes period and repeated after 30 minutes if required.
- **Tenecteplase** is another recombinant tPA with a long half-life and has greater binding affinity for fibrin than alteplase. It can be administered as a single IV bolus dose, whereas other thrombolytic agents (except reteplase) are given by intravenous infusion. It is given as a single IV bolus injection in a dose of 0.5 mg/kg.
- These agents may lyse both normal and pathologic thrombi.

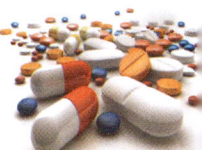

Indications

- Acute myocardial infarction: Streptokinase is given as soon as possible. Alteplase is preferred (in patients who can afford it) due to better efficacy.
- Acute pulmonary embolism.
- Acute ischemic stroke: Alteplase given within 3–6 hours of the transient ischemic attack is beneficial in early recovery.
- Treatment of severe deep vein thrombosis: All agents have equal efficacy in this condition.

Before administering the thrombolytic therapy, a careful assessment of the patient is done keeping in view the relative contraindications as given in Table 10.15.

Adverse Effects

- The major side effect is hemorrhage.
- The other common side effects are fever, hypotension.
- The allergic reaction is common with streptokinase.
- These agents are contraindicated in pregnancy, and in patients with wounds, a history of cerebrovascular accident, brain tumor, head trauma and metastatic cancer.

TABLE 10.15: Absolute and relative contraindications to fibrinolytic therapy

Absolute Contraindications	Relative Contraindications
• Prior intracranial hemorrhage • Known structural cerebral vascular lesion • Known malignant intracranial neoplasm • Ischemic stroke within 3 months • Suspected aortic dissection • Active bleeding or bleeding diathesis (excluding menses) • Significant closed-head trauma or facial trauma within 3 months	• Uncontrolled hypertension (systolic blood pressure >180 mm Hg or diastolic blood pressure >110 mm Hg) • Traumatic or prolonged cardiopulmonary resuscitation or major surgery within 3 weeks • Recent (within 2–4 weeks) internal bleeding • Non-compressible vascular punctures • For streptokinase: Prior exposure (more than 5 days ago) or prior allergic reaction to streptokinase • Pregnancy • Active peptic ulcer • Current use of warfarin and INR >1.7

INR, international normalized ratio.

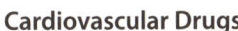

Drug Interactions

- Combined use of aspirin and clopidogrel produces synergistic effect.
- Combined use of anticoagulants and antiplatelet agents increases the bleeding tendencies.
- Dipyridamole enhances the antiplatelet effect of aspirin.
- Dipyridamole enhances the anticoagulant effect of warfarin.

Nursing Implications

Antiplatelets and fibrinolytics

- Assess for any known allergies to these drugs to avoid potential hypersensitivity reactions.
- History of previous administration of streptokinase should be confirmed before administering it.
- The availability of tenecteplase should be ensured as the timing for the administration of tenecteplase is critical to resolve the clot before permanent damage occurs to the myocardial cells in case of myocardial infarction or the nervous tissue in case of transient ischemic attacks.
- Monitor coagulation profile and platelet count to detect thrombocytopenia and increased risk of bleeding.
- Suggest and try to provide the safety measures to decrease the risk of bleeding. Provide increased precautions against bleeding during invasive procedures; use pressure dressings and ice to decrease excessive blood loss caused by anticoagulation.
- Monitor patient response to the drug (increased bleeding time, prevention of occlusive events) and adverse effects (bleeding, GI upset, dizziness, headache).
- Evaluate the effectiveness of the teaching plan (patient can name drug, dosage, adverse effects to watch for, and specific measures to avoid them; patient understands the importance of continued follow-up).

HYPOLIPIDEMIC DRUGS

- The hypolipidemic drugs are used to correct the lipids and lipoproteins abnormalities in the blood.
- The clinically significant abnormalities which need drug interventions are elevated levels of LDL-C and triglycerides and low levels of HDL-C.
  (LDL-C: low-density lipoprotein cholesterol or *"bad" cholesterol"*)
  (HDL-C: high-density lipoprotein cholesterol or *"good" cholesterol"*)
- Cholesterol levels may be elevated due to lifestyle factors such as lack of exercise or diet containing excess saturated fats and some other risk factors such as family history of coronary artery disease, cigarette smoking, hypertension, obesity, diabetes and metabolic syndrome.
- Hyperlipidemias can also result from an inherited defect in lipoprotein metabolism or genetic and lifestyle factors.
- Appropriate lifestyle changes, along with drug therapy, can lead to a 30–40% reduction in congenital heart disease mortality which is a leading cause of deaths worldwide.
- Hypolipidemic drugs retard the accelerated atherosclerosis and prevent cardiovascular disease in hyperlipidemic individuals.

The primary goal of cholesterol-lowering therapy is reduction of LDL-C and keeping the levels of HDL-C on

313

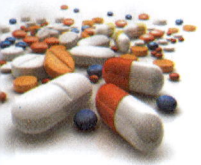

a higher side as this strategy has been associated with a decreased risk for heart diseases.

CLASSIFICATION OF HYPOLIPIDEMIC DRUGS

These drugs have been classified as given in Table 10.16.

HMG-CoA Reductase Inhibitors

(*Lovastatin, Simvastatin, Pravastatin, Atorvastatin, Rosuvastatin, Pitavastatin*)

These drugs are also called '*Statins*'. These are considered first-line treatment for patients with dyslipidemias. In addition to hypolipidemic effects, these drugs also have some other properties such as:

- Vascular antiinflammatory agents.
- Atheromatous plaque stabilizers.
- Endothelial function improving agents.
- Fibrinolysis enhancing agents
- Risk lowering agents for stroke, dementia and Alzheimer's disease.

Mechanism of Action

- These drugs competitively inhibit the enzyme (HMG-CoA) reductase, which is required for conversion of HMG-CoA (3-Hydroxy-3-methyl glutaryl coenzyme A) to mevalonic acid. This is the rate-limiting step in cholesterol synthesis.
- These drugs (except Atorvastatin and Rosuvastatin) should ideally be given at bedtime because maximum cholesterol synthesis in the liver takes place during night-time between midnight and 2:00 AM.

Pharmacokinetics

- All these drugs are same in their pharmacological profile except potency and efficacy. Absorption of the statins varies from 30% to 85% following oral administration.
- All statins are metabolized in the liver and the excretion takes place through bile, feces and urine. The half-lives of different statins are variable.

TABLE 10.16: Classification of hypolipidemic drugs

Drug Class	Drugs
5-hydroxy-3-methylglutaryl-co-enzyme A (HMG-CoA) reductase inhibitors (statins)	Lovastatin, Simvastatin, Pravastatin, Atorvastatin, Rosuvastatin, Pitavastatin
Bile acid sequestrants (resins)	Cholestyramine, Colestipol, Colesevelam
Lipoprotein lipase activators (PPARα activators, Fibrates)	Clofibrate, Gemfibrozil, Bezafibrate, Fenofibrate
Lipolysis and triglyceride synthesis inhibitors	Nicotinic acid
Sterol absorption inhibitor	Ezetimibe
Omega-3-fatty acids	

- All statins are administered in their active form except lovastatin and simvastatin which need to be hydrolyzed to their active form.
- Up to 20–50% reduction in cholesterol is obtained with these drugs.

Atorvastatin

It has good potency and efficacy. It has a longer duration of action with plasma t½ of 18–24 hours. It has additional antioxidant property. It is given orally in a dose of 10–40 mg/day up to a maximum of 80 mg/day.

Rosuvastatin

This is more potent than other statins with a longer t½ of 18–24 hours. Rosuvastatin 10 mg is equivalent to 20 mg atorvastatin. It is given orally in a dose of 5–20 mg/day up to a maximum of 40 mg/day.

Lovastatin

It was the first clinically used statin, but rarely used these days due to availability of better alternatives. Its t½ is only 1–4 hours. It is given in a dose of 10–40 mg/day up to a maximum of 80 mg.

Simvastatin

It is more efficacious than lovastatin. Its t½ is 2–3 hours and is given in a dose of 5–20 mg/day up to a maximum of 80 mg.

Pravastatin

It is equally potent to lovastatin and is given in a dose of 10–20 mg/day.

Pitavastatin

This is the most potent statin and is given in a dose of 1–4 mg/day. The plasma t½ is 12 hours.

Common Indications of Statins

- As a first choice drug for primary hyperlipidemia with raised LDL-C and total cholesterol levels.
- As a first choice drug for secondary hyperlipidemia with or without raise triglyceride levels.
- Dyslipidemia in diabetics.
- As a preventive measure for coronary artery disease in dyslipidemic patients.

Common Adverse Effects of Statins

The common side effects are:

- Myalgia
- Gastrointestinal disturbances
- Mild headache
- Rashes

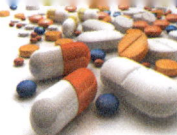

- Sleep disturbances
- Rise in serum transaminase levels (on prolonged therapy)
- Rhabdomyolysis (rare)

BILE ACID SEQUESTRANTS

(Cholestyramine, Colestipol, Colesevelam)

Bile acid sequestrants (resins) have significant LDL cholesterol–lowering effects, but less than those observed with statins.

Mechanism of Action

- These are anion-exchange resins that bind with negatively charged bile acids and bile salts in the small intestine.
- The resin-bile acid complex is unabsorbable and excreted in the feces, thus lowering the bile acid concentration.
- This causes hepatocytes to increase conversion of cholesterol to bile acids, which are essential components of the bile.
- Consequently, the intracellular cholesterol concentration decreases, which activates an increased hepatic uptake of cholesterol-containing LDL particles, leading to a fall in plasma LDL-C.

Pharmacokinetics

These drugs are insoluble in water and after oral administration, they are neither absorbed nor metabolized, but completely excreted in feces.

Therapeutic uses

- For treating, type IIA and type IIB hyperlipidemias. For this indication, these are most often given in combination with meals or niacin.
- *Cholestyramine* helps to provide relief in pruritus due to biliary stasis.
- *Colesevelam* is also given along with other hypoglycemic drugs for type 2 diabetes due to its glucose-lowering effects.
- Cholestyramine: Given in a dose of 4–16 g once daily.
- Colestipol: Given in a dose of 5–30 g once daily
- Colesevelam: Given in a dose of 3.75 g once daily.

Adverse Effects

- The common side effects are GI disturbances, nausea, constipation and flatulence. Incidence of side effects is less with *Colesevelam*.
- These drugs may raise triglyceride levels. Hence, contraindicated in patients with significant hypertriglyceridemia (≥400 mg/dL).
- These drugs also decrease the absorption of the fat-soluble vitamins such as vitamin A, D, E, and K.

LIPOPROTEIN-LIPASE ACTIVATORS

(Fenofibrate, Gemfibrozil, Bezafibrate, Clofibrate)

- *Fibrates* are derivatives of fibric acid that increase HDL-C levels and decrease serum triglyceride levels.
- Some other beneficial effects of fibrates in the patients with coronary artery disease are:
  - Inhibition of coagulation.
  - Promotion of thrombolysis.
  - Decrease in plasma uric acid levels.

Mechanism of Action

- The peroxisome proliferator–activated receptors (PPARs) regulate lipid metabolism. These drugs bind to peroxisome proliferator activated receptor (PPARs) and increase the expression and activity of lipoprotein lipase enzyme, which increases the degradation of very low density lipoprotein (VLDL).
- Fenofibrate is more effective than gemfibrozil in lowering triglyceride levels. These agents also decrease hepatic triglyceride (TG) synthesis.

Therapeutic uses

- In the treatment of hypertriglyceridemias, particularly type III hyperlipidemia.
- Patients of type 2 diabetes and metabolic syndrome with raised TG and low HDL-C levels.
- Gemfibrozil: Given in a dose of 600 mg twice daily before meals.
- Bezafibrate: Given in a dose of 200 mg thrice daily with meals.
- Fenofibrate: Given in a dose of 200 mg once daily with meals.

Pharmacokinetics

- Gemfibrozil and fenofibrate are completely absorbed after oral administration.
- Fenofibrate is a prodrug and is converted to its active form, fenofibric acid. After metabolism, these are excreted in the urine as glucuronide conjugates.
- Clofibrate is rarely used.

Adverse Effects

The common side effects are:
- Mild gastrointestinal (GI) disturbances (*which decrease with time*).
- Predisposition to form gallstones (*as these drugs increase biliary cholesterol excretion*).
- Myopathy and rhabdomyolysis can occur (*if given along with statins*).

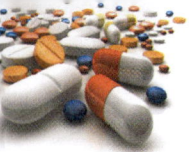

NIACIN (NICOTINIC ACID)

Niacin reduces LDL-C, increases HDL-C and also lowers the triglycerides levels.

Niacin can be used in combination with statins.

Mechanism of Action

- Normally, liver uses circulating free fatty acids as a major precursor for triglyceride synthesis.
- Niacin strongly inhibits the lipolysis in adipose tissues and reduces the production of free fatty acids, which decrease hepatic VLDL production.
- This reduces the plasma concentrations of LDL-C (*IDL and LDL are VLDL degradation products*).

Pharmacokinetics

- Niacin is administered orally.
- It is converted in the body to nicotinamide, which is used up as a cofactor and the metabolites are excreted in the urine.
- Nicotinamide alone does not decrease plasma lipid levels.

Therapeutic uses

- Familial hyperlipidemias and other severe hypercho-lesterolemias. It is given in combination with other hypolipidemic agents.
- Nicotinic acid given immediately after meals in a dose of 100 mg thrice daily initially for a few days then gradually increase to 2–4 gm times/day in divided doses.

Adverse Effects

The most common side effects are:
- An intense cutaneous flush, which is accompanied by pruritus and uncomfortable feeling of warmth and postural hypotension.
- Nausea and abdominal pain.
- Predisposition to hyperuricemia and gout (*due to inhibition of tubular secretion of uric acid*)
- Impaired glucose tolerance
- Hepatotoxicity
- It is contraindicated during pregnancy and in children.

CHOLESTEROL ABSORPTION INHIBITORS

Ezetimibe

Mechanism of Action

- Ezetimibe selectively inhibits absorption of dietary and biliary cholesterol in the small intestine, leading to a decrease in the delivery of intestinal cholesterol to the liver.

- This causes a reduction of hepatic cholesterol stores and an increase in clearance of cholesterol from the blood.

Pharmacokinetics

Ezetimibe is primarily metabolized in the small intestine and liver via glucuronide conjugation, with subsequent biliary and renal excretion.

Therapeutic uses

- It is used as an adjunct to statin therapy or in statin-intolerant patients.
- Ezetimibe is given once daily in a dose of 10mg.

Adverse Effects

- Adverse effects are uncommon with use of ezetimibe.
- Patients with moderate to severe hepatic insufficiency should not be treated with ezetimibe.

OMEGA-3 FATTY ACIDS

- Omega-3 polyunsaturated fatty acids (PUFAs) are found in marine sources such as tuna, halibut, and salmon fish.
- These omega-3 PUFAs [Eicosapentaenoic acid (EPA) and docosahexaenoic acid (DHA)] are essential fatty acids.
- Essential fatty acids inhibit VLDL and triglyceride synthesis in the liver.
- Omega-3 PUFAs are considered as an adjunct to other lipid-lowering therapies for individuals with significantly elevated triglycerides. These can be used as supplements.
- The most common side effects of these agents are GI effects such as abdominal pain, nausea, diarrhea and a fishy aftertaste.

To summarize, the different hypolipidemic drugs have different effects on LDL-c, HDL-c and TGs levels as given in Table 10.17.

TABLE 10.17: Effects of hypolipidemic drugs on LDL-c, HDL-c and TG levels

Drugs	Effects on LDL	Effects on HDL	Effects on Triglycerides
HMG CoA reductase inhibitors (statins)	↓↓↓↓	↑↑	↓↓
Fibrates	↓	↑↑↑	↓↓↓↓
Niacin	↓↓	↑↑↑↑	↓↓↓
Bile acid sequestrants	↓↓↓	↑	↑
Cholesterol absorption inhibitor	↓	↑	↓

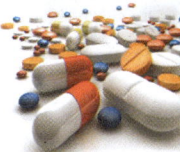

Drug Interactions

- Concurrent use of statins and some other drugs like nicotinic acid, gemfibrozil, ketoconazole, erythromycin, protease inhibitors, etc. should be avoided as chances of occurance of myopathy (rhabdomyolysis) increase many folds.
- Statins and fenofibrate combination has synergistic effect in lowering the lipid levels.
- Nicotinic acid increases the chances of postural hypotension when given to the patients already on antihypertensive drug treatment.

Nursing Implications

- **Hypolipidemic drugs**
    - Assess for any known allergies to these drugs to avoid potential hypersensitivity reactions.
    - Monitor serum cholesterol and high density lipoproteins (HDL) and low-density lipoprotein (LDL) levels before and periodically during therapy to evaluate the effectiveness of the drug.
    - Educate the patient about cholesterol lowering diet and exercise program to decrease the risk of coronary artery disease and to increase the effectiveness of drug therapy.
    - Suggest the use of barrier contraceptives for women of childbearing age because there is a risk of severe fetal abnormalities if these drugs are taken during pregnancy.
    - Monitor for adverse effects (headache, dizziness, blurred vision, cataracts, GI upset, liver failure, rhabdomyolysis, etc.).
    - Evaluate the effectiveness of the teaching plan.

Assess Yourself

Long and Short Answer Questions

1. Classify β-blockers. Describe metoprolol in detail.
2. What are antihypertensive drugs? Classify them, with at least two examples each.
3. What are hypolipidemic agents? Classify them, with at least two examples each.
4. Describe the role of nurses in the management of digitalis toxicity.
5. Why low dose aspirin is used in the prophylaxis of myocardial infarction?
6. Write short on:
    a. Statins
    b. Cardiotonic
    c. Iron preparations
    d. Nitrates
    e. ACE inhibitors
    f. Plasma expanders
    g. Antiplatelets
    h. Thrombolytics
    i. Anticoagulants

Multiple Choice Questions

1. **Heparin is**
    a. Only *in vivo* anticoagulant
    b. Only in vitro anticoagulant
    c. Oral anticoagulant
    d. Parenteral anticoagulant

2. **Which of the following is a thrombolytic agent:**
    a. Aspirin
    b. Streptokinase
    c. Clopidogrel
    d. Ticlodipine

3. **Renin is secreted from:**
    a. Juxtaglomerular apparatus
    b. PCT
    c. DCT
    d. Collecting ducts

4. **The most significant adverse effect of ACE inhibition is:**
    a. Hypotension
    b. Hypertension
    c. Hypocalcemia
    d. Hypercalcemia

5. **ACE inhibitors should not be used with:**
    a. Amiloride
    b. Calcium channel blockers
    c. Chlorthalidone
    d. Spironolactone

Answer Key

1. d.	2. b.	3. a.	4. a.	5. a and b.

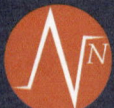
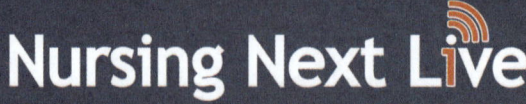
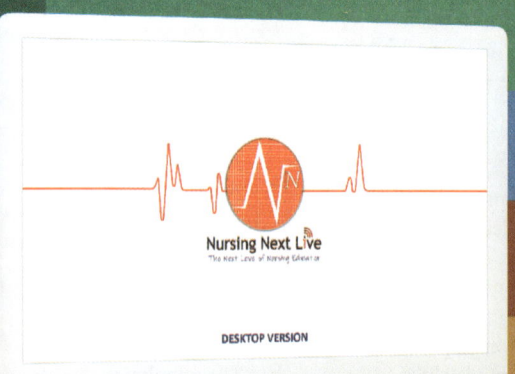

Drugs used for Hormonal Disorders and Supplementation, Contraception and Medical Termination of Pregnancy

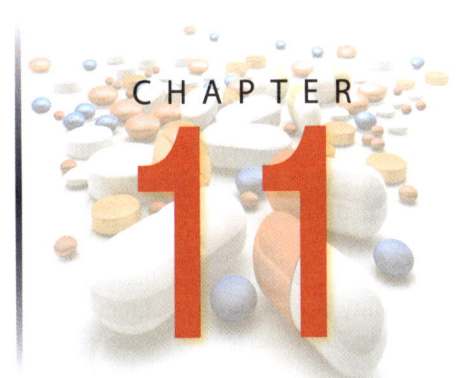

C H A P T E R

11

 CHAPTER OUTLINE

- Insulin and Oral Hypoglycemics
- Diagnosis of Diabetes Mellitus
- Thyroid Supplements and Suppressants
- Steroids and Anabolic Steroids
- Uterine Stimulants and Relaxants
- Contraceptives
- Estrogen and Progesterone Preparations
- Hormones
- Calcium Salts
- Calcium Regulators

INSULIN AND ORAL HYPOGLYCEMICS

- The pancreas produces three peptide hormones. These are insulin, glucagon and somatostatin. These peptide hormones are secreted from cells in the islets of Langerhans in pancreas.
- Insulin is produced by β-cells, glucagon by α-cells and somatostatin is produced by δ cells. The 'P cells' of islets of Langerhans produce pancreatic polypeptide.
- These hormones play an important role in regulating metabolic activities of the body.
- Diabetes mellitus is a chronic metabolic disorder characterized by hyperglycemia and altered metabolism of carbohydrates, lipids and proteins. This may occur due to a relative or absolute lack of insulin. If this disorder is not timely treated, various problems like retinopathy, nephropathy, neuropathy and cardiovascular complications can occur.
- The morbidity and mortality associated with diabetes can be reduced by timely administration of insulin preparations or other glucose-lowering agents.

Clinically, the diabetes mellitus can be of following types:
- **Type 1-diabetes** or insulin dependent diabetes mellitus.
- **Type 2-diabetes** or non-insulin-dependent diabetes mellitus.
- **Other types of diabetes:** Gestational diabetes, maturity onset diabetes of young (MODY), diabetes due to drugs, pancreatectomy, endocrine abnormalities or due to other causes such as genetic defects, etc.

DIAGNOSIS OF DIABETES MELLITUS

It is diagnosed according to the following criteria:
- Clinical features of the disease.
- Laboratory findings of blood glucose and the levels of HbA1c (Table 11.1).

TABLE 11.1: Variables for diagnosis of diabetes mellitus

Variables	Normal Glucose Tolerance	Impaired Glucose Tolerance	Diabetes Mellitus
Fasting serum glucose mg/dL (mmol/L)	<100 (5.6)	100–125 (5.6–6.9)	≥126 (7.0)
Two hours after glucose load mg/dL (mmol/L)	<140 (7.8)	≥140–199 (7.8–11.0)	≥200 (11.1)
HbA1c (%)	<5.7	5.7–6.4	≥6.5

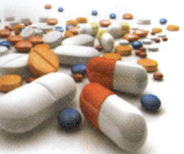

TYPE 1 DIABETES

- Type 1-diabetes appears clinically when more than 90% of β-cells of pancreas are destroyed due to autoimmune-mediated processes or other environmental toxins.
- Patients with type 1-diabetes show classic symptoms of insulin deficiency such as polydipsia, polyphagia, polyuria, and weight loss.
- In type 1-diabetes, the basic abnormality lies in the inability of pancreas to maintain basal and bolus levels of insulin. *The basal level of insulin secretion is 0.5–1.0 unit/hr and the bolus secretion after meals may go up to 6 units/hr.*
- In type 1-diabetics, the primary mode of treatment is administration of exogenous insulin. This is necessary to prevent severe life threatening hyperglycemia and ketoacidosis.
- The goal of *insulin* therapy is to maintain blood glucose as close to normal as possible and to avoid marked variations in glucose levels.
- These days, self-monitoring of blood glucose levels at home is advocated with the help of glucometer for better control.

TYPE 2 DIABETES

- Type 2-diabetes accounts for greater than 90% of cases.
- The main causes of type 2-diabetes are genetic factors, aging, obesity, and peripheral insulin resistance, rather than autoimmune processes.
- The pancreas retains some β-cell function, but insulin secretion is not sufficient to maintain glucose homeostasis.
- Type 2-diabetes also lacks of sensitivity of target organs to insulin known as *peripheral insulin* resistance.
- The goal in treating type 2-diabetes is to maintain blood glucose within normal limits and to prevent the development of long-term complications.
- The stepwise approach in the management is as follows:
  - Weight reduction, exercise, and dietary modification decrease insulin resistance and correct hyperglycemia in some patients with type 2-diabetes.
  - Most patients require pharmacologic intervention with oral glucose-lowering agents.
  - As the disease progresses, β-cell function declines and insulin therapy is often needed to achieve satisfactory glucose levels.

Some clinical studies show that initiating early insulin therapy in the management of type-2 diabetes is more beneficial than waiting for the progression of the disease. Probably, this helps in rejuvenation of fatigued β-cells or maintains the remaining β-cells function for a longer time.

INSULIN AND INSULIN ANALOGUES

- Insulin was discovered by **Banting and Best** in 1921.
- It contains two polypeptide chains (chain-A and chain-B) connected by connecting peptide (C-peptide).
- Insulin is made up of a total of **51 amino acids** (chains-A has 21 amino acids and chain-B has 30 amino acids).
- Both C-peptide and insulin are synthesized and secreted in blood in equal amounts.
- The measurement of C-peptide plasma levels provides a better index of insulin production.
- The plasma insulin levels may not accurately reflect insulin production as it is immediately used up and degraded.

Normal Physiological Regulation of Insulin Secretion

Insulin secretion is regulated by:

- **Chemical mechanisms:** The levels of glucose, fatty acids and amino acids stimulate secretion of insulin from β-cells.
- **Hormonal influences:** Growth hormone, thyroxine, steroidal hormones, glucagon, gastrin, sectretin, etc. influence the secretion of insulin.
- **Neural mechanisms:** Parasympathetic stimulation increases and sympathetic stimulation decreases the insulin secretion. Sympathetic stimulation increases the glycogenolysis in liver.

Actions of Insulin

Insulin has a major anabolic role:

- It promotes uptake of glucose, amino acids and fatty acids from plasma.
- It promotes glycogenesis, protein synthesis and lipogenesis.
- It inhibits hepatic glycogenolysis, gluconeogenesis and lipolysis.
- Insulin helps in the entry of glucose in nearly all body tissues. However, entry and utilization of glucose into RBCs, WBCs, liver and brain can occur independently. Muscular exercise facilitates entry and utilization of glucose into the muscle cells without the help of insulin.

GLUCOSE TRANSPORTERS (GLUT)

- These are the glycoproteins involved in glucose transportation mechanisms.
- There are 14 subtypes of GLUT expressed on different tissues. GLUT-4 is present in muscles and adipose tissues.

Pharmacokinetics

- Insulin cannot be given by oral route as proteolytic enzymes destroy it.

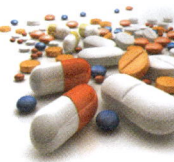

- It is administered by subcutaneous route in routine and by intravenous route in emergencies.
- Both endogenous and exogenous insulins are metabolized in liver, kidney and muscles.
- It is broken down to amino acids and these amino acids are recycled and reutilized.

Insulin Preparations

Insulin preparations differ in their source, onset and duration of action.

Based upon source, these can be grouped as bovine, porcine, human or recombinant insulin.

- **Conventional insulin**
  - These are obtained from ox and pig pancreas and known as bovine and porcine insulins.
  - These are mostly immunogenic in nature.
  - They are purified by gel filtration and ion exchange chromatography.
  - Monocomponent and single peak insulin are purified form of insulin.
- **Human insulin**
  - Examples of human insulin are human regular insulin, human lente insulin, human isophane insulin and a mixture of human regular insulin and isophane insulin (30:70), etc.
- **Newer Insulin analogues**
  - Insulin lispro, insulin aspart, insulin glulisine, insulin glargine and insulin detemir are insulin analogues and are prepared by recombinant DNA technology.

Dose of Insulin

- The insulin dose is individualized according to the blood glucose level and HbA1c level.
- Several regimens including mixture of different insulin preparations are used.
- The combinations of different insulin preparations are administered preferably in multiple doses to simulate the physiologic insulin secretion.
- In Type 1-diabetes patients, the insulin requirement varies between 0.2 and 1 U/kg/day.
- In Type 2-diabetes patients, the insulin requirement varies between 0.2 and 1.6 U/kg/day.
- Slightly higher doses are required in obese patients.

Indications of Insulin Therapy

- Type 1 and 2 diabetes mellitus
- Gestational diabetes
- Diabetic ketoacidosis
- Hyperosmolar or non-ketotic diabetic coma
- During acute exacerbations of different diseases (stressful conditions) in patients on oral hypoglycemic agents.

Types of Insulin

Various types of insulins are given in Table 11.2.

Adverse Effects to Insulin Therapy

- The most common and serious side effect of insulin therapy is hypoglycemia.
- Other side effects are injection site reactions, weight gain and lipodystrophy, which can be managed by alteration of injection sites.
- Adjustment of dose is advocated in case of renal impairment.

Insulin Delivery Devices

- Insulin is delivered through different devices for accurate glycemic control.
- These devices are:
  - Insulin syringes
  - Pen devices

TABLE 11.2: Class, drugs, onset of action and duration of action of insulin

Class	Drugs	Onset of action	Duration of action
Ultra short or rapid acting insulin	Lispro-Insulin	0.2–0.3 hours	3–5 hours
	Aspart-Insulin	0.2–0.3 hours	3–5 hours
	Glulisine-Insulin	0.2–0.4 hours	3–5 hours
Short acting insulin	Regular soluble insulin	0.5–1 hours	5–8 hours
	Semilente	1–2 hours	12–14 hours
Intermediate acting insulin	Insulin zinc or Lente	1–2 hours	20–24 hours
	Neutral protamine hagedorn or isophane insulin	1–2 hours	20–24 hours
Long acting insulin	Insulin detemir	1–4 hours	20–24 hours
	Insulin glargine	2–4 hours	24 hours
Ultra-long acting insulin	Degludec	30–90 minutes	24–40 hours
	Ultralente	6 hours	20–36 hours

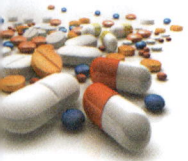

- Inhaled insulin (available in the USA and Europe only)
- Insulin pump
- Implantable insulin pump
- Oral insulin (under developmental stage)

ORAL HYPOGLYCEMIC AGENTS (OHAs)

- The drugs, which are given by oral route and produce lowering of blood sugar levels are known as oral hypoglycemic agents (OHAs).
- These are given mostly in type 2-diabetes during initiation and maintenance of anti-diabetic therapy.
- These are also given as adjuvant to insulin therapy.
- Complete understanding of the pathophysiology of diabetes at molecular level has helped to develop different types of OHAs.

> **Classification of Oral Hypoglycemic Agents (OHAs)**
> **Insulin Secretagogues**
> - **Sulfonylureas**
>   - **First generation:** Tolbutamide, Chlorpropamide
>   - **Second generation:** Glibenclamide, Glipizide, Glimepiride and Gliclazide
> - **Meglitinide analogues:** Nateglinide and Repaglinide
> **Insulin sensitizers**
> - **Biguanide:** Metformin
> - **Thiazolidinediones:** Pioglitazone, Rosiglitazone (banned)
> *Others*
> - **α-Glucosidase inhibitors:** Voglibose, Acarbose and Miglitol
> - **Amylin analogue:** Pramlintide
> - **Sodium-glucose cotransport-2 inhibitor (SGLT-2 inhibitor):** Empagliflozin, *Canagliflozin* and Dapagliflozin
> - **Glucagon-like peptide-1 (GLP-1) receptor agonists:** Liraglutide, Albiglutide and Exenatide
> - **Dipeptidyl peptidase-4 (DPP-4) inhibitors:** Sitagliptin, Saxagliptin, Vildagliptin, Alogliptin, Linagliptin.

INSULIN SECRETAGOGUES

Sulfonylureas

- **First generation:** Tolbutamide, chlorpropamide
- **Second generation:** Glibenclamide, glipizide, glimepiride and gliclazide
- These agents are classified as insulin secretagogues, because they promote insulin release from the β cells of the pancreas.
- Currently, 2nd generation sulfonylureas are used clinically.

Mechanism of Action

- The main mechanism of action includes stimulation of insulin release from the β cells of the pancreas.

- In addition, sulfonylureas may reduce hepatic glucose production.
- They also increase the sensitivity of peripheral tissues to insulin.
- Glimepiride and gliclazide also have antioxidant property.

Pharmacokinetics

- All sulfonylureas are well absorbed when given by oral route.
- The metabolism occurs in liver and excretion occurs in kidneys and feces.
- They have high plasma protein binding (90–95%).
- The duration of action ranges from 12 hours to 24 hours (Table 11.3).

Adverse Effects

- Commonly seen side effects are hypoglycemia, nausea, vomiting, photosensitivity and hyperinsulinemia.
- Weight gain (on prolonged use).
- Dose adjustment is advocated in renal and hepatic impairment.
- They are teratogenic in nature.

Meglitinide Analogues (Nateglinide and Repaglinide)

- Like the sulfonylureas, the meglitinides also stimulate insulin secretion by binding to the α cell but on a different site.
- In contrast to the sulfonylureas, the meglitinides have a rapid onset and a short duration of action.
- They are known as postprandial glucose regulators because their main effect is in early release of insulin that occurs after a meal.
- Meglitinides should not be used in combination with sulfonylureas due to same mechanism of action and synergistic effect that may cause severe hypoglycemia.

Pharmacokinetics

- Meglitinides should be taken before meal and are well absorbed after oral administration.
- The metabolism occurs in liver and excretion through bile.

TABLE 11.3: Dose and duration of action of sulfonylureas

Drug	Dose	Duration of action
Glibenclamide	2.5–10 mg once daily	12–24 hours
Glipizide	5–20 mg once daily	12–18 hours
Glimepiride	1–4 mg once daily	24 hours
Gliclazide	30–240 mg once daily	12–24 hours

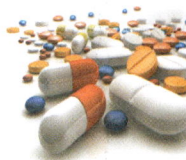

TABLE 11.4: Dose and duration of action of meglitinides

Drug	Dose	Duration of action
Nateglinide	60–120 mg, 30 minutes before every meal	4–5 hours
Repaglinide	0.25–4 mg, 30 minutes before every meal	4–5 hours

Dose and duration of action of meglitinides are given in Table 11.4.

Adverse Effects

- Commonly seen side effects are hypoglycemia, weight gain, mild headache and arthralgia.
- Hypersensitivity reaction (incidence is lower than sulfonylureas).
- Dose adjustment is advocated in hepatic impairment.

INSULIN SENSITIZERS

Biguanide (Metformin)

- *Metformin* is the only clinically important biguanide.
- It is considered better than sulfonylureas as the risk of hypoglycemia is not there.

Mechanism of Action

- The main mechanism of action of metformin is increased peripheral glucose uptake and its utilization.
- It causes reduction in hepatic gluconeogenesis.
- It also slows intestinal absorption of sugars.
- Weight loss may occur because it causes loss of appetite.

Pharmacokinetics

- It is well absorbed orally and is not bound to serum plasma proteins.
- It is not metabolized and excretion occurs through kidneys in unchanged form.

Dose: 500–2000 mg daily in 1–2 divided doses.

Indications

- Metformin is the initial drug of choice for type 2-diabetes.
- It is also a drug of choice in diabetic obese individuals as it causes anorexia and weight loss.
- Non-diabetic uses:
  - Metformin is effective in the treatment of polycystic ovary syndrome. It increases insulin sensitivity and may enhance fertility in these women and also improves hirsutism by decreasing the androgen levels.

Adverse Effects

- The common side effects are flatulence, anorexia, metallic taste, weight loss and diarrhea.
- Rarely, potentially fatal lactic acidosis can occur.
- Long-term use may interfere with vitamin B_{12} absorption.

Thiazolidinediones (Pioglitazone)

- The thiazolidinediones (TZDs) are also known as insulin sensitizers.
- Pioglitazone and rosiglitazone are the two drugs in this class.
- Rosiglitazone has been banned since 2010 due to cardiotoxic effects.

Mechanism of Action

- The TZDs act as agonists for the peroxisome proliferator activated receptor-γ (PPARγ), a nuclear hormone receptor and lower insulin resistance.
- They increase glucose transport by increasing the number of GLUT4 and thereby increase insulin sensitivity in adipose tissues, liver, and skeletal muscle.
- Pioglitazone decreases triglycerides and increases HDL cholesterol levels also.
- Pioglitazone can be used as monotherapy or in combination with other glucose-lowering agents or insulin.
- Pioglitazone is a second- or third-line agent for type 2 diabetes.

Pharmacokinetics

- Pioglitazone is well absorbed after oral administration and is highly bound to serum albumin.
- It undergoes extensive metabolism in liver and excretion occurs in the bile and feces.
- No dosage adjustment is required in renal impairment.
- It is given once daily in a dose of 15–45 mg.

Adverse Effects

- Some side effects are liver toxicity, edema, weight gain, osteopenia with increased risk of fractures.
- Pioglitazone may also increase the risk of bladder cancer.

OTHER ORAL HYPOGLYCEMIC AGENTS

α-Glucosidase Inhibitors

(Acarbose, Voglibose, and Miglitol)

Acarbose, Voglibose, and Miglitol are oral agents used for the treatment of type 2-diabetes.

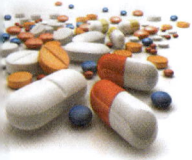

Mechanism of Action

- α-glucosidase enzyme is located in the intestinal brush border and breaks down carbohydrates into glucose and other simple sugars for better absorption.
- These agents reversibly inhibit α-glucosidase enzymes and delay the digestion of carbohydrates, resulting in lower postprandial glucose levels.
- These agents do not cause hypoglycemia when used as monotherapy. However, when used with insulin secretagogues or insulin, hypoglycemia may develop.

Pharmacokinetics

- Acarbose and Voglibose are poorly absorbed by oral route and are metabolized primarily by intestinal bacterial flora, and some of the metabolites are absorbed and excreted into the urine.
- Miglitol is very well absorbed but has no systemic effects. It is excreted unchanged by the kidney.
- Acarbose is given in a dose of 50–100 mg in the beginning of every meal.
- Voglibose is given in a dose of 0.2–0.3 mg in the beginning of every meal.
- Miglitol is given in a dose of 25–100 mg in the beginning of every meal.

Adverse Effects

- The main side effects are flatulence, diarrhea, and abdominal cramps.
- Patients with inflammatory bowel disease, colonic ulceration, or intestinal obstruction should not use these drugs.

Amylin Analogue *(Pramlintide)*

- Amylin is a neuroendocrine hormone that is co-secreted with insulin from β-cells of pancreas immediately after food intake.
- Pramlintide is a synthetic amylin analogue and acts as hypoglycemic agent by following mechanisms:
  - It delays gastric emptying.
  - It decreases postprandial glucagon secretion.
  - It improves satiety and suppresses appetite.
- It is given by subcutaneous injection immediately prior to meals.
- In patients with type 1 and 2 diabetes, it is indicated as an adjuvant to mealtime insulin therapy.
- The dose of insulin should be decreased to avoid a risk of severe hypoglycemia.
- It is given in a dose of 60–120 μg subcutaneously before meals.
- The common side effects are anorexia, nausea and vomiting.

Sodium-Glucose Cotransport-2 (SGLT-2) Inhibitors *(Dapagliflozin, Empagliflozin and Canagliflozin)*

- The sodium–glucose cotransporter-2 (SGLT-2) is responsible for reabsorbing filtered glucose in the tubular lumen of the kidney.
- The mechanism responsible for lowering blood glucose is by inhibition of SGLT-2 by these agents, which causes decrease in the reabsorption of glucose. This increases the excretion of urinary glucose and causes glycosuria.
- In addition, osmotic diuresis also occurs due to inhibition of sodium absorption. Hence, reduction of systolic blood pressure may also be seen.

Pharmacokinetics

- They are well absorbed by oral route and are given once daily in the morning.
- The metabolism occurs in the liver and excretion occurs through feces and also by kidneys.

Dose and Route

- **Canagliflozin:** Given in a dose of 100–300 mg orally, empty stomach in the morning.
- **Dapagliflozin:** Given in a dose of 5–10 mg orally, empty stomach in the morning.
- **Empagliflozin:** Given in a dose of 10–25 mg orally, empty stomach in the morning.

Adverse Effects

- Commonly seen adverse effects are urogenital infections in females, increased frequency, vulvovaginal candidiasis, weight loss and hypotension.
- These side effects are due to increased glucose in urine and diuresis.

Glucagon-Like Peptide-1 (GLP-1) Receptor Agonists

(Liraglutide, Albiglutide and Exenatide)

- GLP-1 (incretin-hormone) is released from the gut after oral glucose administration and is responsible for 60–70% of postprandial insulin secretion.
- GLP-1 receptor agonists are also called incretin-mimetics as they behave like incretin hormone.
- Exenatide and liraglutide are injectable incretin-mimetics used for the treatment of type 2-diabetes.

Mechanism of Action

- These agents act by following mechanisms:
  - Improvement in glucose dependent insulin secretion.
  - Slow gastric emptying time, reduce food intake by enhancing satiety (a feeling of fullness).

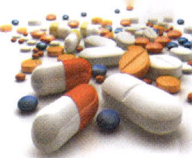

- Decrease postprandial glucagon secretion.
- Promote β-cell proliferation.
- Reduction in HbA1c, postprandial hyperglycemia and weight.

Pharmacokinetics

These agents are administered subcutaneously in once daily dose, irrespective of meal timings.

- Liraglutide and Albiglutide have a long half-life and given once daily.
- Exenatide has a short half-life and given twice daily.

A once-weekly extended-release preparation is also available.

Indications

Resistant type 2 diabetes mellitus and postprandial hyperglycemia.

Dose and Route

- **Exenatide:** Given in a dose of 5–10 μg subcutaneously, twice daily, preferably 30–60 minutes before meals.
- **Liraglutide:** Given in a dose of 0.6–1.8 mg subcutaneously once a day.
- **Albiglutide:** Given in a dose of 30–50 mg subcutaneously once a day.

Adverse Effects

- Commonly seen side effects are nausea, vomiting, diarrhea, constipation.
- Pancreatitis is rare.

Dipeptidyl Peptidase-4 (DPP-4) Inhibitors

(Sitagliptin, Saxagliptin, Vildagliptin, Alogliptin, Linagliptin)

All dipeptidyl peptidase-4 (DPP-4) inhibitors are given orally for the treatment of type 2 diabetes mellitus.

Mechanism of Action

- Incretin hormones (GLP-1) are metabolized by DPP-4 enzymes.
- These drugs act by inhibiting the DPP-4 enzyme, allow incretin-hormone to act for a longer time and increase insulin release in response to meals and also reduce inappropriate secretion of glucagon.
- These drugs are used as monotherapy or in combination with sulfonylureas, metformin, TZDs, or insulin.

Pharmacokinetics

- They are well absorbed after oral administration and food does not affect the extent of absorption.

TABLE 11.5: Doses of DPP-4 inhibitors

Drugs	Dose
Sitagliptin	25–100 mg orally, once daily
Saxagliptin	2.5–5 mg orally, once daily
Vildagliptin	50 mg orally, once daily
Alogliptin	6.25–25 mg orally, once daily
Linagliptin	50 mg orally, once daily

- The metabolism occurs in liver and excretion mostly occurs in unchanged form via kidneys.
- Linagliptin undergoes enterohepatic circulation.
- Dose adjustment is advocated in renal impaired patients the usual doses of DPP-4 inhibitors are given in Table 11.5.

Adverse Effects

- These drugs are well tolerated.
- The common side effects are nasopharyngitis and headache.
- Pancreatitis is an uncommon side effect.

Drug Interactions

- β adrenergic blockers should not be given to patients on insulin therapy as the warning signs of hypoglycemia (like palpitation, tremor and anxiety) are suppressed and fatal hypoglycemia can occur.
- The effectiveness of insulin is decreased by drugs like diuretics (furosemide, thiazides), oral contraceptives, corticosteroids, nifedipine and salbutamol. These drugs have a tendency to raise the blood sugar levels.
- Theophylline, lithium and high dose aspirin enhance the insulin secretion and peripheral glucose utilization. This may produce additional hypoglycemia.
- Some drugs such as phenylbutazone, sulfinpyrazone, salicylates, sulfonamides displace sulfonylureas from protein binding and may accentuate hypoglycemia
- Some drugs such as ketoconazole, sulfonamides, warfarin, chloramphenicol inhibit metabolism and excretion of sulfonylureas and may accentuate hypoglycemia
- Some drugs such as phenobarbitone, phenytoin, rifampicin induce the metabolism of sulfonylureas and may diminish their efficacy.

Nursing Implications

- **Insulin and oral hypoglycemics**
  - Assess for contraindications or cautions and any known allergy to any insulin and current status of pregnancy or lactation so that appropriate monitoring and dose adjustments can be completed.

Contd...

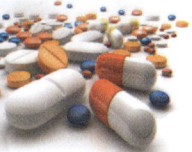

 ## Nursing Implications

- ☞ Educate the patient to follow a proper dietary and exercise regimen to improve the effectiveness of the insulin and OHAs and maintain good hygiene.
- ☞ Educate the patient about changing the injection sites regularly to avoid damage to muscles and to prevent subcutaneous atrophy.
- ☞ Monitor the patient for signs and symptoms of hypoglycemia during insulin therapy.
- ☞ Provide the consultation of dietician to all admitted diabetic patients and provide the diet accordingly.
- ☞ Ensure that all the investigations ordered to the diabetic patients are carried out timely as these are required for fine control of diabetes.
- ☞ Always verify the name of the insulin being given because each insulin has a different peak and duration, and the names can be confused.
- ☞ The mixtures of regular and NPH insulin should be administered within 15 minutes after combining them to ensure appropriate suspension and therapeutic effect.
- ☞ Store insulin in a cool place away from direct sunlight to ensure effectiveness.
- ☞ Monitor for adverse effects (hypoglycemia, ketoacidosis, and injection-site irritation).
- ☞ Evaluate the effectiveness of the teaching plan (patient can name drug, dosage, adverse effects to watch for, specific measures to avoid them, and proper administration technique).
- ☞ Administer a single daily dose of L-thyroxine before breakfast (preferably at 06:00 am) each day to ensure consistent therapeutic levels.

THYROID SUPPLEMENTS AND SUPPRESSANTS

- The thyroid gland is located in the middle of the neck and surrounds the trachea like a shield. Its name has been derived from the Greek words *thyros* (shield) and *eidos* (gland).
- The thyroid gland produces three different hormones naming thyroxine, or tetra-iodothyronine (T_4), levo-thyroxine or tri-iodothyronine (T_3) and calcitonin.
- The thyroid hormones play many important roles in regulating nearly all bodily systems. These hormones regulate the rate of metabolism in almost all the cells of the body. The thyroid hormones affect heat production and body temperature, enzyme system activity, metabolism of carbohydrates, fats, and proteins. Thyroid hormone is also an important regulator of growth and development, especially within the reproductive and nervous systems.

REGULATION OF THYROID HORMONE SECRETION

- The production and release of thyroid hormones is regulated by thyroid-stimulating hormone (TSH), which in turn is produced by the anterior lobe of pituitary gland.
- The secretion of TSH is regulated by thyrotropin-releasing hormone (TRH), which is released by hypothalamus (Fig. 11.1).
- A delicate balance exists among the thyroid, the pituitary, and the hypothalamus in regulating the levels of thyroid hormone.

TSH, thyroid stimulating hormone; TRH, thyroid releasing hormone.

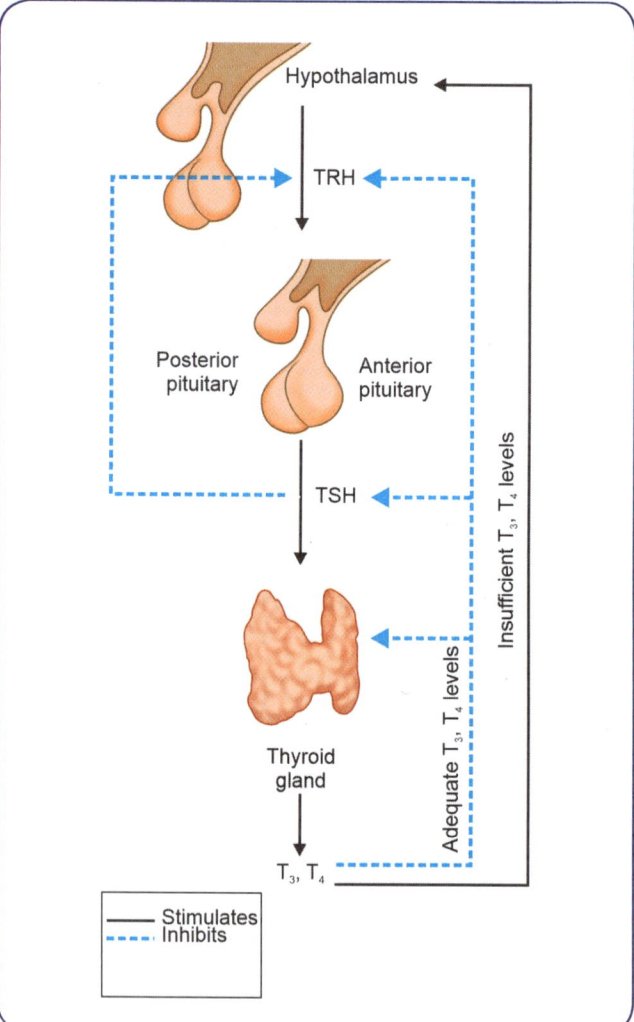

FIG. 11.1: Regulation of thyroid hormone secretion

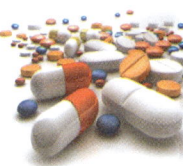

THYROID DYSFUNCTION

- Thyroid dysfunction involves either under-activity (hypothyroidism) or over-activity (hyperthyroidism). These dysfunctions can affect any age group.
- Hypothyroidism is the most common type of thyroid dysfunction.
- **Hypothyroidism** is a condition in which there is a lack of sufficient levels of thyroid hormones to maintain a normal metabolism. Deficiency of thyroid hormone in children results in cretinism, and in adults it causes myxedema. This condition is treated mainly by *drug replacement therapy* or supplementation with thyroid hormones. This condition occurs in a number of pathophysiological states such as:
  - Lack of sufficient iodine in the diet to produce the required level of thyroid hormones.
  - Lack of sufficient functioning thyroid tissue due to tumor or autoimmune disorders.
  - Lack of TSH due to pituitary disease.
  - Lack of TRH related to a tumor or disorder of the hypothalamus.
  - Absence of the thyroid gland after surgery (thyroidectomy).

- **Hyperthyroidism** occurs due to the over-activity of thyroid gland resulting in hypersecretion of thyroid hormones. The resultant effect is a group of symptoms and signs, known as hyperthyroidism, Grave's disease or thyrotoxicosis. Drugs used for the treatment of hyperthyroidism are known as antithyroid drugs.

THYROID HORMONES

The thyroid gland produces three different hormones naming thyroxine, or tetra-iodothyronine (T_4), levo-thyroxine or tri-iodothyronine (T_3) and calcitonin.

T_4 and T_3 are involved in various bodily functions as described above and calcitonin is primarily involved in the regulation of calcium metabolism.

Synthesis, Storage and Release of Thyroid Hormones

- The thyroid hormones are synthesized and stored in the thyroid follicles. Iodine is essentially required for its synthesis and diet is the major source of iodine.
- The principal steps involved in the synthesis of thyroid hormones are as follows (Fig. 11.2).

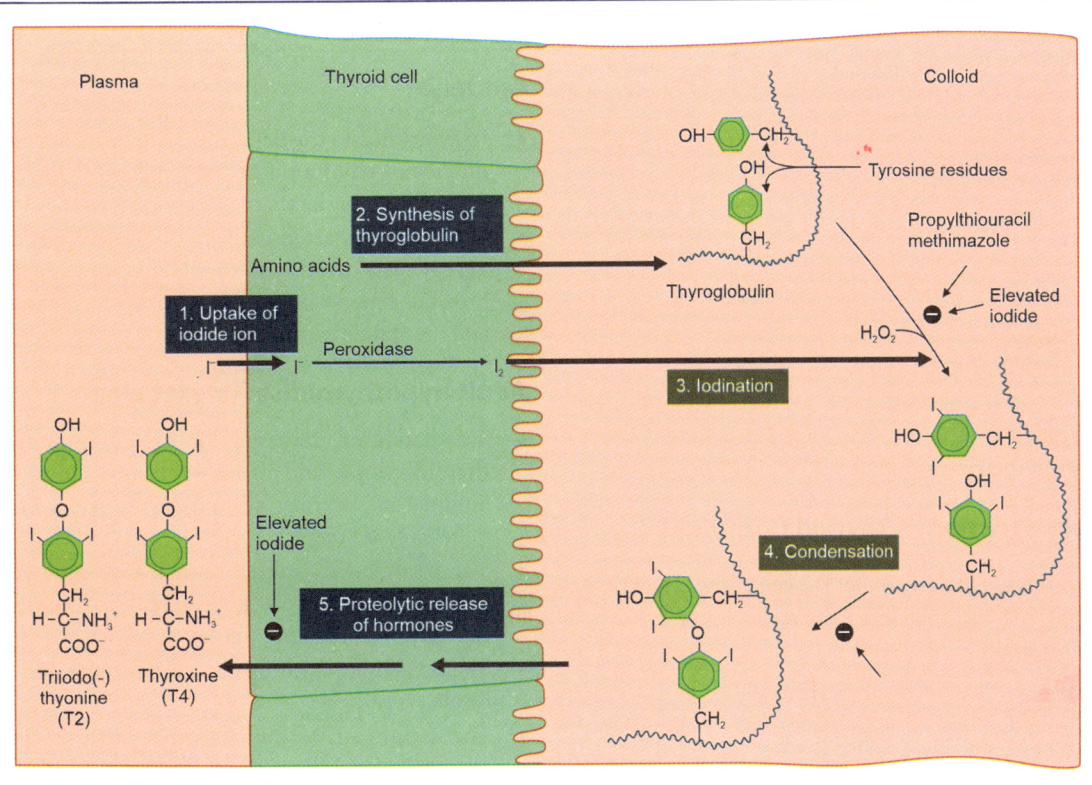

FIG. 11.2: Synthesis, storage and release of thyroid hormones

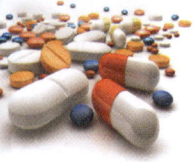

Iodide Trapping or Iodine Uptake

- The iodide ions are taken up by the follicular cells of thyroid gland by an active transport mechanism with the help of sodium iodide transporter.
- Thiocyanates and perchlorates can inhibit this process.

Oxidation and Iodination

- The iodide ions are oxidized to iodinium (I^+) ions by the membrane bound thyroid peroxidase enzyme (TPO).
- These forms of iodine combine with tyrosine residues of thyroglobulin to form monoiodotyrosine (MIT) and diiodotyrosine (DIT).
- This reaction does not require any enzymatic intervention.

Coupling

- This is the final step in the synthesis of thyroid hormones.
- It is an oxidative reaction and the same thyroid peroxidase enzyme (TPO) catalyzes this reaction.
- In this reaction, two molecules of DIT couple to form T_4 and one molecule of MIT couples with one molecule of DIT to form T_3.
  - DIT + DIT= T_4, DIT + MIT= T_3

Storage and Release

Thyroglobulin containing iodinated tyrosine residues are stored in the follicles and are released under the influence of TSH.

Peripheral Conversion of T_4 to T_3

- Most of the hormone released in the circulation by thyroid gland is T_4.
- T_4 is converted to T_3 in liver and kidneys.
- T_3 is the active form of thyroid hormone.
- T_4 is less potent than T_3.
- Most of the body tissues utilize T_3 for their metabolic needs except brain and pituitary, which take up T_4 and convert it to T_3 within their own cells.

Mechanism of Action of Thyroid Hormones

- The hormones (T_3 and T_4) enter the cell of the target tissues by active transport, then enter the nucleus and attaches to specific receptors.
- The activation of these receptors promotes the formation of RNA and subsequent protein synthesis, which is responsible for the effects of these hormones.

Preparations of Thyroid Hormones

- Levothyroxine sodium (T_4) tablet and IV preparation.

- Liothyronine (T_3) tablets and IV preparations.
- Combination of T_4 and T_3 (4:1) tablets form.

Intravenous preparations are used only in emergencies.

Pharmacokinetics

- Both T_4 and T_3 are absorbed after oral administration.
- Food, calcium preparations, and aluminum-containing antacids can decrease the absorption of T_4.
- De-iodination is the major route of metabolism of T_4.
- T_3 also undergoes sequential de-iodination.
- The hormones are also metabolized in liver via conjugation with glucuronides and sulfates and excreted into the bile.
- The plasma t½ of T_4 is 6–7 days and that of T_3 is 1–2 days.
- T_3 is fast acting and 3–5 times more potent than T_4.

Therapeutic uses of Thyroid hormones

- Thyroid hormones are used therapeutically as supplementation or replacement therapy in deficiency states.
- Oral formulations are used for long-term use and parenteral preparation in emergencies. The dose is guided by the serum levels of T_3, T_4 and TSH. The common uses are as follows:

PROBLEMS ASSOCIATED WITH THYROID DYSFUNCTION

Cretinism

- It occurs due to the deficiency of thyroid hormones during infancy or childhood and may be in the form of sporadic cretinism or endemic cretinism.
- Treatment is started with thyroxine in a dose of 8–12 μg/kg/day. The treatment should be started at the earliest possible time to prevent further deterioration of physical and mental development.

Adult Hypothyroidism (Myxedema)

- This condition develops due to autoimmune thyroiditis, thyroidectomy, and drugs such as iodides, lithium and amiodarone or may accompany simple goiter, if iodine deficiency is severe.
- The treatment is started with L-thyroxine (T_4) in a low dose of 50 μg per day and increased every 2–3 weeks to maximum of 100–200 μg/day.
- The dose is adjusted by clinical response and serum TSH levels.
- The treatment of subclinical hypothyroidism cases is optional depending upon the clinical features if the TSH level is between 6 and 10 mU/L. In subclinical hypothyroidism with TSH level >10 mU/L, patients should be treated with T_4.

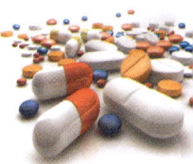

Myxedema Coma

- It is an emergency condition due to acute hypothyroidism and rapid thyroid hormone replacement therapy is life saving.
  L-thyroxine (T$_4$) is administered intravenously in a dose of 200–500 µg stat and followed by 100-µg IV once daily till oral therapy can be initiated. T$_3$ is not given as it can cause fatal cardiac arrhythmias. Besides administering T$_4$, the general management of the patient is done as follows:
- Rewarming the patient with the help of blankets or direct heat.
- Corticosteroids (hydrocorticosone) by IV route.
- Intravenous antibiotics are given if any evidence of infection is there.
- Correction of electrolyte imbalance such as hyponatremia.
- Correction of hypoglycemia.
- Ventilatory support may be required.
- Cardiovascular support, if required

Nontoxic Goiter

- It could be endemic (due to iodine deficiency) or sporadic (due to defect in hormone synthesis).
- Patients present with enlarged thyroid gland known as goiter.
- Clinically, patient may be euthyroid or hypothyroid.
- Iodine deficiency needs to be corrected in these cases with the help of iodized salt and other measures.
- Treatment with T$_4$ is given in the form of replacement therapy and most of the recently enlarged gland regresses. Old fibrosed gland may not regress.
- Thyroxine therapy may be withdrawn after a year or so in some cases and some may need life-long therapy.

GOITRINS

These are goiter-causing agents and found in plants such as cabbage, turnip, mustard, etc. Consumption of these goitrins may contribute to endemic goiter in certain iodine deficient regions. Goitrins are the cause of goiter in cattle who feed on these plants.

- **Benign thyroid nodule and TSH responsive thyroid carcinomas:** These thyroid enlargements may regress when TSH is suppressed by T4 therapy.
- **Miscellaneous uses:** Infertility, menstrual disorders refractory anemias (*hypothyroidism may be a cause of these disorders*).

HYPERTHYROIDISM AND ANTITHYROID DRUGS

- The over–activity of thyroid gland results in hypersecretion of thyroid hormones, which is known as hyperthyroidism.

- It may manifest in the form of thyrotoxicosis. The cause of thyrotoxicosis may be Grave's disease or thyroid nodule or toxic nodular/multinodular goiter.
- In these situations, TSH levels are reduced due to negative feedback.
- Drugs used for the treatment of hyperthyroidism are known as antithyroid drugs.
- The goal of antithyroid therapy is to decrease synthesis and/or release of additional hormone. This can be accomplished by removing part or all of the thyroid gland, by inhibiting synthesis of the hormones, or by blocking release of the hormones from the follicles.

Classification of Antithyroid Drugs

- **Thyroid hormone synthesis inhibitors or antithyroid drugs:** Propylthiouracil, Methimazole, Carbimazole.
- **Inhibitors of iodide trapping or Ionic inhibitors:** Thiocyanates ($^-$SCN), Perchlorates ($^-$ClO$_4$), Nitrates ($^-$NO$_3$).
- **Hormone release inhibitors**: Iodine, Iodides of Na and K, Organic iodide.
- **Thyroid tissue destroying agents:** Radioactive iodine (^{131}I, ^{125}I, ^{123}I).
- **As a side effect of some drugs:** Lithium amiodarone sulfonamides, phenytoin, rifampicin, etc.

Thyroid Hormone Synthesis Inhibitors or Antithyroid Drugs: *(Propylthiouracil, Methimazole, Carbimazole)*

- These drugs inhibit the synthesis of thyroid hormone.
- These drugs bind to the thyroid peroxidase and prevent oxidation of iodide/iodo-tyrosyl residues. This causes inhibition of iodination of tyrosine residues in thyroglobulin and also inhibition of coupling of iodo-tyrosine residues to form T$_3$ and T$_4$.
- In addition, Propylthiouracil also inhibits the peripheral conversion of T$_4$ to T$_3$.

Pharmacokinetics

- These drugs have good oral absorption and are widely distributed in all the compartments of body.
- The metabolism occurs in liver and excretion via kidneys.
- These drugs attain good concentration in thyroid tissue, cross placental barrier and are also secreted in the milk also.
- Carbimazole gets converted to methimazole after absorption and has a longer t ½.
- **Propylthiuracil** is most rapidly absorbed and has a short half-life, so it has to be given 6–8 hourly. Propylthiouracil is given in a dose of 50–150 mg thrice daily in the starting and it is followed by 25–50 mg twice to thrice daily for maintenance therapy.

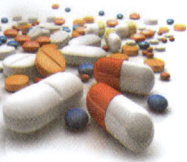

- **Methimazole** is given in a dose of 5–10 mg thrice daily in the starting and it is followed by 5–15 mg once or twice daily for maintenance therapy.
- **Carbimazole** is given in a dose of 5–15 mg thrice daily in the starting and it is followed by 2.5–10 mg once or twice daily for maintenance therapy.

Therapeutic Uses

Antithyroid drugs are used in following conditions:
- Hyperthyroid states like thyrotoxicosis in both Graves' disease (diffuse toxic goiter) and toxic nodular goiter.
- Thyroid storm.
- Hyperthyroidism in pregnancy because in pregnancy radioactive iodine ^{131}I and thyroidectomy both are contraindicated.
- Along with radioactive iodine ^{131}I and propranolol to improve recovery in thyrotoxicosis.
- Preoperatively before surgery.

Maintenance doses are titrated on the basis of clinical status and laboratory findings of the patient.

Adverse Effects

- Reversible hypothyroidism and goiter (occurs due to overtreatment only).
- Some other side effects are GI disturbances, skin rashes and joint pain, loss or greying of hair, aguesia, pyrexia and mild hepatotoxicity can occur.
- Rarely reversible agranulocytosis can also occur.

INHIBITORS OF IODIDE TRAPPING OR IONIC INHIBITORS

(Thiocyanates, Perchlorates, Nitrates)
- These drugs inhibit iodide trapping and block synthesis of thyroid hormones.
- Due to their highly toxic nature, they are not used clinically.

HORMONE RELEASE INHIBITORS

(Iodine, Iodides of Na and K, Organic iodide)
- Iodides have a paradoxical effect in thyroid hormone synthesis when given in therapeutic dose.
- The symptoms of thyrotoxicosis subside within 2–3 days and the gland starts shrinking within 2 weeks period. Higher concentrations of iodides inhibit almost all steps of synthesis of thyroid hormone and its release.
- It is given orally in the form of solution.
- Iodide is given in a dose of 100–300 mg/day therapeutically and 5–10 mg/day prophylactically in the patients of endemic goiter.

Therapeutic Uses

- Preoperative preparation for thyroidectomy in Graves' disease.
- Thyroid storm.
- Prophylaxis of endemic goiter, it is generally used as iodized salt.
- Antiseptic and mucolytic agent, in the form of tincture iodine, povidone iodine and as potassium iodide in cough syrup preparations.

Adverse Effects

- **Acute effects** are seen due to hypersensitivity to iodine and present as fever, arthralgia, swelling of lips and eyelids, angioedema of larynx and petechial hemorrhages, etc.
- **Chronic effects** are seen due to overdose and the patient presents in the form of a syndrome known as iodism.
  - The presenting features are flu-like symptoms like headache, rhinorrhea, sneezing, lacrimation, swelling of eyelids, inflammation of all mucous membranes, etc.
  - The symptoms are reversible on stopping the drug. Higher doses for long-term can cause hypothyroidism and goiter also.

THYROID TISSUE DESTROYING AGENTS

(Radioactive Iodine$^{(131}$I$^{, 125}$I$^{, 123}$I$^{)}$)

^{131}I is the only radioactive isotope of Iodine which has therapeutic importance.
- After oral administration, it gets concentrated in thyroid follicles and emits β-particles.
- These β-particles penetrate 0.5–2.0 mm of thyroid tissue and ablate it.
- The hyperthyroid state is corrected.
- It has a physical half-life of 8 days.
- Radioactive iodine is given in a dose of 25–100 μ curie for diagnostic purpose and 3–6 m curie in therapeutic doses.
- The response starts after 2 weeks and gradually reaches to a peak at 3 months time.

Advantages

- Treatment is economical, is given on outpatient basis and the cure is permanent.
- There is no risk of surgical scar or injury to parathyroid glands or recurrent laryngeal nerves.

Disadvantages

- Not suitable for young patients
- Hypothyroidism
- Long latent period of response
- Contraindicated during pregnancy

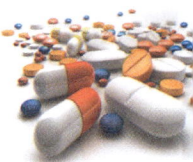

β-ADRENERGIC BLOCKERS

- They improve the symptoms of thyrotoxicosis, which are due to sympathetic over-activity.
- These symptoms are palpitations, tremors, nervousness, and sweating.
- Propranolol has an inhibitory effect on the peripheral conversion of T_4 to T_3.
- Propranolol is the most commonly used beta-blocker for this purpose.

AS A SIDE EFFECT OF SOME DRUGS

(Lithium, Amiodarone, Sulfonamides, Phenytoin, Rifampicin, etc.)
The above listed drugs and many more produce antithyroid effects when given for prolonged durations.

Drug Interactions

- The absorption of L-thyroxine is reduced by proton pump inhibitors, sucralfate, calcium and iron. Hence, concurrent use should be avoided or dose should be adjusted.
- Carbamazepine, phenytoin and rifampicin increase the metabolism of T_4. Hence, dose of L-thyroxine needs to be adjusted accordingly.

Nursing Implications

- **Thyroid supplements and suppressants**
  - Educate the patient about the importance of long-term treatment and continuous follow-up.
  - Educate the patients about diet and not to take goitrogenous substances.
  - Assess patient carefully to detect any potential drug–drug interactions if giving thyroid hormone in combination with other drugs.
  - Monitor for adverse effects (tachycardia, hypertension, anxiety, and skin rash).
  - Evaluate the effectiveness of the teaching plan (patient can name drug, dosage, adverse effects to watch for, and specific measures to avoid them).

STEROIDS AND ANABOLIC STEROIDS

- The adrenal gland (suprarenal gland) consists of cortex and medulla.
- The cortex secretes two types of corticosteroids (glucocorticoids and mineralocorticoids) and the adrenal androgens.
- The medulla secretes catecholamines (adrenaline and nor-adrenaline).

- The adrenal cortex has three zones, and each zone synthesizes a different type of steroid hormone from cholesterol.
- **The outer zona glomerulosa** produces mineralocorticoids (aldosterone) that is responsible for regulating salt and water metabolism. Production of aldosterone is regulated primarily by the renin–angiotensin system.
- **The middle zona fasciculata** synthesizes glucocorticoids (cortisol) that are involved in metabolism and response to stress.
- **The inner zona reticularis** secretes adrenal androgens.
- Adrenocorticotropic hormone (ACTH) released from the pituitary gland in response to hypothalamic corticotropin-releasing hormone (CRH) controls the secretions of adrenal gland by a feedback system (Fig. 11.3).
- There is a diurnal variation in the rate of secretion of ACTH and cortisol (circadian rhythm). Their levels are highest in the early morning and lowest in the evening hours.

MECHANISM OF ACTION

- The glucocorticoid receptors are widely distributed throughout the body.
- The mineralocorticoid receptors are present in excretory organs, such as the kidney, colon, salivary glands and sweat glands.

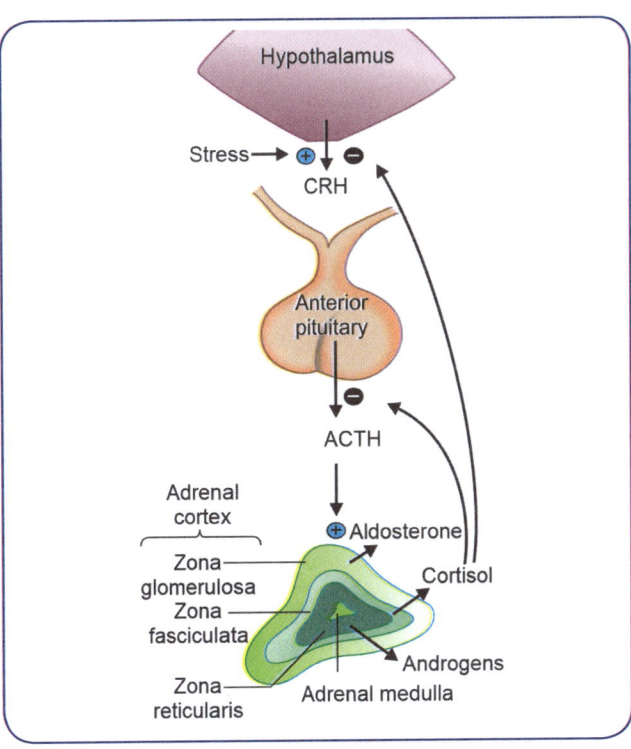

FIG. 11.3: Regulation of corticoids synthesis

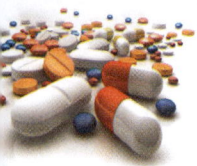

- The brain has both types of receptors.
- The corticosteroids bind to specific intracellular cytoplasmic receptors in target tissues and the receptor hormone complex translocates into the nucleus and produces the effects.

The term corticosteroids is synonymous to corticoids and it includes all the natural glucocorticoids and mineralocorticoids and their synthetic analogues.

Some clinically useful corticoids are given in Table 11.6.

The dosage, route and special features of common corticosteroids are given in Table 11.7.

TABLE 11.6: Clinically useful corticoids

Compound	Duration of action	Drugs	Relative potency
Glucocorticoids	Short (half-life: ≤12 hours)	Hydrocortisone	20 mg
	Intermediate (half-life: 12-36 hours)	Prednisolone	5 mg
		Methylprednisolone	4 mg
		Triamcinolone	4 mg
		Deflazacort	6 mg
	Long (half-life: ≥36 hours)	Dexamethasone	0.75 mg
		Betamethasone	0.75 mg
Mineralocorticoids	Desoxycortico-sterone acetate (DOCA)	2.5 mg (sublingual)	
	Fludrocortisone	0.2 mg	

TABLE 11.7: Dose, route and special features of common corticosteroids

Drug	Dose and route	Special features
Hydrocortisone	For replacement therapy: 20 mg morning + 10 mg afternoon orally In emergencies:100 mg IV bolus + 100 mg 8 hourly IV infusion	• Fast acting with short duration of action • Has both glucocorticoid and mineralocorticoid activities • Used in acute adrenal insufficiency, shock and status asthmaticus
Prednisolone	5–60 mg/day oral, or 1 mg/kg/day	• Four times more potent than hydrocortisone with intermediate duration of action • Glucocorticoid activity is more. • Mineralocorticoid activity occurs at high doses and causes fluid retention • Single morning dose or alternate day treatment causes less pituitary-adrenal axis suppression • Used for allergic, autoimmune, inflammatory diseases and malignancies
Methyl-prednisolone	4–32 mg/day orally. For Pulse therapy 1 gm IV in the form of infusion is given after every 6–8 weeks	• More potent than prednisolone • Minimal suppression of pituitary adrenal axis • Used in ulcerative colitis, active rheumatoid arthritis, pemphigus, renal transplant, etc. • Used in high doses in spinal cord injuries and pulse therapy
Triamcinolone	4–32 mg/day oral, 5–40 mg IM, intra-articular injection	• More potent than prednisolone • Highly selective glucocorticoid activity • Also used as topical preparation
Dexamethasone	0.5–5 mg/day oral, 4–20 mg/day IV infusion or IM injection	• Very potent and long-acting • Highly selective glucocorticoid • Marked pituitary-adrenal suppression occurs with its use • It is used for shock, cerebral edema, allergic and inflammatory conditions • Topical preparations are also used in steroid responsive skin conditions
Betamethasone	0.5–5 mg/ day oral, 4–20 mg IM/IV injection	• Similar to dexamethasone • Preferred in cerebral edema

Contd...

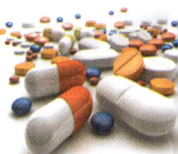

Drug	Dose and route	Special features
Deflazacort	Initially: 60–120 mg/day Maintenance: 6–18 mg/day Children: 0.25–1.5 mg/kg daily or on alternate days	• Less potent than prednisolone • No mineralocorticoid activity • Causes lesser adverse effects • Used inflammatory and immunological disorders and preferred in children
Desoxy-corticosterone Acetate (DOCA)	2–5 mg sublingual 10–20 mg IM once or twice weekly	• Has good mineralocorticoid activity • Used for replacement therapy in Addison's disease
Fludrocortisone	50–200 µg daily as replacement therapy 50–200 µg/day for congenital adrenal hyperplasia 100–200 µg/day for postural hypotension	• A potent mineralocorticoid with some glucocorticoid activity • Used in Addison's disease (as Replacement therapy), congenital adrenal hyperplasia and idiopathic postural hypotension
Aldosterone		• Most potent mineralocorticoid • Not used clinically due to low oral bioavailability

Main Hormones and their Actions

Summary of special features, dose and route of administration of main hormones is given in Table 11.8.

Glucocorticoids (Systemic Effects)

Factors such as stress and levels of the circulating steroids influence their secretion. The cortisols have so many effects such as:

- **Promotion of normal intermediary metabolism:** Glucocorticoids favor gluconeogenesis, stimulate protein catabolism (except in the liver) and lipolysis.
- **Increase resistance to stress:** By raising plasma glucose levels, glucocorticoids provide the body with energy to combat stress caused by trauma, fright, infection, bleeding, or debilitating disease.
- **Alter blood cell levels in plasma:** Glucocorticoids also increase hemoglobin, erythrocytes, platelets, and polymorphonuclear leukocytes. Glucocorticoids cause a decrease in eosinophils, basophils, monocytes, and lymphocytes by redistributing them from the circulation to lymphoid tissue.
- **Anti-inflammatory action:** Glucocorticoids possess potent anti-inflammatory and immunosuppressive activities due to lowering of circulating lymphocytes. Glucocorticoids also decrease the production and release of proinflammatory cytokines. They inhibit phospholipase A_2, which blocks the release of arachidonic acid (the precursor of the prostaglandins and leukotrienes) from membrane-bound phospholipid. The decreased production of prostaglandins and leukotrienes produces anti-inflammatory action.
- **Effect on other systems:** Adequate cortisol levels are essential for normal glomerular filtration. High levels of glucocorticoids serve as feedback inhibitors of ACTH production and affect the endocrine system by suppressing further synthesis of glucocorticoids and thyroid-stimulating hormone.

Mineralocorticoids (Systemic Effects)

- Mineralocorticoids help to control fluid status and concentration of electrolytes, especially sodium and potassium.
- Aldosterone acts on distal tubules and collecting ducts in the kidney, causing reabsorption of sodium, bicarbonate, and water.

TABLE 11.8: Summary of effects of main hormones

Hormones	Minerelocorticoid (aldosterone, desoxy-corticosterone)	Glucocorticoids (hydrocortisone)
Action	Regulate water and electrolyte balance.	Metabolic (carbohydrate, protein and fat) anti-inflammatory, immunosuppressant and anti-allergic action
Hypersecretion	Primary hyperaldosteronism (Conn's disease)	Cushing disease
Deficiency	Addison's disease	

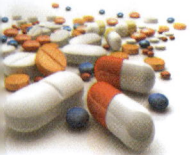

Therapeutic Uses of the Corticosteroids

- Several semisynthetic derivatives of corticosteroids are available.
- Different agents differ in anti-inflammatory potency, mineralocorticoid activity and duration of action.
- Corticosteroids are used in replacement therapy and in the treatment of severe allergic reactions, asthma, rheumatoid arthritis, other inflammatory disorders, and some cancers.
- Some common uses of corticosteroids are as follows:
  - As a replacement therapy for adrenal corticoid disorders
    - **For primary adrenocortical insufficiency (Addison's disease):** Hydrocortisone and fludrocortisone are given in Addison's disease.
    - **For secondary or tertiary adrenocortical insufficiency:** Hydrocortisone is used for treatment of these deficiencies.
    - **For congenital adrenal hyperplasia (CAH):** Treatment of the condition requires administration of sufficient corticosteroids to normalize hormone levels.
  - **Diagnosis of Cushing's syndrome**
    - Cushing's syndrome is caused by hypersecretion of glucocorticoids (hypercortisolism) that results from excessive release of ACTH by the anterior pituitary or an adrenal tumor. Testing cortisol levels in urine, plasma, and saliva and the dexamethasone suppression test are used to diagnose Cushing's syndrome.
  - **For relief of inflammatory symptoms**
    - Corticosteroids provide symptomatic relief and prevent the damage due to the inflammatory mediators. These are not curative in these disorders. Corticosteroids significantly reduce the manifestations of inflammation associated with:
    - Rheumatoid arthritis
    - Inflammatory skin conditions (redness, swelling, heat, and tenderness).
    - Persistent asthma, as well as management of asthma exacerbations (for early and better symptom control)
    - Active inflammatory bowel disease.
  - **In non-inflammatory disorders** (osteoarthritis), intra-articular corticosteroids may be used for treatment.
  - **For treatment of allergies:** By preventing the formation of inflammatory mediators, these drugs provide a beneficial effect in the treatment of allergic rhinitis, as well as drug, serum, and transfusion allergic reactions.
  - **For acceleration of lung maturation:** Betamethasone or dexamethasone is administered intramuscularly to the mother within the 48 hours before premature delivery can accelerate lung maturation in the fetus.
  - **Gouty arthritis:** These drugs provide dramatic relief in acute gouty arthritis, not responding to other modes of therapy.
  - **Collagen vascular disorders:** These drugs are life saving in diseases such as systemic lupus erythematosus (SLE), nephrotic syndrome, glomerular nephritis, polyarteritis nodosa, etc.
  - **Autoimmune disorders:** Autoimmune diseases such as idiopathic thrombocytopenic purpura, autoimmune hemolytic anemia, etc. respond to steroids (prednisolone is preferred).
  - **Eye diseases:** These drugs can prevent blindness in certain inflammatory ocular diseases but, should not be used in routine.
  - **Cerebral edema:** These drugs decrease the cerebral edema and prevent the neurological complications.
  - **Malignancies, organ transplantation and skin grafting.**

Adverse Effects

- The side effects of glucocorticoids are due to use of these drugs for more than 2–3 weeks in supraphysiological doses. Otherwise, these drugs are life saving in many dreadful conditions.
- **Side effects due to Mineralocorticoids activity:** Edema, and rise in blood pressure occurs due to sodium and water retention.
- **Side effects due to Glucocorticoid activity:**
  These are:
  - Metabolic effects: Hyperglycemia and precipitation of diabetes.
  - Cushing's habitus: Presents as moon face, obesity of trunk with relatively thin limbs, small mouth and buffalo hump.
  - Skin becomes fragile with purple striae, telangiectasia, hirsutism and easy bruising. With topical preparations, skin atrophy can also occur.
  - Decrease in immune status causes susceptibility to various opportunistic infections. Flaring up of latent tuberculosis may occur.
  - Muscular weakness in the form of myopathy can occur.
  - Delayed wound healing of minor wounds.
  - Dyspeptic and peptic ulcers may develop.
  - Corticosteroids can be a cause of 'corticosteroid induced osteoporosis' and 'corticosteroid induced avascular necrosis' of head of femur, humerus or knee joint.
- In the eye, glaucoma and development of posterior subcapsular cataract may occur.

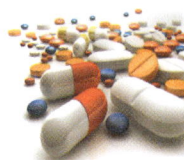

- Growth retardation can occur in children.
- Due to teratogenic effects there is always a risk to mother (gestational diabetes, pregnancy induced hypertension [PIH] and preeclampsia) and fetus (abortion, stillbirth and fetal abnormalities).
- Psychiatric disturbances may be seen after long-term use.

Hypothalamo-pituitary-adrenal (HPA) Axis Suppression

- When the corticoids are used for long-term and in higher doses (more than physiological limits), the suppression of HPA axis occurs due to negative feedback mechanisms. This is most dangerous side effect of corticoids.
- The adrenal cortex atrophies and stops the synthesis of natural corticoids.
- Sudden withdrawal of corticoids exhibits withdrawal syndrome in the form of anorexia, nausea, malaise, fever, postural hypotension, weakness, pain in muscles, joints and electrolyte imbalance.
- Whenever these patients are subjected to stress, they may go into acute adrenal insufficiency and cardiovascular collapse occurs.

To prevent this condition, following measures provide help:

- A scheme of gradual withdrawal is employed in which the corticoids are given in tapered doses so that HPA axis gets enough time to revive. This is must in any patient who has received >20–25 mg/day hydrocortisone, or ≥5 mg prednisolone/day or during stressful situations, within one year of steroid withdrawal or equivalent for longer than 2–3 weeks.
- Whenever possible, topical preparations should be used for dermatological conditions.
- A single morning dose at 6.00–8.00 am causes least hypothalamic pituitary adrenal (HPA) axis suppression as this time matches with circadian rhythm of corticoids secretion.
- In chronic conditions, alternate day therapy can be employed.
- Preferably, shorter acting steroids (hydrocortisone, prednisolone) at the lowest possible dose should be given.
- If a patient on steroid therapy develops an infection, the steroid should not be discontinued *but* the dose should be increased to meet the stress of infection. In these patients, the surgery should be covered by intra-operative and post-operative IV hydrocortisone till the condition stabilizes. This should be invariably followed by oral prednisolone therapy for an appropriate period.

The Contraindications to Corticoids use

- All the contraindications of steroid use are relative, as corti-coids are mostly used in compelling situations.
- A cautious use is advocated in following associated conditions:
  - Hypertension
  - Infections such as viral and fungal infections, tuberculosis, herpes simplex keratitis, etc.
  - Peptic ulcer
  - Osteoporosis
  - Diabetes mellitus
  - Renal failure
  - Psychosis
  - Epilepsy
  - Congestive heart failure.

ANABOLIC STEROIDS

- Anabolic steroids are synthetic androgens with higher anabolic and comparatively low androgenic activity.
- These are believed to increase the muscle mass by enhancing the protein anabolism. Basically, these drugs behave similar to androgens.
- Combination of these drugs with any other drug is not allowed and banned legally also.
- The various anabolic steroids are Nandrolone, Stanozolol, Oxymetholone, and Methandienone (Table 11.9).

Therapeutic Uses of Anabolic Steroids

- **Catabolic states:** Anabolic steroids may provide some beneficial effects in debilitated and elderly patients after surgery, trauma and weakness due to prolonged illness. During the period of convalescence, these drugs may improve the appetite, help in weight gain and provide some sense of well-being. All these effects are due to the positive nitrogen balance provided by these drugs.

TABLE 11.9: Dose of anabolic steroids

Drug	Dose
Nandrolone decanoate	25–100 mg by IM route every 3 weeks
Nandrolone phenyl propionate	10–50 mg by IM route once or twice weekly
Stanozolol	2–6 mg daily by oral route
Oxymetholone:	5–10 mg once daily
Methandienone	2–5 mg once or twice orally or 25 mg by IM route weekly

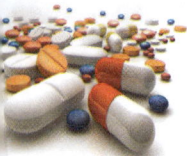

- **Senile osteoporosis:** In elderly males, these drugs may help in new bone formation and bone mineralization. Otherwise, bisphosphonates are the preferred agents.
- **Refractory anemia associated with hemolysis and malignancy:** Some gain in Hb% is obtained in some selected patients only. Erythropoietin therapy is more selective and preferred as compared to anabolic steroids.
- **To enhance the physical ability in athletes:** These drugs can help in increasing the strength of exercised muscles, increase in the stamina, and muscle mass. Anabolic steroids have been included in the list of 'dope test' performed on athletes before any competitive games. Use of anabolic steroids is not advocated medically for this purpose.

Adverse Effects

Main side effects seen are masculinization and acne in females, precautious puberty in young boys, jaundice and worsening of lipid profile in elderly patients.

 Drug Interactions

- Glucocorticoids antagonize the action of insulin and other OHAs. Hence, concurrent use should be avoided.
- Glucocorticoids antagonize the action of antihypertensive drugs. Hence, concurrent use should be avoided or dose should be adjusted accordingly.

Nursing Implications

- **Steroids and anabolic steroids**
  - The corticosteroids should be administered between 8 am and 9 am to minimize suppression of the hypothalamic–pituitary axis.
  - Patient should be educated about tapering the doses of corticosteroids when discontinuing from high doses or from long-term therapy to give the adrenal glands a chance to recover and prevent acute adrenal insufficiency.
  - Arrange for increased dose when the patient is under stress to supply the increased demand for corticosteroid associated with the stress reaction.
  - Do not give live virus vaccines when the patient is immunosuppressed because there is an increased risk of infection.
  - Protect the patient from unnecessary exposure to infection and invasive procedures because the steroids suppress the immune system and the patient is at increased risk for infection.
  - Assess the patient carefully for any potential drug to drug interactions to avoid adverse effects.
  - Monitor for adverse effects (increased susceptibility to infections, skin changes, endocrine dysfunctions, fatigue, fluid retention, peptic ulcer, psychological changes).
  - Evaluate the effectiveness of the teaching plan.

UTERINE STIMULANTS AND RELAXANTS

- Uterine stimulants are the drugs, which stimulate the uterine contractions. These agents are also known as *oxytocics* or *ecbolics*. These drugs are also known as abortifacients as these can also be used to induce abortions.
- These drugs are usually employed to augment uterine contractions during labor to assist the delivery or to induce abortion.
- Uterine relaxants are the drugs, which produce a relaxant effect on the uterus or slow down the uterine contractions/activity. These agents are known as **tocolytics**.

The various drugs used as uterine stimulants or oxytocics are as follows:

- **Oxytocin** (hormone secreted by Posterior pituitary)
- **Ergot alkaloids derivatives:** Ergometrine (Ergonovine), Methylergometrine
- **Prostaglandins:** PGE_2, $PGF_{2\alpha}$, 15-methyl $PGF_{2\alpha}$ and Misoprostol.
- **Miscellaneous:** Ethacridine, and Quinine.

OXYTOCIN

- Oxytocin is a peptide hormone secreted by the posterior pituitary.
- It is released by stimuli such as parturition, suckling and coitus.
- The amount of secretion depends upon the nature of the stimulus.
- Commercially available oxytocin is produced synthetically.

Pharmacokinetics

- It is given by intramuscular or intravenous route in infusion only and is ineffective orally.
- The metabolism occurs in liver and excretion occurs through kidneys by an enzyme called oxytocinase.
- The plasma t ½ is 8–15 minutes.

Pharmacological Actions

- **Uterus:**
  - Oxytocin increases the force and frequency of uterine contractions. This effect is seen more vividly in pregnant uterus after >24 weeks pregnancy as estrogens sensitize the uterus to oxytocin.
  - Oxytocin acts through oxytocin receptors and the number of these receptors is increased by estrogens.
  - Non-pregnant uterus and that during early pregnancy is resistant to the effect of oxytocin.
- **Breast:** Oxytocin facilitates milk ejection by contraction of the mammary glands. Suckling (nipple and areolar region) stimulates the release of oxytocin.

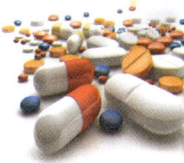

- **CVS:** Higher doses may cause vasodilatation and may produce hypotension with flushing and reflex tachycardia.
- **Kidney:** Higher doses of oxytocin produce antidiuretic effect and cause fluid retention. This effect is rarely seen at conventional doses.

Physiological Roles

Oxytocin plays an essential role in labor, milk ejection reflex and formation of love bonding between mother and infant.

Therapeutic Uses

- **Induction of labor:** For induction of labor, the following schedule is employed: 5 IU is diluted in 500 mL of glucose or saline solution (10 milli IU/ml) and the intravenous infusion is started at a low rate of 0.2–2.0 ml/min and progressively accelerated according to response. Usually a total of 2–4 IU is needed before starting infusion; obstetric contraindications should be evaluated thoroughly.
- **Postpartum hemorrhage (PPH):** Oxytocin can be used as an alternative to ergometrine when it is contraindicated. For this purpose, 5 IU of oxytocin may be injected intramuscularly or may be administered by intravenous infusion for immediate control of PPH.
- **Breast engorgement:** Intranasal oxytocin spray is useful when milk ejection is impaired in nursing mothers.
- **Uterine inertia:** If uterine contractions are feeble and there is no cephalopelvic disproportion, oxytocin can be used.

Adverse Effects

- Excessive doses of oxytocin can cause rupture of uterus, fetal hypoxia and even fetal death.
- Prolonged oxytocin infusion can lead to water intoxication due to anti-diuretic like action.

Desamino-oxytocin

It is a buccal formulation of oxytocin and is given in a dose of:

- 50 IU buccal tablet to be repeated every 30 minutes up to a maximum of 10 tabs, for induction of labor
- 25 IU every 30 minutes for uterine inertia,
- 25–50 IU just before breastfeeding for breast engorgement cases.

Carbetocin is another long-acting analogue of oxytocin.

ERGOMETRINE, METHYLERGOMETRINE

- Ergometrine is an alkaloid.
- Methylergometrine is a semisynthetic derivative.
- Both have similar pharmacological actions, but methylergometrine is more potent than ergometrine.

Pharmacological Actions

- **Uterus:**
  - These drugs increase force, frequency and duration of uterine contractions.
  - These actions are evident on both upper and lower uterine segments and uterus passes into a state of sustained tonic contractions.
  - This uterotonic action is due to partial agonistic action on 5-HT$_2$ and α adrenergic receptors.
  - **CVS:** These drugs can raise blood pressure in higher doses but not in therapeutic doses used in obstetrics.

Pharmacokinetics

- Ergometrine is rapid and short acting.
- It can be given by oral, IM or IV route.
- The onset of uterine action is 15 minutes by oral route, 5 minutes by IM route and almost immediately by IV route.
- These drugs are partly metabolized in liver and excreted in urine with a plasma t½ of 1–2 hours, and the effect of a single dose remains up to 3–4 hours.

Adverse Effects

Nausea, vomiting and occasional rise in blood pressure.

Therapeutic Uses

- **Postpartum hemorrhage (PPH):**
  - 0.2–0.3 mg of ergometrine is given by IM route at delivery of anterior shoulder. It reduces the blood loss and chances of PPH.
  - In active PPH: 0.5 mg ergometrine by IV route or a combination of 0.5 mg ergometrine with oxytocin 5 IU IM or IV may be used.
- To prevent **uterine atony after cesarean** section or instrumental delivery.
- **To hasten uterine involution:** 0.125 mg of ergometrine or methylergometrine is given thrice daily orally for 7 days.

PROSTAGLANDINS AND UTERUS

- Prostaglandins are synthesized by the uterus and play an important role in menstruation and parturition.
- PGE2, PGF2α and 15-methyl PGF2α stimulate the contraction of both pregnant and non-pregnant uterus. (sensitivity is higher in the later part of pregnancy).
- They also cause ripening of cervix.
- PGE2 (Dinoprostone) is used intravaginally or extra-amniotically, 15-methyl PGF2α (carboprost) by deep IM and misoprostol by intravaginal route.

Ethacridine is used for:

- Extra-amniotic infusion for medical termination of pregnancy in the second trimester.

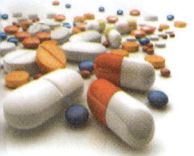

- For this purpose, 150 mL (containing 150 mg) is injected slowly extra-amniotically, which produces uterine contractions and expulsion of fetus with membranes.

UTERINE RELAXANTS

- These drugs (tocolytics) decrease the uterine motility or contractions and produce relaxation of uterus.
- These are used to delay or postpone labor to arrest the progress of threatened abortion and in dysmenorrhea.

The following drugs are used as tocolytics:

- **Adrenergic agonists:** Ritodrine, Isoxpurine, Salbutamol and terbutaline.
- **Oxytocin antagonist:** Atosiban
- **Prostaglandin synthesis inhibitors:** Aspirin, Indomethacin, mefenamic acid, etc.
- **Miscellaneous drugs:** Magnesium sulfate, Nifedipine.

Adrenergic Agonists

- The β_2 selective agonist have more prominent uterine relaxant action and they have the ability to suppress premature labor in a large number of cases.
- Ritodrine is most preferred agent and is given as 50 µg/min IV infusion. According to the response, the rate can be titrated and is increased every 10 minutes till the cessation of uterine contractions or the maternal heart rate rises to 120/minute. This is followed by either 10 mg IM or orally for a period of 48 hours at the most.
- Salbutamol and terbutaline are also used as alternatives to ritodrine. Isoxsuprine can be used by both oral and IM route in cases of threatened abortion.
- Main side effects are headache, anxiety, hypotension, tachycardia, hyperglycemia and hypokalemia.

Oxytocin Antagonist

- **Atosiban** acts as antagonist at the oxytocin receptors.
- It is used for inhibition of labor between 24 and 33 weeks of gestation.
- It is used as an alternative to β_2 adrenergic agonists.

Prostaglandin Synthesis Inhibitors

- Aspirin, indomethacin, mefenamic acid, etc.
- NSAIDs produce tocolytic effect by inhibiting prostaglandin synthesis.
- These drugs are not used as tocolytics primarily because of their propensity to cause premature closure of ductus arteriosus and subsequently pulmonary hypertension in the infant.
- These can be used for the relief of dysmenorrhea, but not to delay labor.

Miscellaneous Drugs

Magnesium sulfate, Nifedipine

Magnesium Sulfate

- It is used to suppress convulsions and control of BP in preeclampsia and eclampsia.
- It also acts as a tocolytic.
- Not preferred nowadays, due to availability of better alternative drugs.

Calcium Channel Blockers (Nifedipine)

These drugs are also having tocolytic effects but not a preferred agent, due to adverse effects of decrease reduction in placental perfusion.

Indications of Tocolytic Agents

Tocolytic agents are useful in:

- To delay the premature labor.
- To inhibit the uterine contractions in threatened abortion.
- To suppress the painful uterine contractions in dysmenorrhea.

Nursing Implications

- **Uterine stimulants and relaxants**
  - Assess for contraindications or cautions and history of allergy to oxytocics to avoid hypersensitivity reactions.
  - Ensure fetal position and cephalopelvic proportions before starting the oxytocin infusion to prevent serious complications.
  - Regularly check the number of drops being administered in the oxytocin drip and change the rate if required.
  - Monitor blood pressure and fetal heart rate frequently during and after administration to monitor for adverse effects. Discontinue the drug if blood pressure rises dramatically.
  - The partograph (record of progress of labor) should be maintained properly in neat and clean handwriting
  - Discontinue the drug at any sign of uterine hypertonicity to avoid potentially life-threatening effects; provide life support as needed.
  - Monitor for adverse effects (blood pressure changes, uterine hypertonicity, water intoxication, ergotism).
  - Evaluate the effectiveness of the teaching plan

CONTRACEPTIVES

- Contraceptives are the agents, which are used for the reversible suppression of fertility.
- Many types of contraceptives are available such as oral, parenteral and others.

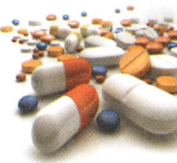

- These agents are mostly hormonal in nature whereas non-hormonal contraceptives are also there.

ORAL CONTRACEPTIVES

- Oral contraception is the most popular and effective method of contraception.
- The following types of oral contraceptives are available:
  - Combined hormonal oral contraceptives:
    - Monophasic, biphasic, triphasic
  - Progestin only pill or minipill.
  - Post coital oral contraceptives.
  - Others (Centchroman).

COMBINED HORMONAL ORAL CONTRACEPTIVES

- These oral contraceptives contain low doses of estrogens and progestins.
- The estrogen used is ethynylestradiol and the progestins used are norethisterone, levonogestrel, desogestrel, norgestrel, etc.
- These are highly efficacious with success rate of 99%.

Mechanism of Action of Combined Oral Contraceptives

- The combination pill suppresses the ovulation by inhibiting the release of follicular stimulating hormone (FSH) and luteinizing hormone (LH). Therefore, the proliferative and secretory phase of menstrual cycle is interrupted. These are mainly estrogenic effect.
- Progesterogenic effects include increase in the viscosity of cervical mucus, which makes the sperm penetration difficult and to ensure withdrawal bleeding after stopping the medication.

Monophasic Combination Pills

- These pills contain *fixed amount* of estrogen and progesterone.
- The pill is given orally for 21 consecutive days, beginning on the day 5th of the menstrual cycle, followed by a gap of 7 days (pill-free period) and the next course starts on the day 5th of the menstrual cycle.
- The pack contains 28 tablets (21 hormonal and 7 iron tablets) and these are numbered/arrowed so that a woman takes the tablet in continuation.
- The menstruation starts in the pill-free period like a normal menstrual cycle.
- The pills should be taken every day at a fixed time, preferably before going to bed at night.
- If the woman forgets to take the pill, on the next day two pills should be taken and the cycle of taking pills should be continued as usual.

- If pills are missed for 2–3 days or more, then the course should be stopped and additional precautionary measures like condoms, diaphragm or spermicidal sponge/jelly should be used and the next course should start from the day 5th of menses as usual.
- The combined hormonal pills are available in following low dose combinations:

COMBINED PILLS		
PROGESTIN		ESTROGEN
Norgestrel 300 µg	+	Ethinylestradiol 30 µg
Norgestrel 500 µg	+	Ethinylestradiol 50 µg
Levonorgestrel 250 µg	+	Ethinylestradiol 50 µg
Levonorgestrel 150 µg	+	Ethinylestradiol 30 µg
Levonorgestrel 100 µg	+	Ethinylestradiol 20 µg
Desogestrel 150 µg	+	Ethinylestradiol 30 µg
Desogestrel 150 µg	+	Ethinylestradiol 20 µg

Biphasic Combination Pills

- These pills mimic the natural physiological hormonal changes during the menstrual cycle.
- These pills have a fixed dose of estrogen for 21 days and progesterone is given concurrently in increasing doses in two successive phases, i.e., from day 1–10, then days 11–21. Next seven days are pill-free days.
- These pills are not preferred.

Triphasic Combination Pills

- These pills contain higher dose of estrogen near midcycle but with increasing doses of progesterone for three successive phases, i.e., for days 1–6, 7–11, 12–21. Next seven days are pill-free days.
- These pills are recommended for the women over 35 years or when other risk factors are present and monophasic pills cannot be given.

Progestin Only Pill or Minipill

- These pills contain only progesterone in low dose and are recommended in women in whom estrogen is contraindicated.
- These are taken daily without any gap in between.
- The menstrual cycle may become irregular and its efficacy is lower as compared to combined pills.
- These pills are less preferred nowadays.

Post Coital Oral Contraceptives (Emergency Pills)

- This method is recommended to be followed after the unprotected sexual intercourse to prevent the risk of pregnancy.

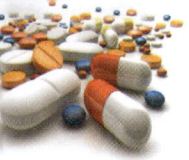

- This method has high failure rate and more side effects as compared to regular contraceptives; hence, this method should be reserved for emergency contraception only in cases like rape, condom failure, etc.
- There are five regimens:
  1. 0.75 mg levonorgestrel tablet, two doses at 12-hours interval within 72 hours of unprotected intercourse.
  2. Alternatively, 1.5 mg single tablet can be taken as soon as possible, but before 72 hours of unprotected intercourse.
  3. Yuzpe method: 0.5 mg levonorgestrel + 0.1 mg ethinyl-estradiol, two doses at 12-hours interval within 72 hours of unprotected intercourse.
  4. Single dose of 600 mg mifepristone (anti-progesterone) taken within 72 hours of unprotected intercourse and follow it up 48 hours later by a single 400 mg oral dose of misoprostol.
  5. Single dose of 30 mg ulipristal (selective progesterone receptor modulator) as soon as possible, but within 5 days of unprotected intercourse.

Common Side Effects of Oral Contraceptives

- The incidence of adverse effects with oral contraceptives is determined by the specific compounds and combinations used.
- The most common adverse effects with estrogens are breast fullness, fluid retention, headache, and nausea. Increased blood pressure may also occur. Progestins may be associated with depression, changes in libido, hirsutism, and acne. Thromboembolism, thrombophlebitis, myocardial infarction, and stroke may occur rarely with use of oral contraceptives.
- These severe adverse effects are most common among women who are over the age of 35 yrs and are heavy smokers.
- The incidence of cervical cancer may be increased with oral contraceptives, because these women are less likely to use additional barrier methods of contraception that reduce exposure to human papillomavirus (the primary risk factor for cervical cancer).
- Oral contraceptives themselves are associated with a decreased risk of cervical and ovarian cancer.

Contraindications of Oral Contraceptives

- Oral contraceptives are contraindicated in the presence of cerebrovascular and thromboembolic disease, estrogen-dependent neoplasms, liver disease, and pregnancy.
- Combination oral contraceptives should not be used in patients over the age of 35 years who are heavy smokers.

- Drugs that induce the CYP3A4 isoenzyme (for example, rifampicin) may significantly reduce the efficacy of oral contraceptives.
- Concurrent use of these agents with oral contraceptives should be avoided, or an alternate barrier method of contraception should be utilized.
- Antibiotics that alter the normal gastrointestinal flora may reduce enterohepatic recycling of the estrogen component of oral contraceptives, thereby diminishing their effectiveness.
- Patients should be warned about the possible interaction between antibiotics and oral contraceptives, along with the potential need for an alternate method of contraception during antibiotic therapy.

OTHERS (CENTCHROMAN)

- Centchroman (Ormeloxifene) is non-hormonal, non-steroidal selective estrogen receptor modulator (SERM).
- It is having estrogen-antagonizing effect.
- It prevents the implantation of zygote by inhibiting the proliferation of endometrium.
- The advantages of centchroman over steroidal contraceptive agents are:
  - No weight gain
  - No incidence of nausea, vomiting and vertigo.
  - No thrombotic episodes.
  - Does not alter secretion of pituitary, thyroid and adrenal hormones.
  - Does not alter the lipid profile.
  - It does not produce carcinogenic, mutagenic or teratogenic effects.

Dose

- **As contraceptive following schedule is adopted:** 30 mg twice a week for 12 weeks followed by once a week as long as required.
- **In dysfunctional uterine bleeding (DUB)**, it is given in a dose of 60 mg twice a week for 12 weeks, then once a week for next 12 weeks.

Side Effects and Precautions

- The only known side effect of centchroman is prolonged duration of menstrual cycle.
- The protection from pregnancy begins only after one month; hence, in the first month, other protection measures (like condom, jelly, spermicidal sponge) are advised.

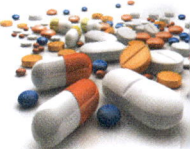

ESTROGEN AND PROGESTERONE PREPARATIONS

ESTROGENS

- The estrogens are naturally occurring sex hormones and are produced by the ovaries, placenta and in small amounts by adrenals and testes by peripheral aromatization of androgens.
- The natural levels of these hormones are under feedback control of both hypothalamus and anterior pituitary.

Estrogens are both natural and synthetic in nature.

- **Natural estrogens:** Estradiol, estrone, estriol.
- **Synthetic estrogens:** Ethinyl estradiol, stilbesterol (diethyl stilbesterol), mestranol, tibolone, dienestrol, etc.

Pharmacokinetics

Naturally occurring estrogens are readily absorbed through the gastrointestinal tract, skin, and mucous membranes. Taken orally, estradiol is rapidly metabolized (and partially inactivated) by the microsomal enzymes of the liver. Bioavailability is low due to first pass metabolism. Micronized form of estradiol has better bioavailability.

Synthetic estrogens are also well absorbed after oral administration and metabolized by the liver and peripheral tissues. Metabolism of synthetic estrogens occur more slowly than the naturally occurring estrogens. Being fat soluble, they are stored in adipose tissue, from which they are slowly released. Therefore, the synthetic estrogen analogues have a prolonged action and a higher potency as compared to those of natural estrogens.

To reduce first-pass metabolism, the drugs may be administered via the transdermal route (patch, topical gel, topical emulsion, or spray), intravaginally (tablet, cream, or ring), or by injection.

After absorption, metabolism occurs in liver and excretion in bile. Then, these are reabsorbed through the enterohepatic circulation and inactive products are excreted in urine.

Estrogen Receptors (ER)

- Estrogens exert their actions through two types of receptors: ERα and ERβ receptors.
- **ERα-receptors** are present in female reproductive tract, breast, blood vessels and hypothalamus.
- **ERβ-receptors** are present in ovaries and prostrate.

Mechanism of Action

- Hormones diffuse across the cell membrane and bind with high affinity to specific nuclear receptor proteins and initiate hormone-specific RNA synthesis.
- This results in the synthesis of specific proteins that mediate a number of physiological functions.

Actions of Estrogens

Estrogens have following effects on different body sites:

- Estrogens are required for the normal maturation of female reproductive tract.
- These are required for development of secondary sexual characters in females.
- These are required for stimulation of pre-ovulatory endometrium.
- They promote rhythmic contractions of fallopian tubes and myometrium.
- They make the cervical secretions thin and watery and facilitate entry of spermatozoa.
- Estrogens are important for maintenance of normal structure of skin and blood vessels in women.
- Estrogens decrease bone resorption, increase high density lipoproteins (HDL) and decrease low density lipoproteins (LDL) cholesterol, promote retention of sodium, nitrogen and fluid in the tissues and enhance coagulability of blood.

Therapeutic uses

Estrogens have following uses:

- **Contraception:** The combination of an estrogen and progestrogen provides effective contraception via the oral, transdermal, or vaginal route.
- **Postmenopausal syndrome and hormone replacement therapy (HRT):** The primary indication for estrogen therapy in postmenopausal women is menopausal symptoms, such as vasomotor (hot flashes or hot flushes) and vaginal atrophy. The amount of estrogen used in replacement therapy is substantially less than the doses used in oral contraception.
- In women with an intact uterus with premature menopause or premature ovarian failure, a progestrogen is always included with the estrogen therapy, *(to decrease the risk of endometrial carcinoma associated with unopposed estrogen)*.
- The women who have undergone a hysterectomy, only estrogen therapy alone is recommended.
- **As a replacement therapy in primary hypogonadism:** Estrogen therapy mimicking the natural cyclic pattern, and usually in combination with a progestrogen, is instituted to stimulate development of secondary sex characteristics in young women with primary hypogonadism. Continued treatment is required after growth is completed
- **Senile vaginitis:** Topical estrogen therapy is recommended.
- **Dysmenorrhea:** Estrogens in combination with progesterone suppress ovulation and make the cycle painless.
- **Carcinoma prostate:** In androgen dependent tumors of prostate, estrogens act by antagonizing the androgenic effects and provide palliation.

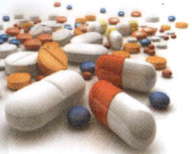

Adverse Effects

- The most common adverse effects are nausea and breast tenderness.
- In addition, the risk of thromboembolic events, myocardial infarction, breast and endometrial cancer is increased with use of estrogen therapy, which can be decreased by including a progestrogen along with the estrogen therapy.

Tibolone is a synthetic steroid, having estrogenic, progestrogenic with weak androgenic properties. It is used in a dose of 2.5 mg daily to reduce the symptoms of estrogen deficiency in menopausal syndrome. It is helpful in controlling the vasomotor symptoms and osteoporosis but can cause weight gain.

ANTIESTROGENS

Clomiphene Citrate

Clomiphene citrate has antiestrogenic activity. It acts as a competitive inhibitor of endogenous ERα and ERβ receptors. It also acts as a partial estrogen agonist and interferes with the negative feedback of estrogens on the hypothalamus. This effect increases the secretion of gonadotropin-releasing hormone (GnRH) and gonadotropins (FSH and LH), thereby leading to stimulation of ovulation.

Therapeutic uses

- **Infertility:** It is used in the treatment of infertility due to anovulation. It is given orally, 50 mg daily for 5 days starting from 5th day of cycle. Treatment is given on monthly basis. If the response is not seen in 3 months, dose may be increased to 100 mg daily for 5 days for next 2–3 cycles.
- **For male infertility:** 25 mg daily for a period of maximum 6 months in case of oligozoospermia has some beneficial effects.
- It is also used for **in vitro fertilization(IVF), gamete intra fallopian transfer (GIFT) technique** and **assisted reproduction therapy (ART).**

Side Effects

- Hot flushes, nausea, vomiting, polycystic ovaries, vertigo, allergic dermatitis.
- Clomiphene increases the risk of twins or triplets.

FULVESTRANT

- It is an estrogen receptor antagonist and blocks both ERα and ERβ receptors.
- It also degrades and down regulates the estrogen receptors. Therefore, it is also called 'selective estrogen receptor down-regulators' (SERDs).

- It is given as IM depot preparation of 250 mg once a month in patients of breast cancer resistant to tamoxifen.
- It can cause headache, hot flushes and nausea.

SELECTIVE ESTROGEN RECEPTOR MODULATORS (SERMs)

- SERMs are a class of estrogen-related compounds that display selective agonism or antagonism for estrogen receptors depending on the tissue type.
- The SERMs include Tamoxifen, Raloxifene, Toremifene, Clomiphene, and Ospemifene.

Tamoxifen

Actions of Tamoxifen

- **Estrogenic actions:**
  - Uterus: It causes endometrial proliferation.
  - Bone: It decreases bone resorption.
  - Plasma lipids: It decreases cholesterol and LDL levels.
- **Antiestrogenic actions:**
  - Breast: It decreases tumor size.
  - Peripheral sites: It causes hot flushes.

Indications and Dose

It is given orally in a dose of 20 mg per day in OD or BD doses.

- It is indicated in ER +ve breast cancer patients specially for palliation of advanced breast cancer in post- menopausal patients.
- It can also be used as prophylactic therapy to reduce the risk of breast cancer in high-risk patients.

Side Effects

They include nausea, vomiting, anorexia, vaginal dryness, bleeding and increase in the risk of endometrial cancer and thromboembolism.

Raloxifene

Actions of Raloxifene:
- **Estrogenic actions:**
  - Bone: It decreases bone resorption.
  - Plasma lipids: It decreases cholesterol and LDL levels.
  - Blood: It increases risk of deep vein thrombosis and pulmonary embolism.
- **Antiestrogenic actions:**
  - Breast: It decreases tumor size by antiproliferative effects.

Indications and Dose

- It is given orally in a dose of 60 mg per day.
- It is used for prevention and treatment of postmenopausal osteoporosis.

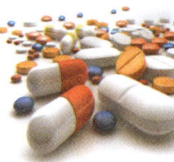

Side Effects

They include hot flushes, leg cramps and increases the risk of endometrial cancer and thromboembolism. It does not increase the risk of endometrial cancer.

Toremifene has similar actions, and side effects to tamoxifen and is indicated in the treatment of metastatic breast cancer in postmenopausal women.

AROMATASE INHIBITORS

(Letrozole, Anastrozole, Exemestane)
- Aromatase enzyme converts testosterone to estrogen.
- These agents inhibit the aromatase enzyme and the levels of estrogen are declined.
- These drugs are useful in suppressing the growth of breast cancer cells even in the patients resistant to tamoxifen therapy.
- Letrozole is given orally in a dose of 2.5 mg once daily and anastrazole 1 mg daily.
- These are used as:
  - First line drug in Ca breast.
  - Adjuvant following mastectomy.
  - For palliation of advanced breast cancer in postmenopausal woman.
  - Alternative therapy in CA breast patients resistant to tamoxifen therapy.
- These are preferred over tamoxifen as they do not increase the risk of thromboembolism or endometrial cancer.
- These drugs are given orally.
- Commonly seen side effects are hot flushes, nausea, diarrhea, arthralgia, etc.
- It also increases the risk of osteoporosis.

PROGESTOGENS

The natural progestogen, is secreted by corpus luteum of the ovary and by placenta during pregnancy by the influence of luteinizing hormone (LH).

Progesterone are both natural and synthetic in nature.
- **Natural Progesterone:** Progesterone.
- **Synthetic Progesterone:**
  - Progesterone derivatives: Medroxyprogesterone, hydroxyprogesterone, Megestrol.
  - 19-nortestosterone derivatives: Norethindrone, Norgestrel, Levonorgestrel, Desogestrel, Norgestimate.

Mechanism of Action

- Progesterone promotes the development of a secretory endometrium that can accommodate implantation of a newly forming embryo.
- The high levels of progesterone in luteal phase of menstrual cycle inhibit the production of gonadotropins and, therefore, prevent ovulation.

- During pregnancy, progesterone maintains the endometrium in a favorable state for the continuation of the pregnancy and reduces the uterine contractions.
- In the absence of pregnancy, the corpus luteum degenerates and the production of progesterone ceases abruptly. The menstruation starts due to sudden withdrawal of progesterone.

Actions of Progesterone

- **Uterus:** It facilitates the secretory changes in uterus and is very important for maintenance of pregnancy.
- **Cervix:** Progesterone converts the watery secretions to viscid secretions.
- **Vagina:** Pregnancy like changes occur.
- **Mammary glands:** It is responsible for the development of secretory glands in breast and prepares the glands for lactation.
- **Body temperature:** It increases the body temperature from 0.5°C to 1°C during luteal phase at the beginning of ovulation.

Pharmacokinetics

- Natural progesterone is rapidly absorbed after oral administration but undergoes high first pass metabolism.
- Natural progesterone has a short half-life in the plasma and is almost completely metabolized by the liver.
- The synthetic progesterone orally effective; less metabolized and has longer half-life.
- The metabolism occurs in liver and excretion primarily occurs via kidneys.
- Oral medroxyprogesterone acetate has a half-life of 30 days. When injected intramuscularly or subcutaneously, it has a half-life of about 40–50 days and provides contraceptive activity for approximately 3 months.
- The other progesterone have half-lives of 1–3 days, allowing for once-daily dosing.

Therapeutic Uses of Progestogens

- **Contraception:** For contraception, they are often used in combination with estrogens.
- **Postponement of menstrual cycle:** Given in the second half of menstrual cycle, it prolongs the luteal phase and thus postpones the menstruation.
- **Hormone replacement therapy:** In women with an intact uterus with premature menopause or premature ovarian failure, a progestogen is always included with the estrogen therapy, *(to decrease the risk of endometrial carcinoma associated with unopposed estrogen action)*.
- **Suppression of ovarian function:** Progesterone suppress the ovulation in dysmenorrhoea, endometriosis, dysfunctional uterine bleeding, etc.

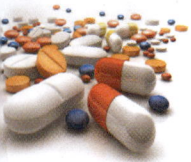

- **Threatened abortion:** Progesterone deficiency induced threatened abortion responds to the treatment well.
- **To delay premature labor:** Progesterone have a beneficial role in preventing the premature labor pains.
- **Diagnostic purpose:** To test the estrogen secretions in women with amenorrhea. Progesterone for 5 days should be followed by withdrawal bleeding, if estrogen levels are normal.

Adverse Effects

- Commonly seen side effects are headache, depression, weight gain, and changes in libido.
- 19-nortestosterone derivatives exhibit some androgenic activity because of their structural similarity to testosterone and can cause acne and hirsutism.
- Less androgenic progesterone, such as norgestimate and drospirenone, may be preferred in women with acne.

PROGESTERONE DERIVATIVES

Danazol

- It is primarily used in the treatment of endometriosis, menorrhagia, fibrocystic disease of breast and gynecomastia.
- It inhibits the midcycle surge of FSH and LH and causes atrophic changes in endometrium.
- It is given orally in a dose of 200–600 mg once daily.
- The commonly seen side effects are hot flushes, edema, weight gain, headache, adrenal suppression and hepatotoxicity.

Antiprogestin

Mifepristone

- Mifepristone binds to the progesterone receptors and antagonizes the action of progesterone. It also has antiglucocorticoid and antiandrogenic activity.
- Mifepristone induces menstruation by sensitizing the myometrium to prostaglandins.
- It blocks the progesterone activity, which is essential for the maintenance of pregnancy. Hence, when given in early pregnancy, it causes abortion.

Pharmacokinetics

- It is given by oral route and the bioavailability is only 25%.
- The metabolism occurs in liver and excretion occurs via bile.
- It undergoes enterohepatic circulation.
- The plasma t½ is 20–36 hours.

Indications

- **Termination of pregnancy:** Up to 49 days: It is given orally in a single dose of 600 mg followed 48 hours later by a single oral dose of 400 mcg of misoprostol to facilitate the expulsion of conceptus. This is preferred method for early first trimester abortion. Gemeprost (1 mg) pessary can be inserted intravaginally in place of oral misoprostol.
- **Postcoital contraception:** It can be used as an emergency contraceptive measure. Mifepristone 600 mg interferes with implantation, if given within 72 hours of unprotected sexual intercourse.
- **Cervical ripening and induction of labor:** It facilitates cervical ripening during normal vaginal delivery and is also helpful in expulsion of fetus that died in utero (IUD).
- **Cushing's syndrome:** Due to its anti-glucocorticoid activity, it is helpful in ameliorating the symptoms of Cushing's syndrome.

Adverse Effects

- Commonly seen side effects are nausea, diarrhea, abdominal cramps and prolonged vaginal bleeding for 1–2 weeks.
- The vaginal bleeding may have to be treated with drugs.

Ulipristal

- It is a newer 'selective progesterone receptor modulator' (SPRM) and has been approved for as emergency contraceptive in a dose of 30 mg to be taken preferably within 72 hours and maximum up to 5 days of unprotected sexual intercourse.
- The commonly seen side effects are GI disturbance and headache.

Drug Interactions

- Oral contraceptives and other estrogen and progesterone preparations:
  - There are chances of contraceptive failure if the following microsomal enzyme inducer drugs are used concurrently:
    - a. Rifampicin
    - b. Ritonavir
    - c. Phenytoin
    - d. Carbamazepine
    - e. Phenobarbitone
  - Some antibiotics such as ampicillin suppress the intestinal microflora and decrease the effectiveness of oral contraceptive by interfering their enterohepatic circulation. Normal intestinal microflora is essentially required for the deconjugation of estrogens (a step necessary for enterohepatic circulation for OCPs).

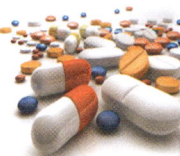

 Nursing Implications

⇨ **Oral contraceptives and progesterone preparations**
- ☞ Nurse should educate the patient regarding regular intake of oral contraceptive pills (OCPs) and the possible signs and symptoms of side effects.
- ☞ Nurse should educate the patient for self breast examination every month.
- ☞ Nurse should educate the patient using OCPs about the missed doses.
- ☞ Females should be advised to use alternative methods of contraception if pills are missed for >2 days.
- ☞ Nurses should study the indications, contraindications and precautions of OCPs and other methods of contraception.
- ☞ Strongly urge the patient to stop smoking to reduce the risk of thromboemboli.
- ☞ Monitor for swelling and changes in vision or fit of contact lenses to monitor for fluid retention and fluid changes.
- ☞ Arrange for at least an annual physical examination, including pelvic examination, pap smear, and breast examination, to reduce the risk of adverse effects and to monitor drug effects.
- ☞ Evaluate the effectiveness of the teaching plan.

HORMONES

Hormones are chemical substances, produced in the specialized cells of body(endocrine glands). These are secreted directly into blood to act on target tissues for specific function. The target tissues are usually away from the site of their secretion. **Hormones have been divided into two types based upon their chemical nature. These are:**

- **Peptide hormones:** Thyrotropin releasing hormone (TRH), Corticotropin releasing hormone (CRH), gonadotropin releasing hormone (GnRH,) etc.
- **Steroid hormones:** Cortisols, estrogens, progesterone, etc.

ACTION OF HORMONES

- Hormones act through certain specific receptors located on the target tissues.
- These receptors are present either on cell membranes, cytoplasm or nucleus of the cells.
- The pituitary gland is called the 'master gland of the body' as it releases the stimulating hormones for various endocrine glands.
- The secretary function of pituitary gland is regulated by hypothalamus through releasing hormone or release inhibitory hormones (Fig. 11.4 and Table 11.10).
- The hypothalamic hormones reach anterior pituitary through portal circulation and posterior pituitary through neurohypophysis system.
- The various hormones secreted by hypothalamus are:
  - Growth hormone releasing and release inhibiting hormone.
  - Thyrotropin releasing and release inhibiting hormone.
  - Corticotropin releasing and release inhibiting hormone.
  - Gonadotropin releasing and release inhibiting hormone.
  - Prolactin releasing and release inhibiting hormone.

CORTICOTROPHINS

- Adrenocorticotropic hormone (ACTH) is also known as *corticotrophin* as it stimulates the adrenal cortex of adrenal gland.
- ACTH secretion follows a characteristic circardian (diurnal) rhythm pattern.
- ACTH is released from the pituitary in pulses with an overriding diurnal rhythm, with the highest concentration occurring in the early morning and the lowest in the late evening.
- Stress stimulates its secretion, whereas cortisol or externally given steroids suppress its release by negative feedback mechanism.

Mechanism of Action

- ACTH binds to receptors on the surface of the adrenal cortex and starts the synthesis of corticoids through adrenocorticosteroid-synthetic pathway.
- This pathway ends with the synthesis and release of the adrenocorticosteroids and the adrenal androgens.
- Excessive production of ACTH leads to adrenal hypertrophy and conditions like Cushing's syndrome.
- Absence or deficiency of ACTH results in adrenal atrophy and condition like Addison's disease.

Therapeutic uses

- **As diagnostic:** It is used as a diagnostic tool for differentiating between primary adrenal insufficiency (Addison's disease, associated with adrenal atrophy) and secondary adrenal insufficiency (caused by the inadequate secretion of ACTH by the pituitary).
Cosyntropin (synthetic human ACTH) is used for diagnostic purpose.

345

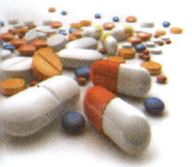

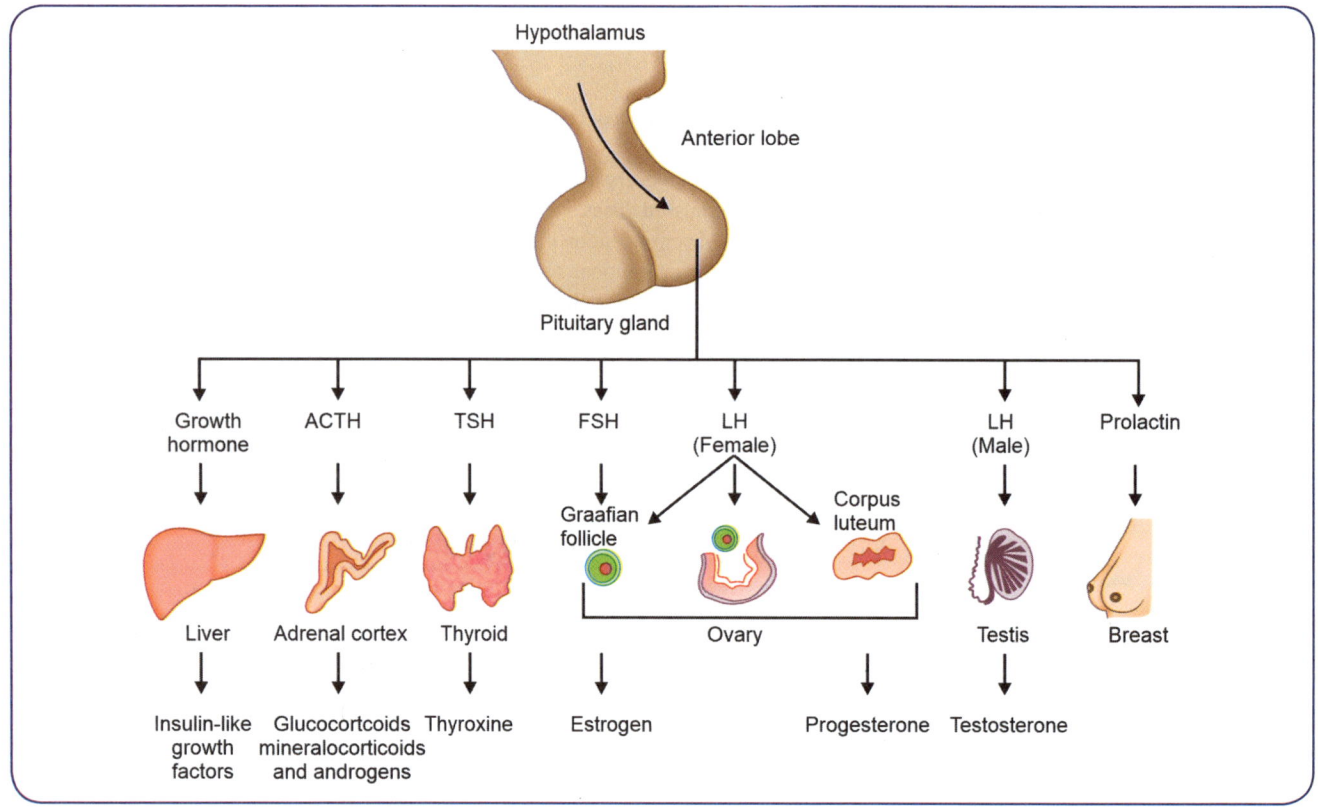

FIG. 11.4: Hormones secreted by anterior pituitary and their target glands

TABLE 11.10: Target glands and specific actions of pituitary hormones

Hormones secreted by hypothalamus	Hormones secreted from anterior pituitary	Target gland	Specific actions
Growth hormone releasing hormone (GHRH)	Growth hormone (GH)	Liver and all body tissues	Produces insulin like growth factor-1 and also acts directly on all body tissues.
Thyrotropin releasing hormone (TRH)	Thyroid stimulating hormone (TSH)	Thyroid gland	T_3 and T_4
Corticotropin releasing hormone (CRH)	Adrenocorticotrophic hormone (ACTH)	Adrenal gland	Glucocorticoids, mineralocorticoids and androgens
Gonadotropin releasing hormone (GnRH)	Follicle stimulating hormone (FSH) Luteinizing hormone (LH)	Ovaries and testis	Estrogen, progesterone and testosterone
Prolactin release inhibitory hormone (PRIH)	Prolactin	Mammary glands	Production of milk

- **As therapeutic:**
  - It is not used for therapeutic purpose in routine as it stimulates the secretion of mineralocorticoids and androgens beside glucocorticoids.
  - ACTH is only used in the treatment of infantile spasm (West syndrome).

Adverse Effects

- It is well tolerated in the doses given for diagnostic purpose.
- On prolonged use, it produces glucocorticoids like side effects such as hypokalemia, hypertension, peripheral edema, emotional disturbances, Cushing's syndrome,

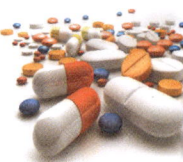

osteoporosis, hyperglycemia, increased risk of infection and delayed wound healing. Suppression of adrenal cortex does not occur with ACTH.

GONADOTROPINS

- Gonadotropins are the hormones, which stimulate the gonads to produce gonadal hormones.
- The gonadotropins (FSH and LH) are produced in the anterior pituitary.
- The pattern of secretion of gonadotropins is in discrete pulses every 60–120 minutes.
- The secretion of gonadotropins is controlled by levels of estrogens, progesterone and testosterone by negative feedback mechanism.
- Functions of FSH and LH are given in Table 11.11.

Natural Gonadotropins and Preparations

Gonadotropins are obtained as follows:
- **From urine of postmenopausal women**
  - **Menotropins or human menopausal gonadotropins** *(hMG)* contains both FSH and LH.
  - **Urofollitropin** or urinary FSH (uFSH) contains only FSH and is devoid of LH activity.
- **From the urine of pregnant women:**
  Human chorionic gonadotropin (hCG) is a placental hormone that is excreted in the urine of pregnant women.
  The above hormones are administered by intramuscular route.
- **Recombinant preparations:**
  - Recombinant FSH (rFSH): *Follitropin-*α and *follitropin* β are two different human FSH products manufactured using recombinant DNA technology.
  - Recombinant hCG (rhCG): The effects of *hCG* and *choriogonadotropin* α are essentially identical to those of LH. It is prepared by using recombinant DNA technology.

The above hormones are administered by subcutaneous route.

Therapeutic Uses

- To treat infertility in both females and males.
- Cryptorchidism
- To facilitate in-vitro-fertilization (IVF).

Adverse Effects

- The adverse effects are ovarian enlargement and ovarian hyperactive stimulation syndrome, which may be life threatening. Multiple births are common.
- hCG can induce precocious puberty, abdominal pain and gynecomastia in males.

ADRENALINE

- Adrenaline is also known as epinephrine and is a major neurotransmitter of sympathetic nervous system.
- It is one of the endogenous catecholamines (adrenaline, noradrenaline and dopamine) synthesized from amino acid phenylalanine.
- Under physiological conditions, adrenaline functions largely as a hormone as it is secreted from the adrenal medulla into the blood and then it acts on distant body tissues.
- Adrenaline exhibits its actions via α and β adrenergic receptors.

The details of adrenaline have been described in the chapter 'adrenergic system and drugs'.

PROSTAGLANDINS (PGS)

The word 'Prostaglandin' (PG) has been derived from the word **prosta- prostate + glandin- gland,** as first of all, it was isolated from the prostatic fluid in semen.

Synthesis of Prostaglandins

- The PGs are synthesized from cell membrane phospholipids of nearly all body tissues (Fig. 11.5).

TABLE 11.11: Functions of FSH and LH

Functions of follicle stimulating hormone (FSH)		Functions of luteinizing hormone (LH)	
Females	**Males**	**Females**	**Males**
• Gametogenesis • Production of estrogen and progesterone • Development of follicles • Regulation of menstrual cycle	• Stimulation and maintenance of spermatogenesis	• Regulation of menstrual cycle • Induction of ovulation • Formation and maintenance of corpus luteum • Promotion of estrogen and progesterone production	• Biosynthesis of androgens and testosterone

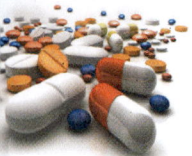

- There are no prostaglandin stores in the body and these are synthesized locally in response to appropriate stimuli (external, internal, mechanical, chemical, etc).
- These stimuli activate the phospholipase-A_2 enzyme, which converts membrane phospholipids to arachidonic acid (AA).
- Arachidonic acid is converted to different prostaglandins (PGG_2, PGH_2) via cyclooxygenase (COX) pathway.
- PGG_2 and PGH_2 are unstable compounds and are converted to:
  - PGE_2, PGD_2 and $PGF_{2\alpha}$ in the tissues where isomerase enzyme is present.
  - PGI_2 in the tissues where prostacyclin synthase is present.
  - TXA_2 in the tissues where thromboxane synthase is present.
- The Phospholipsae-A_2 inhibitors (glucocorticoids) and COX inhibitors (NSAIDs), inhibit the synthesis of prosta-glandins; thereby produce anti-inflammatory actions.

Natural Prostaglandins

The various prostaglandins in different tissues are PGG_2 and PGH_2, PGE_2, PGD_2, $PGF_{2\alpha}$ and PGI_2.

Pharmacokinetics

- The prostaglandins can be given by oral, intravaginal, intra-amniotic, extra-amniotic and intravenous route depending upon the preparation and the indication of use.
- Most of the prostaglandins have plasma t½ of a few seconds to a few minutes.
- These are converted to inactive metabolites, which are excreted in urine.
- PGI_2 is catabolized mainly in the kidneys.

Actions of Prostaglandins

- As all the cells and tissues of body are capable of forming one or more type of prostaglandins, the prostaglandins have an important role in a number of normal physiological processes and pathological states of body.
- Some important actions of PGs in different body systems are given in Table 11.12.

Therapeutic Uses

- The PGs are less commonly used due to limited availability, short lasting action, cost and frequent side effects. Nevertheless, these are very frequently used in the management of glaucoma and in obstetrics. The common indications of PGs are as follows (Table 11.13).

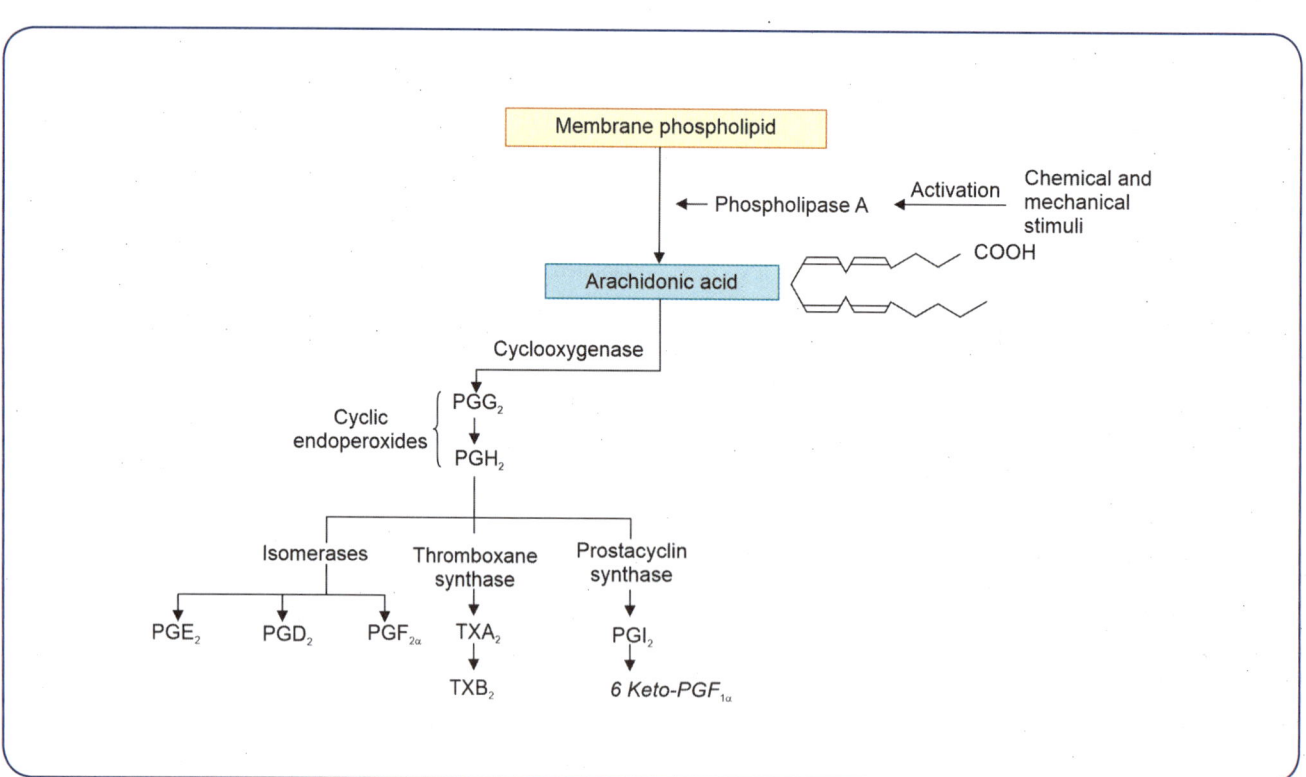

FIG. 11.5: Synthesis of prostaglandins

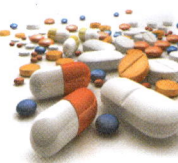

TABLE 11.12 Preparations of prostaglandins or Prostaglandin analogues

Prostaglandin type	PG analogue	Preparation and route of administration	Therapeutic uses
PGE$_1$	Misoprostol	200 mcg tablet, 1–3 tablets oral	Medical Abortion
PGE$_1$	Gemeprost	1 mg vaginal pessary	Cervical priming and mid-trimester abortion
PGE$_2$	Alprostil	2.5–25 mcg inj	Erectile dysfunction , maintenance of patency of ductus arteriorus
PGF$_{2\alpha}$	Dinoprostone	0.5 mg vaginal gel, vaginal tab, extra-amniotic solution	Induction and facilitation of labor, mid-trimester abortion
PGF$_{2\alpha}$	Dinoprost	5 mg/mL intra-amniotic injection	Induction and facilitation of labor, mid-trimester abortion
PGF$_{2\alpha}$	Latanoprost, Bimatoprost	0.0005% eye drops	Glaucoma treatment
PGI$_2$	Epoprostanol	0.5 mg injection	For prevention of platelet aggregation in cardiopulmonary bypass, pulmonary hypertension

TABLE 11.13: Actions of prostaglandins on various sites

Site of action	PGE$_2$	PGF$_{2\alpha}$	PGI$_2$
Cardiovascular system	Vasodilatation, and weak inotropic effect	Vasodilatation, larger veins constrict and weak inotropic effect	Vasodilatation is marked and decrease in BP occurs
Platelets	–	–	Anti-aggregatory effect
Inflammation and immunity	Mediate inflammation and pain	–	Mediate inflammation and pain
Eye	Reduce intraocular pressure	Reduce intraocular pressure	–
Female reproductive system	Contraction of uterus and softening of cervix	Contraction of uterus and softening of cervix	–
Male reproductive system	Facilitate movement of sperm and thereby fertility.	–	Facilitate movement of sperm and also have a role in penile erection by causing vasodilatation
Respiratory system	Relaxation of bronchi	Constriction of bronchi	Relaxation of bronchi
Stomach	Decreases acid secretion and increases mucous secretion	–	Decreases acid secretion and increases mucous secretion
Intestines	Increase peristalsis or spasmogenic effects	Increase peristalsis or spasmogenic effect	Weak spasmogenic effect
Kidneys	Vasodilation, diuretic effect and renin release	–	Vasodilation, diuretic effect and renin release
Endocrine	Release of ant. pituitary hormones, steroids, insulin; TSH like action	Release of gonadotropins and prolactin hormone.	–

- **Obstetric and gynecological uses:**
  - **Abortion:**
    - PGE$_2$ and PGF$_{2\alpha}$ are used in 1st and 2nd trimester abortion and ripening of cervix during abortion.
    - Intravaginal PGE$_2$ pessary minimizes trauma to the cervix by reducing resistance to dilatation.
    - A single oral dose of misoprostol 400 mcg is given 2–3 days after mifepristone (antiprogestin) 600 mg for medical abortion up to 49 days of pregnancy.
    - Intravaginal misoprostol can also be given as the side effects are less with this route.
    - PGs are also useful in midterm abortion, missed abortion and molar gestation.
  - **For facilitation of labor** (Induction or augmentation purpose):
    - PGE$_2$ and PGF$_{2\alpha}$ can be used in toxemic and renal failure patients in the place of oxytocin as PGs do not cause fluid retention.

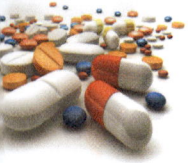

- ◆ PGE_2 may also be used by intravaginal route for this purpose.
  - ▪ **Cervical priming** (cervical ripening): PGE_2 in low doses administered intravaginally or in the cervical canal, makes the cervix soft and more compliant for induction of labor.
  - ▪ **Postpartum hemorrhage** (PPH): PPH due to atony of uterus can be treated by intramuscular Carboprost (15-methyl $PGF_{2\alpha}$) injection in ergometrine and oxytocin resistant patients.
- **Gastrointestinal uses**: In the patients of NSAIDs induced peptic ulcers, PGE_1 (misoprostol) and PGE_2 (enprostil) are helpful in early healing of the ulcers.
- **Eye:** In the patients of glaucoma, $PGF_{2\alpha}$ analogues like Latanoprost, Travoprost, Bimatoprost are used topically. These days, PG analogues are used as the first choice drugs in wide angle glaucoma.
- **Cardiovascular uses:** PGE_1 (Alprostadil) is used to maintain patency of ductus arteriosus in neonates with congenital heart defects, till surgery is undertaken. PGI_2 (Epoprostenol) is used to prevent platelet aggregation and damage during hemodialysis or cardiopulmonary bypass.
- **Erectile dysfunction or impotence:** 2.5–5.0 mcg of PGE_1 (alprostadil) as uretheral suppository or injection into the penis causes erection lasting 1–2 hours and may be used as an alternative to sildenafil or tadalafil.
- **Pulmonary hypertension:** PGI_2 (epoprostenol) infusion is also helpful in management of primary pulmonary hypertension.
- **Peripheral vascular diseases:** In the patients of Raynaud's disease and other peripheral vascular diseases, the intravenous infusion of PGI_2 (or PGE_1) provides relief from rest pain, intermittent claudications and promotes healing of ischemic ulcers due to vasodilatory effects of these PGs.

Adverse Effects

- The adverse effects of PGs depend upon the type of preparation, route used and the dose in which these have been used.
- Commonly seen side effects are nausea, vomiting, abdominal cramps causing watery diarrhea, painful uterine cramps and vaginal bleeding. Feverish feeling, hypotension and palpitations are also seen.

CALCITONIN

- Calcitonin is a peptide hormone produced by parafollicular 'C' cells of thyroid gland.
- It was discovered by Copp in 1962.
- It is a hypocalcemic hormone.

- It is also secreted by parathyroids, thymus and cells of medullary carcinoma of thyroid.
- Synthesis and secretion of calcitonin is regulated by plasma calcium levels.
- A rise in the serum plasma levels of calcium increases and a fall in plasma calcium levels decrease calcitonin release.
- Calcitonin plays a very minor physiological role in the regulation of plasma calcium levels.
- It has a plasma $t\frac{1}{2}$ of 10 minutes, but the duration of action is very prolonged and may last for several hours.

Mechanism of Action

- Calcitonin binds to the calcitonin receptors and enhances the production of vitamin D producing enzymes and leads to greater calcium retention and enhanced bone mineral density.
- Calcitonin receptors are found in osteoclasts.

Actions of Calcitonin

Calcitonin acts opposite to parathyroid hormone. It lowers serum calcium and phosphate levels by acting on bone and kidneys.

- **Actions on bone:** It inhibits the osteoclastic activity and decreases the bone resorption.
- **Actions on kidneys:** It decreases the reabsorption of both calcium and phosphate from the proximal tubules of kidneys and thus their excretion is increased.

Preparations of Calcitonin

- Natural human calcitonin and synthetic (salmon) calcitonin , both are available for therapeutic purposes.
- Synthetic (salmon) calcitonin is more potent and longer acting.
- Both preparations are given by either subcutaneous or intramuscular route.

Synthetic salmon calcitonin is given subcutaneous or intramuscular route in a dose of 100 IU/mL (1 IU = 4 µg of the standard preparation).

Indications and Doses

- **In hypercalcemic states** like hypercalcemia of malignancy, osteolytic bony metastasis, hyperparathyroidism, hypervitaminosis D.
  - ▪ It is given intramuscularly in a dose of 4–8 IU/kg, BD-QID for 2 days.
  - ▪ Its action starts within four hours and the peak response is seen in 2 days, i.e., 48 hours.
- **For emergency treatment of hypercalcemia:** It is given in a slow infusion form after diluting 5–10 IU/kg in 500 mL of saline. The infusion should be administered slowly over a period of 6–8 hours.

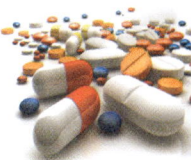

- **Paget's disease:** It is given by subcutaneous or intramuscular route in a dose of 100 IU daily or on alternate days. **Bisphosphonates are the first line drugs**.
- **Postmenopausal osteoporosis:** Nasal spray of 200 IU/actuation increases the bone mineral density and reduces the risk of pathological vertebral fractures.
- **Diagnosis of medullary carcinoma of thyroid:** High levels of calcitonin are diagnostic of medullary carcinoma of thyroid.

CALCIUM SALTS

- Calcium constitutes approximately 2% of the body weight, i.e., in an average adult, 1–1.5 kg calcium is present. Out of this, 99% of calcium is present in bone and teeth.
- Calcium is required for various physiological functions in body.
  - It is essential for tissue excitability, excitation-contraction-coupling (nerve conduction, muscular contraction).
  - In addition, it acts as an intracellular messenger for hormones, autacoids and transmitters as well as controls impulse generation and A-V conduction in heart
  - It is required for the smooth functioning of clotting mechanism.
  - It is an integral part of bone and teeth.
- The calcium homeostasis is regulated by vitamin D, parathormone (PTH) and calcitonin.
- The normal plasma level of calcium is 9–11 mg/dL. The normal levels of calcium are regulated by vitamin D, parathyroid hormone and calcitonin.
- Hypocalcemia may lead to tetany, which is presented as muscle spasms. Deficiency in children causes rickets and in adults osteoporosis. Chronic hypercalcemia may cause nephrolithiasis.
- Calcium salt supplementation is usually required in these above-mentioned states.

PREPARATIONS OF CALCIUM SALTS

Calcium preparations are available in both oral and parenteral forms.

Oral Preparations

- **Calcium citrate**
  - It provides 40% of calcium.
  - It is tasteless and insoluble in nature.
  - It is best absorbed in acidic medium and absorption decreases in patients taking H_2 blockers and proton pump inhibitors (PPIs).
  - It is most economical calcium preparation and widely available.

- **Calcium citrate**
  - It provides 21% of calcium.
  - It is tasteless and slightly soluble in nature.
  - It is best absorbed in acidic medium and absorption occurs to some extent in patients taking H_2 blockers and PPIs also.
- **Calcium gluconate**
  - It provides 9% of calcium.
  - It is available as 500 and 1000 mg tablets form and available in various flavors also.
  - It is non-irritating in nature.
- **Calcium lactate**
  - It provides 13% of calcium.
  - It is well-tolerated and non-irritating in nature.
- **Calcium dibasic phosphate**
  - It provides 23% of calcium.
  - It is tasteless and insoluble in nature.
  - It is best absorbed in acidic medium and absorption decreases in patients taking H_2 blockers and PPIs.
- **Calcium aspartate**
  - It is an organic calcium compound based on L-aspartic acid.
  - The major source of calcium aspartate is green plant and vegetables extract.
  - It has a good oral absorption.
- **Calcium orotate**
  - It is the best bioavailability enhancer and the calcium given in the form of calcium orotate directly reaches the cells.
- **Coral calcium**
  - It is obtained from fossilized coral reefs.
  - It has good bioavailability.
  - It is composed of calcium carbonate with small amount of magnesium and other trace elements.
- **Calcium chloride**
  - It provides 27% of calcium but not used frequently due to its highly GI irritating nature.

Parenteral Preparations

- **Calcium gluconate**
  - It is available as 10% injection in 5 mL ampoules.
  - It is the most preferred IV preparation of calcium salt.
  - It can be given safely by slow IV route, as it is non-irritating to the vascular endothelium. Extravasation should be avoided.
  - It is most commonly used in management of acute hypocalcemia.
  - It produces a sensation of warmth on IV injection.
- **Calcium chloride**
  - It is not preferred as it is highly irritating in nature and causing tissue necrosis.

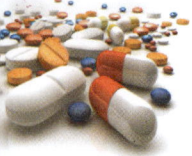

INDICATION OF CALCIUM SALTS

- For immediate treatment of tetany (parenteral preparation is preferred).
- As dietary supplement in pregnancy, lactating mother, postmenopausal women and growing children.
- It is also given both therapeutically and prophylactically in all age groups, mostly in combination with vitamin-D.
- It is given in the treatment of osteoporosis, in addition to other treatment such as bisphosphonates, raloxifene and hormone replacement therapy (HRT).
- As a constituent of many antacid preparations.

ADVERSE EFFECTS

- Commonly seen side effects are constipation, bloating, GI disturbance.
- Nephrolithiasis can occur when given in higher doses and for longer duration.

CALCIUM REGULATORS

The calcium homeostasis is chiefly regulated by parathyroid hormone (PTH), vitamin-D and calcitonin.

PARATHYROID HORMONE (PTH)

- Parathyroid hormone is secreted by parathyroid glands.
- The secretion of parathyroid hormone is regulated by the plasma calcium levels. The PTH has a role in maintaining the calcium levels.
- Low plasma calcium levels stimulate the PTH secretion, whereas high calcium levels inhibit its secretion.
- Prolonged hypocalcemia causes hypertrophy and hyperplasia of parathyroid glands, whereas prolonged hypercalcemic states have opposite effects.

Actions of PTH

It increases the serum calcium levels by acting on the following organs:
- **Actions on bone:**
  - It increases the osteoclastic activity and bone remodelling; thereby increases the bone resorption and serum calcium levels.
  - This effect is seen in prolonged higher levels of PTH. When PTH is given in intermittently low doses, it also promotes new bone formation.
- **Actions on kidneys:** It increases the reabsorption of calcium from the distal tubules of kidneys and increases the serum calcium levels. Simultaneously, it promotes phosphate excretion also.

- **Actions on intestines:** PTH enhances the calcium absorption from intestine indirectly by stimulating/enhancing the formation of calcitriol in the kidneys.

PTH Dysfunctions

- **Hypoparathyroidism:**
  - It is characterized by the low serum calcium levels and may be due to accidental removal of parathyroid glands during thyroidectomy.
  - Clinically, PTH is not used to treat hypoparathyroidism as the normal levels of calcium can be achieved/maintained by vitamin-D therapy also.
- **Hyperparathyroidism:** It is characterized by high levels of calcium and presents as nephrolithiasis, myalgia, constipation and pathological bone fractures. It is treated by:
  - Surgical removal of parathyroid tumors.
  - By low calcium, high phosphate diet along with plenty of oral fluids.
  - **Cinacalcet** inhibits the secretion of PTH and is given for the treatment of secondary hyperparathyroidism due to renal disease and in parathyroid tumor also.

Uses of PTH

It is not used for therapeutic purpose but used only for diagnostic purpose in pseudohypoparathyroidism.

TERIPARATIDE

- It is a recombinant PTH, used for the management of severe osteoporosis.
- It is injected subcutaneously in a dose of 20 mcg once daily and it increases the bone mineral density.
- It is used for differentiating pseudohypoparathyroidism from true hypoparathyroidism. In pseudohypoparathyroidism, plasma levels of calcium fail to rise even after IV teriparatide.

VITAMIN-D

- Vitamin D is a fat-soluble vitamin. It is also a pre-hormone produced in the skin from 7-dehydrocholesterol under the effect of UV rays.
- It is converted to active metabolites in the body, which regulate plasma calcium levels and various functions of the cells.

Uses of Vitamin-D

- **As therapeutic and prophylaxis:**
  - **Vitamin-D deficiency:** For prophylaxis: 400 IU oral, daily and for therapeutic purpose 3000–4000 IU oral,

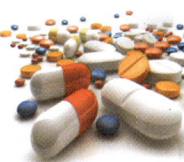

daily or alternatively 3–6 lac IU every 3–6 month orally/ intramuscularly can be given.

- **Obstructive jaundice:** 6,00,000 IU intramuscularly.
- **Nutritional rickets and osteomalacia:** 6,00,000 IU intramuscularly then repeat after 4–6 weeks.
- **Vitamin-D resistant rickets:** Phosphate supplementation with high dose of vitamin-D is helpful.
- **Vitamin-D dependent rickets:** Occurs due to inability of body to convert vitamin-D to its active form, calcitriol. Calcitriol or 1-α-calcidiol is effective in the treatment.
- **Senile osteoporosis or postmenopausal osteoporosis:** Oral vitamin-D with calcium supplementation is helpful.
- **Hypoparathyroidism:** Calcitriol with calcium supplementation is helpful.

Calcium supplementation should be invariably done along with vitamin-D therapy.

Calcitonin (Described in calcitonin chapter).

OTHER DRUGS USED IN BONE DISODERS

Bisphosphonates

- These agents are analogs of pyrophosphate and they inhibit the bone resorption.
- These are the most effective antiresorptive drugs useful in preventing osteoporosis and treating hypercalcemia and metabolic bone diseases.
- They have been grouped according to their potency and efficacy into three generations (Table 11.14).

Mechanism of Action

- Bisphosphonates decrease osteoclastic bone resorption, which results in a small increase in bone mass and a decreased risk of fractures in patients with osteoporosis.
- Bisphosphonates increase the apoptosis of osteoclastic cells.

TABLE 11.14: Classification of bisphosphonates

Generations	Potency	Drugs
1st generation bisphosphonates	Least potent	• Etidronate • Tiludronate
2nd generation bisphosphonates	10–100 times more potent than 1st gen	• Alendronate • Pamidronate • Ibandronate
3rd generation bisphosphonates	10,000 times more potent than 2nd gen	• Risedronate • Zoledronate

Pharmacokinetics

- The oral bisphosphonates (alendronate, risedronate) can be given on a daily, weekly, or monthly basis depending on the drug.
- These are poorly absorbed after oral administration and the bioavailability is even <1%.
- Bisphosphonates are rapidly cleared from the plasma, primarily because they bind to hydroxyapatite in the bone. After binding to the bone, they are cleared over a period of hours to years.
- These are eliminated mainly by the renal route.
- Patients should be instructed to follow strict guidelines to maximize its absorption as food and other medications significantly interfere with their absorption. Hence, these agents should always be given empty stomach.
- The patients, who are unable to tolerate oral bisphosphonates due to any reason, alternatively intravenous pamidronate or zoledronate can be given.

Dose, routes and special features of common bisphosphonates are given in Table 11.15.

TABLE 11.15: Individual drugs bisphosphonates and their features

Drugs	Dose and Route	Special features
Etidronate	5–7.5 mg/kg daily, both oral and IV	• It was the first bisphosphonate used clinically • Not in use nowadays due to its side effects (osteomalacia)
Tiludronate	1 mg/kg, intravenously	• Used in animal only • Not available in India
Alendronate	5–10 mg once daily or 35–70 mg once weekly	• It is orally effective • Should be given empty stomach • Weekly treatment is preferred • The terminal elimination plasma half-life is 10.5 years
Ibandronate	150 mg once a month, orally 3 mg IV given over 15–30 seconds and repeat every 3 months	• Should be taken 60 minutes before meals
Pamidronate	30–90 mg intravenously given over 2–4 hours	• Used only as IV infusion • Not given orally • Thrombophebitis may occur

Contd...

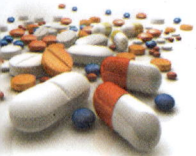

Drugs	Dose and Route	Special features
Risedronate	35 mg oral, weekly	• It is orally effective • Should be given empty stomach with full glass of water
Zoledronate	**Method of administration** • Intravenous infusion of 4 mg to be diluted in the 100 mL of saline/glucose and given over 15 minute. (It can be repeated after 7 days then after 3–4 weeks intervals for osteolytic bony metastasis) • Intravenous infusion of 4 mg yearly (osteoporosis in postmenopausal women)	• Most potent bisphosphonate • Most preferred agent for hypercalcemia • Least irritating effect to the vein • Flu like symptoms, nausea, vomiting may be seen • Renal toxicity may occur, which can be prevented by liberal fluid intake

Therapeutic uses of Bisphosphonates

- **Osteoporosis:** Bisphosphonates are given along with calcium and vitamin D. These are effective in preventing and treating postmenopausal osteoporosis. These are also effective in steroid-induced, age related and idiopathic osteoporosis in both men and women. Aledronate and risedronate are preferred.
- **Paget's disease:** These drugs provide pain relief and induce remission.
- **Hypercalcemia of malignancy:** Intravenous preparations are preferred as hypercalcemia of malignancy requires immediate management.
- **Osteolytic bony metastasis:** Parenteral bisphosphonates reduce the bone pain by arresting the osteolytic bone lesions.

Adverse Effects

- Oral preparations are associated with esophagitis and esophageal ulcers. To minimize esophageal irritation, patients should remain upright after taking oral bisphosphonates.
- Other side effects include retrosternal pain due to esophagitis, dyspepsia, headache, generalized body aches due to initial fall in serum calcium levels.
- Flu-like symptoms are seen with the parenteral preparation only.
- Osteonecrosis of the jaw has been reported with bisphosphonates but is usually associated with higher intravenous doses used for hypercalcemia of malignancy.

Special Precautions and Advise for Oral Bisphosphonate Therapy

- These drugs should be taken empty stomach with plenty of water.
- The tablets should not be chewed; it should be swallowed in whole.
- These medications should not be taken with mineral water, juice, tea, coffee, etc.

- The patients should be advised not to take any other medication or food within 60 minutes of taking these drugs.
- Patients should not lie down after taking these drugs and should maintain an up-right posture for 30–60 minutes after ingesting the medication.
- If there is any retrosternal pain, worsening of heartburn or any swallowing difficulty, these drugs should be discontinued immediately.
- These drugs are not recommended for patients below 18 years of age.
- These drugs should not be given in pregnancy, lactation and uncorrected hypocalcemic patients.

 ## Drug Interactions

- Vitamin D absorption is decreased by liquid paraffin and cholestyramine. Hence, the concurrent use should be avoided.
- Prolonged use of phenobarbitone and phenytoin can cause rickets and osteomalacia by decreasing the effect of calcitriol.

Nursing Implications

- **Calcitonin, calcium salts and calcium regulators**
  - Assess for history of allergy to any components of the drugs being used.
  - Monitor serum calcium concentration periodically before and during treatment to allow for adjustment of dose to maintain calcium levels within normal limits.
  - Arrange for a nutritional consultation if GI effects are severe to ensure nutritional balance.
  - Monitor patient response to the drug (return of serum calcium levels to normal).
  - Monitor for adverse effects (weakness, headache, GI effects).
  - Evaluate the effectiveness of the teaching plan (patient can name drug, dosage, adverse effects to watch for, and specific measures to avoid them).

Contd...

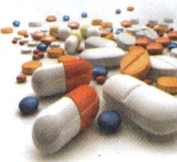

Assess Yourself

Long and Short Answer Questions

1. What is insulin? Classify the various types of insulin preparations, with at least two examples each.
2. Classify oral hypoglycemic agents, describe sulfonylureas.
3. What is glucocorticoids, describe their side effects and therapeutic uses.
4. Write short notes on:
   a. Metformin
   b. Anabolic steroids
   c. Thyroxine
   d. Oral contraceptives
   e. Bisphosphonates
   f. Calcium preparations
   g. Tocolytic agents
   h. Prostaglandins
   i. Non-steroidal oral contraceptives
   j. Progesterone

Multiple Choice Questions

1. **Oxytocin is given by which route?**
   a. Oral
   b. Infusion
   c. Inhalation
   d. Subcutaneous

2. **Anti-diabetic drug given subcutaneously is:**
   a. Vildagliptin
   b. Metformin
   c. Pramlintide
   d. Acarbose

3. **Oral anti-diabetic drug not having severe hypoglycemic effect is:**
   a. Metformin
   b. Glibenclamide
   c. Glimipride
   d. Gliclazide

4. **Bisphosphonates act by:**
   a. Increasing osteoid formation
   b. Increasing mineralization of osteoid
   c. Decreasing osteoclast mediated resorption of bone
   d. Decreasing PTH secretion

5. **Parathyroid hormone:**
   a. Decreases bone resorption
   b. Increases bone resorption
   c. Enhances phosphate reabsroption from kidney
   d. Decreases calcium reabsroption from kidney

Answer Key

| 1. | b. | 2. | a. | 3. | b. | 4. | c. | 5. | b. |

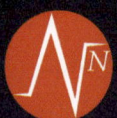
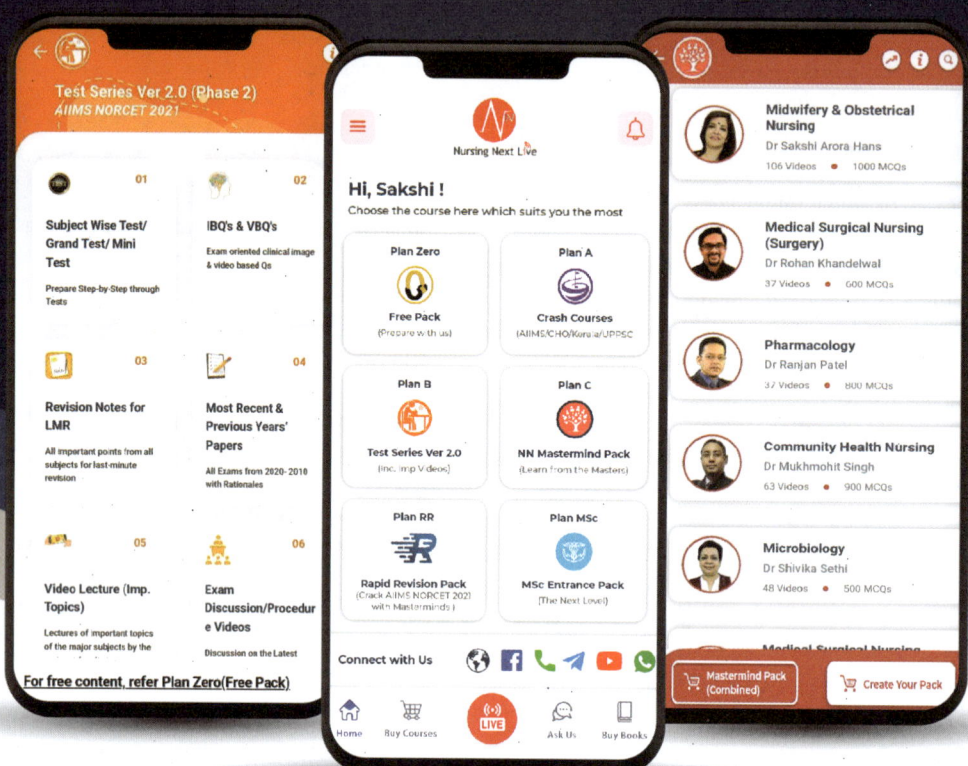

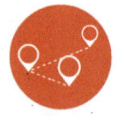

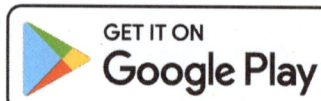
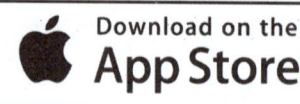
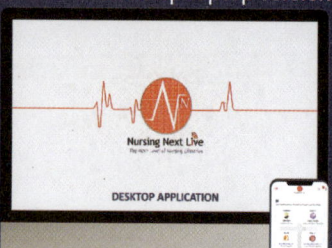

Introduction to Drugs used in Alternative Systems of Medicine

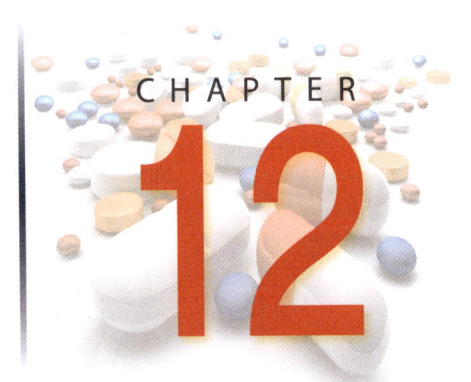

ALTERNATIVE SYSTEM OF MEDICINES

In India, the Central Council of Indian Medicines (CCIM) a statutory body established in 1971 under Department of Ayurveda, Yoga and Naturopathy, Unani, Siddha and Homeopathy (AYUSH), Ministry of Health and Family Welfare, Government of India, monitors higher education in areas of Indian medicine including, Ayurveda, Unani and Siddha.

AYURVEDA

- Ayurveda (*Ayur-life, Veda-knowledge*) is a system of medicine with historical roots in the Indian subcontinent. Ayurveda is considered as one of the oldest systems of medicine in the world. Globalized and modernized practices derived from Ayurveda traditions are a type of complementary or alternate medicine.
- The oldest record of documents regarding use of plants as medicines in India is found in Rigveda (during 2000 BC).
- Atharvaveda (1500–1000 BC), described many more plants for medicinal use and introduced more concepts of ayurveda.
- The original texts of ayurveda have been documented in Charaka Samhita (1000 BC) and Sushruta Samhita (1000 BC).

- The practical knowledge and training of these concepts was imparted to students by Punarvasu Atreya and Dhanvantari.
- In Hindu mythology, the origin of ayurvedic medicines is credited to Dhanvantari, *the physician of the Gods.*

AYURVEDIC CONCEPT OF HEALTH

- According to ayurveda, the body is composed of five elements and three doshas.
- The health is defined as the state of equilibrium of these following elements and doshas:
  - Five elements [Earth, Water, Fire, Air and Universe (ether)]
  - Three doshas (Vata, Pitta, Kapha)
- The five elements (*panch-mahabhootha*) denote earth, water, fire, air and universe (ether).
Ayurvedic concept of health is shown in Figure 12.1.
- Ayurveda names seven basic tissues (saptadhatu), which are:
  - Plasma or rasa dhatu
  - Blood or rakta dhatu
  - Muscles or mamsa dhatu
  - Fat or meda dhatu
  - Bone or asthi dhatu
  - Marrow or majja dhatu
  - Semen or shukra dhatu

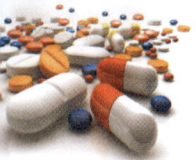

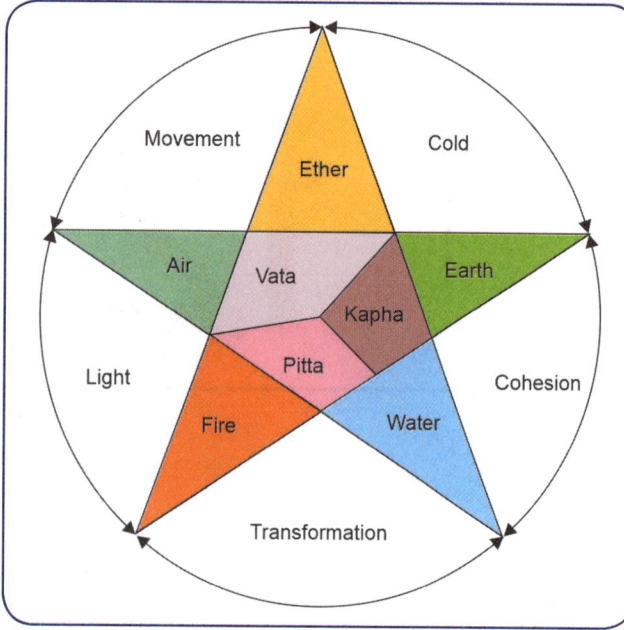

FIG. 12.1: Ayurvedic concept of health

The diseases are caused by abnormalities between these above-mentioned dhatus.

THREE DOSHAS

Vata or Vatha (Airy Element)

- It is characterized by properties of dry, cold, light, minute, and movement.
- All movements in the body are due to the property of vata.
- Pain is the characteristic feature of deranged vata.

- Some of the diseases due to vata are wind humur, flatulence, gout, rheumatism, etc.

Pitta

- It is the fiery element or bile that is secreted between the stomach and bowels and flows through the liver and permeating spleen, heart, eyes, and skin.
- It is characterized by hotness, moist, liquid, sharp and sour.
- Its main quality is heat.
- It is the energy principle, which uses bile to direct digestion and enhance metabolism.
- It is primarily characterized by body heat or burning sensation and redness.

Kapha

- It is the watery element.
- It is characterized by heaviness, cold, tenderness, softness, slowness, lubrication, and the carrier of nutrients.
- It is nourishing element of the body.
- All the soft organs are made by kapha.
- It plays an important role in taste perception, joint nourishment and lubrication.

THE PRINCIPLE OF AYURVEDA

- The fundamental theory of ayurveda is that a balance between panchmahabhoot, saptadhatu and three doshas is necessary for the normal physiological functions of the body. The imbalance between these elements causes disease.
- The balance between panchmahabhoot, saptadhatu and doshas are maintained by the procedure of treatment depicted in Figure 12.2.

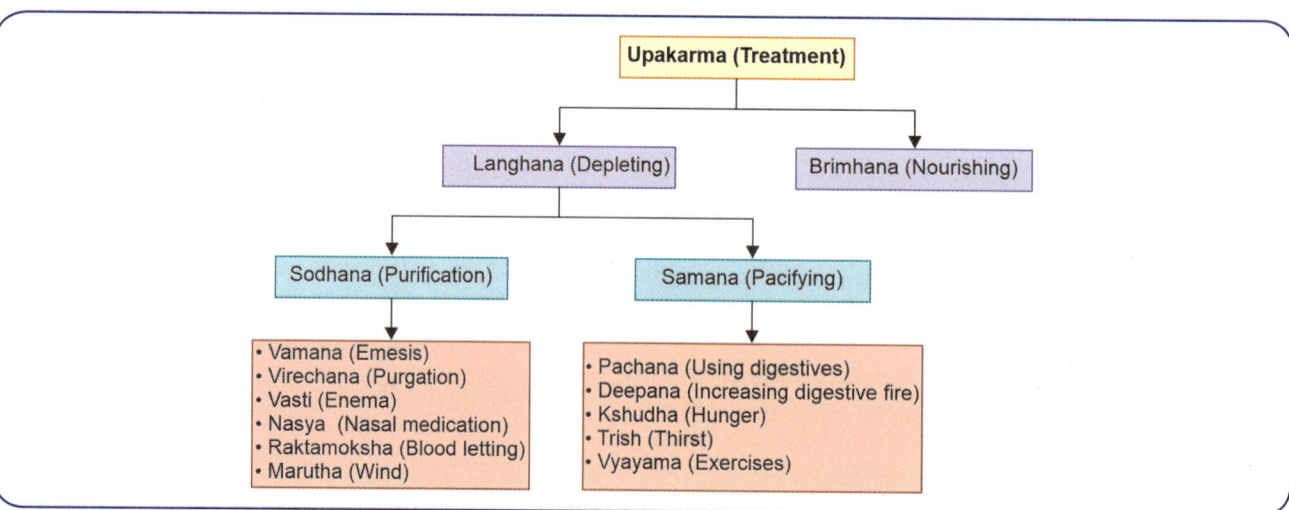

FIG. 12.2: Procedure of treatment in Ayurveda

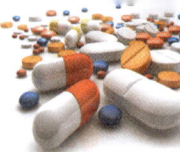

Drugs in Ayurveda

Ayurvedic drugs are of natural origin, including:

- **Plants:** Whole plants or their parts such as Ajawain, Saunff, Haldi, Banafsa, Mullathi, Safed Musali, Isabgol, etc.
- **Animals:** Animal parts and their products such as Ghee, Milk, Bones, etc.
- **Minerals:** Minerals either alone or in combinations such as Sulfur, Copper, Arsenic, Gold, Iron, etc.

  All of the above mentioned ayurvedic drugs might be given alone or in combinations.

  Phanchakarma therapy is an important part of Ayurveda.

HOMEOPATHY

- Dr Samuel Hahnemann, a German physician, introduced the system of Homeopathy in 1796.
- Homeopathy is defined as the therapeutic method based on the law, *similia similibus curentur*, usually translated as "let likes be cured by likes", that states that if any substance causes a symptom in healthy people it can be used to treat the same symptom in sick people.
- Dr Hahnemann penned down his experiences and the guidelines for practicing the system of medicine in "Organon of Medicine", which guides how a physician should proceed while treating the patients.

Principles of Homeopathy

- Homeopathy is based on the following three primary principles:
  1. Law of Similia, which states that only that substance can treat a particular disease which has a capability of producing similar symptoms in healthy individuals
  2. Law of Simplex, which states that only one single, simple medicinal substance is to be administered to a patient in a given point of time.
  3. Law of Minimum, which states that medicine should be administered in minute doses. The quantity is minimum, yet appropriate, for a gentle remedial effect.
- Individualization is yet another foundation stone of homeopathy that means that the characteristics of the chosen medicine should be as similar as possible to the characteristics of the illness in the patient.
- An example will clarify the concept of homeopathy. If coffee keeps you awake, then according to homeopathy, diluted coffee will put you to sleep. The more dilute, the stronger the effect. If you keep diluting it until there isn't a single molecule of coffee left, it will be even stronger.

Drug Proving

- Apart from the primary 3 principles stated above, drug proving forms an important principle of homeopathy. To find out which remedy does what, they are tested—not by controlled scientific studies but instead by "provings."
- Healthy people ingest the substance and report everything that happens to them (for example, "my big toe itched at midnight, I got heartburn after eating a big meal, I felt angry"). There is no attempt to separate the ordinary changes of everyday life from symptoms caused by the substance.
- These reports are then compiled as an index, which is called Repertory, where the practitioner can look up a patient's symptoms or characteristics to find out the remedies associated with a particular symptom in the provings.

Homeopathic Remedies

- Homeopathic remedies are prepared from various sources. Anything could be a homeopathic remedy. The primary sources of homeopathic remedies are:
  - Plants (like digitalis, poison ivy, belladonna, etc.)
  - Animals (snake venoms, ants, spiders, etc.)
  - Minerals (silver, gold, phosphorus, common salt, etc.)
  - Healthy secretions (milk of various mammals)
  - Unhealthy secretions (secretion from cancerous tissue in breast cancer)
  - Various energy sources (magnetic poles, eclipsed moonlight, etc.)
- Soluble materials could be diluted in water or alcohol. Non-soluble materials could be ground into powder (triturated) and diluted with sugar (lactose powder).
- Homeopathic remedies are usually labeled with the notation X or C, corresponding to ten and one hundred. 15 C would mean that one part of remedy was diluted in 100 parts of water, one part of the resulting solution was again diluted in 100 parts of water, and the process was repeated fifteen times.
- Hahnemann typically used 30 C remedies. At 30 C, it would take a container thirty million times the size of Earth to hold enough of the remedy to make it likely that it would contain a single molecule of the original substance.
- There are higher potencies available as well and they depend on the amount of dilution done.
- The practitioner consults Materia Medica for a list of symptoms that are associated with each remedy. For example, for Lachesis, the remedy made from the venom of bushmaster snake, the book lists symptoms in all the following areas: mind, head, eyes, ears, nose, face, stomach, abdomen, rectum, urine, male/female, respiratory, heart, extremities, sleep, skin, fever, and modalities.
- The symptoms are then matched to the most similar remedy and it is then prescribed to the patient.

359

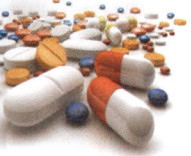

DOCTRINE OF DRUG POTENTIZATION

Potentization is a process, by which the medicinal/ curative properties of a substance are increased and the negative/ toxic properties are negated. This is done by two methods known as:

- Succussion (the substance is diluted with alcohol with distal water and shaken vigorously).
- Trituration (the insoluble solids are diluted by grinding them with lactose).

CURRENT SCENARIO OF HOMEOPATHY IN INDIA

- The Central Council of Homeopathy was established in 1973 to monitor higher education in homeopathy, and National Institute of Homeopathy in 1975.
- A minimum of a recognized diploma in homeopathy and registration on a state register or the Central Register of Homeopathy is required to practice homeopathy in India.
- Use of homeopathy is widely accepted nowadays.

UNANI MEDICINE

- **Yunani** or **Unani** medicine is the term for Perso-Arabic traditional medicine as practiced in Mughal India during 13th century.
- It is based on the concept of the four humors:
  - Blood
  - Phlegm
  - Yellow bile
  - Black bile

BASIS OF DISEASE ACCORDING TO UNANI MEDICINE

- Unani medicine has similarities to Ayurveda. Both are based on theory of the presence of the elements in the human body.
- According to followers of Unani medicine, these elements are present in different fluids and their balance leads to health and their imbalance leads to illness.
- The abnormal humor leads to pathological changes in the tissues anatomically and physiologically at the affected site and exhibits the clinical manifestations.

DIAGNOSIS OF DISEASE ACCORDING TO UNANI MEDICINE

- In the diagnosis, clinical features, i.e., signs, symptoms, laboratory features and *mizaj* (temperament) are important.

- Any cause and/or factor is countered by *Quwwat-e-Mudabbira-e-Badan* (the power of body responsible to maintain health), the failing of which may lead to quantitatively or qualitatively derangement of the normal equilibrium of *akhlat* (humors) of body, which constitute the tissues and organs.

PRINCIPLES OF MANAGEMENT

- After diagnosing the disease, *Usool-e-Ilaj* (principle of management) of disease is determined on the basis of etiology in the following pattern:
  - **Izalae Sabab** (elimination of cause)
  - **Tadeele Akhlat** (normalization of humors)
  - **Tadeele Aza** (normalization of tissues/organs)
- According to Unani medicine, management of any disease depends upon the diagnosis of disease.
- These medicines help to restore body functions and cure the disease.

CURRENT SCENARIO OF UNANI MEDICINE IN INDIA

- As an alternative form of medicine, Unani has found favor in India where popular products like Roghan Baiza Murgh (Egg Oil) and Roghan Badaam Shirin (Almond Oil) are commonly used for hair care.
- Unani practitioners can practice as qualified doctors in India, as the government approves their practice.

SIDDHA MEDICINE

- It is a traditional medicine first developed in Tamilakam in Tamil Nadu, India.
- According to the Palm leaf manuscripts, "Siddha system was first described by Lord Shiva to his wife Parvati". Parvati explained all this knowledge to her son Lord Muruga. He taught this knowledge to his disciple sage Agasthya.
- Agasthya is considered as the first siddha and the guru of all Siddhars.

BASIS OF DISEASE ACCORDING TO SIDDHA MEDICINE

- According to Siddha, the normal functioning of the body depends upon seven elements, namely;
  - Blood
  - Plasma
  - Fat tissues
  - Bone
  - Brain

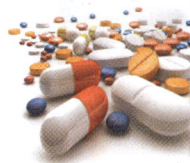

- Muscles
- Semen
- Generally, the basic concepts of the Siddha medicine are similar to Ayurveda.
- It is assumed that when the normal equilibrium of the three humors; Vaadham, Pittham and Kabam is disturbed, disease is caused.
- Under normal conditions, the ratio between Vaadham, Pittham, and Kabam are 4:2:1, respectively.

PRINCIPLES OF TREATMENT IN SIDDHA MEDICINE

- According to the Siddha medicine system, diet and lifestyle play a major role in health and in curing diseases.
- This concept of the Siddha medicine is termed pathiyam and apathiyam, which is essentially a list of "do's and don'ts".
- The principle treatment in siddha medicine is keeping the three humors in equilibrium and maintenance of seven elements.
- Treatment is classified into three categories:
  - *Devamaruthuvum* (Divine method)
  - *Manudamaruthuvum* (Rational method)
  - *Asuramaruthuvum* (Surgical method)

DRUGS IN SIDDHA MEDICINE

- The drugs used by the Siddhars could be classified into three groups:
  - *Thavaram* (herbal substances)
  - *Thadhu* (inorganic substances)
  - *Jangamam* (animal substances)
- The siddha medicines have been divided into two classes according to their site of application:
  - *Internal medicine* (used through the oral route and classified into 32 categories).
  - *External medicine* is used topically and classified into 32 categories.

CURRENT SCENARIO OF SIDDHA MEDICINE IN INDIA

- Siddha medicine is practiced by Siddha family doctors (traditional practitioners), and medically certified Siddha doctors who have studied in government Siddha medical colleges.
- Internationally 14 April is celebrated as 'World Siddha Day'.

Assess Yourself

Long and Short Answer Questions

1. Describe alternative systems of medicine.
2. Write short notes on:
   a. Ayurveda
   c. Homeopathy
   b. Siddha
   d. Unani

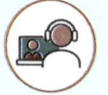

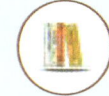

Glossary

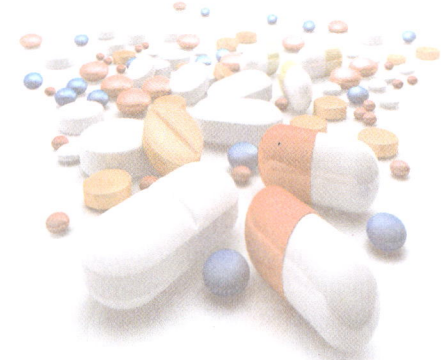

- **Agonist:** The drug having both affinity and intrinsic activity is called an agonist.
- **Analgesic:** Analgesics are the drugs having the property to provide relief from pain.
- **Antagonist:** The drug, which opposes the action of other drug, when given together or in combination, is called antagonist. The net response obtained by the combination of these drugs is always on the lesser side.
- **Antibiotics:** These are substances produced by microorganisms (fungi, bacteria, and actinomycetes, etc. which selectively suppress the growth of or kill other microorganisms at very low concentrations.
- **Antidote:** The drug or chemical which counteracts the harmful effects of other drug or chemical is called antidote.
- **Antiseptics:** These are the agents, which are used to inhibit or kill the microbes *on living tissue*. These agents are applied topically on skin, mucous membranes, or wounds. In concentrated form, some of the antiseptics can be used as disinfectants also.
- **Bactericidal agents:** These are the antimicrobial agents which irreversibly damage and kill the microorganisms. These drugs act better on the fast multiplying microorganisms. Examples: Cephalosporins, aminoglycosides and penicillin, etc.
- **Bacteriostatic agents:** These are the antimicrobial agents who do not kill the microorganisms but inhibit only the growth and multiplication of susceptible microorganisms. This inhibition is reversible in nature. Examples: Tetracyclines, Sulfonamides, etc.
- **Bioavailability:** It is a measure or fraction of administered dose of a drug that reaches the systemic circulation in the unchanged or active form. Bioavailability of the drug injected intravenously is 100%.
- **Disinfectants:** These are the chemical agents which are used to inhibit or kill the microbes *on inanimate objects*

such as surgical instruments/tables, floor, etc. These agents should never be applied on living tissue.
- **Drug allergy:** It is an abnormal individual immunologic response to a drug.
- **Drug dependence:** It means the state of a person arising after repeated and continuous use of a substance in which all-detrimental effects and craving appears. There is a psychological and physical need to continue the drug for the fear of getting the withdrawal symptoms.
- **Drug efficacy:** It refers to the maximum response, which can be elicited by a particular drug.
- **Drug interaction:** Refers to modification of response to one drug by another when they are administered simultaneously or in quick succession.
- **Drug potency:** It refers to the amount of drug needed to produce a certain response. Relative potency is a more meaningful term in which we compare the dose of two similar drugs at which they produce the same response.
- **Drug:** Any substance, which is synthetic, semisynthetic, natural, biotechnological used for diagnosis, prevention, treatment or cure of a disease or disorder is known as Drug.
- **Essential drugs:** According to the WHO essential drugs are defined as "those drugs that satisfy the basic healthcare need of the majority of the population". These drugs should be available at the affordable price, in adequate amounts and at all the times.
- **Half-life:** It is the time taken for the amount of drug in the body to decrease to one half its peak levels.
- **Hofmann elimination:** This is the inactivation of drug in the body, where no enzyme is involved in the inactivation of the drug, but spontaneous molecular rearrangement occurs. Examples: atracurium, cistracurium.
- **Inverse agonist:** An agent which activates a receptor to produce opposite effect to that of an agonist.

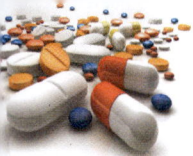

- **Loading dose:** Administering drug at a dose higher than the routinely used dose is called loading dose. It is given to achieve the required peak levels in blood.

- **Orphan drugs:** The drugs or biological products, which are meant for diagnosis, treatment or prevention of a rare disease or condition. From the sale of these drugs, pharmaceutical companies may or may not be able to recover the cost of developing and marketing of these drugs. Examples: liothyronine (T3), liposomal amphotericin-B, miltefosine, rifabutin, somatropin, etc.

- **Partial agonist:** An agent which activates a receptor to produce submaximal effect and antagonizes the action of an agonist.

- **Pharmacodynamics** (*What the drug does to the body):* It is a branch of pharmacology, which deals with the effects of drugs on the different body systems and includes mechanism of action of drugs at the molecular, cellular and organ level.

- **Pharmacokinetics** (*What the body does to the drug*): It is a branch of pharmacology, which deals with the journey or movements of drug *in, through and out* from the body. In other words, its deals with the scientific study of the administration, absorption, distribution, biotransformation (metabolism), and excretion (AADME) of drugs.

- **Pharmacology:** It is derived from the Greek word *Pharmacon* that means *Drugs* and *Logos* that means *study or knowledge*. It deals with the detailed knowledge about drugs including their history, sources, physical, chemical properties and their effects on the various body systems.

- **Pharmacopeia** (*Pharmacon-* Drug, *Poeia-* is to make)**:** is the official publication, which contains all details about the established drugs, being in use in a particular country. It is one of the official drug information sources. All countries have their own pharmacopeias such as Indian pharmacopeia (IP), British Pharmacopeia (BP), United States pharmacopeia (USP).

- **Pharmacovigilance:** It deals with the detection, assessment, understanding and prevention of various drug-related problems.

- **Placebo action:** Placebo (Latin word) means *I Shall Please*. It is inert and harmless substance, which physically resembles the actual medicine.

- **Plasma half-life:** The Plasma half-life (t½) of a drug is the time taken for its plasma concentration to be reduced to half of its original value.

- **Side effects:** Any undesirable actions, which occurs to the patient after administering the therapeutic dose levels.

- **Synergism** (Greek: *Syn*—together; *ergon*—work): When the action of one drug is potentiated or increased by the other, they are said to be synergistic.

- **Teratogenicity:** It is the study of the harmful effect of various drugs on fetus. This study guides us on safe use of various drugs in pregnancy.

Appendices

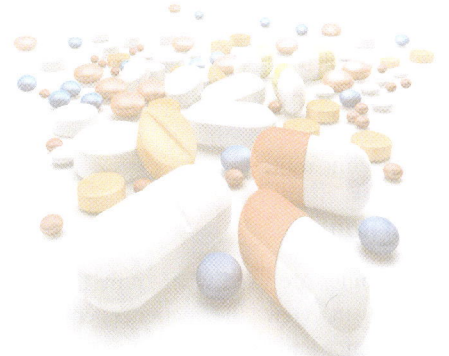

Appendix I: General Pharmacological Concepts

1. SOURCES OF DRUGS

The drugs are obtained from various sources such as:
- **Natural sources**
  - **Plants:** The drugs can be obtained from all parts of a plant such as roots, stem, leaves and fruits. Examples:
    - Dhatura—a source of Atropine.
    - Cinchona bark—a source of Quinine.
  - **Animals and human:** The drugs can be obtained from animals and human beings also. Examples: Heparin-liver, insulin from the pancreas of cows and pigs, serum from animal source (horse) and human gonadotropin hormone from pregnant women.
  - **Microorganisms:** The bacteria and fungi are also the sources of various drugs, such as penicillin and streptomycin.
  - **Heavy metals, minerals and mineral oils:** Aluminium, fluoride, iron, gold and liquids paraffin are also used to treat various conditions.

Metals	Medicinal uses
Iron	Treatment of iron deficiency anemia
Calcium	Treatment of diseases due to calcium deficiencies. Such as rickets in children and osteoporosis in adults
Aluminium and magnesium	As a part of various antacid combinations
Fluorine	Prevention of dental cavities Prevention of osteoporosis

Contd...

Metals	Medicinal uses
Radioisotopes	Radioactive Iodine for diagnosis and treatment of various thyroid disorders
Gold	Treatment of rheumatoid arthritis

- **Synthetic and semisynthetic sources**
  - The drugs synthesized from various chemical substances are called synthetic drugs. Examples: paracetamol, aspirin, diclofenac sodium, sulphonamides, calcium channel blockers, etc.
  - The drugs obtained by changing the structure of naturally obtained substances are called semisynthetic drugs. Examples: penicillin ampicillin, amoxicillin dicloxacillin, etc.
- **Engineered sources:** Some drugs are obtained by using modern technology methods. Such as human insulin by recombinant DNA technology, monoclonal antibodies and various vaccines for rabies and hepatitis, etc.

2. ROUTES AND PRINCIPLES OF ADMINISTRATION OF DRUGS

There are various routes available through which the drugs can be administered in the body, for their appropriate action. A detailed knowledge of exact route of drug administration is must for prescribing physician and nurses as well. The responsibility of administering various drugs lies on the shoulders of nurses, when the patient have been admitted indoor, day care centers or as an advisor to the outdoor patients.

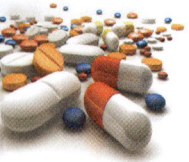

The decision about the choice of route in a particular patient lies largely on the patient's requirement, condition as well as the drug preparation available.

The routes of drug administration can be divided into:

- Local routes
- Systemic routes

Local Routes

These routes are used where only the local action is desired keeping in view the patient's conditions, requirements, convenience and tolerability to systemic drugs. The following are the commonly used local routes for drug administration:

Topical

Here the drug is applied topically/externally on skin and mucous membranes to get the local effects only. The various preparations to be applied on skin and mucous membrane are: creams, gel, ointments, lotion, liniments, paints, jellies, paste, passaries, suppositories, drops, sprays, etc.

Local Injections

When we do not want to expose whole of the body to a particular medication. This is unnecessary when the patient is suffering from local disease only. We prefer local injection at a particular site as the drug remains confined to that particular diseased tissue. For example: intra-articular corticosteroid injection in arthritis, intramedullary anti-cancerous drugs in some bone cancers, intrafemoral or intrabrachial anti cancerous drug infusion in some limb malignancies.

Systemic Routes

These routes are used, when the systemic action is desired keeping in view the patient's conditions, requirements, convenience and tolerability to systemic drugs. The drug administered by systemic routes reaches the blood circulation and it is distributed all over the body tissues including site of its action. The following are the commonly used systemic routes for drug administration:

Oral Route

- It is also called as enteral route.
- It is the oldest, the most common and considered to be safest route of drug administration.
- Administering drug through this route does not need any assistance for adults. Pediatric and geriatric patients may need assistance.
- The oral formulations are usually cheaper than other formulations.

- The following forms of drugs can be given by oral route: tablets, capsules, spansules, caplets, powders, drops, syrup, gel, mixtures, suspensions, emulsions, elixirs, GITS (gastrointestinal therapeutic system), etc.

GITS

There are some special preparations made for convenient dosing such as slow/sustained/extended/delayed/controlled/continuous release form of capsules or tablets. This is done to delay the absorption of the drug, so that frequency of dosing can be reduced. The enteric coated tablets protect the tablet from the acidic pH (HCl) of the stomach and the drug can safely pass into small intestine for better absorption.

Only scored tablets can be broken into the pieces. The unscored tablets should never be broken before administration.

This route is not suitable when

- The patient is uncooperative, unconscious and vomiting constantly.
- The patient has been brought in emergency.
- The drugs are irritant and unpalatable. Example: chloramphenicol
- The drugs are destroyed by gastric juice or enzyme. Example: Trypsin, chymotrypsin
- The drugs are having high first pass metabolism in liver. Example: Nitroglycerine
- The drugs cannot be absorbed. Example: Streptomycin

Sublingual (S/L) Route

- The tablet or pellet containing the drug is placed under the tongue or crushed in the mouth to be spread over the buccal mucosa for absorption.
- Absorption is relatively rapid and action can be produced in minutes.
- The drug can be spit out once the desired effect has been obtained.
- Drugs given sublingually are—GTN, buprenorphine, desamino-oxytocin.
- This route is generally employed in emergencies. Example GTN in MI patients.

Rectal

- This route is used when the patient is having recurrent vomitings or is unconscious.
- The irritant and unpleasant drugs can be put into the rectum as suppositories or retention enemas for systemic effects.
- The absorption is slow and irregular by this route and the effect is unpredictable.
- Examples: Rectal diazepam for treating epilepsy in children, indomethacin, paracetamol, etc.

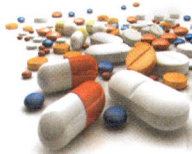

Cutaneous

- When slow and prolonged absorption of a drug is required for its systemic action, this route is preferred.
- The drug has to be highly lipid soluble.
- These drugs are presented in various forms like skin patches, etc.

Transdermal Therapeutic Systems (TTS)

These are devices in the form of adhesive patches of various shapes and sizes (5–20 cm²) which deliver the contained drug at a constant rate into systemic circulation via the stratum corneum layer of skin. The patch is to be peeled off just before application. The drug is delivered at the skin surface by diffusion for percutaneous absorption into the circulation. The usual sites for applying patches are chest, abdomen, upper arm, lower back, buttock and mastoid regions. Transdermal patches of GTN, fentanyl, nicotine, etoricoxib and estradiol are available in India. TTS have been designed to last for 1–3 days. Local irritation and erythema can occurs in some patients, but is generally mild. This can be minimized by changing the site of application each time by rotation.

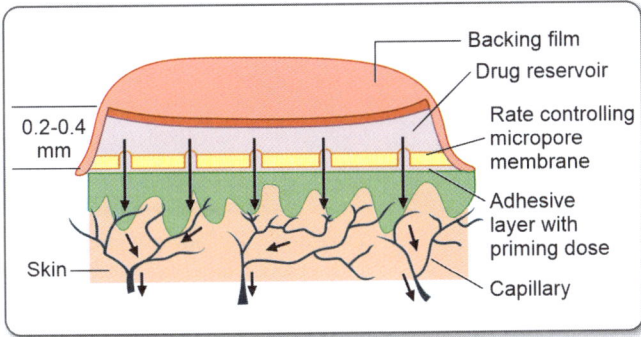

Illustration of a transdermal drug delivery system

Inhalational Route

- Drugs given by this route are absorbed through respiratory tract.
- The drugs are either volatile liquids, aerosol form or gases used to produce general anesthesia.
- This route is also use for the treatment for some local lung diseases.
- Drugs are presented in the form of inhalers, rotahalers and nebulizers.

Parenteral

(*Par*—beyond, *enteral*—intestinal):
- It refers to administration of drug by injection.
- The action of the drug is faster and useful in emergency.
- This routes is employed in unconscious, uncooperative or vomiting patient.

- The preparation is costlier and has to be sterilized.
- The technique is painful as it is invasive.

The Various Parenteral Routes are:

Intravenous (IV) route

The drugs are directly injected in to the superficial veins in the form of injection or infusion.

The drug
- Reaches directly into the blood stream.
- The onset of action is the fastest.
- Effects are produced immediately.
- Very useful in emergency.
- The bioavailability is 100%.
- Response is accurately measurable.
- Highly irritant drugs can be injected by this route *as the intima of veins is insensitive to pain and the drug gets diluted with blood.*
- Titration of the dose with the response is possible.

Disadvantages
- The technique is invasive and painful.
- The formulations are usually costlier.
- Strict aseptic measures need to be followed.
- Self-administration is usually not possible.
- Once the drug is injected, it cannot be withdrawn.
- Sometimes, thrombophlebitis of the injected vein and necrosis of adjoining tissues can occur if extravasation of the drug occurs. This can be minimized by diluting the drug or injecting it into a running IV line.
- Chances of causing air embolism is another risk.
- The vital organs like heart, brain, etc. get exposed to high concentrations of the drug, so it can prove to be a risky route also.

Precautions
- Drug sensitivity test should be performed before administration (where indicated).
- Make sure that needle is in the vein by withdrawl methods.
- Drug should be injected slowly.
- Oil based preparations should not be injected by this route.

Intramuscular (IM) Route
- The site of injection of drug is one of the large skeletal muscles like, gluteus maximus, deltoid, triceps, rectus femoris, etc.
- The drug is deposited in the muscles mass and from there it is absorbed gradually into the systemic circulation taking some time.
- The time taken for action of drug is slightly more than the time taken by the IV route.

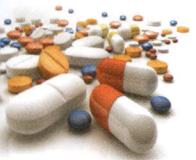

This route is preferred as

- Muscles are more vascular and absorption of drugs is faster than oral.
- Even the mild irritant drugs can be injected as muscles are less richly supplied with sensory nerves.
- The vital organs like heart, brain, etc. are not exposed to very high concentrations of the drug.
- Chances of causing air embolism are not there.

Disadvantages

- It can produce local hematoma in patients with blood coagulation disorders
- Self-injection impracticable
- Assistant require in case of children
- Chances of local abscess formations are there, if strict aseptic measures are not followed.
- Inaccurate administration can lead to nerve injury sometimes (sciatic nerve injury).

Subcutaneous (S/C) Route

- This route is used where, very prolonged action is required.
- The drug is deposited in the loose subcutaneous area.
- Self-injection is possible because deep penetration is not needed.

Disadvantages

- The absorption is slower than intramuscular route as the subcutaneous area is less vascular.
- Irritant drugs cannot be injected as it is richly supplied by nerves.
- Only small volume of the drug can be injected.
- It is not a preferred route in shock patients as the absorption is delayed due to vasoconstriction.
- Preparations are expensive.

Intradermal Injection (I/D) Route

- The drug is injected under the epidermis raising a bleb.
- This route is employed for specific purposes only.
- Use for sensitivity testing of various drugs such as penicillin testing, montoux test.
- Use for BCG vaccination.

Other Routes

- **Intra-arterial:** Direct injection in arteries.
- **Intracardiac:** Direct injection in chamber of heart.
- **Intrathecal:** Direct injection in sub arachnoid space
- **Intraperitoneal:** Direct injection in peritoneal cavity.
- **Epidural:** Direct injection in Epidural space.

Various parenteral route

Route	Absorption pattern	Special utility	Limitations and precautions
Intravenous	Absorption circumvented Potentially immediate effects Suitable for large volumes and for irritating substances, or complex mixtures, when diluted	Valuable for emergency use Permits titration of dosage Usually required for high-molecular-weight protein and peptide drugs	Increased risk of adverse effects Must inject solutions slowly as a rule Not suitable for oily solutions or poorly soluble substances
Subcutaneous	Prompt, from aqueous solution Slow and sustained, from repository preparations	Suitable for some poorly soluble suspensions and for instillation of slow-release implants	Not suitable for large volumes Possible pain or necrosis from irritating substances
Intramuscular	Prompt, from aqueous solution Slow and sustained, from repository preparations	Suitable for moderate volumes, oily vehicles, and some irritating substances Appropriate for self-administration (e.g., insulin)	Precluded during anticoagulant therapy May interfere with interpretation of certain diagnostic tests (e.g., creatine kinase)
Oral ingestion	Variable, depends on many factors	Most convenient and economical; usually more safe	Requires patient compliance Bioavailability potentially erratic and incomplete

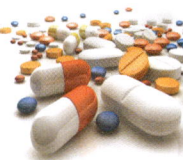

3. SPECIAL DRUG DELIVERY SYSTEM

- **Dermojet:** In this method no needle is used. A high velocity jet of drug solution is projected through a micro-fine orifice using a gun-like device. The solution gets deposited in the subcutaneous tissue. It is painless method.
- **Pellet implantation:** The drug is presented in the form of solid pellet. It is introduced surgically with the help of trochar and cannula. The drug keeps on releasing for weeks and month. Example: DOCA, testosterone
- **Implants:** Crystalline drug packed in tube and capsule made of suitable material are implanted under the skin.

Uniform and slow a release of a drug occurs for months together.

- **Liposomes:** This are minute vesicles made of phospholipids into which the drug is incorporated. Used for targeted drug delivery. Example: Some anticancer drug and amphotericin B.
- **Monoclonal antibodies:** These are antibodies which selectively react with specific antigen. These are produced using bio technology and cell culture methods. Used for targeted drug delivery. Example: Rituximab, Cetuximab, etc.

4. METABOLISM OR BIOTRANSFORMATION

Biotransformation means chemical alteration of the drug in the body to change it into easily excretable forms.

Sites of Metabolism or Biotransformation

These are liver kidneys, intestine, lungs and plasma

Mechanism of Metabolism or Biotransformation

It occurs by two methods
- Nonsynthetic or Phase-I or Fictionalization reactions.
- Synthetic or Phase-II or Conjugation reactions.

Differences between phase 1 and phase 2 metabolic reactions

Phase I reactions	Phase II reactions
It changes functional group of drug molecule and uses cytochrome P450 monooxygenase	It attach a conjugate to the drug molecule
Reaction are: • Oxidation (most common) • Reduction • Hydrolysis • Decyclization • Cyclization	Reactions are: • Glucuronide conjugation (most common) • Acetylation • Methylation • Sulfate conjugation • Glycine conjugation • Glutathione conjugation

5. KINETICS OF ELIMINATION

Differences between first order and zero order kinetics

First order kinetics	Zero order kinetics
Rate of elimination of a drug is directly proportional to its plasma concentration	Rate of elimination is constant irrespective of its plasma concentration
Accumulation of drug does not occur	Accumulation of drug occurs
Level of drug remains constant, in spite of increase in dose	Toxicity can occur if dose of the drug is increased
Drug follows first order kinetics till the saturation of various elimination mechanisms	Drug follows zero order kinetics after the saturation of various elimination mechanisms
Example: Most of the drugs	Examples: Phenytoin, warfarin, theophylline, tolbutamide

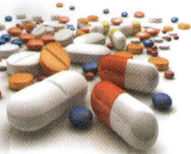

6. COMMONLY USED DRUGS WITH THEIR THERAPEUTIC INDEX

Drugs with very narrow therapeutic index	Drugs with narrow therapeutic index	Drugs with wide therapeutic index
• Vancomycin	• Warfarin	• Almost all Antibiotics
• Amphotericin B	• Levothyroxine	• NSAIDS
• Polymyxin	• Carbamazepine	• Hypnotics/ Sedatives
	• Lithium Carbonate	• Beta- blockers
	• Digoxin	• Benzodiazepines
	• Phenytoin	
	• Theophylline	
	• Morphine	

7. LIST OF MICROSOMAL ENZYME INDUCERS AND INHIBITORS

Microsomal enzymes properties
• All anti-fungals are microsomal enzyme inhibitors except Griseofulvin.
• All anti-epileptics are microsomal enzyme inducers except valproate.
• Acute alcoholism is a microsomal enzyme inhibitor, while chronic alcoholism is microsomal enzyme inducer.

Microsomal enzyme inducer drugs (Garimas)	Microsomal enzyme inhibitor drugs
• G—Griseofulvin, glucocorticoids	• Ketoconazole, Itraconazole
• A—Anti Epileptics (Phenobarbitone, Phenytoin and carbamazepine)	• Metronidazole
• R—Rifampin	• Valproate, Verapamil
• I—Isoniazid	• Protease Inhibitor (M/C Ritonavir)
• M—Meat	• Selective Serotonin Reuptake Inhibitor
• A—Alcohol	• C—Ciprofloxacin, Clarithromycin
• S—Smoking	• O—Oral contraceptive pills
• Others: Omeprazole, DDT, phenylbutazone	• C—Cimetidine, Chloramphenicol
	• A—Allopurinol, Amiodarone
	• E—Erythromycin

8. LIST OF PRODRUGS

The drug, which is inactive as such and need conversion in the body to one or more active metabolites. Such a drug is called a "prodrug".

List of prodrugs and their active forms are as follows:

Prodrug	Active form
Acyclovir	Acyclovir triphosphate
Fluorouracil	Fluorouridine monophosphate
Bacampicillin	Ampicillin
Prednisone	Prednisolone
Sulindac	Sulfide metabolite
Enalapril	Enalaprilat
Alfa-Methyldopa	α-methyl norepinephrine
Fosphenytoin	Phenytoin

9. DRUGS AND THEIR DEPOSITIONS IN THE VARIOUS BODY TISSUES

Body tissues where deposition occurs	Drugs
Bone and teeth	Tetracycline, heavy metals (bound to mucopolysaccharides of connective tissue)
Retina	Chloroquine (bound to nucleoproteins)
Liver	Chloroquine, tetracycline, emetine, digoxin.
Thyroid	Iodine.
Kidney	Digoxin, Chloroquine, emetine
Skeletal muscle, heart	Digoxin, emetine (bound to muscle proteins).

Appendix II: Systemic Pharmacology

1. CLASSIFICATIONS OF DRUGS

Diuretics

High efficacy diuretics	Medium efficacy diuretics	Weak or adjunctive diuretics
Na$^+$ K$^+$2Cl cotransport Inhibitors	Na$^+$Cl$^-$ symport Inhibitors	• Inhibitors of carbonic anhydrase enzyme: Acetazolamide • Potassium sparing diuretics

• Furosemide
• Torasemide
• Bumetanide
• Indacrinone
• Ethacrynic acid
	Thiazides diuretics:
	• Hydrochlorothiazide
	• Chlorthiazide
	• Benzthiazide,
	• Hydroflumethiazide, Bendroflumethiazide
	Thiazide like diuretics:
	• Chlorthalidone
	• Indapamide
	• Xipamide
	• Metolazone
	• Quinethazone
		▪ Aldosterone receptor antagonist:
		  ♦ Spironolactone
		  ♦ Eplerenone
		▪ **Na$^+$ channel inhibitors (at collecting duct):**
		  ♦ Triamterene
		  ♦ Amiloride
		• **Osmotic diuretics:**
		• Mannitol
		• Glycerol
		• Isosorbide

Penicillins

- **Acid-labile (Natural) Penicillin:** Penicillin G, Procaine Penicillin G, Fortified Penicillin G, Benzathine Penicillin G.
- **Acid-resistant alternative to penicillin G:** Phenoxymethyl penicillin (Penicillin V).
- **Penicillinase-resistant penicillins:** Methicillin, Cloxacillin, Dicloxacillin.
- **Extended spectrum penicillins:**
  - Aminopenicillins: Ampicillin, Bacampicillin, Amoxicillin.
  - Carboxypenicillins: Carbenicillin.
  - Ureidopenicillins: Piperacillin, Mezlocillin.
- **β-lactamase inhibitors:** Clavulanic acid, Sulbactam, Tazobactam.

Cephalosporins

Cephalosporins have been conventionally divided into five generations:

Generation	Oral	Parenteral
First generation cephalosporins	Cephalexin Cefadroxil	Cefazolin
Second generation cephalosporins	Cefaclor Cefprozil Cefuroxime axetil	Cefuroxime Cefoxitin
Third generation cephalosporins	Cefixime Cefpodoxime proxetil Cefdinir Ceftibuten Ceftamet pivoxil	Cefotaxime Ceftizoxime Ceftriaxone Ceftazidime Cefoperazone
Fourth generation cephalosporins	–	Cefepime Cefpirome
Fifth generation cephalosporins	–	Ceftobiprole Ceftaroline Ceftolozane

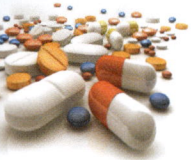

Fluoroquinolones

Generation	Drugs
First generation Fluoroquinolones	Norfloxacin, Ofloxacin, Ciprofloxacin, Pefloxacin
Second generation Fluoroquinolones	Levofloxacin, Moxifloxacin, Lomefloxacin, Gemifloxacin, Sparfloxacin, Prulifloxacin etc.

Macrolides

Group	Drugs
Macrolides	Erythromycin, Clarithromycin, Azithromycin Roxithromycin, Telithromycin, Spiramycin

Opioids

Based upon their nature of origin, opioids have been classified into following three types:

Natural opium alkaloids (Opiates)	Semisynthetic opiates	Synthetic opioids
• Morphine • Codeine	• Diacetylmorphine (Heroin) • Pholcodeine • Ethylmorphine • Hydromorphone* • Oxymorphone* • Hydrocodone* • Oxycodone*	• Pethidine (Meperidine) • Fentanyl • Methadone • Dextropropoxyphene • Tramadol • Tapentadol • Levorphanol* • Dextromoramide* • Dipipanone* • Alfentanil* • Sufentanil* • Remifentanil*

Not available in India.

Antihypertensive Drugs

Antihypertensive drugs have been classified as follows:

- **Diuretics**
  - **Thiazides:** Hydrochlorothiazide, Chlorthalidone, Indapamide
  - **High ceiling diuretics:** Furosemide etc.
  - **K^+ Sparing diuretics:** Spironolactone, Amiloride
- **Drugs acting on RAAS**
  - **ACE inhibitors:** Captopril, Enalapril, Lisinopril, Perindopril, Ramipril, Fosinopril, etc.
  - **Angiotensin (AT_1 receptor) blockers:** Losartan, Candesartan, Irbesartan, Valsartan, Telmisartan
  - **Direct renin inhibitor:** Aliskiren, Ramikiren
- **Calcium channel blockers:**
  - **Dihydropyridines (DHPs):** Nifedipine, Amlodipine, Felodipine, Nitrendipine, Nimodipine, Lacidipine, Lercanidipine, Benidipine
  - **Others:** Verapamil, Diltiazem
- **Sympatholytics drugs**
  - **β Adrenergic blockers:** Propranolol, Metoprolol, Atenolol, etc.
  - **β + α Adrenergic blockers:** Labetalol, Carvedilol
  - **α Adrenergic blocker:** Prazosin, Terazosin, Doxazosin, Phentolamine, Phenoxybenzamine
  - **Central sympatholytics:** Clonidine, Methyldopa
- **Vasodilators:**
  - **Arteriolar dilator:** Hydralazine, Minoxidil, Diazoxide
  - **Arteriolar and venous dilator:** Sodium nitroprusside

Antiarrhythmic Drugs

Class of anti-arrhythmic drugs	Moa	Drugs

I (Na$^+$ channel blockers)	Act on phase- 0, depolarization.
	Subdivided into : IA
	           : IB
	           : IC
		Quinidine, Procainamide, Disopyramide
		
		Lignocaine, Mexiletine
		Propafenone, Flecainide

II (β blockers)	Act on phase –II and IV	Propranolol, Esmolol, Sotalol
III (K$^+$ channel blockers)	Act on phase –III and prolong repolarization	Amiodarone, Dronedarone, Dofetilide, Ibutilide
IV (Ca^{2+} channel blockers)	Act on phase –II	Verapamil, Diltiazem
Others	• PSVT: Adenosine, Digoxin are used. • A-V block: Sympathomimetics (isoprenaline, etc), Anticholinergics (atropine) are used. • In atrial flutter and fibrillation and PSVT digitalis is used to control ventricular rate.	

Antitubercular Drugs

First-line drugs	Second-line drugs		
		Fluoroquinolones	**Injectable drugs**
Rifampin (R)	Rifabutin	Moxifloxacin	Kanamycin
Isoniazid (H)	Thiacetazone	Ciprofloxacin	Amikacin
Ethambutol (E)	Ethionamide Prothionamide	Ofloxacin	Capreomycin
Pyrazinamide (Z)	Cycloserine	Levofloxacin	
Streptomycin (S)	Para-aminosalicylic acid		

Antifungal Agents

- **Antifungal Antibiotics**
  - **Polyenes:** Nystatin, Amphotericin B (AMB) and Hamycin.
  - **Echinocandins:** Micafungin, Caspofungin and Anidulafungin.
  - **Heterocyclic benzofuran:** Griseofulvin.
- **Azoles**
  - **Imidazoles**
    Topical: Miconazole, Clotrimazole, Oxiconazole and Econazole.
    Systemic: Ketoconazole.
  - *Triazoles* (systemic): Fluconazole, Itraconazole, Iuliconazole, Posaconazole and Voriconazole.
- **Allylamine:** Terbinafine and Butenafine, etc.
- **Other topical agents:** Butenafine, Tolnaftate, Benzoic acid, Quiniodochlor, Ciclopiroxolamine, Selenium sulfide, etc.

Commonly used Antimalarial Drugs

The various drug used in the treatment of malaria can be classified according to their clinical structure as follows:

- **Cinchona alkaloid:** Quinine, Quinidine.
- **Quinoline-methanol:** Mefloquine.
- **4-Aminoquinolines:** Chloroquine (CQ), Amodiaquine (AQ), Piperaquine.
- **8-Aminoquinoline:** Primaquine, Tafenoquine.
- **Biguanide:** Proguanil (Chloroguanide).
- **Diaminopyrimidine:** Pyrimethamine.
- **Sulfonamides and sulfone:** Sulfadoxine, Sulfamethopyrazine.
- **Antibiotics:** Tetracycline, Doxycycline, Clindamycin.
- **Sesquiterpinelactones:** Artesunate, Artemether, Arteether, Arterolane.
- **Amino alcohols:** Halofantrine, Lumefantrine.
- **Naphthyridine:** Pyronaridine.
- **Naphthoquinone:** Atovaquone.

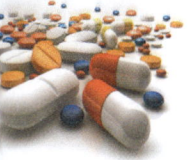

Prostaglandins and Leukotrienes Synthesis Pathway with the Site of Action of Some Related Drugs

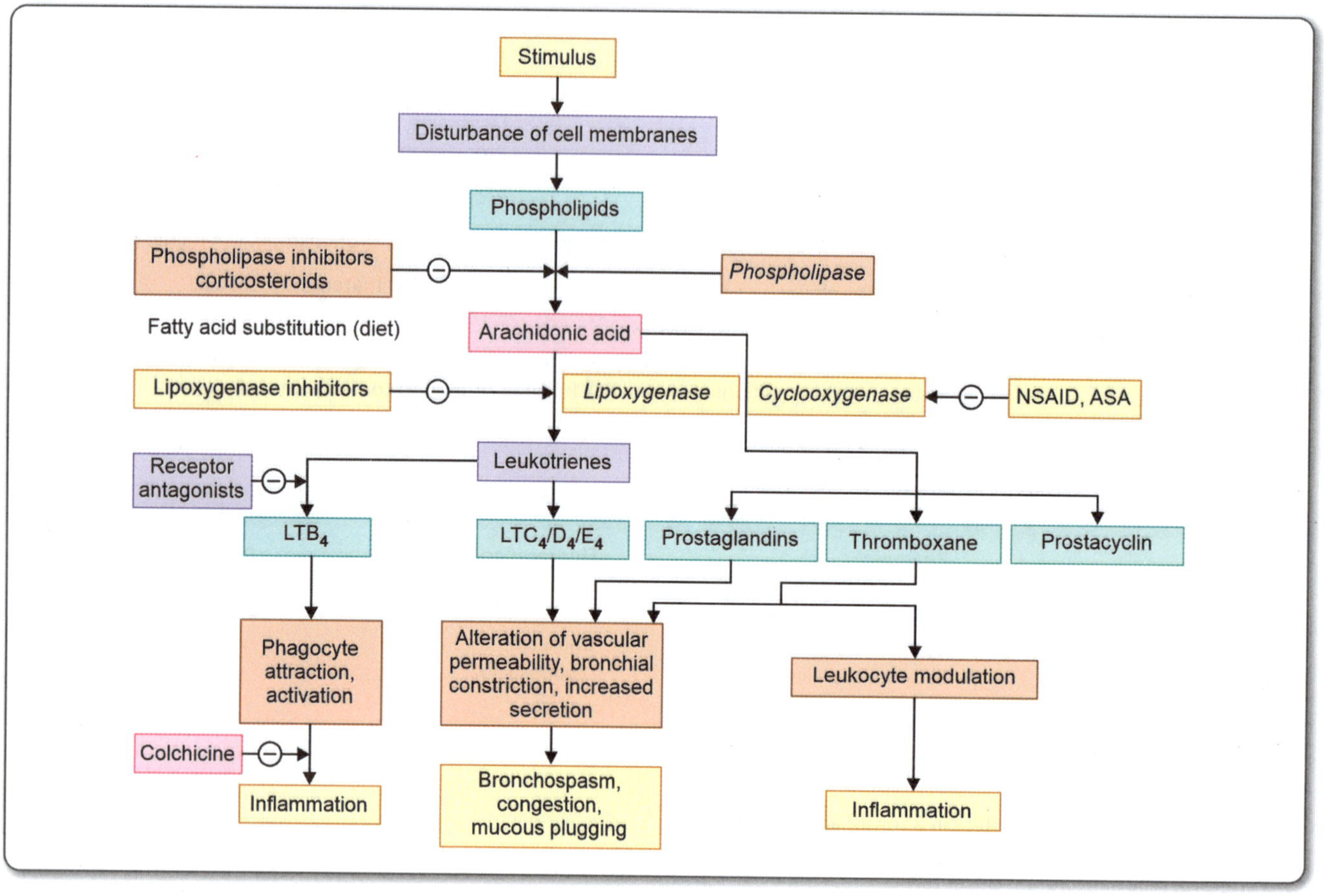

```
                              ┌───────────┐
                              │ Stimulus  │
                              └─────┬─────┘
                                    ↓
                    ┌───────────────────────────────┐
                    │ Disturbance of cell membranes │
                    └───────────────┬───────────────┘
                                    ↓
                            ┌───────────────┐
                            │ Phospholipids │
                            └───────┬───────┘
                                    ↓
┌─────────────────────────┐       ┌─┐              ┌──────────────┐
│ Phospholipase inhibitors│──────⊖│ │──────────────│ Phospholipase│
│    corticosteroids      │       └─┘              └──────────────┘
└─────────────────────────┘

 Fatty acid substitution (diet)    ┌─────────────────┐
                                   │ Arachidonic acid │
                                   └─────────────────┘

┌─────────────────────┐    ┌──────────────┐   ┌──────────────┐      ┌───────────┐
│Lipoxygenase inhibitors│──⊖│ Lipoxygenase │   │Cyclooxygenase│──⊖───│ NSAID, ASA│
└─────────────────────┘    └──────────────┘   └──────────────┘      └───────────┘

┌──────────────┐   ┌──────────────┐
│  Receptor    │──⊖│ Leukotrienes │
│ antagonists  │   └──────────────┘
└──────────────┘
```

| LTB₄ | LTC₄/D₄/E₄ | Prostaglandins | Thromboxane | Prostacyclin |

- Phagocyte attraction, activation
- Alteration of vascular permeability, bronchial constriction, increased secretion
- Leukocyte modulation

Colchicine ──⊖──→ Inflammation

Bronchospasm, congestion, mucous plugging

Inflammation

NSAIDs

Depending upon the specificity of COX inhibition, the NSAIDs have been broadly classified as follows:

- **Nonselective COX inhibitors (traditional NSAIDs):** Aspirin, Ibuprofen, Ketoprofen, Naproxen, Flurbiprofen, Mephenamic acid, Piroxicam, Tenoxicam, Ketorolac, Indomethacin, Nabumetone, Phenylbutazone, Oxyphenbutazone.
- **Preferential COX-2 inhibitors:** Nimesulide, Diclofenac, Aceclofenac, Etodolac, Meloxicam etc.
- **Selective COX-2 inhibitors:** Celecoxib, Etoricoxib, Parecoxib.
- **Analgesic-antipyretics with poor anti-inflammatory action:** Paracetamol (Acetaminophen), Metamizol, Nefopam, Propiphenazone etc.
- **Both COX and LOX inhibitors:** Licofelone

Anticancer Drugs

A. Cytotoxic drugs	
• Alkylating agents	Mechlorethamine, Cyclophosphamide, Ifosfamide, Chlorambucil, Melphalan, Busulfan, Carmustine, Lomustine, Dacarbazine, Temozolomide, Procarbazine
• Platinum analogues	Cisplatin, Carboplatin, Oxaliplatin
• **Antimetabolites** ▪ **Folate antagonist:** Methotrexate (Mtx), Pemetrexed ▪ **Purine antagonist:** 6-Mercaptopurine (6-MP), 6-Thioguanine (6-TG), Azathioprine, Fludarabine ▪ **Pyrimidine antagonist:** 5-Fluorouracil (5-FU), Capecitabine, Cytarabine	

Contd...

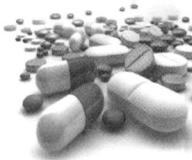

- Microtubule damaging agents
  - **Vinca alkaloids:** Vincristine, Vinblastine, Vinorelbine
  - **Taxanes:** Paclitaxel, Docetaxel

• Topoisomerase-2 inhibitors	Etoposide, Tenipocite
• Topoisomerase-1 inhibitors	Topotecan, Irinotecan
• Antibiotics	Actinomycin D (Dactinomycin), Doxorubicin, Daunorubicin, Epirubicin, Mitoxantrone, Bleomycins, Mitomycin C
• Miscellaneous	Hydroxyurea, L-Asparaginase, Tretinoin, Arsenic trioxide

B. Targeted drugs

• Tyrosine protein- kinase inhibitors	Imatinib, Nilotinib
• Endothelial growth factor [EGF] receptor inhibitors	Gefitinib, Erlotinib, Cetuximab, Panitumumab, Sorafenib
• Angiogenesis inhibitors	Bevacizumab, Sunitinib
• Proteasome inhibitor	Bortezomib
• Unarmed monoclonal antibody	Rituximab, Trastuzumab

C. Hormonal drugs

• Glucocorticoids	Prednisolone and others
• Estrogens	Fosfestrol, Ethinylestradiol
• Selective estrogen receptor modulators	Tamoxifen, Toremifene
• Selective estrogen receptor down regulators	Fulvestrant
• Aromatase inhibitors	Letrozole, Anastrozole, Exemestane
• Antiandrogen	Flutamide, Bicalutamide
• 5-α reductase inhibitor	Finasteride, Dutasteride
• GnRH analogues	Nafarelin, Leuprorelin Triptorelin
• Progestins	Hydroxyprogesterone acetate, etc.

Insulins and OHAs

Class, drugs, onset of action and duration of action of insulin

Class	Drugs	Onset of action (Hours)	Duration of action (Hours)
Ultra short or rapid acting insulin	Lispro-Insulin	0.2–0.3	3–5
	Aspart-Insulin	0.2–0.3	3–5
	Gluilisine-Insulin	0.2–0.4	3–5
Short acting insulin	Regular soluble insulin	0.5–1	5–8
	Semilente	1–2	12–14
Intermediate acting insulin	Insulin zinc or Lente	1–2	20–24
	Neutral protamine hagedorn or isophane insulin	1–2	20–24
Long acting insulin	Insulin detemir	1–4	20–24
	Insulin glargine	2–4	24
Ultra-long acting insulin	Degludec	30–90 minutes	24–40
	Ultralente	6	20–36

375

Contd...

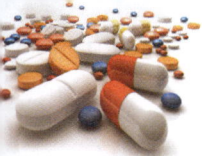
Classification of oral hypoglycemic agents (OHAs)

- Insulin secretagogues
  - **Sulfonylureas**
    - First generation: Tolbutamide, Chlorpropamide
    - Second generation: Glibenclamide, Glipizide, Glimepiride and Gliclazide
  - **Meglitinide analogues:** Nateglinide and Repaglinide
- Insulin sensitizers
  - Biguanide: Metformin
  - Thiazolidinediones: Pioglitazone, Rosiglitazone (banned)
- Others
  - α-Glucosidase inhibitors: Voglibose, Acarbose and Miglitol
  - Amylin analogue: Pramlintide
  - Sodium-glucose cotransport-2 inhibitor (SGLT-2 inhibitor): Empagliflozin, Canagliflozin and Dapagliflozin
  - Glucagon-like peptide-1 (GLP-1) receptor agonists: Liraglutide, Albiglutide and Exenatide
  - Dipeptidyl peptidase-4 (DPP-4) inhibitors: Sitagliptin, Saxagliptin, Vildagliptin, Alogliptin, Linagliptin.

Bisphosphonates

Generations	Potency	Drugs
First generation Bisphosphonates	Least potent	Etidronate Tiludronate
Second generation Bisphosphonates	10–100 times more potent than first gen	Alendronate Pamidronate Ibandronate
Third generation Bisphosphonates	10,000 times more potent than second gen	Risedronate Zoledronate

Drugs Used in Management of Bronchial Asthma

Drugs used in the treatment of bronchial asthma are of following types:

- **Bronchodilators**
  - **Sympathomimetics:** Salbutamol, Terbutaline, Salmeterol, Formoterol, Bambuterol and Ephedrine
  - **Methylxanthines:** Theophylline, Aminophylline, Doxophylline, Acebrophylline
  - **Anticholinergics:** Tiotropium bromide and Ipratropium bromide
- **Leukotriene antagonists:** Zafirlukast and Montelukast
- **Mast cell stabilizers:** Ketotifen and Sodium cromoglycate
- **Corticosteroids**
  - **Systemic:** Prednisolone, Hydrocortisone and Deflazacort, etc.
  - **Inhalational:** Budesonide, Fluticasone, Beclomethasone and ciclesonide
- **Anti-IgE antibody:** Omalizumab

Second Generation Antihistaminics

These are none sedating in nature.
Examples are Rupatadine Desloratadine Fexofenadine, Loratadine, Levocetirizine, Azelastine, and Cetirizine.

Drugs Used in Management of Acute and Chronic Gout

Acute gout		Chronic gout	
- NSAIDs - Colchicine - Corticosteroids	- Uricosurics - Probenecid - Sulfinpyrazone	- Uric acid synthesis inhibitors - Allopurinol - Febuxostat	

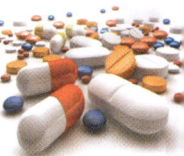

2. MOST COMMONLY ASKED TREATMENTS

Mushroom Poisoning

It occurs due to accidental consumption of poisonous mushrooms *Amanita muscaria* and Inocybe species. Due to the presence of *muscarine alkaloid in these species*, the muscarinic actions are seen.

Three types of mushroom poisonings are known. The symptoms depend upon the toxic principle present in the particular species.

1. **Early mushroom poisoning (Muscarine type):** It occurs due to consumption of Inocybe and related species. Symptoms appear within an hour of eating the mushroom, and are promptly reversed by atropine.
2. **Hallucinogenic type:** It occurs due to consumption of A. muscaria and related mushrooms. These compounds produce hallucinogenic symptoms due to muscarinic receptors blockade in the brain. There is no specific treatment and atropine is contraindicated.
3. **Late mushroom poisoning (Phalloidin type):** It occurs due to consumption of A. phalloides, galerina and related species. Symptoms are due to damage to the gastrointestinal mucosa, liver and kidney and appear after many hours of consumption of poisonous mushrooms. Supportive measures need to be given and in some cases Thioctic acid may be given as antidote.

Organophosphate Poisoning

Acute Organophosphate Poisoning or Anticholinesterase Poisoning

The various agricultural and household insecticides are cholinomimetic agents, as these are anticholinesterases. The poisoning with these agents can be accidental, suicidal or homicidal. The symptoms observed are due to persistence action of acetylcholine on the cholinomimetic receptors. The various symptoms observed are:

- **Eye:** Irritation of eye, lacrimation, salivation, sweating, copious tracheo-bronchial secretions, miosis, blurring of vision,
- **Cardiovascular system (CVS):** Fall in BP, bradycardia or tachycardia, cardiac arrhythmias, vascular collapse
- **Respiratory, GIT and urinary system:** bronchospasm, breathlessness, colic, involuntary defecation and urination.
- **Skeletal system:** Muscular fasciculations, weakness, respiratory paralysis (central as well as peripheral).
- **Central nervous system (CNS):** Irritability, disorientation, unsteadiness, tremors, ataxia, convulsions, coma and death.

   Death is generally due to respiratory failure.

Treatment

Treatment should be started as early as possible (within few hours). The patients are managed by following general management and specific management guidelines.

- General management
  - Prevention of further exposure to the poison: Area of contact should be cleaned with soap and water. The further absorption is prevented by gastric lavage.
  - Maintains of airway patency and oxygenation.
  - Supportive measures: To maintain BP and prevention/ treatment convulsions.
- Specific management
  - Atropine (Dose: 2 mg IV, repeat every 10 minutes until signs of atropinization such as mydriasis and tachycardia appear.)
  - Cholinesterase reactivators: Pralidoxime, obidoxime and diacetyl-monoxime (DAM). These drugs reactivate the cholinesterase enzyme by blocking the action of anticholinesterases.

Chronic Organophosphate Poisoning

- Repeated exposure to certain organophosphates manifest as polyneuritis and demyelination after a latent period of days to weeks.
- Clinically, sensory disturbances, muscle weakness, tenderness and depressed tendon reflexes occur due to lower motor neurone paralysis.
- Later on, spasticity and upper motor neurone paralysis occur gradually.
- There is no specific treatment. Avoidance of further exposure to organophosphates along with symptomatic management are the only measures which can be taken.
- Recovery may take quite a long time.

Management of Status Asthmatics
Status Asthmaticus/Refractory Asthma

- It is also known as acute severe asthma.
- It is a life-threatening condition and mostly occurs due to precipitation of chronic asthma by acute respiratory infection.

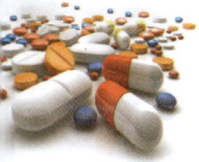

Signs and Symptoms

- Unable to speak a sentence due to severe dyspnea.
- Severe cyanosis.
- Pulsus paradoxus (inspiratory fall in systolic blood pressure ≥10 mm Hg).
- Silent chest (No pathological sign during auscultation).
- Encephalopathy, seizure, coma and death if not treated appropriately within the golden period.

Management of Status Asthmaticus

- Hydrocortisone 100 mg intravenously given stat, then 100–200 mg 4–8 hourly infusion (or equivalent dose of another glucocorticoid). The onset of action of hydrocortisone takes about 6 hours.
- 2.5–5 mg of nebulized salbutamol + 0.5 mg of ipratropium bromide.
- Administration of humidified oxygen in high flow.
- Salbutamol/terbutaline 0.4 mg intramuscularly or subcutaneously can be given for its better therapeutic effect.
- In severe respiratory distress, intubation and mechanical ventilation is advocated.
- Broad-spectrum antibiotic therapy is required to control the chest infection.
- Correction of electrolyte imbalance.
- Correction of acidosis with Sod. Bicarbonate/lactate infusion.
- If hypokalemia is detected, correct with potassium chloride infusion.
- Recording and maintenance of vitals.

Drugs used by Inhalational Route for Asthma Treatment

Drugs used by Inhalational Route for Asthma Treatment

- *The following types of antiasthmatic drugs are available in inhalational forms.*
  - *Glucocorticoids (Beclomethasone, Fluticasone, Budesonide, Ciclesonide)*
  - *β_2 agonists (Salbutamol, Terbutaline, Salmetrol, etc.)*
  - *Anticholinergics (Ipratropium bromide, Tiotropium bromide)*
  - *Cromoglycate sodium*

- *Currently, inhalational agents are the preferred drugs for both short and long-term management of asthma.*
- *Drugs given by inhalational route have following advantages over that given by oral route:*
  - *The drug is delivered directly at the site of action.*
  - *Prompt action is achieved.*
  - *Minimal systemic side effects than oral antiasthamatics.*
  - *Inhalational doses are lower than oral doses of the same drug.*

Management of Status Epilepticus

Status Epilepticus

- It is an emergency condition, which can prove fatal if not treated timely.
- It is defined as the condition when the seizures occur repeatedly without any evidence of recovery in between the seizures.
- The period of seizure activity is mostly more than 30 minutes. If proper and timely intervention is not done, it can lead to permanent brain damage and death.
- The management of patients suffering from status epilepticus is as follows:
- Initial general management includes
  - Hospitalization
  - Maintenance of the airways.
  - Maintenance of fluid and electrolytes.
  - Monitoring of cardiac rhythm and BP.

Drug Management

- Diazepam in a dose of 0.2–0.3 mg/kg or 10mg IV is given.
- Alternatively, lorazepam can be given in a dose of 0.1 mg/kg or 4 mg injected IV slowly.
- If available, fosphenytoin can be given in a dose of 15–20 mg/kg in the form of IV infusion.
- Alternatively, phenytoin sodium is given in a loading dose of 500–1000 mg followed by IV infusion at the rate of 25–50 mg/min.
- Phenobarbitone sodium can be given in a dose of 10–15 mg/kg IV, if previous mentioned drugs do not control the seizure activity. Respiratory depression is major side effects; hence, should be watched carefully.
- If the seizures are not controlled with above-mentioned management or drugs, the last resort is giving general anesthesia with propofol or **thiopentone** sodium.

After the control of seizures, long-term antiepileptic therapy is mandatory.

Types of epilepsy and indicated drugs			
Types of epilepsy	Drugs of 1st choice	Drugs of 2nd choice	Add-on drugs
GTCS	Carbamazepine, Phenytoin	Valproic acid Phenobarbitone	Topiramate Lamotrigine Levetiracetam Gabapentin
Absence seizures	Valproic acid	Ethosuximide Lamotrigine	Clonazepam
Myoclonic seizures	Valproic acid	Topiramate Lamotrigine	Clonazepam Levetiracetam
Atonic seizures	Valproic acid	Clonazepam	Lamotrigine
Febrile seizure	Diazepam	Lorazepam	–

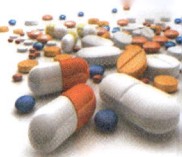

Drugs for Angina Pectoris

Class of drugs	Drugs
For treatment of Acute anginal attack	• **Nitrates** (short acting): Gliceryltrinitate (GTN) • **Nitrates** (long acting): Isosorbide dinitrate (short acting by sublingual route)
For chronic prophylaxis of anginal attack	• **Nitrates** (long acting): Isosorbide dinitrate, Isosorbide mononitrate, Erythrityltetrani-trate, Pentaerythritoltetranitrate • **β-Blockers**: Propranolol, Metoprolol, Atenolol and others. • **Calcium channel blockers** • **Phenyl alkylamine:** Verapamil • **Benzothiazepine:** Diltiazem • **Dihydropyridines:** Nifedipine, Felodipine, Amlodipine, Nitrendipine, Nimodipine, Lacidipine, Lercanidipine, Benidipine • **Potassium channel opener:** Nicorandil • **Others:** Dipyridamole, Trimetazidine, Ranolazine, Ivabradine,

Management of Myocardial Infarction (MI)

- Immediately on the suspicion of myocardial infarction, the patient should be administered 4 tablets of Aspirin (75 mg each) or one tablet of aspirin (325 mg) and 4 tablets of clopidogrel (75 mg each) without wasting any time. It should be followed by Tablet GTN (sublingual), to be repeated after 5 minutes but, not more than 3 doses.
- Injection Morphine (4–8 mg) is given to relieve pain, anxiety and apprehension.
- Oxygen inhalation and assisted respiration, if required.
- Slow IV infusion of saline or low molecular weight dextran to maintain tissue perfusion.
- Intravenous sodium bicarbonate infusion to correct acidosis.
- Intravenous infusion of a β-blocker (metoprolol 5 mg every 5 minutes, maximum 3 doses) for the prevention and treatment of arrhythmias.
- Bradycardia and heart block is managed with atropine or electrical pacing.
- Intravenous infusion of dopamine or dobutamine, if there is a pump failure.
- Furosemide should be given if there is evidence of overload or edema.
- Streptokinase/urokinase/alteplase is given as thrombolytic therapy.
- Surgical intervention in the form of PTCA or CABG may be needed.
- After the successful management of MI, patient is prescribed ACE inhibitors/ARBs, aspirin and clopidogrel, β blockers, nitrates, diuretic and stat in to reduce the risk of reinfarction and mortality.

DRUGS USED FOR ANAPHYLAXIS

- Injection Adrenaline (0.3–0.5 mL 1:1000 sol) is given by Intramuscular route
- Injection Hydrocortisone 100 mg IV
- Injection Chlorpheniramine maleate 20–50 mg IV

The general management is done on the basis of cause and the signs and symptoms.

DRUGS THERAPY FOR MIGRAINE

Extent or severity of migraine	Drug therapy recommended
Mild migraine attack	Simple analgesics/NSAIDs or their combinations (± antiemetic) Example: Paracetamol ± Domperidone/ metochlopramide
Moderate migraine attack	NSAIDs combinations/a triptan/ergot alkaloids (+ antiemetic) Example: Paracetamol + Ibuprofen, or naproxen/sumatriptan/ergotamine (Domperidone/ metochlopramide)
Severe migraine attack	Triptan/ergot alkaloids (+ antiemetic); Example: Sumatriptan/ergotamine (Domperidone/ metochlopramide) + Prophylaxis (any one of these) Propranolol or Amitriptyline or Flunarizine or Nifedipine or Valproate/topiramate/divalproex

Management of Hypothyroidism

- The treatment is started with L-thyroxine (T4) in a low dose of 50 µg per day and increased every 2–3 weeks to maximum of 100–200 µg/day.
- The dose is adjusted by clinical response and serum TSH levels.
- The treatment of subclinical hypothyroidism cases is optional depending upon the clinical features if the TSH level is between 6–10 mU/L. In subclinical hypothyroidism with TSH level >10 mU/L, patients should be treated with T_4.

Management of Hypoglycemia

- Hypoglycemia is a metabolic disorder in which the blood sugar levels become low than normal. The symptoms of hypoglycemia begin at 60 mg/dL and impairement of brain function starts at 50 mg/dL.
- The final plan of management of these patients depends upon the cause of hypoglycemia in a particular patient.
- The immediate management is to start the infusion of Dextrose 50% or 25% or whichever concentration is available.

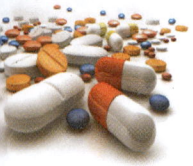

- Alternatively, if IV infusion is not possible/available, one can give sugar, juice, chocolate or sweets, etc. by oral route to rescue the patient.

CALCULATION OF IRON REQUIREMENT IN IRON DEFICIT INDIVIDUAL

The total iron requirement is calculated by the following formula:
Iron requirement (mg) = 4.4 × body weight (kg) × Hb deficit (g/dL)

CONSTITUENTS OF ORS

New formula WHO-ORS	
Content	**Concentrations**
NaCl: 2.6 g	Na⁺—75 mM
KCl: 1.5 g	K⁺—20 mM
Trisod. citrate: 2.9 g	Cl⁻—65 mM
Glucose: 13.5 g	Citrate—10 mM
Water: 1 L	Glucose—75 mM
Total osmolarity 245 mOsm/L	

Drugs Therapy in Diarrhea

Drug therapy (Antidiarrhoeal Agents) is used in addition to ORS therapy in the cases where the evidence of bacterial or amoebic infection is there.

Antimicrobial therapy should be considered when the suspected cause of diarrhea/dysentary is bacterial, protozoal or mixed.

The oral drugs of choice for empiric treatment are:
- Fluoroquinolones (ciprofloxacin 500 mg, ofloxacin 200 mg, or norfloxacin 400 mg, twice daily) for 5–7 days.
- Rifaximin, 200 mg three times daily for 3 days, is approved for empiric treatment of noninflammatory traveller's diarrhea.
- Nitroimidazoles (metronidazole 400 TDS, Tinidazole 500 BD, Ornidazole 500 mg BD) for 5–7 days and Secnidazole 2 Gm stat.
- Nitazoxanide 500 mg BD for 5–7 days. (Covers both protozoal and helminths)
- Quiniodochlor 250 mg TDS for 7 days.
- Furazolidone 100 mg TDS for 5–7 days
- Loperamide 4 mg orally initially, followed by 2 mg after each loose stool (maximum: 16 mg/24 h).
- Rececadotril decreases the fluid loss in diarrhea.
- Combination of Prebiotics and Probiotics is also useful in diarrhea.

Use of Zinc in pediatric diarrhea decreases the frequency and severity of diarrhea in future for three months.

3. DRUGS OF CHOICE IN DIFFERENT DISEASES

Conditions	Drugs of choice
Acute migraine attack	Sumatriptan
Acute gout	NSAIDs, Colchicine
Acute spinal cord injury	Methyl prednisolone sodium succinate
Alopecia	Minoxidil (topical), biotin (oral)
Amebiasis	Metronidazole, Tinidazole, Ornidazole
Anaphylactic shock	Adrenaline
Anginal pain	Nitroglycerine
Anorexia	Cyproheptadine
Anxiety	Alprazolam, Etizolam
Bacillary dysentery	Ciprofloxin, Norfloxin, or Ofloxin
Bell's palsy	Prednisolone
Belladonna poisoning	Atropine
Benzodiazepine overdose	Flumazenil
Cheese reaction	Phentolamine
Chemotherapy-induced vomiting	Ondansetron, Granisetron, Aprepitant
Chronic simple glaucoma	Timolol and Latanoprost

Contd...

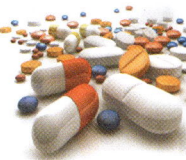

Conditions	Drugs of choice
Chronic gout	Allopurinol, Febuxostat
Closure of ductus arteriosus	Indomethacin
Day care surgery	Propofol
Diabetes insipidus	Vasopressin
Diarrhea	ORS, Probiotics, Rececadotril
Dysmenorrhea	Mephenamic acid + Dicyclomine
Emergency contraception	Levo- norgestrel
Erectile dysfunction	Sildenafil
Esophageal spasm	Nitrates
Febrile seizures	Diazepam
Filariasis	Diethyl carbamazine citrate
Hepatitis induced Pruritus	Deoxycholic acid, hydroxyzine
Hyperkalemia	Insulin, glucose and acetazolamide
Hyperpyrexia	Paracetamol
Hypertension with diabetes	ACEIs & ARBs
Hyperthyroidism	Carbamizole or Propylthiouracil
Hypothyroidism	l- thyroxine
Insomnia	Zolpidem
Leprosy	Dapsone
Lithium induced diabetes insipidus	Thiazide
Mania	Lithium
MI induced pain	Morphine
Morning sickness	Doxylamine succinate
Motion sickness	Hyoscine
Nocturnal enuresis	Imipramine
Non specific headache	Paracetamol (650 mg)
Nonspecific abdominal colic	Dicyclomine, Drotaverine
Peptic ulcer disease	Omeprazole, Rabeprazole, Pantoprazole
Pheochromocytoma	Phentolamine
Pneumocystis jeroveci (AIDS patients)	Cotrimoxazole
Pregnancy induced hypertension	Alfa-methyldopa, hydralazine, labetalol
Pruritis	Cetirizine, levocetrizine, fexofenadine
PSVT	Adenosine
Rheumatic fever	Aspirin, Amoxicillin, PPF
Rheumatic heart disease	Benzathine Penicillin
Rickettsia disease (scrub typhus)	Doxycycline, azithromycin, ceftriaxone injection
Scabies	Ivermectin (oral), Permethrin (topical)
Thrombophlebitis	Heparin topical application
Toxoplasmosis	Spiramycin
Vaginal candidiasis	Cotrimoxazole (local vaginal pessaries) fluconazole (oral)

Contd...

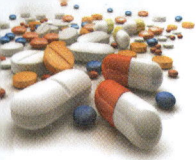

Textbook of Pharmacology for BSc Nursing Students for KUHS

Conditions	Drugs of choice
Vertigo	Cinnarizine
Vomiting	Domperidone, Metoclopramide
Worm infestation	Albendazole + Ivermectin
Xeropthalmia	Vitamin A
Zollinger Ellison syndrome	Lansoprazole, levosupride

4. LIST OF COMMONLY USED ANTIDOTES, THEIR DOSE, ROUTE AND MECHANISM OF ACTION

Toxicity causing agents	Antidotes	Dose and route	Mechanism of action
Iron	Desferrioxamine	10–15 mg/kg/hr IV (max 75 mg/day) or 50 mg/kg IM	Chelates ferrous ions and enhances its elimination in the urine
Streptokinase overdose	Epsilon-Aminocaproic acid (EACA)	5 g oral/iv, followed by 1 g hourly till bleeding stops (max 30 g in 24 hours)	Inhibits plasminogen activation
Methotrexate overdose	Leucovorin or folinic acid	3.0 mg iv to be repeated as required	Being active coenzyme form protects the healthy cells from the effects of methotrexate
Methanol poisoning	Fomepizole	Loading dose: 15 mg/kg IV Maintenance dose: 10 mg/kg every 12 hours till serum methanol falls below 20 mg/dL	A competitive inhibitor of the enzyme alcohol dehydrogenase and prevents toxic metabolites formation
Cyanide poisoning	Sodium nitrite or amyl nitrite and sodium thiosulfate	Sod. Nitrite: 10 mL of 3% sol. IV then, Sod. Thiosulfate: 50 mL 25% sol. IV	Sod. Nitrite forms met hemoglobin, which binds to cyanide & forms cyano-methemoglobin, which is converted to easily excretable form sod thiocyanate by sod. Thiosulfate
Lead poisoning	Calcium disodium edetate	1 g is diluted to 200–300 mL in saline or glucose solution and infused IV over 1 hour twice daily for 3–5 days	Chelation of lead ions
Heparin overdose	Protamine sulfate	1 mg IV for every 100 units of heparin	Protamine forms a stable complex with heparin and neutralizes it
Copper	d-Penicillamine	100 mg/kg/day orally in 4 divided doses for 3–7 days	Chelation of copper ions
Organophosphate poisoning	Atropine Oximes	**Atropine:** 2 mg IV repeat every 10 minutes **Pralidoxime:** 30 mg/kg IV loading dose, followed by 8–10 mg/kg/hr continuous infusion till recovery	**Atropine:** Anti-muscarinic **Oximes:** Reactivation of ChE enzyme. (No role in carbamate poisoning)
Morphine overdose	Naloxone	0.4–0.8 mg IV every 2–3 minutes: max 10 mg	Competitive antagonist on all types of opioid receptors
Warfarin overdose	Vitamin-K or Fresh Frozen plasma	10 mg IM followed by 5 mg 4 hourly for one day then 5 mg OD to be titrated with response	Induces synthesis of clotting factors
As, Hg, Au, Bi, Ni, Sb poisoning	Dimercaprol (British antilewisite; BAL)	5 mg/kg *stat* followed by 2–3 mg/kg every 4–8 hours for 2 days, then once or twice a day for 10 days	Chelation of ions

382

Contd...

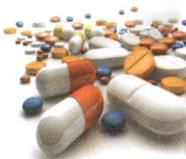

Toxicity causing agents	Antidotes	Dose and route	Mechanism of action
Belladona poisoning (Atropine)	Physostigmine	0.5–2 mg IV repeated as required	Reversible anti-cholinesterase effect
Paracetamol poisoning	Acetylcysteine	Orally 140 mg/kg, followed by 70 mg/kg every 4 hours for 17 doses. Or IV 150mg /kg infusion over 15 minutes may be repeated; if required	Restores depleted glutathione stores
Benzodiaze-pines	Flumazenil	1 mg over 1–3 minutes; maximum dose 1–5 mg given over 2–10 minutes	Competitive benzodiazepine inhibitor
Curare [arrow poison]	Neostigmine	0.5–2.0 mg IV, preceded by atropine or glycopyrrolate 10 µg/kg	Anti-cholinesterase at neuromuscular junction
Digitalis	Digoxin immune fab	Parenteral: 38 or 40 mg per vial with 75 mg sorbitol lyophilized powder to reconstitute for IV injection. Each vial will bind approximately 0.5 mg digoxin or digitoxin	Binds free glycosides in plasma, complex excreted in urine easily
Carbon monoxide	Oxygen	100% oxygen by high flow non breathing mask	Competitive displacement of carbon monoxide

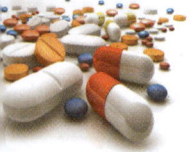

Appendix III: Other Important Topics

1. NORMAL BIOCHEMICAL PARAMETERS

Parameters	Normal values
Hemoglobin (male)	14.0–17.4 g/dL
Hemoglobin (female)	12.3–15.7 g/dL
White Blood Cell Count	$4.0–10.0 \times 10^3/mm^3$
Erythrocyte Sedimentation Rate (male)	≤6 mm/hr
Erythrocyte Sedimentation Rate (female)	≥10 mm/hr
International Normalized Ratio (INR)	0.9–1.2
Platelet Count	$130–400 \times 10^3/mm^3$
Iron	60–178 µg/dL
Blood Glucose (fasting)	70–100 mg/dL
Blood Glucose (post prandial)	70–140 mg/dL
HbA1c Nondiabetic Prediabetic Diabetic ADA target Action suggested	 <5.7 5.7–6.4 ≥6.5 7.0 >8.0
Blood urea nitrogen (BUN)	17–43 mg/dL
Serum Creatinine	0.67–1.17 mg/dL
Uric acid	3.5–7.2 mg/dL
Sodium	136.0–146.0 mEq/L
Potassium	3.50–5.10 mEq/L
Chloride	101.0–109.0 mEq/L
Bicarbonate (HCO_3)	18–30 mEq/L
Calcium	8.80–10.20 mg/dL
Phosphorus	2.30–3.70 mg/dL
Alkaline Phosphatase	30–120 U/L
Bilirubin (Total)	0.20–1.10 mg/dL
Bilirubin (Direct)	<0.20 mg/dL
Amylase	53–123 U/L
Lipase	10–150 U/L
Aspartate Aminotransferase (AST)	0–35 U/L
Alanine Aminotransferase (ALT)	3–36 U/L
Total cholesterol Desirable Borderline high High	 ≤200 mg/dL 201–239 mg/dL ≥240 mg/dL
Triglyceride Desirable Borderline high High	 ≤150 mg/dL 150–199 mg/dL ≥200 mg/dL

Contd...

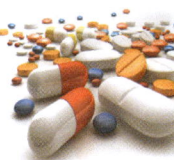

Parameters	Normal values
HDL-C	
Desirable	≥60 mg/dL
Borderline low	35–45 mg/dL
Low	≤35 mg/dL
LDL-C	
Optimal	≤100 mg/dL
Near optimal	100–129 mg/dL
Borderline high	130–159 mg/dL
High	≥160 mg/dL
VLDL	2–30 mg/dL
Total Protein	6.4–8.10 g/dL
Albumin	3.20–4.60 g/dL
Globulin	2.50–3.50 g/dL
Albumin: Globulin ratio	0.8–2.0
Ammonia	20–70 µg/dL
Vitamin-D (1,25-Dihydroxy-Cholecalciferol)	24–65 pg/mL
Vitamin-B12	100–700 pg/mL
C-reactive protein	≤1.0
TSH	0.4–5.0 µU/mL
T3	0.61–1.81 ng/mL
T4	5.01–12.45 µg/dL
Insulin	5–25 µU/L
Oxygen pressure, arterial – PaO_2	85–105 mm Hg
Carbon dioxide pressure, arterial ($PaCO_2$)	35–45 mmHg
pH (arterial)	7.35–7.45
pH (venous)	7.31–741
Serum osmolality	280–300 mOsm/kg

2. DRUGS USED DURING PREGNANCY

Drugs safe in pregnancy (Drugs, which do not cross placenta)	Drugs contraindicated in pregnancy (Drugs, which cross placenta) or teratogenic drugs
• Heparin	• Lithium
• Insulin	• Ciprofloxacin
• Desmopressin	• Tetracycline
• Chloroquine	• Aminoglycosides
• Isoniazid, Rifampicin, Ethambutol	• Angiotensin converting enzyme inhibitors
• Methyldopa, Hydralazine	• Atropine
• Acyclovir	• Metronidazole
• Penicillin	• Theophylline
• Macrolides, most cephalosporins	• Chloramphenicol
• Quinine	• Diazepam, corticosteroids,
• Warfarin (can be given in 2nd trimester)	• Phenytoin, valproate
• Prophylthiouracil	• Retinoid, tamoxifen, busulfan

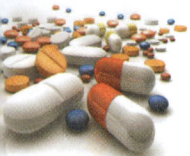

3. DRUGS USED DURING BREASTFEEDING

Safe during breastfeeding	Contraindicated
• Prophylthiouracil	• Antithyroid drugs and radioiodine
• Insulin	• Lithium
• Erythromycin, Cephalosporin	• Tetracycline
• Warfarin	• Phenindione
• Digoxin	• Ergotamine, gold salt
• Antacid	• Anticancer/cytotoxic drugs, e.g., methotrexate, cyclophosphamide

4. LIST OF ANTIBIOTICS TO BE AVOIDED IN RENAL DISEASE

Level of renal failure	Dose adjustment required
Mild renal failure	Cephalosporins, Aminoglycosides, Ethambutol, Flucytosine, Amphotericin B, Vancomycin
Moderate-severe renal failure	Fluoroquinolones, Cotrimoxazole, Imipenem, Carbenicillin, Clarithromycin, Meropenem, Metronidazole, Aztreonam
Drug to be avoided in renal disease	
Severe renal failure	Nitrofurantoin, Nalidixic acid, Tetracyclines,but doxycycline can be used

5. LIST OF ANTIBIOTICS TO BE AVOIDED IN LIVER DISEASE

Dose adjustment required	Clindamycin, Isoniazid, Rifampin, Chloramphenicol, Metronidazole
Drug to be avoided in liver disease	Tetracyclines, Erythromycin, Pyrazinamide, Nalidixic acid

Annexure

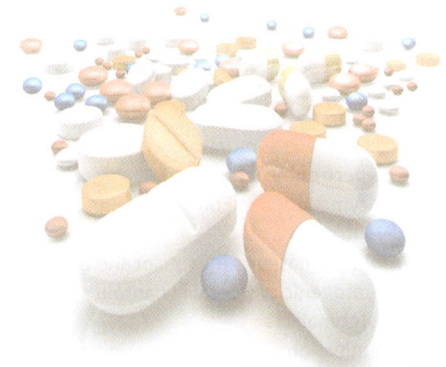

Most Important Mnemonics

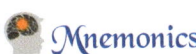 **Mnemonics**

Mnemonics for easy remembrance of certain important terminologies/clinical uses/adverse effects of various drugs

Essential Drugs (Important Points, Remember 'ESSENTIAL')

E : Effective and economical
S : Safe
S : Single drug formulation
E : Environmental factor
N : Needed by the majority of population
T : They must be available all the time
I : In proper dosage form
Aim is to optimal use the limited financial resources
L : List of essential drugs

Pharmacokinetics (Steps of Pharmacokinetics, Remember 'AADME')

A : Administration
A : Absorption
D : Distribution
M : Metabolism
E : Excretion

Atropine

It is a prototype of anticholinergic drugs obtained from Atropa balladona. Remember clinical uses of atropine by ATROPA

A : As mydriatric-cycloplegic
T : Traveller's diarrhoea
R : Rapid onset mushroom poisoning
O : Organophosphate poisoning
P : Preanaesthetic medication
A : Arrhythmias (Brady arrhythmia)

Atropine Side Effects (Remember DHATURA)

D : Dry mouth
H : Hypotension and Hot dry skin
A : Accommodation paralysis
T : Tachycardia
U : Urinary retention
R : Respiratory depression
A : Ataxia and acute congestive glaucoma

Organophosphate Poisoning Clinical Symptoms (remember SLUDGE syndrome)

S : Salivation
L : Lacrimation
U : Urination
D : Diaphoresis
G : GI symptoms
E : Emesis

Clinical uses of Adrenaline (Remember ABCDE)

A : Anaphylactic shock
B : Bronchial Asthma
C : Cardiac resuscitation
D : Duration prolongation of LAs
E : Epistaxis control by local action

Side Effects of Lithium (Remember LITHIUM)

LI : Leukocyte Increased (Leukocytosis)
T : Tremors and Thirst increased
H : Hypothyroidism

Contd...

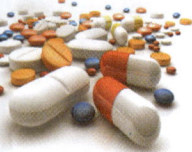

IU : Increased Urine output (Diabetes incipidus)

M : Mother to child transmission (teratogenicity causing fetal goiter and cardiac anomalies)

Side Effects of Phenytoin (Remember PHENYTOIN)

P : Plasma level is monitoring is must due to its zero order kinetics

H : Hypertrophy of gum and Hypersensitivity reactions

E : Enzyme inducer, Epigastric pain

N : Neutropenia

Y : Younger patients (hirsutism and acne may occur)

T : Teratogenicity (foetal hydantoin syndrome)

O : Osteomalacia

I : IV injection causes Hypotension and Cardiac arrhythmia

N : Neurological manifestations such as ataxia, vertigo and nystagmus

Side Effects of ACE Inhibitors (Remember CAPTOPRIL)

C : Cough (Dry cough)

A : Angioedema, allergy

P : Potassium level increase

T : Taste alteration (disgeusia), Teratogenicity

O : On first dose Hypotension

P : Pregnancy (contraindicated)

R : Rashes, renal artery stenosis (contraindicated)

I : Itching

L : Loss of appetite

Uses of Benzodiazepines (remember AC-DIAZEPAM)

A : Alcohol withdrawal syndrome

C : Conscious sedation

D : Diagnostic and minor operative procedure

I : Insomnia

A : Adjuvant to antiemetic

Z : Zig-Zag movements of tardive dyskinesia

E : Epilepsy

P : Preanaesthetic medication

A : Anti-anxiety

M : Muscles relaxant

Actions of Morphine (Remember MARPHINE-CVS)

M : Miosis

A : Analgesia

R : Respiratory depression

P : Psychological and physical dependence

H : Histamine release, Hypotension and Hypothermia

I : Itching

N : Nausea and vomiting

E : Euphoria

C : Cough suppression, Constipation

V : Vagal stimulation (bradycardia)

S : Sedation and hypnosis

Side Effects of Opioids (Remember BAD-AMERICANS)

B : Bradycardia and Hypotension

A : Anorexia

D : Depression of vasomotor and respiratory centre

A : Apnea of newborn

M : Mental clouding, Miosis

E : Euphoria

R : Respiratory depression

I : Increase smooth muscle activity (Biliary sphincter constriction)

C : Constipation

A : Ameliorate cough reflex

N : Nausea and Vomiting

S : Sedation

Side Effects of Corticosteroids (Remember GLUCOCORTICOID)

G : Glaucoma, Glucose level increases (precipitation of diabetes mellitus),

L : Long time to heal

U : Ulcer (GI)

C : Cushing's syndrome (moon like face and buffalo hump)

O : Osteoporosis

C : Cataract

O : Obesity

R : Retardation of growth in children and Retention of fluid

T : Thin and fragile skin

I : Immunosuppressant

C : CNS disorders and CHF

O : Oedema and opportunistic infections

I : Increase in BP

D : Depression of hypothalamic pituitary adrenal (HPA) axis

Therapeutic Uses of Corticosteroids (Remember ABCDEFGHI)

A : Arthritides

B : Bronchial asthma

C : Collagen vascular disorders

D : Dermatological inflammatory conditions

E : Eye diseases

F : Functional testing of HPA axis

G : GI inflammatory condition

H : Hormone replacement therapy

I : Immunosuppressant

Uses of Chloroquine (Remember MALARIA)

M : Malaria (all types)

A : Amebiasis (hepatic)

L : Lepra reaction

A : Anti-photogenic reactions

R : Rheumatoid arthritis

I : Infectious mononucleosis

A : Autoimmune disorders (DLE)

Drugs Causing Gynecomastia (Remember DISCO)

D : Digitalis

I : Isoniazid

S : Spironolactone

C : Cimetidine

O : Oestrogen

Drugs Increasing K+ levels (Remember K- BANK)

K : K+ sparing diuretics

B : beta-blocker

Contd...

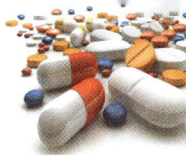

A : ACEIs

N : NSAIDs

K : K+ supplement

Side Effects of First Line Antitubercular Drugs

INH

I : Insanity (mental disturbance)

N : Neuritis

H : Hepatitis

RIFAMpicin

R : Red discoloration of urine

I : Induction of liver enzyme

F : Flu-like symptoms

A : Abdominal symptoms (nausea, vomiting, abdominal cramps)

M : Malaise

PyRAzInamide

Py : Problem in liver (Hepatotoxicity)

R : Rashes

A : Arthralgia

I : Increase in uric acid levels

ETHambutol

E : Eye toxicity

T : Toxicity dose and duration dependent

H : Hyperuricemia

Streptomycin

S : Side effects similar to aminoglycosides

Drugs Causing Disulfiram Like Reaction (Remember MSC³)

M : Metronidazole

S : Sulfonylureas

C : Cefoparazone

C : Cefotetan

C : Cefomandole

First Line Antihypertensive Drugs (Remember ABCD)

A : ACE inhibitors

B : Beta-blockers

C : Calcium channel blockers

D : Diuretics

Side Effects Of Diuretics (Remember DIURETICS)

D : Dehydration and Decrease in potassium, sodium, calcium, magnesium levels

I : Increase in glucose levels

U : Uric acid level rise

R : Rashes

E : Electrolyte disturbance

T : Toxicity to ear

I : Increase in lipids levels

C : Cramps in muscles

S : Skin photosensitivity increased

Drugs Used in CHF (Remember 5-Ds)

D : Digitalis (digoxin; digitoxin)

D : Dopamine and Dobutamine

D : Diesterase (Phosphodiesterase inhibitors) Amrinone, Milrinone

D : Dilators of both arterioles and venules (ACEIs Nitrates)

D : Diuretics

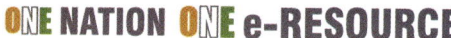

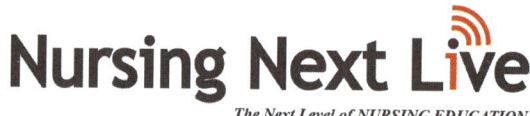

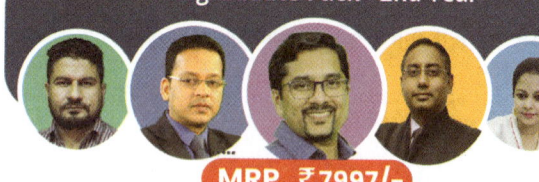
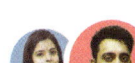 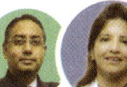 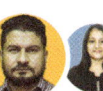
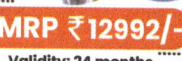

Index

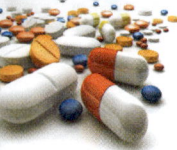

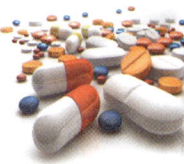

Index

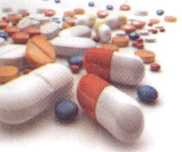

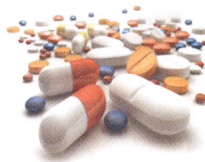

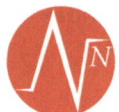

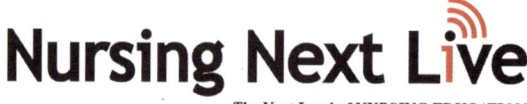

Nursing Next Live
The Next Level of NURSING EDUCATION

PREPARE ANYTIME, ANYWHERE FOR
Nursing Officer/Staff Nurse/CHO/ Nursing Undergraduate & Postgraduate Exams

AIIMS NORCET 2020

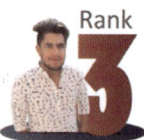 Rank **3**
Rahul Dahiya
Roll No. 9016060

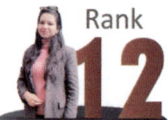 Rank **12**
Nisha Singla
Roll No. 9101820

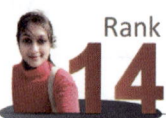 Rank **14**
Arushi Mittal
Roll No. 9079646

 Rank **51**
Komal Dhull
Roll No. 9024458

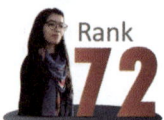 Rank **72**
Shivani Bourai
Roll No. 9092877

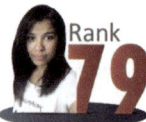 Rank **79**
Nivedita Saini
Roll No. 9004587

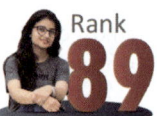 Rank **89**
Rupali Garg
Roll No. 9054544

CHO 2020

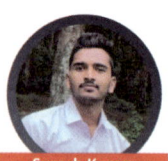
Suresh Kumsr
Rank- 1
Roll No. 12090
MP

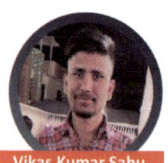
Vikas Kumar Sahu
Rank- 14
Roll No. 10011
MP

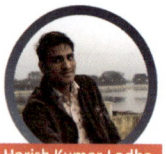
Harish Kumar Lodha
Rank- 18
Roll No. 7930
MP

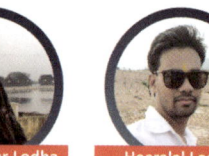
Heeralal Lodha
Rank- 33
Roll No. 10009
MP

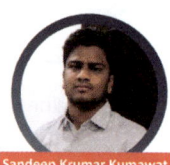
Sandeep Krumar Kumawat
Rank- 44
Roll No. 12585
MP

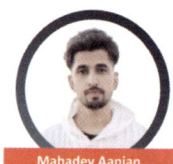
Mahadev Aanjan
Rank- 50
Roll No. 10130
MP

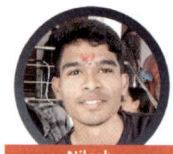
Nilesh
Rank- 81
Roll No. 10572
MP

BFUHS 2021

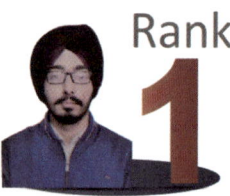 Rank **1**
Harjeet Singh
Roll No- 472478

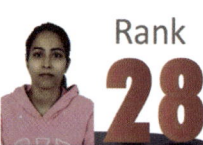 Rank **28**
Kuljit Kaur
Roll No. 473956

 Rank **32**
Karan Sharma
Roll No. 469134

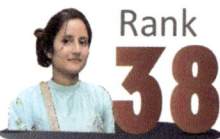 Rank **38**
Smriti Rana
Roll No. 463342

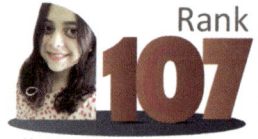 Rank **107**
Harpreet Kaur
Roll No. 474125

AIIMS MSc ENTRANCE EXAM 2021

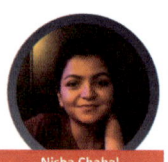
Nisha Chahal
AIIMS AIR-18

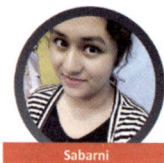
Sabarni
AIIMS AIR-21

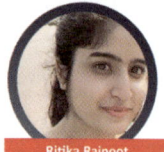
Ritika Rajpoot
AIIMS AIR-23

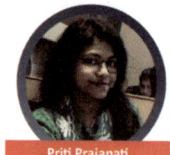
Priti Prajapati
AIIMS AIR-39

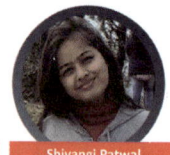
Shivangi Patwal
AIIMS AIR-64

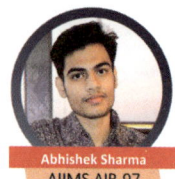
Abhishek Sharma
AIIMS AIR-97

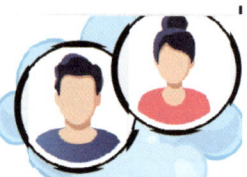
You Will Be The Next...

Follow us:

CALL US +91- 999-911-7411
w w w . n u r s i n g n e x t l i v e . c o m

Scan the QR Code to download the app

Nursing Knowledge Tree
An Initiative by CBS Nursing Division

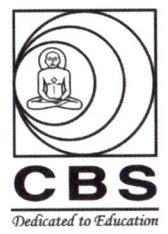

Nursing Books Catalogue 2021-22

Books for All

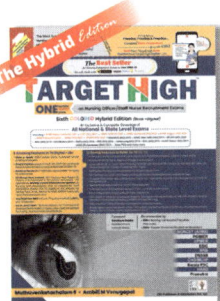

Target High
Muthuvenkatachalam S et al.
978-93-90619-55-9
6/e, 2022
MRP: ₹1499/-

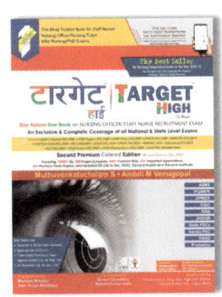

Target High (In Hindi)
Muthuvenkatachalam S et al.
978-81-94025-65-8
2/e, 2020
MRP: ₹1299/-

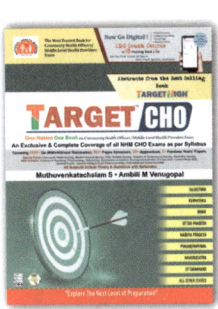

Target CHO
Muthuvenkatachalam S et al.
978-81-940256-0-3
1/e, 2020
MRP: ₹495/-

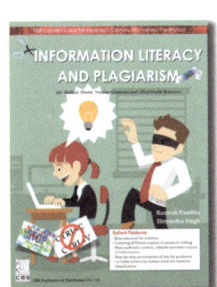

Information Literacy and Plagiarism
for Medical, Dental, Nursing Graduates
and Allied Health Sciences
Ramesh Pandita et al.
978-93-86827-13-5
1/e, 2018
MRP: ₹370/-

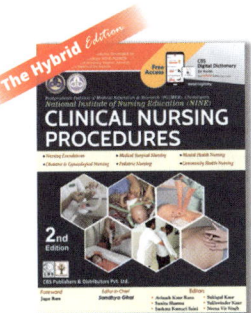

PGI NINE
Clinical Nursing Procedures
Sandhya Ghai
978-93-89261-97-4
2/e, 2020
MRP: ₹1295/-

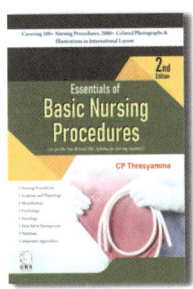

Essentials of
Basic Nursing Procedures
CP Thresyamma
978-81-94523-47-5
2/e, 2020
MRP: ₹795/-

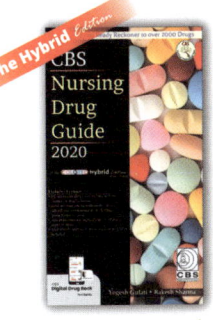

CBS Nursing Drug Guide
2020-2021
Yogesh Gulati et al.
978-93-88178-53-2
1/e, 2020
MRP: ₹1050/-

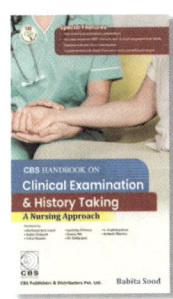

CBS Handbook on
Clinical Examination & History Taking
A Nursing Approach
Babita Sood
978-81-948693-9-9
1/e, 2021
MRP: ₹350/-

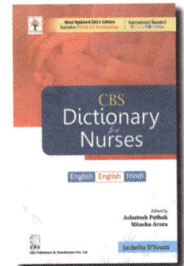

CBS Dictionary for Nurses
Jacintha D'Souza
978-93-90619-06-1
1/e, 2021
MRP: ₹595/-

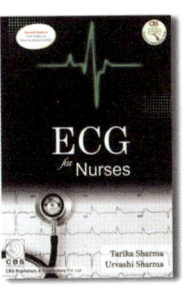

ECG for Nurses
Tarika Sharma et al.
978-93-89261-88-2
1/e, 2019
MRP: ₹350/-

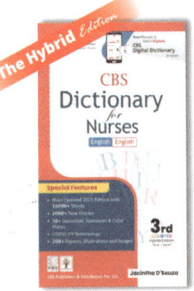

CBS Dictionary for Nurses
Jacintha D'Souza
978-93-90619-29-0
3/e, 2022
MRP: ₹450/-

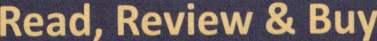
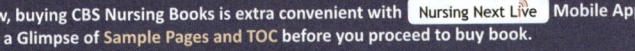

Community Health Nursing

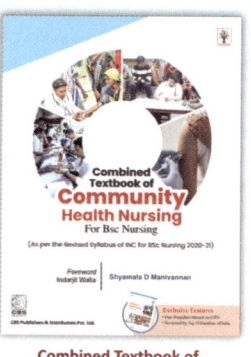

Combined Textbook of Community Health Nursing
For BSc Nursing
Shyamala D Manivannan
978-93-90619-37-5
1/e, 2022
TBA

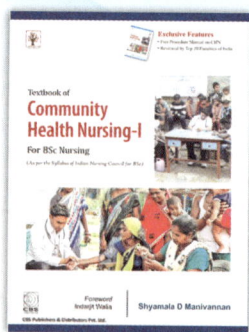

Textbook of Community Health Nursing-I
For BSc Nursing
Shyamala D Manivannan
978-81-23927-01-5
1/e, 2018
MRP: ₹750/-

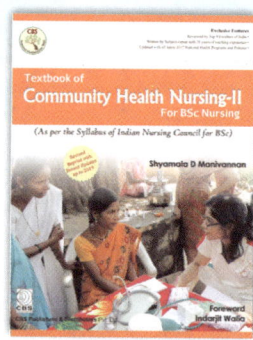

Textbook of Community Health Nursing-II
For BSc Nursing
Shyamala D Manivannan
978-93-86827-22-7
1/e, 2018
MRP: ₹450/-

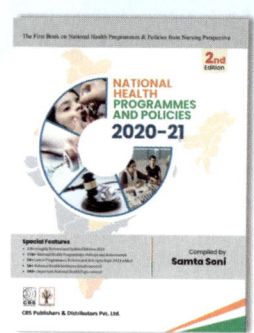

National Health Programmes & Policies 2020-21
Samta Soni
978-93-90619-13-9
2/e, 2022
MRP: ₹695/-

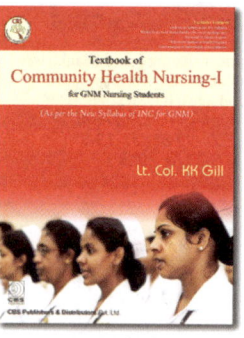

Textbook of Community Health Nursing-I
For GNM Nursing Students
Lt. Col. KK Gill
978-93-86827-17-3
1/e, 2018
MRP: ₹550/-

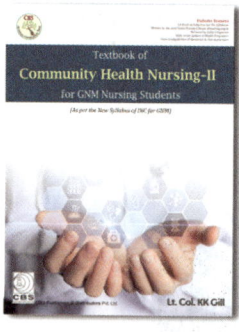

Textbook of Community Health Nursing-II
for GNM Nursing Students
Lt. Col. KK Gill
978-93-88178-57-0
1/e, 2019
MRP: ₹525/-

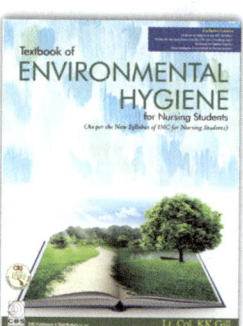

Textbook of Environmental Hygiene for Nursing Students
Lt. Col. KK Gill
978-93-88178-56-3
1/e, 2018-19
MRP: ₹225/-

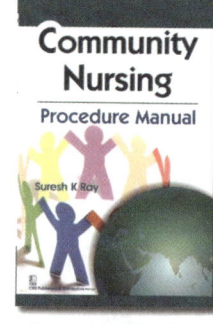

Community Nursing Procedure Manual
Suresh K Ray
978-81-23929-35-4
1/e, 2017
MRP: ₹265/-

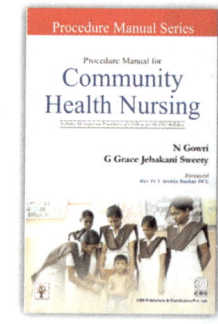

Procedure Manual for Community Health Nursing
N Gowri et al.
978-81-948693-6-8
1/e, 2021
MRP: ₹195/-

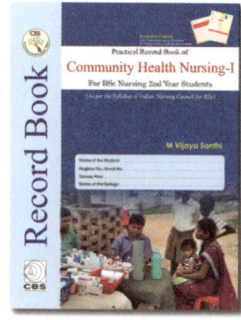

Practical Record Book of Community Health Nursing-I
for BSc Nursing 2nd Year Students
M Vijaya Santhi
978-81-23926-84-1
1/e, 2016
MRP: ₹450/-

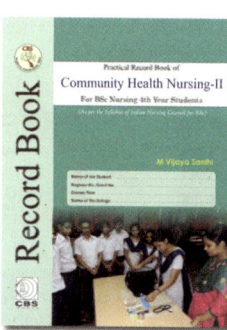

Practical Record Book of Community Health Nursing-II
for BSc Nursing 4th Year Students
M Vijaya Santhi
978-93-88108-77-5
1/e, 2018-19
MRP: ₹575/-

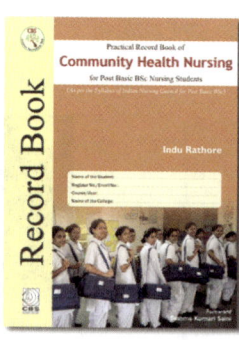

Practical Record Book of Community Health Nursing
for Post Basic BSc Nursing Students
Indu Rathore
978-93-86827-06-7
1/e, 2017
MRP: ₹475/-

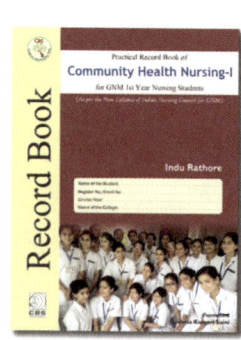

Practical Record Book of Community Health Nursing-I
for GNM 1st Year Nursing Students
Indu Rathore
978-93-86827-07-4
1/e, 2018-19
MRP: ₹350/-

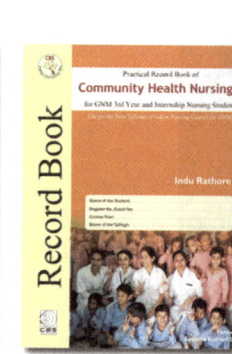

Practical Record Book of Community Health Nursing
for GNM 3rd Year and Internship Nursing Students
Indu Rathore
978-93-86827-30-2
1/e, 2018-19
MRP: ₹395/-

 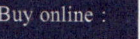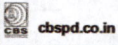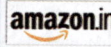 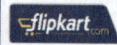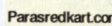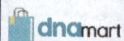

Nursing Foundation

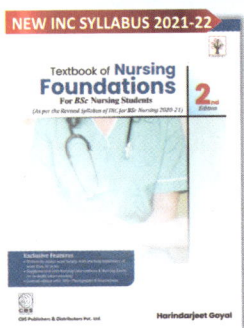

NEW INC SYLLABUS 2021-22

**Textbook of
Nursing Foundations
for BSc Nursing Students**
Harindarjeet Goyal
978-93-90619-12-2
2/e, 2022

MRP: ₹950/-

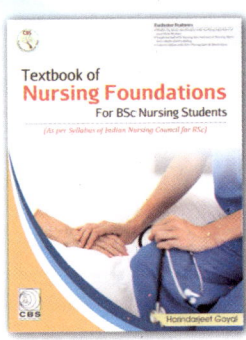

**Textbook of
Nursing Foundations
for BSc Nursing Students**
Harindarjeet Goyal
978-93-88108-94-2
1/e, 2020

MRP: ₹950/-

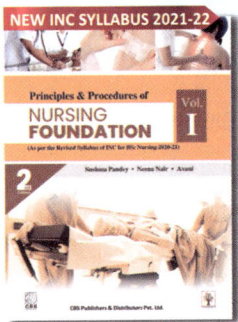

NEW INC SYLLABUS 2021-22

**Principles & Procedures of
Nursing Foundation Vol-I
for BSc Nursing**
Sushma Pandey et al.
978-93-90619-57-3
2/e, 2022

TBA

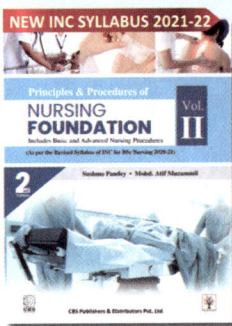

NEW INC SYLLABUS 2021-22

**Principles & Procedures of
Nursing Foundation Vol-II
for BSc Nursing**
Sushma Pandey et al.
978-93-90619-19-1
2/e, 2022

TBA

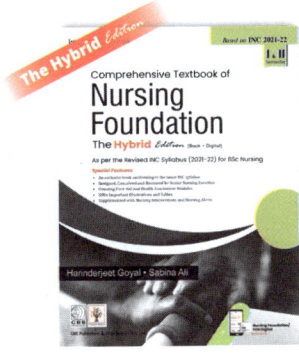

**Textbook of
Nursing Foundations
for GNM Nursing Students**
Harindarjeet Goyal
978-93-90619-70-2
1/e, 2022

MRP: ₹850/-

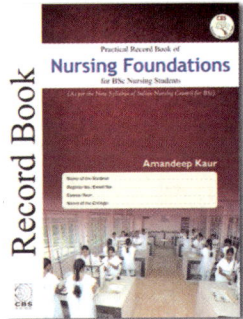

**Practical Record Book of
Nursing Foundations
for BSc Nursing Students**
Amandeep Kaur
978-93-88108-96-6
1/e, 2018-19

MRP: ₹425/-

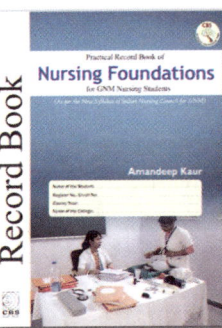

**Practical Record Book of
Nursing Foundations
for GNM Nursing Students**
Amandeep Kaur
978-93-88178-50-1
1/e, 2018-19

MRP: ₹350/-

Medical Surgical Nursing

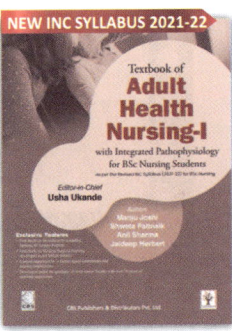

NEW INC SYLLABUS 2021-22

**Textbook of
Adult Health Nursing-I
with Integrated Pathophysiology
for BSc Nursing Students**
Usha Ukande
978-93-90619-20-7
1/e, 2022

TBA

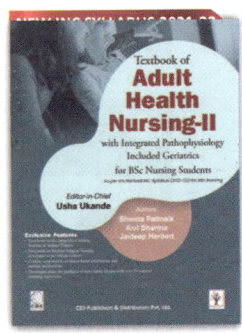

**Textbook of
Adult Health Nursing-II
with Integrated Pathophysiology
Included Geriatrics for BSc Nursing Students**
Usha Ukande
978-93-90619-86-3
1/e, 2022

TBA

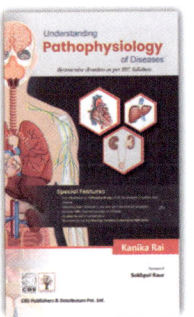

**Understanding
Pathophysiology of Diseases**
Kanika Rai
978-93-90619-11-5
1/e, 2022

MRP: ₹395/-

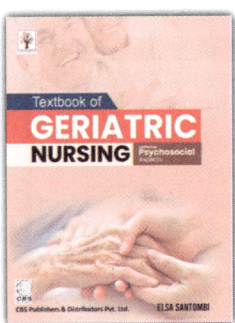

**Textbook of
Geriatric Nursing
Including Psychosocial Aspects**
Elsa Santombi
978-93-90619-79-5
1/e, 2022

TBA

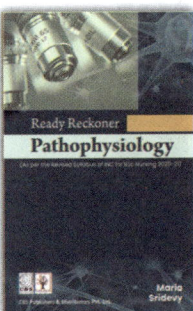

**Ready Reckoner
Pathophysiology
for Nurses**
Maria et al.
978-93-90619-05-4
1/e, 2022

TBA

MSN/Pharmacology/Pathology

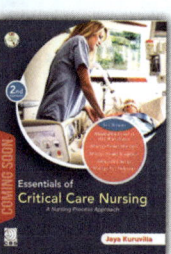

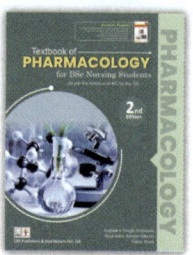

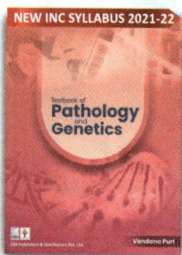

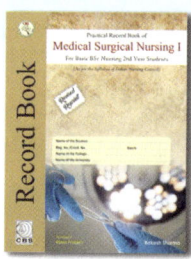

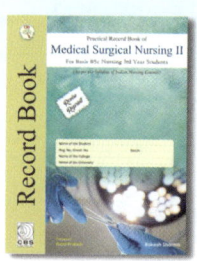

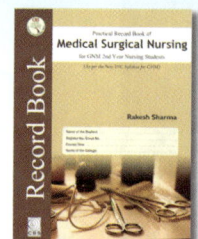

Essentials of
Critical Care Nursing
A Nursing Process Approach
Jaya Kuruvilla
978-93-90619-61-0
2/e, 2022
TBA

Textbook of
Pharmacology
For BSc Nursing Students
Joginder Singh Pathania et al.
978-93-90619-27-6
2/e, 2022
MRP: ₹650/-

Textbook of
Pathology and Genetics
Vandana Puri
978-93-90619-87-0
1/e, 2022
TBA

Practical Record Book of
Medical Surgical Nursing I
for Basic BSc Nursing 2nd Year Students
Rakesh Sharma
978-81-23928-00-5
1/e, 2018-19
MRP: ₹550/-

Practical Record Book of
Medical Surgical Nursing II
for Basic BSc Nursing 3nd Year Students
Rakesh Sharma
978-81-23928-01-2
1/e, 2018-19
MRP: ₹475/-

Practical Record Book of
Medical Surgical Nursing
for GNM 2nd Year Nursing Student
Rakesh Sharma
978-93-86827-04-3
1/e, 2017
MRP: ₹475/-

Child Health Nursing & Pediatric Nursing

Exclusive Marketing & Distribution Rights

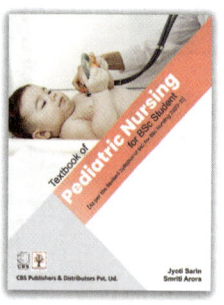

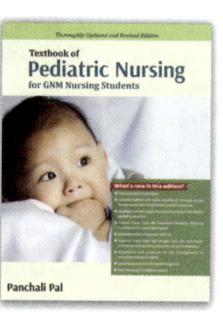

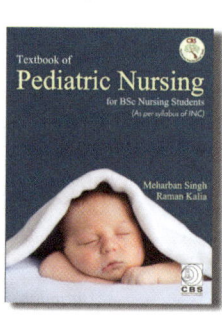

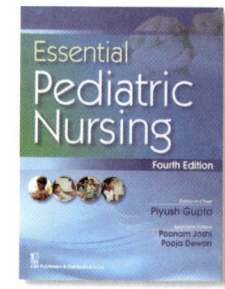

Textbook of
Pediatric Nursing
for BSc Nursing Students
Panchali Pal
978-81-948693-2-0
2/e, 2021
MRP: ₹795/-

Textbook of
Pediatric Nursing
for BSc Nursing Students
Jyoti Sarin et al.
978-93-90619-78-8
1/e, 2022
TBA

Textbook of
Pediatric Nursing
for GNM Nursing Students
Panchali Pal
978-93-90619-71-9
1/e, 2022
TBA

Textbook of
Pediatric Nursing
for BSc Nursing Students
Meharban Singh et al.
978-93-88108-72-0
1/e, 2018
MRP: ₹725/-

Essential
Pediatric Nursing
Piyush Gupta
978-93-86217-87-5
4/e, 2017
MRP: ₹750/-

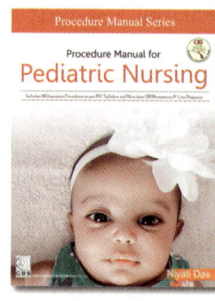

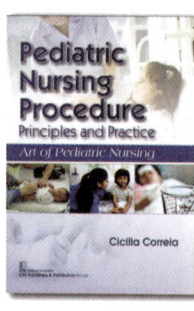

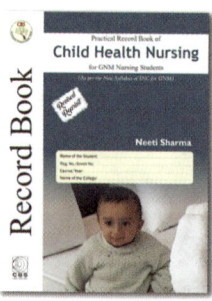

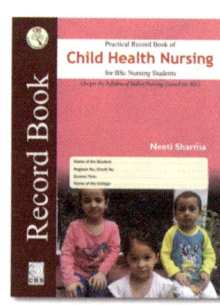

Procedure Manual for
Pediatric Nursing
Niyati Das
978-93-88108-86-7
1/e, 2018
MRP: ₹325/-

Pediatric Nursing Procedure
Principles and Practice
Cicilia Correia
978-93-86310-74-3
1/e, 2017
MRP: ₹450/-

Practial Record Book of
Child Health Nursing
for GNM Nursing Students
Neeti Sharma
978-93-86827-53-1
1/e, 2017
MRP: ₹325/-

Practial Record Book of
Child Health Nursing
for BSc Nursing Students
Neeti Sharma
978-93-86827-05-0
1/e, 2017
MRP: ₹310/-

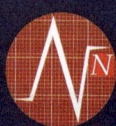

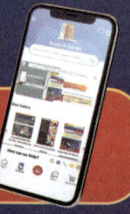

Mental Health Nursing & Psychiatric Nursing

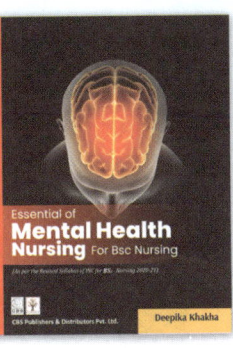

Essential of Mental Health Nursing
for BSc Nursing
Deepika Khakha
978-93-90619-73-3
1/e, 2022

TBA

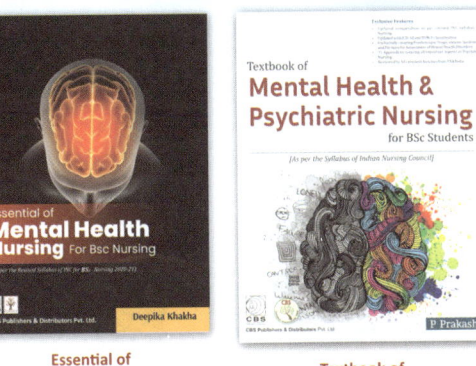

Textbook of Mental Health & Psychiatric Nursing
P Prakash
978-93-89261-91-2
1/e, 2019

MRP: ₹625/-

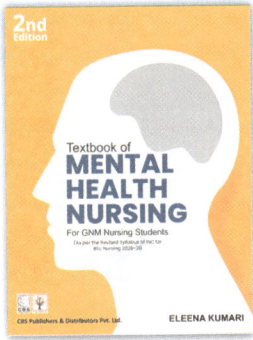

Textbook of Mental Health Nursing
for GNM Nursing Students
Eleena Kumari
978-93-90619-72-6
2/e, 2022

MRP: ₹395/-

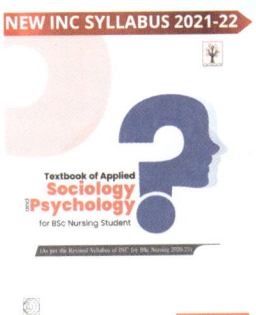

NEW INC SYLLABUS 2021-22

Textbook of Applied Sociology and Psychology
for BSc Nursing Students
P Prakash
978-93-90619-54-2
1/e, 2022

MRP: ₹395/-

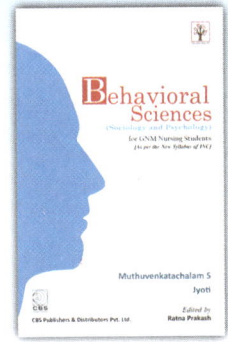

Behavioral Sciences
(Sociology and Psychology)
Muthuvenkatachalam S et al.
978-93-90619-04-7
1/e , 2021

MRP: ₹350/-

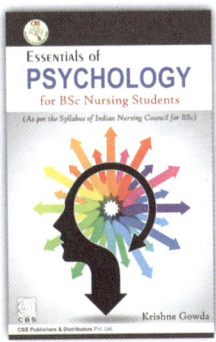

Essentials of Psychology
for BSc Nursing Students
Krishne Gowda
978-81-23927-11-4
1/e, 2017

MRP: ₹340/-

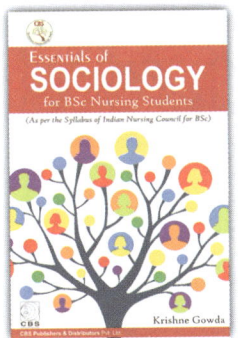

Essentials of Sociology
for BSc Nursing Students
Krishne Gowda
978-93-86217-51-6
1/e, 2017

MRP: ₹395/-

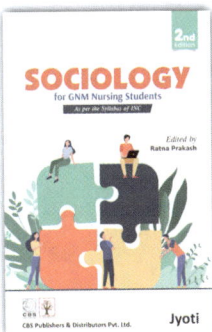

Sociology
for GNM Nursing Students
Jyoti
978-81-948693-1-3
2/e, 2022

MRP: ₹210/-

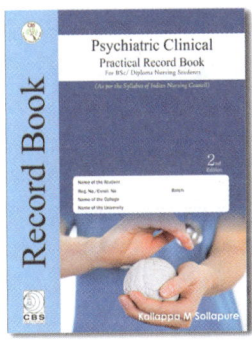

Psychiatric Clinical Practical Record Book
for BSc/Diploma Nursing Students
Kallappa M Sollapure
978-93-88108-81-2
2/e, 2018-19

MRP: ₹395/-

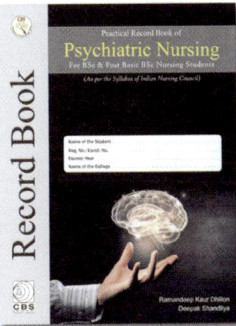

Practial Record Book of Psychiatric Nursing
for BSc & Post Basic BSc Nursing Students
Ramandeep Kaur Dhillon
978-93-88108-80-5
1/e, 2019

MRP: ₹415/-

Midwifery, Obstetrical & Gynecological Nursing

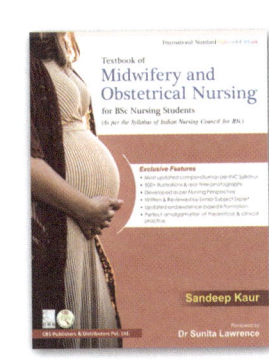

Textbook of Midwifery & Obstetrical Nursing
for BSc Nursing Students
Sandeep Kaur
978-93-89261-90-5
1/e, 2020

MRP: ₹995/-

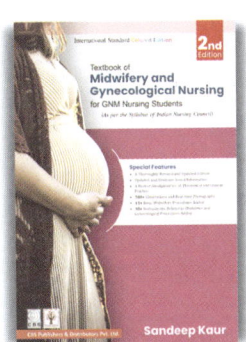

Textbook of Midwifery & Gynecological Nursing
for GNM Nursing Students
Sandeep Kaur
978-93-90619-18-4
2/e, 2022

MRP: ₹895/-

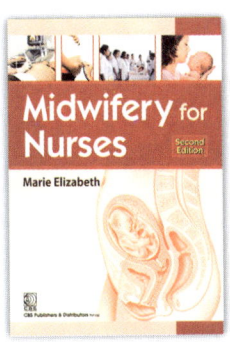

Textbook of Midwifery for Nurses
Marie Elizabeth
978-81-23922-14-0
2/e, 2018

MRP: ₹650/-

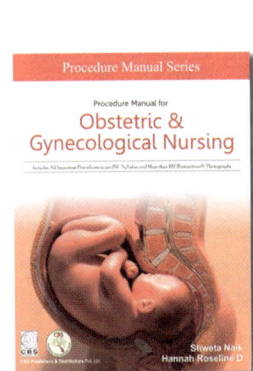

Procedure Manual for Obstetric & Gynecological Nursing
Sheweta Naik et al.
978-93-88178-60-0
1/e, 2018-19

MRP: ₹235/-

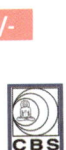

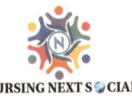

Midwifery, Obstetrical & Gynecological Nursing

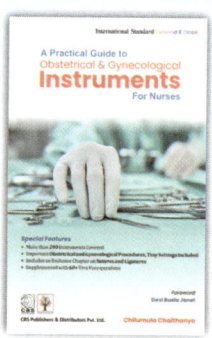

**A Practical Guide to
Obstetric & Gynecological
Instruments for Nurses**
Chilumula Chaithanya
978-93-90619-03-0
1/e, 2022

MRP: ₹250/-

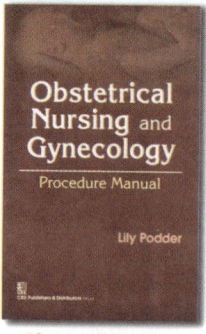

**Obstetrical Nursing
and Gynecology
Procedure Manual**
Lily Podder
978-81-23925-81-3
1/e, 2017

MRP: ₹265/-

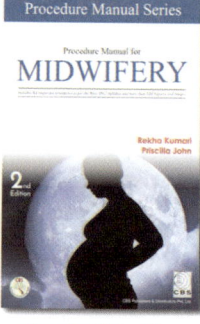

**Procedure Manual for
Midwifery**
Rekha Kumari et al.
978-93-89261-94-3
2/e, 2019

MRP: ₹225/-

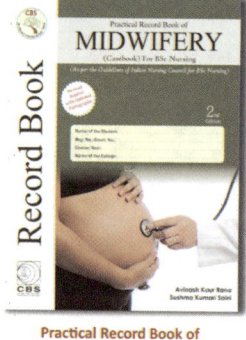

**Practical Record Book of
Midwifery**
(Casebook) for BSc Nursing
Avinash Kaur Rana et al.
978-93-88178-65-5
2/e (R/R), 2018-19

MRP: ₹675/-

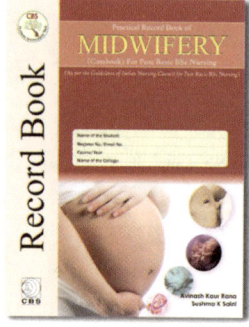

**Practical Record Book of
Midwifery**
(Casebook) for Post Basic BSc Nursing
Avinash Kaur Rana et al.
978-81-23927-07-7
1/e, 2016

MRP: ₹375/-

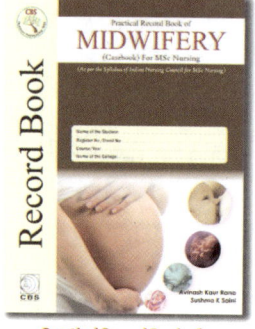

**Practical Record Book of
Midwifery**
(Casebook) for MSc Nursing
Avinash Kaur Rana et al.
978-93-86217-97-4
1/e, 2017

MRP: ₹625/-

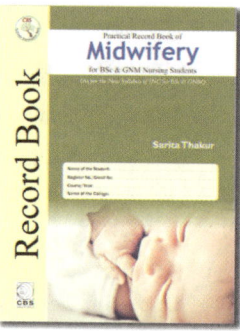

**Practical Record Book of
Midwifery**
for BSc & GNM Nursing Students
Sarita Thakur
978-93-86827-33-3
1/e, 2017

MRP: ₹415/-

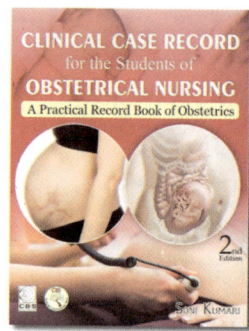

Clinical Case Record
for the Students of
Obstetrical Nursing
A Practical Record Book of Obstetrics
Soni Kumari
978-93-88178-51-8
2/e, 2018

MRP: ₹475/-

Nursing Research/Biostatistics

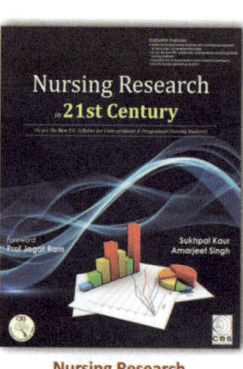

Nursing Research
in 21st Century
Sukhpal Kaur et al.
978-93-89261-89-9
1/e, 2020

MRP: ₹725/-

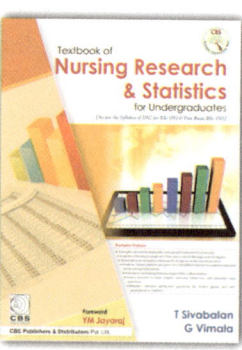

**Textbook of
Nursing Research & Statistics
for Undergraduates**
T Sivabalan et al.
978-93-88178-61-7
1/e, 2018

MRP: ₹525/-

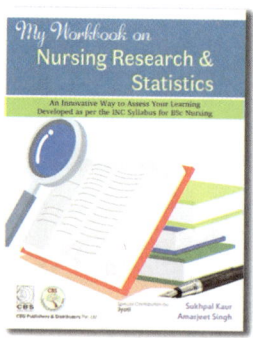

**My Workbook on
Nursing Research & Statistics**
Sukhpal Kaur et al.
978-93-88108-75-1
1/e, 2019

MRP: ₹150/-

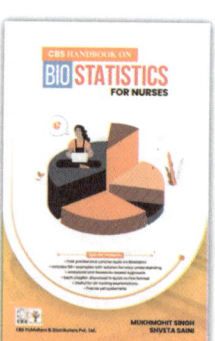

**CBS Handbook on
Biostatistics for Nurses**
Mukhmohit Singh et al.
978-93-90619-10-8
1/e, 2022

MRP: ₹195/-

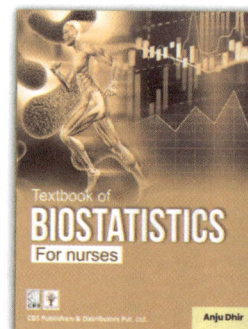

**Textbook of
Biostatistics for Nurses**
Anju Dhir
978-93-90619-47-4
1/e, 2022

TBA

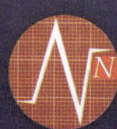

Read, Review & Buy
Now, buying CBS Nursing Books is extra convenient with Nursing Next Live Mobile App.
Get a Glimpse of Sample Pages and TOC before you proceed to buy book.

**Download the App from
Google Playstore or scan
here to download**

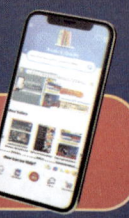

CET/Nursing Education

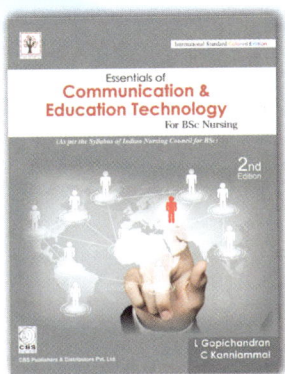

Essentials of
Communication & Education Technology
for BSc Nursing
L Gopichandran et al.
978-93-88178-58-7
2/e, 2019

MRP: ₹495/-

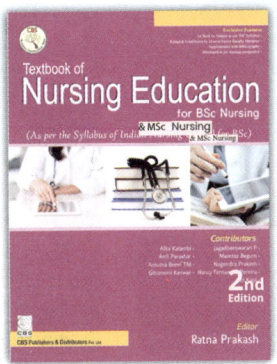

Textbook of
Nursing Education
for BSc & MSc Nursing
Ratna Prakash
978-93-86827-34-0
1/e, 2018

MRP: ₹450/-

Nursing Management & Services

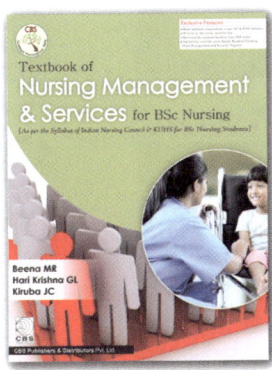

Textbook of
Nursing Management & Services
for BSc Nursing
Beena MR et al.
978-93-88178-62-4
1/e, 2019

MRP: ₹625/-

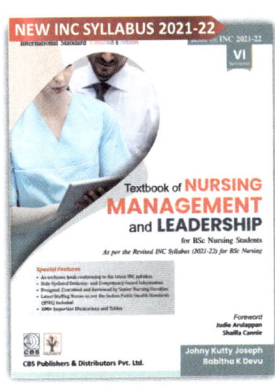

Textbook of Nursing
Management & Leadership
Johny Joseph Kutty
978-93-90619-40-5
1/e, 2022

MRP: MRPV

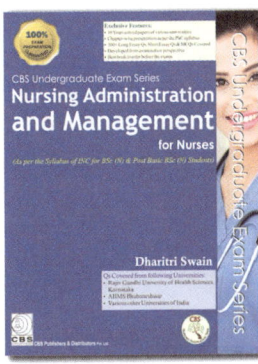

CBS Undergraduate Exam Series
Nursing Administration
and Management for Nurses
Dharitri Swain
978-93-86827-42-5
1/e, 2018

MRP: ₹350/-

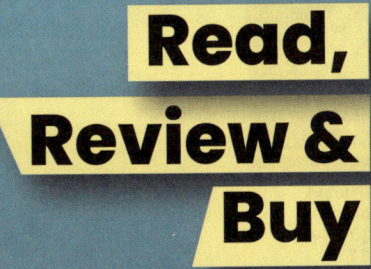
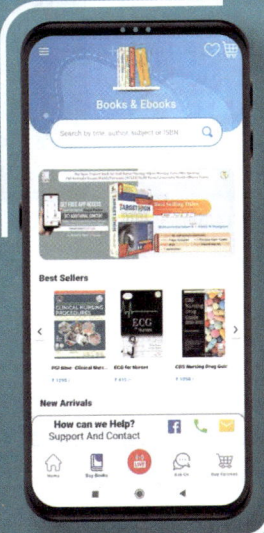
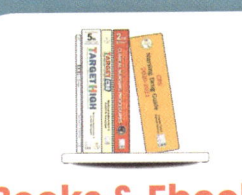

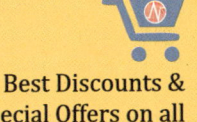

Microbiology

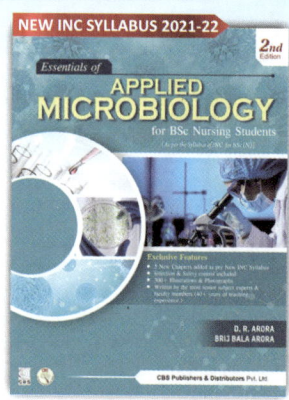

**Essentials of
Applied Microbiology
for BSc Nursing Students**
D.R. Arora et al.
978-81-945234-4-4
2/e, 2020

MRP: ₹575/-

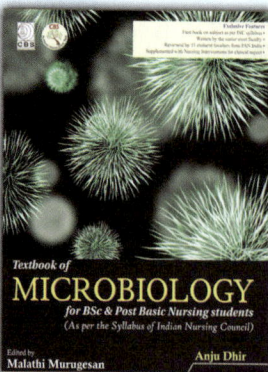

**Textbook of
Microbiology
for BSc & Post Basic Nursing Students**
Anju Dhir
978-93-88108-82-9
1/e, 2018

MRP: ₹725/-

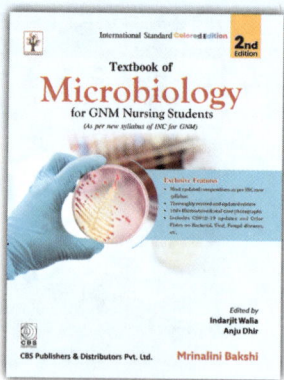

**Textbook of
Microbiology
for GNM Nursing Students**
Mrinalini Bakshi
978-93-90619-12-2
2/e, 2021

MRP: ₹225/-

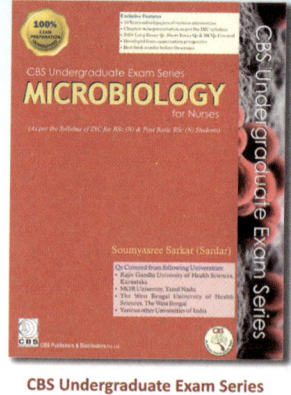

**CBS Undergraduate Exam Series
Microbiology for Nurses**
Soumyasree Sarkar
978-93-86310-49-1
1/e, 2017

MRP: ₹275/-

English/First Aid/Computer

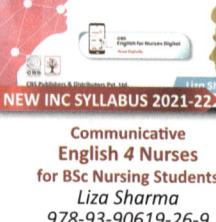

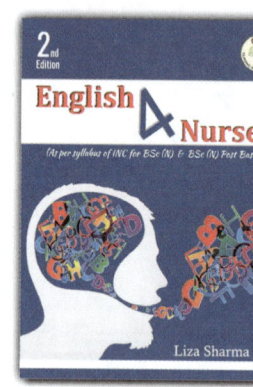

**Communicative
English 4 Nurses
for BSc Nursing Students**
Liza Sharma
978-93-90619-26-9
1/e, 2022

TBA

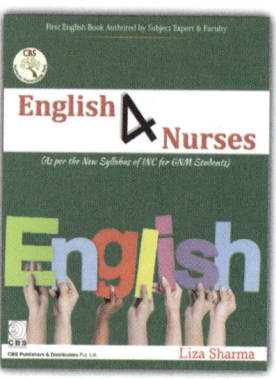

English 4 Nurses (BSc)
Liza Sharma
978-93-89261-95-0
2/e, 2019

MRP: ₹415/-

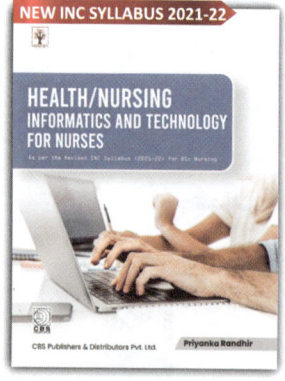

English 4 Nurses (GNM)
Liza Sharma
978-93-86827-09-8
1/e, 2017

MRP: ₹350/-

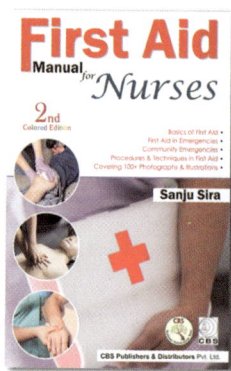

First Aid Manual for Nurses
Sanju Sira
978-93-88178-55-6
2/e, 2019

MRP: ₹310/-

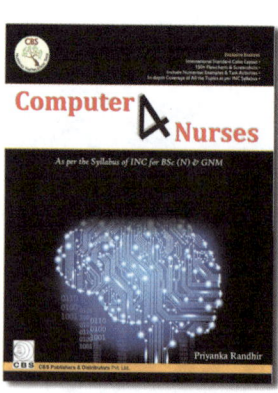

**Health/Nursing Informatics and
Technology for Nurses**
Priyanka Randhir
978-93-90619-21-4
1/e, 2022

TBA

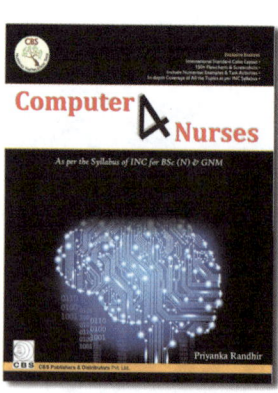

Computer 4 Nurses
Priyanka Randhir
978-93-86310-48-4
1/e, 2017

MRP: ₹370/-

Read, Review & Buy

Now, buying CBS Nursing Books is extra convenient with Nursing Next Live Mobile App.
Get a Glimpse of Sample Pages and TOC before you proceed to buy book.

**Download the App from
Google Playstore or scan
here to download**

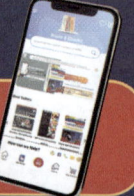

Anatomy & Physiology/Biochemistry & Nutrition

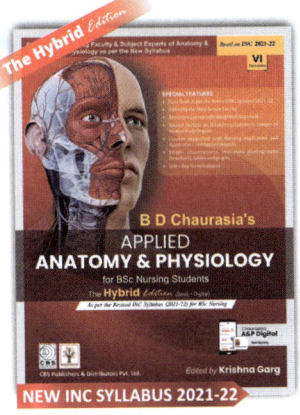
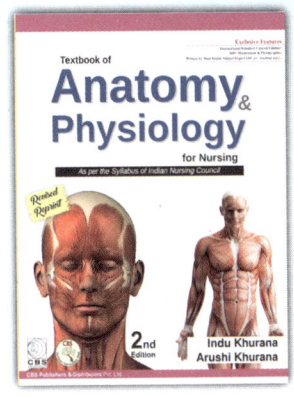

**Tortora's Principles of
Anatomy & Physiology**
Gerard J. Tortora
978-81-26567-61-4
GLOBAL Edition, 2017

MRP: ₹3495/-

**BD Chaurasia's
Applied Anatomy and Physiology
for BSc Nursing Students**
Krishna Garg
978-93-90619-65-8
1/e, 2022

TBA

**Textbook of
Anatomy & Physiology for Nursing**
Indu Khurana et al.
978-93-86827-12-8
2/e, 2018

MRP: ₹995/-

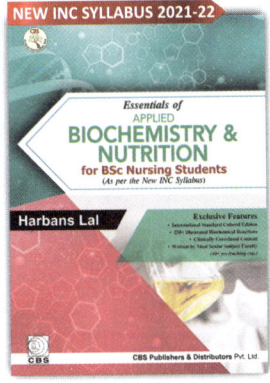
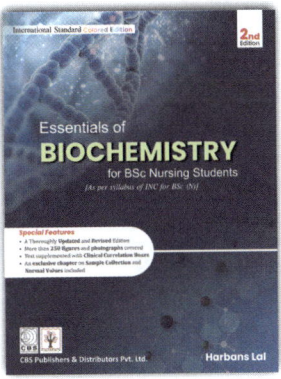
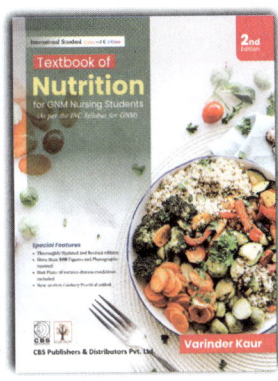

**Essentials of APPLIED
Biochemistry & Nutrition
for BSc Nursing Students**
Harbans Lal
978-93-90619-41-2
1/e, 2022

MRP: ₹450/-

**Essentials of
Biochemistry
for BSc Nursing Students**
Harbans Lal
978-81-948693-3-7
2/e, 2022

MRP: ₹450/-

**Textbook of
Nutrition
for GNM Nursing Students**
Varinder Kaur
978-93-90619-02-3
2/e, 2022

MRP: ₹295/-

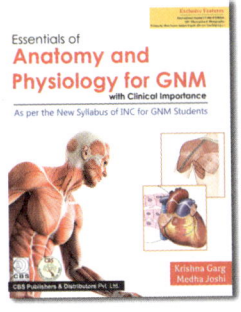
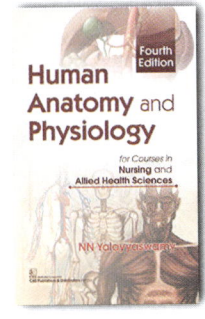
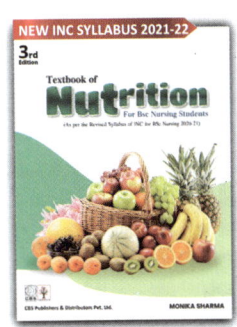
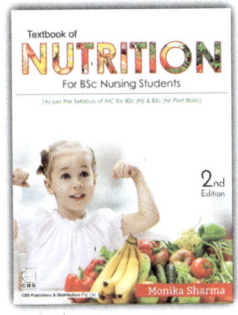

**Essentials of
Anatomy & Physiology for GNM
with Clinical Importance**
Krishna Garg et al.
978-93-86827-11-1
1/e, 2018

MRP: ₹475/-

**Human Anatomy and Physiology
for Nurses**
N.N. Yalayyaswamy
978-93-87085-16-9
4/e, 2018

MRP: ₹395/-

**Textbook of
Nutrition
for BSc Nursing Students**
Monika Sharma
978-93-90619-02-3
3/e, 2022

MRP: ₹370/-

**Textbook of Nutrition
for BSc Nursing Students**
Monika Sharma
978-93-89261-92-9
2/e, 2019

MRP: ₹370/-

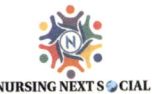
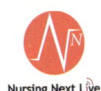

Others

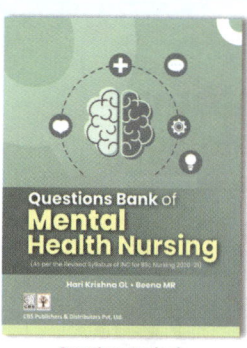

Questions Bank of
Mental Health Nursing
Hari Krishna GL et al.
978-93-90619-46-7
1/e, 2022

TBA

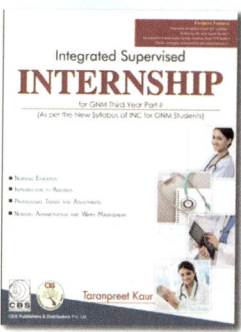

Integrated Supervised
Internship
for GNM Third Year Part-II
Taranpreet Kaur
978-93-88108-89-8
1/e, 2018

MRP: ₹415/-

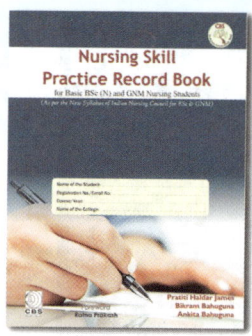

Nursing Skill
Practice Record Book
for Basic BSc (N) and GNM Nursing Students
Pratiti Haldar James et al.
978-93-86827-38-8
1/e, 2018-19

MRP: ₹310/-

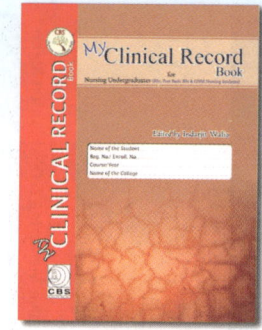

My Clinical Record Book
for Nursing Undergraduates
(BSc, Post Basic BSc & GNM Nursing Students)
Indarjit Walia
978-81-23927-04-6
1/e, 2017-18

MRP: ₹325/-

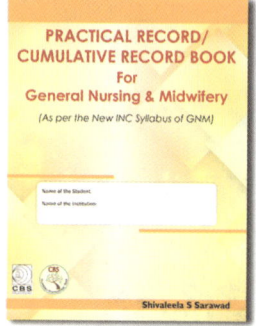

Practical Record/Cumulative Record Book
for General Nursing & Midwifery
Shivaleela S Sarawad
978-93-86827-03-6
1/e, 2018

MRP: ₹225/-

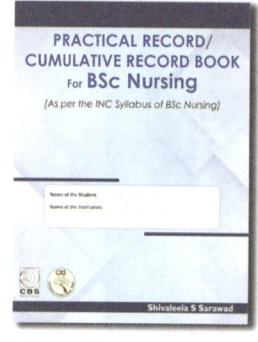

Practical Record/Cumulative Record Book
for BSc Nursing
Shivaleela S Sarawad
978-93-86827-01-2
1/e, 2017

MRP: ₹210/-

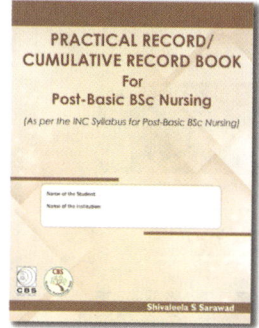

Practical Record/Cumulative Record Book
for Post-Basic BSc Nursing
Shivaleela S Sarawad
978-93-86827-02-9
1/e, 2018

MRP: ₹225/-

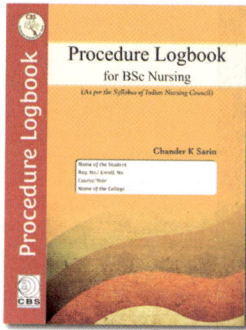

Procedure Logbook
for BSc Nursing
Chander K Sarin
978-93-86310-46-0
1/e, 2017

MRP: ₹210/-

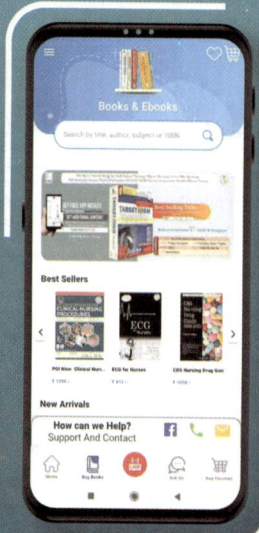
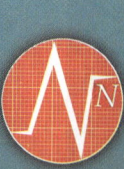
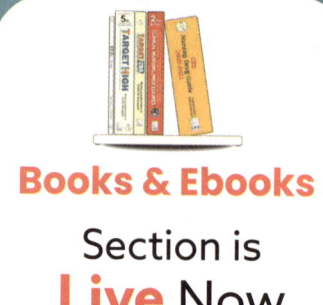

KUHS Series (Kerala University of Health Sciences)

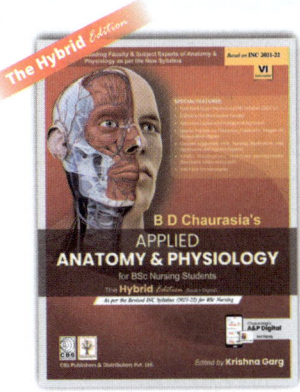

BD Chaurasia's
Applied Anatomy and Physiology
for BSc Nursing Students
Krishna Garg
978-93-90619-65-8
1/e, 2022

TBA

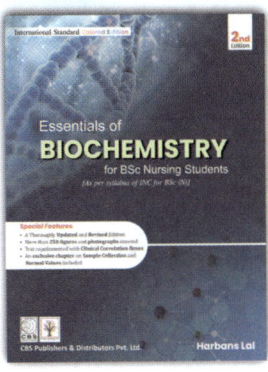

Essentials of Biochemistry
for BSc Nursing Students (As per KUHS)
Harbans Lal
978-81-948693-3-7
2/e, 2022

MRP: ₹450/-

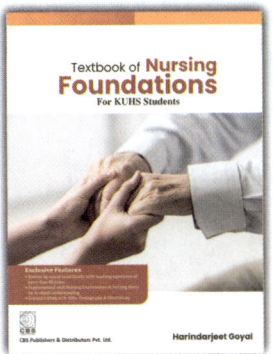

Textbook of
Nursing Foundations
for BSc Nursing (As per KUHS)
Harindarjeet Goyal
978-93-90619-38-2
1/e, 2022

MRP: ₹950/-

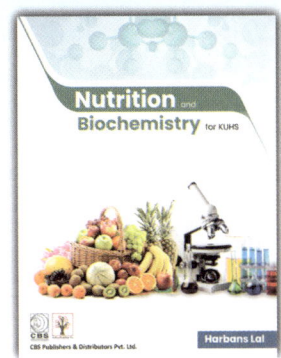

Textbook of
Nutrition & Biochemistry
for BSc Nursing (As per KUHS)
Harbans Lal
978-93-90619-32-0
1/e, 2022

MRP: ₹450/-

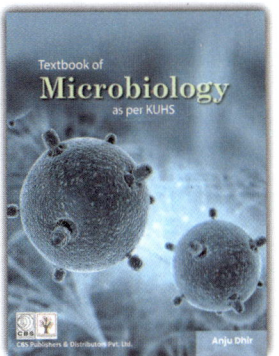

Textbook of
Microbiology
for BSc Nursing (As per KUHS)
Anju Dhir
978-93-90619-49-8
1/e, 2022

MRP: ₹725/-

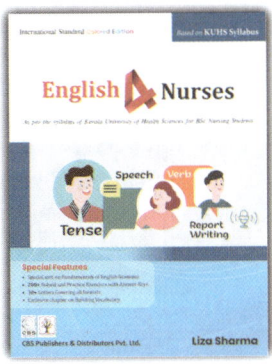

English 4 Nurses
for BSc Nursing (As per KUHS)
Liza Sharma
978-93-90619-33-7
1/e, 2022

MRP: ₹495/-

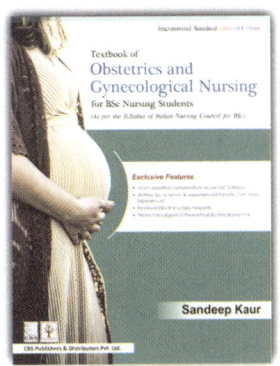

Textbook of
Obstetrics & Gynecological Nursing
for BSc Nursing (As per KUHS)
Sandeep Kaur
978-93-90619-48-1
1/e, 2022

MRP: ₹895/-

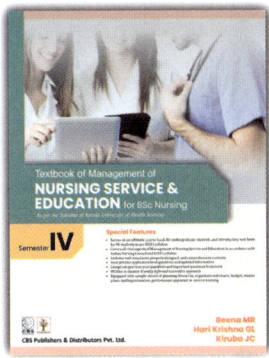

Textbook of
Nursing Management
for BSc Nursing (As per KUHS)
Hari Krishna GL et al.
978-93-90619-39-9
1/e, 2022

MRP: ₹695/-

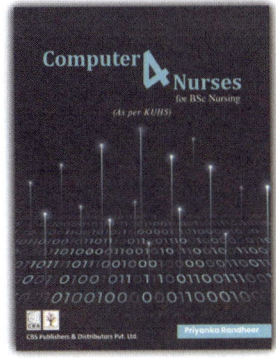

Computer 4 Nurses
for BSc Nursing (As per KUHS)
Priyanka Randheer
978-93-90619-62-7
1/e, 2022

MRP: ₹370/-

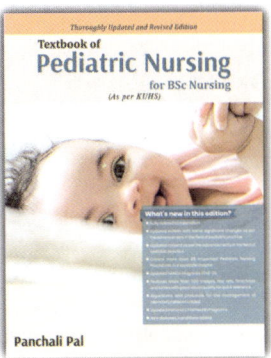

Textbook of
Pediatric Nursing
for BSc Nursing (As per KUHS)
Panchali Pal
978-93-90619-80-1
1/e, 2022

MRP: ₹795/-

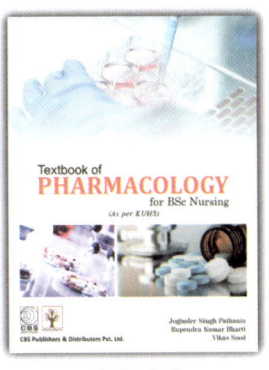

Textbook of
Pharmacology
for BSc Nursing (As per KUHS)
Joginder Singh Pathania et al.
978-93-90619-28-3
1/e, 2022

MRP: ₹650/-

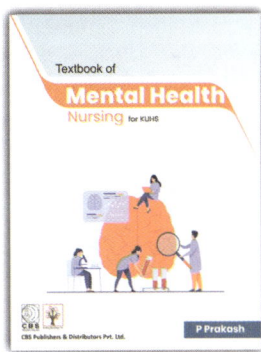

Textbook of
Mental Health Nursing
for BSc Nursing (As per KUHS)
P Prakash
978-93-90619-81-8
1/e, 2022

MRP: ₹625/-

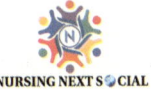

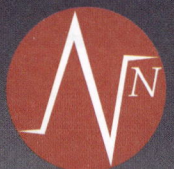
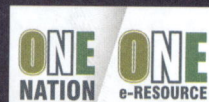
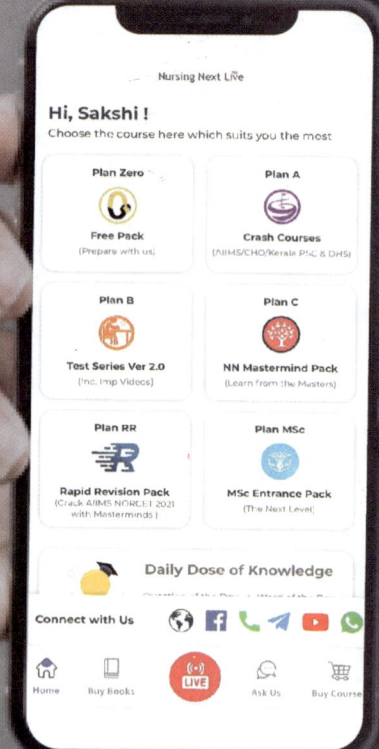 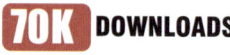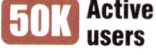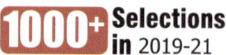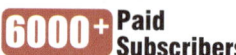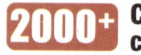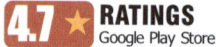

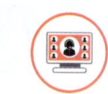

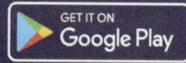
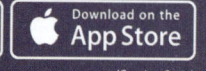